CASE STUDIES IN MODERN DRUG DISCOVERY AND DEVELOPMENT

CASE STUDIES IN MODERN DRUG DISCOVERY AND DEVELOPMENT

Edited by

XIANHAI HUANG
ROBERT G. ASLANIAN

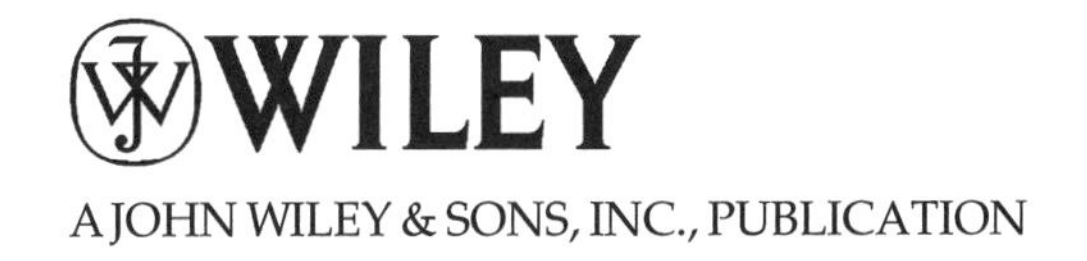

A JOHN WILEY & SONS, INC., PUBLICATION

Published by John Wiley & Sons, Inc., Hoboken, New Jersey
Published simultaneously in Canada

Library of Congress Cataloging-in-Publication Data:

Case studies in modern drug discovery and development / edited by Xianhai Huang, Robert G. Aslanian.
p. ; cm.
Includes bibliographical references and index.
ISBN 978-0-470-60181-5 (cloth)
I. Huang, Xianhai. II. Aslanian, Robert G.
[DNLM: 1. Drug Discovery. 2. Drug Evaluation. QV 744]
615.19–dc23

2011040165

Printed in the United States of America

10 9 8 7 6 5 4 3 2 1

Xianhai is indebted to his wife Dr. Hongmei Li and his kids, Alexander and Angelina for their support and understanding for those numerous weekend absences.

Bob would like to dedicate the book to his wife Antoinette and his boys, Thomas, James and Andrew, who make it all worthwhile.

CONTENTS

PREFACE **xv**

CONTRIBUTORS **xvii**

CHAPTER 1 *INTRODUCTION: DRUG DISCOVERY IN DIFFICULT TIMES* **1**

Malcolm MacCoss

CHAPTER 2 *DISCOVERY AND DEVELOPMENT OF THE DPP-4 INHIBITOR JANUVIA™ (SITA-GLIPTIN)* **10**

Emma R. Parmee, Ranabir SinhaRoy, Feng Xu, Jeffrey C. Givand, and Lawrence A. Rosen

2.1 Introduction **10**
2.2 DPP-4 Inhibition as a Therapy for Type 2 Diabetes: Identification of Key Determinants for Efficacy and Safety **10**
2.2.1 Incretin-Based Therapy for T2DM **10**
2.2.2 Biological Rationale: DPP-4 is a Key Regulator of Incretin Activity **11**
2.2.3 Injectable GLP-1 Mimetics for the Treatment of T2DM **12**
2.2.4 DPP-4 Inhibition as Oral Incretin-Based Therapy for T2DM **12**
2.2.5 Investigation of DPP-4 Biology: Identification of Candidate Substrates **13**
2.2.6 Preclinical Toxicities of In-Licensed DPP-4 Inhibitors **15**
2.2.7 Correlation of Preclinical Toxicity with Off-Target Inhibition of Pro-Specific Dipeptidase Activity **16**
2.2.8 Identification of Pro-Specific Dipeptidases Differentially Inhibited by the Probiodrug Compounds **17**
2.2.9 A Highly Selective DPP-4 Inhibitor is Safe and Well Tolerated in Preclinical Species **19**
2.2.10 A Highly Selective DPP-4 Inhibitor Does Not Inhibit T-Cell Proliferation *in vitro* **19**
2.2.11 DPP-4 Inhibitor Selectivity as a Key Parameter for Drug Development **20**
2.3 Medicinal Chemistry Program **20**
2.3.1 Lead Generation Approaches **20**
2.3.2 Cyclohexyl Glycine α-Amino Acid Series of DPP-4 Inhibitors **20**
2.3.3 Improving Selectivity of the α-Amino Acid Series **22**
2.3.4 Identification and Optimization of the β-Amino Acid Series **22**
2.4 Synthetic and Manufacturing Routes to Sitagliptin **27**
2.4.1 Medicinal Chemistry Route to Sitagliptin and Early Modifications **27**
2.4.2 An Asymmetric Hydrogenation Manufacturing Route to Sitagliptin **28**
2.4.3 A "Greener" Manufacturing Route to Sitagliptin Employing Biocatalytic Transamination **31**
2.5 Drug Product Development **33**
2.5.1 Overview **33**
2.5.2 Composition Development **33**
2.5.3 Manufacturing Process Development **33**
2.6 Clinical Studies **36**

2.6.1 Preclinical PD Studies and Early Clinical Development of Sitagliptin **36**
2.6.2 Summary of Phase II/III Clinical Trials **38**
2.7 Summary **39**
References **39**

CHAPTER 3 *OLMESARTAN MEDOXOMIL: AN ANGIOTENSIN II RECEPTOR BLOCKER* **45**

Hiroaki Yanagisawa, Hiroyuki Koike, and Shin-ichiro Miura

3.1 Background **45**
3.1.1 Introduction **45**
3.1.2 Prototype of Orally Active ARBs **46**
3.2 The Discovery of Olmesartan Medoxomil (Benicar) **47**
3.2.1 Lead Generation **47**
3.2.2 Lead Optimization **49**
3.3 Characteristics of Olmesartan **53**
3.4 Binding Sites of Omlersartan to the AT_1 Receptor and Its Inverse Agonoist Activity **56**
3.4.1 Binding Sites of Olmesartan to the AT_1 Receptor **56**
3.4.2 Inverse Agonist Activity of Olmesartan **56**
3.4.3 Molecular Model of the Interaction between Olmesartan and the AT_1 Receptor **57**
3.5 Practical Preparation of Olmesartan Medoxomil **58**
3.6 Preclinical Studies **58**
3.6.1 AT_1 Receptor Blocking Action **58**
3.6.2 Inhibition of Ang II-Induced Vascular Contraction **59**
3.6.3 Inhibition of the Pressor Response to Ang II **60**
3.6.4 Blood Pressure Lowering Effects **60**
3.6.5 Organ Protection **61**
3.7 Clinical Studies **62**
3.7.1 Antihypertensive Efficacy and Safety **62**
3.7.2 Organ Protection **63**
3.8 Conclusion **63**
References **64**

CHAPTER 4 *DISCOVERY OF HETEROCYCLIC PHOSPHONIC ACIDS AS NOVEL AMP MIMICS THAT ARE POTENT AND SELECTIVE FRUCTOSE-1,6-BISPHOSPHATASE INHIBITORS AND ELICIT POTENT GLUCOSE-LOWERING EFFECTS IN DIABETIC ANIMALS AND HUMANS* **67**

Qun Dang and Mark D. Erion

4.1 Introduction **67**
4.2 The Discovery of MB06322 **69**
4.2.1 Research Operation Plan **69**
4.2.2 Discovery of Nonnucleotide AMP Mimics as FBPase Inhibitors **69**
4.2.3 Discovery of Benzimidazole Phosphonic Acids as FBPase Inhibitors **74**
4.2.4 Discovery of Thiazole Phosphonic Acids as Potent and Selective FBPase Inhibitors **77**
4.2.5 The Discovery of MB06322 Through Prodrug Strategy **80**
4.3 Pharmacokinetic Studies of MB06322 **82**
4.4 Synthetic Routes to MB06322 **83**
4.5 Clinical Studies of MB06322 **83**
4.5.1 Efficacy Study of Thiazole 12.6 in Rodent Models of T2DM **83**
4.5.2 Phase I/II Clinical Studies **84**
4.6 Summary **84**
References **85**

CHAPTER 5 *SETTING THE PARADIGM OF TARGETED DRUGS FOR THE TREATMENT OF CANCER: IMATINIB AND NILOTINIB, THERAPIES FOR CHRONIC MYELOGENOUS LEUKEMIA* **88**

Paul W. Manley and Jürg Zimmermann

5.1 Introduction **88**
5.2 Chronic Myelogenous Leukemia (CML) and Early Treatment of the Disease **89**
5.3 Imatinib: A Treatment for Chronic Myelogenous Leukemia (CML) **92**
5.4 The Need for New Inhibitorts of BCR-ABL1 and Development of Nilotinib **94**
5.5 Conclusion **99**
References **100**

CHAPTER 6 *AMRUBICIN, A COMPLETELY SYNTHETIC 9-AMINOANTHRACYCLINE FOR EXTENSIVE-DISEASE SMALL-CELL LUNG CANCER* **103**

Mitsuharu Hanada

6.1 Introduction **103**
6.2 The Discovery of Amrubicin: The First Completely Synthetic Anthracycline **106**
6.3 Toxicological Profile of Amrubicin **107**
6.4 DNA Topoisomerase II Inhibition and Apoptosis Induction by Amrubicin **110**
6.5 Amrubicin Metabolism: The Discovery of Amrubicinol **113**
 6.5.1 Amrubicinol Functions as an Active Metabolite of Amrubicin **113**
 6.5.2 Tumor-Selective Metabolism of Amrubicin to Amrubicinol **115**
6.6 Improved Usage of Amrubicin **116**
6.7 Clinical Trials **118**
 6.7.1 Clinical Trials of Amrubicin as First-line Therapy in Patients with ED-SCLC **118**
 6.7.2 Clinical Trials of Amrubicin as Second-Line Therapy in Patients with ED-SCLC **121**
6.8 Conclusions **122**
References **123**

CHAPTER 7 *THE DISCOVERY OF DUAL IGF-1R AND IR INHIBITOR FQIT FOR THE TREATMENT OF CANCER* **127**

Meizhong Jin, Elizabeth Buck, and Mark J. Mulvihill

7.1 Biological Rational for Targeting the IGF-1R/IR Pathway for Anti-Cancer Therapy **127**
7.2 Discovery Of OSI-906 **128**
 7.2.1 Summary of OSI-906 Discovery **128**
 7.2.2 OSI-906 Clinical Aspects **129**
7.3 OSI-906 Back Up Efforts **131**
7.4 The Discovery Of FQIT **131**
 7.4.1 Lead Generation Strategy **131**
 7.4.2 Small Molecule Dual IGF-1R/IR Inhibitor Drug Discovery Cascade **133**
 7.4.3 Initial Proof-of-Concept Compounds **134**
 7.4.4 Synthesis of 5,7-Disubstituted Imidazo[5,1-*f*][1,2,4] Triazines **135**
 7.4.5 Lead Imidazo[5,1-*f*][1,2,4] Triazine IGF-1R/IR Inhibitors and Emergence of FQIT **139**
7.5 *In Vitro* Profile of FQIT **140**
 7.5.1 Cellular and Antiproliferative Effects as a Result of IGF-1R and IR Inhibition **140**
 7.5.2 Cellular Potency in the Presence of Plasma Proteins **141**
 7.5.3 *In Vitro* Metabolism and CYP450 Profile **143**
7.6 Pharmacokinetic Properties of FQIT **144**
 7.6.1 Formulation and Salt Study **144**
 7.6.2 Pharmacokinetics Following Intravenous Administration **144**
 7.6.3 Pharmacokinetics Following Oral Administration **145**

7.7 *In Vivo* Profile of FQIT **146**
7.7.1 *In Vivo* Pharmacodynamic and PK/PD Correlation **146**
7.7.2 *In Vivo* Efficacy **146**
7.8 Safety Assessment and Selectivity Profile of FQIT **148**
7.8.1 Effects on Blood Glucose and Insulin Levels **148**
7.8.2 Oral Glucose Tolerance Test **148**
7.8.3 Ames, Rodent, and Nonrodent Toxicology Studies **149**
7.8.4 Selectivity Profile of FQIT **149**
7.9 Summary **150**
Acknowledgments **151**
References **151**

CHAPTER 8 *DISCOVERY AND DEVELOPMENT OF MONTELUKAST (SINGULAIR®)* **154**

Robert N. Young

8.1 Introduction **154**
8.2 Drug Development Strategies **158**
8.3 LTD_4 Antagonist Program **159**
8.3.1 Lead Generation and Optimization **159**
8.3.2 *In Vitro* and *In Vivo* Assays **159**
8.4 The Discovery of Montelukast (Singulair®) **160**
8.4.1 First-Generation Antagonists (Figure 8.3) **160**
8.4.2 Discovery of MK-571 **163**
8.4.3 Discovery of MK-0679 (29) **168**
8.4.4 Discovery of Montelukast (L-706,631, MK-0476, Singulair®) **171**
8.5 Synthesis of Montelukast **174**
8.5.1 Medicinal Chemistry Synthesis **174**
8.5.2 Process Chemistry Synthesis [104, 105] (Schemes 8.5 and 8.6) **176**
8.6 ADME Studies with MK-0476 (Montelukast) **179**
8.7 Safety Assessment of Montelukast **180**
8.8 Clinical Development of Montelukast **180**
8.8.1 Human Pharmacokinetics, Safety, and Tolerability **180**
8.8.2 Human Pharmacology **181**
8.8.3 Phase 2 Studies in Asthma **182**
8.8.4 Phase 3 Studies in Asthma **182**
8.8.5 Effects of Montelukast on Inflammation **185**
8.8.6 Montelukast and Allergic Rhinitis **185**
8.9 Summary **185**
8.9.1 Impact on Society **185**
8.9.2 Lessons Learned **186**
8.10 Personal Impact **187**
References **188**

CHAPTER 9 *DISCOVERY AND DEVELOPMENT OF MARAVIROC, A CCR5 ANTAGONIST FOR THE TREATMENT OF HIV INFECTION* **196**

Patrick Dorr, Blanda Stammen, and Elna van der Ryst

9.1 Background and Rationale **196**
9.2 The Discovery of Maraviroc **199**
9.2.1 HTS and Biological Screening to Guide Medicinal Chemistry **199**
9.2.2 Hit Optimization **200**
9.2.3 Overcoming Binding to hERG **201**
9.3 Preclinical Studies **201**
9.3.1 Metabolism and Pharmacokinetic Characteristics of Maraviroc **201**

9.3.2 Maraviroc Preclinical Pharmacology **202**
9.3.3 Preclinical Investigations into HIV Resistance **202**
9.3.4 Binding of Maraviroc to CCR5 **204**
9.4 The Synthesis of Maraviroc **205**
9.5 Nonclinical Safety and Toxicity Studies **206**
9.5.1 Safety Pharmacology **206**
9.5.2 Immuno- and Mechanistic Toxicity **206**
9.6 Clinical Development of Maraviroc **207**
9.6.1 Phase 1 Studies **207**
9.6.2 Phase 2a Studies **209**
9.6.3 Phase 2b/3 Studies **210**
9.6.4 Development of Resistance to CCR5 Antagonists *In Vivo* **213**
9.7 Summary, Future Directions, and Challenges **214**
Acknowledgments **217**
References **217**

CHAPTER 10 *DISCOVERY OF ANTIMALARIAL DRUG ARTEMISININ AND BEYOND* **227**

Weiwei Mao, Yu Zhang, and Ao Zhang

10.1 Introduction: Natural Products in Drug Discovery **227**
10.2 Natural Product Drug Discovery in China **227**
10.3 Discovery of Artemisinin: Background, Structural Elucidation and Pharmacological Evaluation **228**
10.3.1 Background and Biological Rationale **228**
10.3.2 The Discovery of Artemisinin through Nontraditional Drug Discovery Process **229**
10.3.3 Structural Determination of Artemisinin **231**
10.3.4 Pharmacological Evaluation and Clinical Trial Summary of Artemisinin **231**
10.4 The Synthesis of Artemisinin **232**
10.4.1 Synthesis of Artemisinin using Photooxidation of Cyclic or Acyclic Enol Ether as the Key Step **233**
10.4.2 Synthesis of Artemisinin by Photooxidation of Dihydroarteannuic Acid **236**
10.4.3 Synthesis of Artemisinin by Ozonolysis of a Vinylsilane Intermediate **236**
10.5 SAR Studies of Structural Derivatives of Artemisinin: The Discovery of Artemether **238**
10.5.1 C-10-Derived Artemisinin Analogs **240**
10.5.2 C-9 and C-9,10 Double Substituted Analogs **245**
10.5.3 C-3 Substituted Analogs **246**
10.5.4 C-6 or C-7 Substituted Derivatives **246**
10.5.5 C-11-Substituted Analogs **247**
10.6 Development of Artemether **248**
10.6.1 Profile and Synthesis of Artemether **248**
10.6.2 Clinical Studies Aspects of Artemether **249**
10.7 Conclusion and Perspective **250**
Acknowledgment **250**
References **251**

CHAPTER 11 *DISCOVERY AND PROCESS DEVELOPMENT OF MK-4965, A POTENT NONNUCLEOSIDE REVERSE TRANSCRIPTASE INHIBITOR* **257**

Yong-Li Zhong, Thomas J. Tucker, and Jingjun Yin

11.1 Introduction **257**
11.2 The Discovery of MK-4965 **260**
11.2.1 Background Information **260**
11.2.2 SAR Studies Leading to the Discovery of MK-4965 **262**
11.3 Preclinical and Clinical Studies of MK-4965 (19) **266**

11.4 Summary of Back-Up SAR Studies of MK-4965 Series **266**
11.5 Process Development of MK-4965 (19) **267**
11.5.1 Medicinal Chemistry Route **267**
11.5.2 Process Development **269**
11.6 Conclusion **290**
11.6.1 Lessons Learned from the Medicinal Chemistry Effort of MK-4965 Discovery **290**
11.6.2 Summary and Lessons Learned from the Process Development of MK-4965 **291**
Acknowledgments **291**
References **291**

CHAPTER 12 *DISCOVERY OF BOCEPREVIR AND NARLAPREVIR: THE FIRST AND SECOND GENERATION OF HCV NS3 PROTEASE INHIBITORS* **296**

Kevin X. Chen and F. George Njoroge

12.1 Introduction **296**
12.2 HCV NS3 Protease Inhibitors **298**
12.3 Research Operation Plan and Biological Assays **302**
12.3.1 Research Operation Plan **302**
12.3.2 Enzyme Assay **302**
12.3.3 Replicon Assay **302**
12.3.4 Measure of Selectivity **303**
12.4 Discovery of Boceprevir **303**
12.4.1 Initial Lead Generation Through Structure-Based Drug Design **303**
12.4.2 SAR Studies Focusing on Truncation, Depeptization, and Macrocyclisation **304**
12.4.3 Individual Amino Acid Residue Modifications **307**
12.4.4 Correlations Between P1, P3, and P3 Capping: The Identification of Boceprevir **315**
12.5 Profile of Boceprevir **317**
12.5.1 *In Vitro* Characterization of Boceprevir **317**
12.5.2 Pharmacokinetics of Boceprevir **317**
12.5.3 The Interaction of Boceprevir with NS3 Protease **318**
12.6 Clinical Development and Approval of Boceprevir **319**
12.7 Synthesis of Boceprevir **319**
12.8 Discovery of Narlaprevir **322**
12.8.1 Criteria for the Back-up Program of Boceprevir **322**
12.8.2 SAR Studies **322**
12.8.3 Profile of Narlaprevir **326**
12.8.4 Clinical Development Aspects of Narlaprevir **327**
12.8.5 Synthesis of Narlaprevir **327**
12.9 Summary **329**
References **330**

CHAPTER 13 *THE DISCOVERY OF SAMSCA® (TOLVAPTAN): THE FIRST ORAL NONPEPTIDE VASOPRESSIN RECEPTOR ANTAGONIST* **336**

Kazumi Kondo and Yoshitaka Yamamura

13.1 Background Information about the Disease **336**
13.2 Biological Rational **337**
13.3 Lead Generation Strategies: The Discovery of Mozavaptan **338**
13.4 Lead Optimization: From Mozavaptan to Tolvaptan **347**
13.5 Pharmacological Profiles of Tolvaptan **350**
13.5.1 Antagonistic Affinities of Tolvaptan for AVP Receptors **350**
13.5.2 Aquaretic Effect Following a Single Dose in Conscious Rats **352**
13.6 Drug Development **353**
13.6.1 Synthetic Route of Discovery and Commercial Synthesis [10a] **353**

13.6.2 Nonclinical Toxicology **353**
13.6.3 Clinical Studies **355**
13.7 Summary Focusing on Lessons Learned **356**
Acknowledgments **357**
References **357**

CHAPTER 14 *SILODOSIN (URIEF®, RAPAFLO®, THRUPAS®, UROREC®, SILODIX™): A SELECTIVE α_{1A} ADRENOCEPTOR ANTAGONIST FOR THE TREATMENT OF BENIGN PROSTATIC HYPERPLASIA* **360**

Masaki Yoshida, Imao Mikoshiba, Katsuyoshi Akiyama, and Junzo Kudoh

14.1 Background Information **360**
14.1.1 Benign Prostatic Hyperplasia **360**
14.1.2 α_1-Adrenergic Receptors **361**
14.2 The Discovery of Silodosin **362**
14.2.1 Medicinal Chemistry **362**
14.2.2 The Synthesis of Silodosin (Discovery Route) **363**
14.2.3 Receptor Binding Studies **365**
14.3 Pharmacology of Silodosin **369**
14.3.1 Action Against Noradrenalin-Induced Contraction of Lower Urinary Tract Tissue **369**
14.3.2 Actions Against Phenylephrine-Induced Increase in Intraurethral Pressure and Blood Pressure **371**
14.3.3 Actions Against Intraurethral Pressure Increased by Stimulating Hypogastric Nerve and Blood Pressure in Dogs with Benign Prostatic Hyperplasia **372**
14.3.4 Safety Pharmacology **373**
14.4 Metabolism of Silodosin **373**
14.5 Pharmacokinetics of Silodosin **376**
14.5.1 Absorption **376**
14.5.2 Organ Distribution **377**
14.5.3 Excretion **378**
14.6 Toxicology of Silodosin **379**
14.7 Clinical Trials **382**
14.7.1 Phase I Studies **382**
14.7.2 Phase III Randomized, Placebo-Controlled, Double-Blind Study **383**
14.7.3 Long-Term Administration Study **385**
14.8 Summary: Key Lessons Learned **388**
References **389**

CHAPTER 15 *RALOXIFENE: A SELECTIVE ESTROGEN RECEPTOR MODULATOR (SERM)* **392**

Jeffrey A. Dodge and Henry U. Bryant

15.1 Introduction: SERMs **392**
15.2 The Benzothiophene Scaffold: A New Class of SERMs **394**
15.3 Assays for Biological Evaluation of Tissue Selectivity **394**
15.4 Benzothiophene Structure Activity **395**
15.5 The Synthesis of Raloxifene **401**
15.6 SERM Mechanism **402**
15.7 Raloxifene Pharmacology **405**
15.7.1 Skeletal System **405**
15.7.2 Reproductive System—Uterus **407**
15.7.3 Reproductive System—Mammary **408**
15.7.4 General Safety Profile and Other Pharmacological Considerations **410**

15.8 Summary 411
References 411

APPENDIX I *SMALL MOLECULE DRUG DISCOVERY AND DEVELOPMENT PARADIGM* 417

APPENDIX II *GLOSSARY* 419

APPENDIX III *ABBREVIATIONS* 432

INDEX 443

PREFACE

The discovery of a new drug is a challenging, complicated, and expensive endeavor. Although exact figures are hard to come by, recent published data indicate that it takes about 10 years and close to \$1 billion to develop and bring a new drug to market. Additionally, according to a recent analysis only 11 out of 100 drug candidates entering Phase I clinical trials, and one out of 10 entering Phase III, will become marketed drugs. Many of these drugs will never make back the money invested in their development. These are dismal statistics. Improving the success rate of the discovery and development process is a key factor that will weigh heavily on the success, and perhaps the survival, of the pharmaceutical industry in the future. There are numerous reasons for the current lack of new molecules reaching patients. To address the problem, many large pharmaceutical companies have tried to reinvent themselves over the last 10 to 15 years. The methods employed have included incorporation of what could be described as the latest fads in drug discovery into research operations, internal reorganizations or, as a last resort, mergers. None of these approaches has helped to solve the dearth of new drugs coming from the industry. Another approach to solving this conundrum is to look to the past to see what has previously worked in successful drug discovery programs and try to apply the knowledge gained in those programs to current efforts. Therefore, the critical question becomes how to more efficiently apply proven drug discovery principles and technologies to increase the probability of success for new projects. Knowledge gained from the successful discovery and launch of marketed drugs can provide a very useful template for future drug design and discovery. This rationale was a major factor for compiling *Case Studies in Modern Drug Discovery and Development*.

The primary target audience for *Case Studies in Modern Drug Discovery and Development* is undergraduate and graduate students in chemistry, although all scientists with an interest in the drug discovery process should benefit from these case studies. Most chemists who work in the early stages of drug discovery in the pharmaceutical industry do not train to be medicinal chemists. They train in synthetic organic chemistry, either total synthesis, methodology, or a combination of the two. There is a good reason for this: chemists need to be able to make the compounds they design as quickly as possible so as to drive structure–activity relationships (SAR) to meet project criteria. But prior to starting their careers in the industry, many chemists wonder how they can quickly master the necessary skills and knowledge of the drug discovery process including SAR, pharmacology, drug metabolism, biology, drug development, and clinical studies. Besides providing a roadmap of successful drug development for application to current problems, *Case Studies in Modern Drug Discovery and Development* illustrates these concepts through the use of examples of successful, and not so successful, drug discovery programs. Written by acknowledged leaders in the field from both academia and industry, this book covers many aspects of the drug discovery process with detailed examples that showcase the science and technology that go into drug discovery. We hope that *Case Studies in Modern Drug Discovery and Development* will be suitable for all levels of scientists who have an interest in drug discovery. Additionally, with the comprehensive information included in each independent chapter, it is suitable for professional seminars or courses that relate to drug design. Finally, the drugs collected in this book include some of the most important and life-saving medications currently prescribed, so the information included should be of interest to the public who want to learn more about the drugs that they are taking.

We have to admit that we totally underestimated the amount of work involved in the editing of this case study book. It took more than 3 years from the conception of the book, author recruiting and chapter editing to the publication of the book. During this long process, there are many friends and colleagues who helped to make it happen. We would like to thank Wiley editor Jonathan Rose for initiating the process, giving us the opportunity, and trusting us in editing the book. He always quickly replied to every question that we raised during the process. We would also like to thank all the authors who dedicated their time to contribute to the chapters and their respective companies for permission to publish their work. We believe that all the chapters will have an important impact on future drug discovery programs and benefit future scientists of this field for generations to come. We salute them for their time, effort, and dedication. We would like to thank the reviewers of our book proposal for their valuable suggestions and critiques. Based on their suggestions we have collected examples of drugs that failed to advance to the market to showcase the "dark" side of the drug discovery and development process where huge amounts of work and resources are expended with no obvious return. We would like to thank Drs. Sandy Mills, Ann Webber, William Greenlee, Guoxin Zhu, An-hu Li, David Gray, and Markus Follmann for their assistance in recruiting the chapter authors.

One of our colleagues has said "If you must begin then go all the way, because if you begin and quit, the unfinished business you have left behind begins to haunt you all the time." We as scientists have chosen to make a difference in the improvement of human health, and we need to consistently empower ourselves in knowledge and experience. We hope that this book will help our readers to achieve their goals.

Xianhai Huang
Robert G. Aslanian

New Jersey
July, 2011

CONTRIBUTORS

Katsuyoshi Akiyama, Kissei Pharmaceutical Co., Ltd., Japan

Henry U. Bryant, Lilly Research Laboratories, Eli Lilly and Company, Indianapolis, IN, USA

Elizabeth Buck, OSI Pharmaceuticals, Inc., Broadhollow Bioscience Park, Farmingdale, NY, USA

Kevin X. Chen, Discovery Chemistry, Merck Research Laboratories, Kenilworth, NJ, USA

Qun Dang, Departments of Medicinal Chemistry and Biochemistry, Metabasis Therapeutics, Inc. La Jolla, CA, USA

Jeffrey A. Dodge, Lilly Research Laboratories, Eli Lilly and Company, Indianapolis, IN, USA

Patrick Dorr, Abbott, Abbott House, Vanwall Business Park, Maidenhead, Berkshire, SL6 4XE, UK

Mark D. Erion, Metabasis Therapeutics, Inc., Departments of Medicinal Chemistry and Biochemistry, La Jolla, CA, USA

Jeffrey C. Givand, Delivery Device Development, Merck Research Laboratories, West Point, PA, USA

Mitsuharu Hanada, Pharmacology Research Laboratories, Dainippon Sumitomo Pharma Co., Ltd., Osaka, Japan

Meizhong Jin, OSI Pharmaceuticals, Inc., Broadhollow Bioscience Park, Farmingdale, NY, USA

Hiroyuki Koike, R&D Division, DAIICHI SANKYO Co., Ltd., Shinagawa-ku, Tokyo, Japan

Kazumi Kondo, Qs' Research Institute, Otsuka Pharmaceutical Co., Ltd., Tokushima, Japan

Junzo Kudoh, Department of Urology, Japan Labor Health and Welfare Organization, Kumamoto Rosai Hospital, Japan

Malcolm MacCoss, Bohicket Pharma Consulting LLC, South Carolina, USA

Paul W. Manley, Oncology Department, Novartis Institutes for Biomedical Research

Basel, Switzerland

Weiwei Mao, Synthetic Organic & Medicinal Chemistry Laboratory, Shanghai Institute of Materia Medica, Chinese Academy of Sciences, Shanghai, China 201203

Imao Mikoshiba, Kissei Pharmaceutical Co., Ltd., Japan

Shin-ichiro Miura, Department of Cardiology, Fukuoka University School of Medicine, Fukuoka, Japan

Mark J. Mulvihill, OSI Pharmaceuticals, Inc., Broadhollow Bioscience Park, Farmingdale, NY, USA

F. George Njoroge, Discovery Chemistry, Merck Research Laboratories, Kenilworth, NJ, USA

Emma R. Parmee, Discovery Chemistry, West Point, Merck Research Laboratories, 770 Sumneytown Pike, West Point, PA, USA

Lawrence A. Rosen, Formulation & Basic Pharmaceutical Sciences, Merck Research Laboratories, West Point, PA, USA

Ranabir SinhaRoy, Janssen Research & Development, LLC 920 US Highway 202 South Raritan, NJ 08869

Blanda Stammen, Pfizer Global R&D, Sandwich Laboratories, Kent, CT13 9NJ, UK

Thomas J. Tucker, Discovery Chemistry, Merck Research Laboratories, West Point, PA, USA

Elna van der Ryst, United Therapeutics, Unither House, Curfew Bell Road, Chertsey, Surrey KT16 9FG, United Kingdom.

Feng Xu, Department of Process Research, Merck Research Laboratories, Rahway, NJ, USA

Yoshitaka Yamamura, Department of Clinical Research and Development, Otsuka Pharmaceutical Co., Ltd., Tokyo, Japan

Hiroaki Yanagisawa, R&D Division, DAIICHI SANKYO Co., Ltd., Shinagawa-ku, Tokyo, Japan

Jingjun Yin, Department of Process Research, Merck Research Laboratories, Rahway, NJ, USA

Masaki Yoshida, Department of Medical Informatics, Japan Labor Health and Welfare Organization, Kumamoto Rosai Hospital, Kumamoto, Japan

Robert N. Young, Department of Chemistry, Simon Fraser University, Burnaby, British Columbia, Canada, V5A 1S6

Ao Zhang, Synthetic Organic & Medicinal Chemistry Laboratory, Shanghai Institute of Materia Medica, Chinese Academy of Sciences, Shanghai, China 201203

Yu Zhang, Synthetic Organic & Medicinal Chemistry Laboratory, Shanghai Institute of Materia Medica, Chinese Academy of Sciences, Shanghai, China 201203

Yong-Li Zhong, Department of Process Research, Merck Research Laboratories, Rahway, NJ, USA

Jürg Zimmermann, Oncology Department, Novartis Institutes for Biomedical Research

Basel, Switzerland

CHAPTER 1

INTRODUCTION: DRUG DISCOVERY IN DIFFICULT TIMES

Malcolm MacCoss

At the time of writing (mid-2011), the pharmaceutical industry is facing probably its most difficult time in recent history. As little as a decade ago, the fact that the aging population in the Western world was increasing (i.e., the post-War baby boomer population was reaching retirement age and thus moving into a demographic that requires the use of more medications), coupled with the likelihood of worldwide expansion of modern medicine into large populations of developing countries, led to an assumption that this would move the industry into a golden era of drug discovery and commercial growth [1]. This was expected to be supplemented with the promise of the utilization of the fruits of modern molecular biology and genomics-based sciences following the completion of the Human Genome Project [2,3]. However, despite large increased investments by pharmaceutical companies in research and development (R&D), the number of new molecular entities (NME) approved by the U.S. FDA has not increased at the same rate as the increase in R&D investment [4]. This lack of productivity in the pharma R&D sector has been much analyzed and continues to be a topic of great concern and discussion both within and outside the industry [1,4–13], and ex-heads of research and development at major pharmaceutical companies have joined in the discourse [5,6,8,14,15]. In addition to this lack of productivity, we now find the industry under attack from a number of directions, and this has led to a dramatic reduction in the pharma workforce, at least in the Western world. In fact, since 2000, according to Challenger, Gray, and Christmas, as reported in Forbes [16], the pharmaceutical industry has been under such stress that it has cut 297,650 jobs, that is, about the size of the current Pfizer, Merck, and GlaxoSmithKline combined; thus, the manpower equivalent of three of the largest pharmaceutical houses in the world has been eliminated in a decade. Various mergers and acquisitions, driven by commercial and economic pressures, have led to eradication of a number of well-established pharmaceutical houses that for decades had provided the world with numerous life-saving and quality-of-life-enhancing medicines. The industry that was, for most of the past two decades of the twentieth century, the darling of Wall Street, with Merck, for example, being "America's Most Admired Company" for 7 years in a row, is now under major duress.

So what has gone so badly wrong with this once booming industry? This has been the subject of many editorials, publications, and blogs that are too numerous to mention here, but it all really stems from the coming together of a "perfect storm" of events and an industry that, apparently, was unprepared for the evolving situation.

Patent expirations, in particular, have become an issue for an industry that has been driven by a business model based on blockbuster drugs (generally considered to be a drug molecule that brings in more than $1 billion per year in sales). However, one result of this

Case Studies in Modern Drug Discovery and Development, Edited by Xianhai Huang and Robert G. Aslanian.

model is that the revenue created by a blockbuster drops dramatically overnight when the patent exclusivity expires and generics are allowed to enter the marketplace. This phenomenon, of course, is not new, but what is different now is that in the business model driven by one or two blockbusters per company rather than by a larger number of mid-sized products, the loss of a blockbuster has a much greater impact on any particular company. The research and development divisions of pharmaceutical companies have not been able to produce new replacement products for compounds going off patent in the time frames that the blockbuster products they are replacing have exclusivity in the marketplace. This issue is exacerbated by the increasing cost of research and development [4,5] and, in addition, the time frame that the first-in-class molecules are on the market before the "fast followers" or later entrant "best-in-class" molecules are approved for marketing is rapidly shrinking [5]. This problem has been noted for years. I well remember, in the mid-1980s when I had recently joined the industry, being told by high-level research managers that it was necessary to have a follow-up blockbuster already in place in the late-stage pipeline before the original one was approved, as this seemed to be the best approach to dealing with this conundrum. But the limitations of this approach are readily apparent. First, it is not clear that it is possible to predict with any degree of exactitude which project will lead to a blockbuster and which one will not. The time frame from initiating a project to the launch of an NME from that project is so long that much can change in the biomedical science environment and in the regulatory and commercial space during that period. Thus, companies have had to rely on bigger blockbusters at the expense of working on medicines for some diseases that were likely to bring in less revenues to the company – the inevitable spiral is then started, with more and more effort being put into products based on their commercial viability rather than on the unmet medical need that has driven the industry, and which has served it so well. In a speech made to the Medical College of Virginia in 1950 [17], George W. Merck made this famous comment, ". . . We never try to forget that medicine is for the people. It is not for the profits. The profits follow, and if we have remembered that, they have never failed to appear. The better we have remembered it, the larger they have been . . . How can we bring the best of medicine to each and every person? We cannot rest till the way has been found, with our help, to bring our finest achievement to everyone. . ." Recent trends in the industry (with some notable exceptions) suggest a drift from this mantra.

But the demise of the blockbuster business model is certainly not the only driver of the present situation. Some companies have attempted to overcome the problem of stagnant pipelines by acquiring, or merging with, other pharmaceutical companies that had, apparently, a more robust array of later stage products. The trouble with this approach is that the respite is at best temporary, and the merging of different corporate cultures has usually taken much longer to sort out than even the pessimists had predicted. In addition, there are an inevitable number of lay-offs (as already pointed out) that occur due to redundancies and overlaps in the merging of two large organizations, and such cost cutting is at least partially a result of the need to show a stronger balance sheet after the merger. Each of these acquisitions has left the preponderance of leadership and middle management in the new organization coming from the original company that had the deficient pipeline. It is not always clear whether the reasons for that deficiency had been fully understood – thus, eventually leading down the line to another pipeline crisis and leaving the true problem(s) unsolved. At best, these mergers have bought some time for the company making the acquisition, but several studies have questioned whether in the middle-to-long term they have provided a solution or even whether they have given rise to a stronger and more robust company than what would have been the case if the merger had not occurred and the two companies had progressed independently [4,18]. Altogether, this has resulted in a longer downtime for productivity in the research operations of the new organization than expected and, in particular, the effects on morale have been devastating. How this has impacted the innovation effort is difficult to quantify, but it has to be considerable. It is generally considered that innovation, particularly innovation that often takes years to mature in the extended time lines of drug discovery, needs a stable and secure nonjob-threatening environment to allow appropriate risk taking for the great discoveries to occur. The insidious low morale seen in many pharmaceutical research organizations now makes it very hard for even the most motivated drug researcher to put in the extra hours that were once commonplace and which are often necessary to produce hand-crafted molecules with the right properties to be drug candidates for human use. The loss in productivity of this lost extra time investment is impossible to calculate, but it must be huge.

In the midst of all of this turmoil, companies have been desperately trying to reinvent themselves and to understand why the productivity of their research endeavors has been so poor. All the major pharmaceutical companies have undergone much introspection leading to reorganization and revamping of the way they do things. Mostly, this has been driven by two goals: first, to pinpoint excesses and overspending in their operations and to eliminate them, and second, to highlight better ways of carrying out their operations to become more efficient and streamlined so that they can get to the finish line faster and with a better potential product [19]. Both of these are perfectly laudable and appropriate goals. Unfortunately, it is difficult to quantify precisely the elements that go into making an innovative and creative research environment. These two goals are driven by hard numbers, and Six Sigma-type methods have been extensively used to quantify and then to drive all the excess spending out of the system to give a lean, flexible work environment. Such an environment requires much attention to the process involved and thus a close monitoring of the discovery process. While this undoubtedly has had the desired effect of reducing costs, it is very unclear whether it has at the same time improved the productivity of the research groups. Much innovation and true problem solving goes on "under the radar" and emerges when sufficient information has been gleaned to qualify it for consideration. Unfortunately, this is difficult to justify in the process-driven environment described above. True innovation does require pressure to deliver on time lines, but it also often requires individual freedom to operate and for everyone to live with the consequences. Often, innovation is also enabled by some amount of extra resources over the strict minimum calculated by methods mentioned above to allow researchers to follow-up on unexpected findings.

Any evaluation of a complex research environment requires that the entire operation be broken down into numerous smaller categories, with each of these being closely interrogated. It is often the way these operations are flexibly integrated at the macro level that determines the overall productivity of a complex organization – not necessarily the optimization of the specific parts. Nevertheless, the current paradigm is to break down the drug discovery process, up to the delivery of a candidate for toxicity testing, into target identification and validation, hit identification, hit-to-lead, lead optimization, and candidate selection. It is fair to say that this is a relatively new consideration. A decade ago, it was considered one continuous process with much overlap of the above-mentioned categories. This continuous operation gave a certain amount of autonomy to the scientists involved and certainly gave ownership of projects to the project team members. The more recent breakdown of the drug discovery process into its constituent parts has led to smaller companies being able to specialize in various elements of the overall endeavor, and nowadays the use of specialist contract research organizations (CROs) for various parts of the process is commonplace. A decade ago, such companies would have been based in the United States or Europe and were used primarily to prepare chemical libraries in new areas of research or to supplement in-house research to help with load leveling within the internal operations. However, the past decade has seen a dramatic shift of the preparation of chemical libraries (to supplement and diversify internal repositories that tend to be a footprint of previous in-house programs) to CROs in the emerging nations of China and India where a highly skilled workforce, supplemented by a scientific diaspora of Chinese and Indian scientists trained in the West and returning home, was able to take on these tasks at a reduced full time equivalent (FTE) rate lower than in the United States or Europe. The explosion of science now being witnessed in this area has become transformative, with all companies now associated in some way with out-sourcing of some elements of their research operations. Many consider that the big winners of the future will be those who are the most successful at this venture, and some major pharmaceutical companies have relocated entire research groups and/or therapeutic areas to China or India. This "outsourcing" has greatly increased the complexity of research operations and the operational landscape has changed overnight. The planning, oversight, and monitoring of drug discovery programs with parts of the work going on in different regions of the world, in distant time zones, and sometimes with language issues, has become a huge factor in any pharmaceutical company. Thus, the deep discussions on the last day's results over coffee after work in a close working laboratory environment with friends and colleagues has been replaced with late-night (or early morning) teleconferences with specialist scientists one might never get to meet in person. It remains to be seen if this sea change in the way we do research will be appropriately productive in the long run, but certainly in the short term, because of the financial savings involved, it is a process now taken very seriously by management in pharma operations. My own view is that it will all depend on whether this can deliver the quality drug candidates necessary to sustain the growth of the multibillion dollar pharmaceutical companies, and the ones that will be the most successful are those that will blend the appropriate skill sets of their CRO colleagues with the in-house skills to get the job done quicker and cheaper than it was done previously. But costs in China and India are already starting to rise, and there is always, even in today's electronic world, an issue of turnaround time in the iterative "design – synthesis – assay – redesign – synthesis" drug discovery cycle that is so much an important driver of the productivity and speed of delivery of drug candidates. This point is being addressed now by "full-service" CROs in India and China that are taking on more and more of the early biochemical and biological assays as well as the chemical synthesis, thus, shortening the iterative cycle by having the full cycle performed on the same site.

Of course, there are several other elements to the "perfect storm" that has hit the industry. Certainly, since the voluntary removal of Vioxx from the market because of cardiac issues, there has been an intense scrutiny of other drugs that have been introduced, particularly with regard to cardiovascular issues. Although these have been seen as the Food and Drug Administration (FDA) being more vigilant, it is certainly appropriate that all new medicines are carefully scrutinized for their safety before being approved. New advances and initiatives are ongoing in all companies to consider earlier evaluations of potential toxicity in drug candidates, so that compounds that are likely to fail will do so early on in the process and so save downstream investment from going to waste. While much of this is driven by advances in *in vitro* studies, there remains a need for measures of acute *in vivo* toxicity earlier in the process and this, in turn, brings a need for earlier scale-ups of the active pharmaceutical ingredient (API), which itself can add more time, resources, and costs to the discovery process. The main issue here is that we must be sure that when we kill compounds early, we are indeed killing the appropriate molecules, that is, the introduction of earlier *in vitro* toxicity studies must produce robust "kills," we must not have increased numbers of false positives that throw out the baby with the bath water. We *must* make safer drugs (between 1991 and 2000, $\sim$30% of drug candidates failed for toxicity and clinical safety reasons [6,7]) and when we err, we *must* err on the side of safety, but it has long been known that all xenobiotics have some risk associated with them [20] and the design and discovery of safe drugs is all about the therapeutic ratio and how one assesses the risk involved with any new medicine. There will be any number of iterations of the steps involved at various companies to find the best way forward in this regard, but advances in this area can only lead to a safer armamentarium of medicines for patients.

On the other hand, drugs that are failing in the later phases of development, are not just failing because of toxicities that are being seen in preclinical and clinical studies. Drug candidates are also failing in clinical trials because of lack of efficacy. Despite the recent increase in our biomedical knowledge and our increased understanding of the molecular mechanisms of disease, ~30% of attrition in potential drug candidates is due to lack of efficacy in clinical trials [6,7] although this is somewhat therapeutic area dependent [6]. For instance, some of this might well be due to notoriously unpredictive animal models of efficacy such as in CNS diseases and for oncology [21], both of which have higher failure rates in phase II and III trials. It is disconcerting that positive results in the smaller highly controlled phase II trials don't always replicate in the larger population bases used in phase III trials. But the take-home message is that compounds failing this late in the development process are causing an enormous drain on resources and the "kill early" concept for drug candidates is now the mantra in the pharmaceutical world. In addition, the rate of attrition of compounds working by novel mechanisms is higher than for those working with previously precedented mechanisms [6]. If one makes the assumption that toxicities due to nonmechanism-based side effects (i.e., molecule-specific off-target activities) are likely to be the same across both types of mechanisms, then this implies that the higher attrition rate for novel mechanisms might be due to mechanism-based toxicities that occur because of an incomplete biological understanding of the novel target or due to a lack of efficacy because the target protein is not playing the attributed role in the disease state in humans. One likely outcome of this is that risk-averse organizations might choose to work primarily on precedented mechanisms.

Perhaps more difficult to assess is the commercial need by payers to address the worth of any new treatment that is being proposed. Thus, any new medicine must demonstrate that it provides a measurable increase in value both to the patient and to the payers (governments or insurance companies, or both), not just that it provides a new pill for an old disease, for which older, cheaper medicines might already serve adequately. The question of value will always be somewhat subjective (e.g. cost versus quality of life versus increased life span) and the clinical trials that are sometimes necessary to demonstrate such improvement in a chronic disease, requiring prolonged dosing and being run head-to-head with a current standard of care, in addition to placebo where possible, are often extremely large, long, and expensive. Sometimes, knowing this ahead of time has dissuaded organizations from working in that area. It should be noted that the aging population, and by definition a smaller tax base to support that demographic group, which as mentioned earlier has been a driver for more revenues for the industry, is layered on to the fact that health care systems in the Western world are having a difficult time meeting the financial demands of the increased need for health care in that population – including the costs of new medicines. However, we should not forget that the cost of drugs is still a small percentage of the total healthcare budget and for the large part good medicines allow patients to spend less time in hospitals and other health care institutions.

All these issues have come together in the past decade to increase greatly the cost of drug discovery, despite the industry's efforts to cut costs (see above). The cost to discover a new drug is estimated to be well over $1 billion and there seems to be no end to the increased costs in sight.

Of course, there are other, more scientific issues that over the past decade have changed the playing field upon which we practice our art of medicinal chemistry. Combinatorial chemistry has come and gone, and has now been replaced to a large degree by parallel and high-throughput synthesis of individual molecules. These rapid synthesis methods, along with high-throughput screening (HTS) methods have been major enablers of getting lots of data on lots of molecules. However, I believe a more subtle change is also occurring and that has to do with the nature of the targets that we now address. Before the Human Genome Project, we basically addressed targets such as enzymes, G-protein-coupled receptors (GPCRs), ion channels, and nuclear receptors, targets that had been well studied biochemically prior to the medicinal chemist getting involved on a project. After the Human Genome Project, we were able to associate various proteins with different disease states. Many of these proteins were without any known enzymatic or receptor-driven activity and we have started to attack the problem of making protein–protein interaction inhibitors (PPIs). This new trend has been addressed in a number of ways, but one of the preferred methods has come from using fragment-based hit identification methods coupled with rapid throughput structural biology and chemistry, and computational chemistry methods. Taken together, this has required the preparation of new, hitherto unprecedented, libraries as starting points, as well as improvements in X-ray crystallography and NMR methods to determine how the fragments bind. These developments are taking time to come to full fruition, but there are now numerous examples of these applications in various pipelines. Not too long ago, a medicinal chemistry program could be initiated without a lot of structural information if the correct biochemical assays were in place. Nowadays, the contributions of structural biology to hit identification and hit-to-lead activities can be seen in almost all programs. As we emerge from the postkinase era and more into the PPI era, the companies that are best equipped with these modern methods will benefit the most. There will be a short time lag as these methods get honed, but I believe it will drive us into much newer chemical space and very novel approaches to drug design.

I also feel that the time has come to reassess the very way in which we practice medicinal chemistry. Over the past decade, collectively we have become very good at both solving the problems of acute toxicities (hERG binding, acute liver toxicity, etc.) and solving some of the drug metabolism, absorption, distribution, metabolism, and excretion (ADME) issues while addressing the pharmaceutical properties of the molecules (absorption using Caco-2 cells, metabolic liability using microsomes or hepatocytes, Cyp450 inhibition, brain penetration, log P, polar surface area, solubility, Lipinsky guidelines [22], etc.) and the roles that these all play in *in vivo* readouts and in the big picture of drug discovery and molecule optimization. This is borne out by the much lower attrition rates for drug candidates in the phase I stage than were apparent a decade earlier [6,23]. These improvements occurred because research organizations identified the problem (it was demonstrated that in the 1980s drugs failed primarily because of PK and ADME issues in phase I [6,23]) and drug companies put in place assays and procedures to address the issues. Also, with the advent of high-throughput assays it was possible to get large amounts of data, with a quick turnaround time so that they could meaningfully impact on the next round of synthesis activity, on all these potential issues so the structure–activity relationships (SARs) that drove them were quickly understood. At that time, this represented a sea change from primarily addressing the SAR on just the target protein [23].

However, there is another side to this story. Since the advent of these technologies that allow for rapid evaluation of molecules, there has been a significant trend in the past decade toward making lots of compounds using routine and relatively straightforward chemistries to improve the likelihood of better understanding the numerous (sometimes orthogonal) SARs. This approach has led to many two-dimensional, high molecular weight molecules that often don't explore enough three-dimensional space, and I often wonder if enough time is spent making targeted, three-dimensional molecules to answer specific structural or SAR-related questions. It is this overreliance on "more is better," but with relatively straightforward chemistries involved and where easier metrics can be applied irrespective of the outcome, that has been one of the contributors to the outsourcing phenomenon mentioned earlier. This topic has been discussed by Roughley and Jordan in a paper [24] describing the most frequently used reactions in medicinal chemistry (e.g., amide bond formations, 22%; Suzuki/Sonogoshira reactions, ~10%; and protecting group manipulations, ~20%) and the average number of steps per synthesis (3–4 steps); the publication has stimulated a healthy discussion [25].

Advances in synthesis methods to influence stereo control have made syntheses of chiral molecules from achiral precursors more readily available and the growth of chiral chromatography and SFC methods make access to more complicated (and thus more information-rich) molecules much more feasible. In fact, this issue has recently been discussed in some detail by several authors [26–28] who have clearly demonstrated that molecular complexity and the presence of chiral centers in a candidate drug molecule correlates directly with success as molecules transition from discovery, through clinical testing and to drugs. However, the ability to regularly make meaningful complex molecules, on the shortened timescale we have become used to in medicinal chemistry lead optimization programs, is still some way into the future. Throughout a project we must constantly try to understand all the contacts that a molecule needs to make with its target protein to drive specificity into as small a molecule as possible – this often requires small, complex three-dimensional molecules. Structural biology (X-ray and NMR) and computational chemistry (rational design) can help with the selection of which molecules to make. This understanding of the structural interactions between a target protein and a drug candidate can work well in the early stages of a project with >100 nM potency compounds, before hydration–dehydration effects on binding make the predictions more difficult. This last point is important because one of the drivers of the "more is best" thought process is that, correctly so, most chemists don't want to engage in a long synthesis with only a poor chance of success at the end – better to make a larger number of molecules even if the information obtained from them is less because one sometimes gets surprises that can take the SAR into a completely novel direction. To be sure, I am a believer in making large numbers of molecules by relatively simple chemistries – and weekly, more complex chemistry is being applied to the rapid analogue synthetic armamentarium – but it is important to choose when that particular tool is applied in the drug discovery process. Certainly, in the early hit identification and hit-to-lead space, such methods play an important role, but there comes a clear point in a program where taking time to make the "right" compound(s) is much preferred to making lots more molecules that don't meaningfully advance the understanding of the SAR. Also, it is clear that not all drugs have to be complex molecules, and some good drugs are indeed simple achiral structures. However, because the binding sites on proteins are three-dimensional, it is likely that the more selective small molecules will have more points of contact with the protein surface, and hence have chirality associated with them.

After mentioning above the difficulties that the medicinal chemistry community has had to face in the past decade, it is heartening indeed to see the chapters included in this volume. It is terrific to see the creativity, patience, and innovation needed to design the molecules included in the chapters that follow. It shows again the resilience of the practitioners of our craft who have managed to continue their deep intellectual commitment to drug design and synthesis despite all the difficulties in their work environment. Designing drugs and building them from scratch is one of the most complex tasks that scientists face;

I have heard it said that "... designing a successful drug from the initial, qualitative clinical assessment of the disease, through a complete understanding of the molecular pathways involved, to the delivery of a small molecule which interferes safely with a new biochemical mechanism to change the fate of patients suffering from that disease, is as complex as designing the space shuttle when one considers the number of issues that need to be taken into consideration and the hurdles one has to overcome ..." This process is not something that can be commoditized; although clearly parts of the process can be repetitive, it requires the utmost in intellectual commitment and innovative endeavor.

Thus, it is on this difficult background that the noble endeavor of drug discovery must continue to move forward, even if the path is steep and the costs continue to rise. We must persevere because otherwise our children and their children will be restricted to using only the drugs of their parents to fight their battles with the same devastating diseases, despite all the wonderful discoveries in medicine and the biological sciences that fill academic journals with new understanding of the basic science underlying diseases. This information is derived and published so that those of us who practice medicinal chemistry can use it to design newer and better drugs. This is particularly relevant as we look at a world that is still ravaged by cancer and Alzheimer's disease in a rapidly aging population; in a world where obesity and diabetes are now epidemic; and in a world where humans are still devastated by malaria, tuberculosis, and HIV; and we must do it in a way that patients worldwide can afford and benefit from our endeavors.

REFERENCES

1. PricewaterhouseCoopers., Pharma 2020: The Vision, **2007**.
2. International Human Genome Sequencing, Consortium. Initial sequencing and analysis of the human genome. *Nature* **2001**, *409*, 860–921.
3. Venter J. C. et al. The sequence of the human genome. *Science* **2001**, *291*, 1304–1351.
4. Munos, B. Lessons from 60 years of pharmaceutical innovation. *Nat. Rev. Drug Discov.* **2009**, *8*, 959–968.
5. Paul S. M., Mytelka D. S., Dunwiddie C. T., Persinger C. C., Munos B. H., Lindborg S.R., and Schacht A. L. How to improve R&D productivity: the pharmaceutical industry's grand challenge. *Nat. Rev. Drug Discov.* **2010**, *9*, 203–214.
6. Kola I. and Landis, J. Can the pharmaceutical industry reduce attrition rates? *Nat. Rev. Drug Discov.* **2004**, *3*, 711–715.
7. Schuster, D., Laggner, C., and Langer, T. Why drugs fail: a study on side effects in new chemical entities. *Curr. Pharm. Des.* **2005**, *11*, 3545–3559.
8. Garnier, J.-P. Rebuilding the R&D engine in big pharma. *Harv. Bus. Rev.* **2008**, *8*, 68–70.
9. Accenture. Achieving high performance in pharmaceuticals through sustainable cost reduction, **2009**.
10. Spector, R. A Skeptic's view of pharmaceutical progress. *CSI Skeptical Inquirer* July/August, **2010**, *34*(4). http://www.csicop.org/si/show/a_skepties_view_of_pharmaceutical_progress
11. Douglas, F. L., Narayanan, V. K., Mitchell L., and Litan, R. E. The case for entrepreneurship in R&D in the pharmaceutical industry. *Nat. Rev. Drug Discov.* **2010**, *9*, 683–689.
12. Slater, E. E. and Kaitin, K. *Pharmaceutical Executive*, September **2010**, p. 22.
13. Teague, S. J. Learning lessons from drugs that have recently entered the market. *Drug Discov. Today* **2011**, *16*, 398–411.
14. Cuatrecasas, P. Interview with Pedro Cuatrecasas. *Nat. Rev. Drug Discov.* **2009**, *8*, 446.
15. Cuatrecasas, P. Drug discovery in jeopardy? *J. Clin. Invest.* **2006**, *116*, 2837–2842.
16. Herper, M. **2011**, http://blogs.forbes.com/matthewherper/2011/04/13/a-decade-in-drug-industry-layoffs/#comment-2923.
17. Merck, G. W. (December **1950**), in a speech at the Medical College of Virginia.
18. Grabowski, H. G. and Kyle, M. In *The Economics of Corporate Governance and Mergers* (eds K. Gugler and B. Yurtoglu), Edward Elgar, Cheltenham, **2008**, p. 262.
19. Ullman, F. and Boutellier, R. A case study of lean drug discovery: from project driven research to innovation studios and process factories. *Drug Discov. Today* **2008**, *13*, 543–550.
20. Paracelsus (1493–1541), "All things are poison, and nothing is without poison; only the dose permits something not to be poisonous."

21. Booth, B., Glassman, R., and Ma, P. Oncology's trials. *Nat. Rev. Drug Discov.* **2003**, *2*, 609–610.
22. Lipinsky, C. A., Lombardo, F., Dominy; B. W., and Feeney, P. J. Experimental and computational approaches to estimate solubility and permeability in drug discovery and development settings. *Adv. Drug Deliv. Rev.* **2001**, *46*, 3–26.
23. MacCoss, M. and Baillie, T. A. Organic chemistry in drug discovery. *Science* **2004**, *303*, 1810–1813.
24. Roughley, S. D. and Jordan, A.M. The medicinal chemist's toolbox: an analysis of reactions used in the pursuit of drug candidates. *J. Med. Chem.* **2011**, *54*, 3451–3479.
25. Lowe, D. **2011**, http://pipeline.corante.com/archives/2011/05/09/what_medicinal_chemists_really_make.php.
26. Brooks, W. H., Guida, W. C., and Daniel, K. G. The significance of chirality in drug design and development. *Curr. Top. Med. Chem.* **2011**, *11*, 760–770.
27. Lovering, F., Bikker, J., and Humblet, C. Escape from flatland: increasing saturation as an approach to improving clinical success. *J. Med. Chem.* **2009**, *52*, 6752–6756.
28. Kingwell, K. Medicinal chemistry: exploring the third dimension. *Nat. Rev. Drug Discov.* **2009**, *8*, 931.

CHAPTER 2

DISCOVERY AND DEVELOPMENT OF THE DPP-4 INHIBITOR JANUVIA™ (SITAGLIPTIN)

Emma R. Parmee, Ranabir SinhaRoy, Feng Xu, Jeffrey C. Givand, and Lawrence A. Rosen

2.1 INTRODUCTION

Type 2 diabetes mellitus (T2DM) is a global epidemic characterized by high blood sugar (hyperglycemia) due to insulin deficiency and tissue resistance to insulin-stimulated glucose uptake and utilization. The incidence of T2DM has been exacerbated by increased rates of obesity attributed to a ready availability of high calorie diets and increasingly sedentary lifestyles. It is estimated that at least 170 million people worldwide have diabetes, and this number is expected to double by 2030 [1]. The progressive nature of the disease manifests as a relentless decline in pancreatic islet function, specifically in the β-cells that secrete insulin, exacerbated by increased metabolic stress and secretory demand. Serious complications ensue as consequences of the metabolic derangement, including dyslipidemia, retinopathy, neuropathy, renal failure, and vascular disease. Although several medications are available for the treatment of T2DM, the initial correction of hyperglycemia is usually not sustained beyond a few years. These therapies may also be associated with side effects such as hypoglycemia, GI intolerance, and weight gain. None of these therapeutics is able to reverse or even delay the progressive decline in islet β-cell function. Hence, initial oral monotherapy is inevitably followed by a combination treatment to control blood sugar, and the average patient with type 2 diabetes has to resort to daily insulin injections for glucose control within 6 years of diagnosis [2]. Medications with increased safety and durability in controlling blood glucose levels are key unmet medical needs for this patient population.

2.2 DPP-4 INHIBITION AS A THERAPY FOR TYPE 2 DIABETES: IDENTIFICATION OF KEY DETERMINANTS FOR EFFICACY AND SAFETY

2.2.1 Incretin-Based Therapy for T2DM

Over the past 15 years, considerable research into new therapeutics for T2DM has focused on the physiology and pharmacology of two peptide hormones, glucagon-like peptide 1

Case Studies in Modern Drug Discovery and Development, Edited by Xianhai Huang and Robert G. Aslanian.

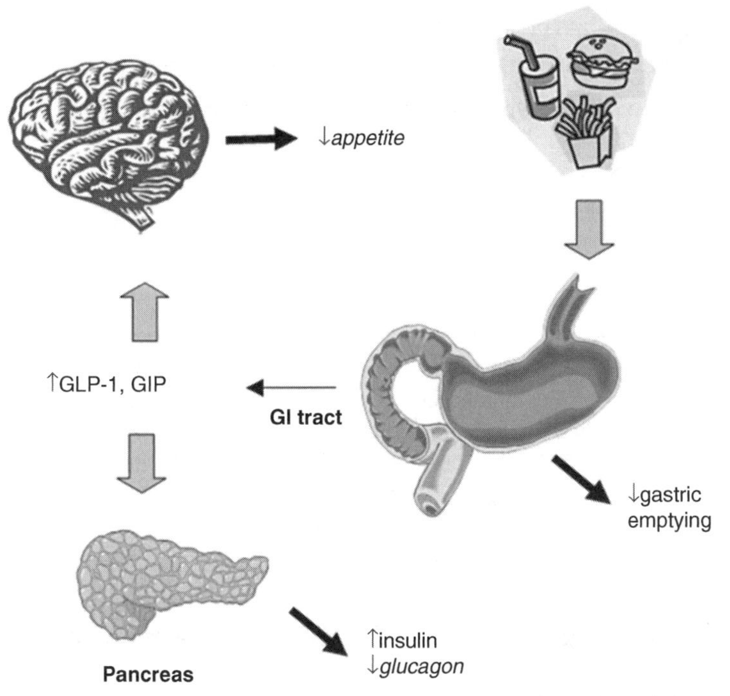

Figure 2.1 Metabolic effects and target organs of action for the incretin hormones GLP-1 and GIP in humans. These hormones are secreted upon the intake of food from enteroendocrine L- and K-cells which line the GI tract. GLP-1-specific effects are indicated in italics.

(GLP-1) [3] and glucose-dependent insulinotropic polypeptide (GIP) [4], which are secreted upon the ingestion of food from specialized enteroendocrine cells lining the GI tract. These "incretin" hormones are so named because they powerfully stimulate insulin secretion and biosynthesis in the islets in response to the delivery of enteric rather than parenteral glucose—the so-called "incretin effect" [5]. The stimulation of insulin secretion occurs in a glucose-dependent manner, which reduces the risk of hypoglycemia. In addition, both incretin hormones exhibit pleiotropic effects that modulate energy homeostasis (Figure 2.1) [6]. GLP-1 in particular decreases circulating levels of glucagon, a hormone that counters the glucose-lowering actions of insulin, and the pharmacology of GLP-1 includes delayed gastric emptying, increased satiety, and reduced food intake. Hence, contrary to the weight gain associated with insulin therapy and with oral antihyperglycemic agents such as sulfonylureas and PPAR-γ agonists, pharmacological activation of the GLP-1 receptor produce modest weight loss, which is of special benefit in treating T2DM patients, many of whom are obese. Unfortunately, GLP-1 and GIP are unstable *in vivo*, which limits their clinical use. Notwithstanding, a 6-week continuous infusion of GLP-1 in patients with type 2 diabetes completely normalized blood glucose levels and caused modest weight loss, underscoring its potential as a therapy for T2DM [7]. In contrast, the actions of GIP appear to be blunted in T2DM patients [8,9].

2.2.2 Biological Rationale: DPP-4 is a Key Regulator of Incretin Activity

The metabolic instability of the incretins GLP-1 and GIP is due to their rapid proteolytic inactivation *in vivo* by the serine ectopeptidase dipeptidyl peptidase IV (DPP-4) [10,11],

```
                   7                                36
GLP-1[7-36]-amide: HA↓EGTFTSDVSSYLEGQAAKEFIAWLVKGR-CONH2
                   7                                37
      GLP-1[7-37]: HA↓EGTFTSDVSSYLEGQAAKEFIAWLVKGRG
                   1                                        42
              GIP: YA↓EGTFISDYSIAMDKIRQQDFVNWLLAQKGKKSDWKHNITQ
```

Figure 2.2 Primary sequences for the incretin hormones GLP-1[9–36] amide and GLP-1[9–37] (collectively comprising "active" GLP-1) and GIP. Residues that are conserved between the two incretins are shaded. Homologous residues are outlined in gray. DPP-4 cleavage sites at the penultimate N-terminal residues are indicated by arrows.

which is ubiquitously expressed in diverse cell types and is also shed from the cell surface as soluble enzyme. As illustrated in Figure 2.2, DPP-4 cleaves N-terminal dipeptides from active GLP-1 (GLP-1[7–36]–amide and GLP-1[7–37]) and active GIP (GIP[1–42]) [11]. The resulting des-dipeptidyl metabolites (GLP-1[9–36]–amide, GLP-1[9–37], and GIP [3–42], respectively) exhibit no incretin activity and are virtually inactive as agonists of the corresponding receptors [11]. It has been estimated that upon subcutaneous administration of GLP-1 to T2DM patients, ~90% of the circulating peptide is inactivated by DPP-4 cleavage [12]. GLP-1 is also rapidly cleared by the kidneys such that the circulating half-life of active peptide is ~1.5 min [13].

2.2.3 Injectable GLP-1 Mimetics for the Treatment of T2DM

The very short half-life of native GLP-1 as a therapeutic has been addressed by the development of protease-resistant GLP-1 mimetics. Exenatide (Byetta™, Amylin/Lilly), a DPP-4 resistant GLP-1 peptide mimetic originally isolated from the saliva of the gila monster [14], and liraglutide (Victoza™, Novo), an acylated palmitoyl-GLP-1 conjugate [15], are marketed therapeutics for T2DM that exemplify this approach. Effective glucose control and modest weight loss are observed in treated patients, especially with liraglutide [16,17]. The efficacy of these agents, however, is tempered by the need for twice-daily and daily injections, respectively, and by adverse GI events (nausea, emesis, and diarrhea), especially at the onset of therapy. These adverse events occur due to supraphysiological (pharmacological) activation of the GLP-1 receptor and appear to be dose limiting for the class [18].

2.2.4 DPP-4 Inhibition as Oral Incretin-Based Therapy for T2DM

The second approach to incretin-based therapy and one that is amenable to oral administration is based upon the stabilization of endogenous GLP-1 and GIP by blocking DPP-4 cleavage with a small molecule inhibitor. The increase in endogenous incretin tone, especially following meals, improves glycemic control with reduced risk of hypoglycemia due to augmented insulin secretion, which occurs only under conditions of high blood glucose. Genetic proof-of-concept for this approach was obtained in 2000 by the characterization of DPP-4 deficient ($Cd26^{-/-}$) mice, which are healthy, fertile, and exhibit improved glucose tolerance with elevated circulating active GLP-1 levels [19]. The same report described mechanism-based efficacy of small molecule DPP-4 inhibitors, which improved glucose tolerance in wild-type mice but not in DPP-4 deficient animals. Since DPP-4 is identical to the T-cell surface antigen marker CD26 present on $CD4^+$ helper T cells, which had been proposed to play a costimulatory role in T-cell receptor activation [20], the absence of immune dysfunction in DPP-4-deficient mice was especially encouraging.

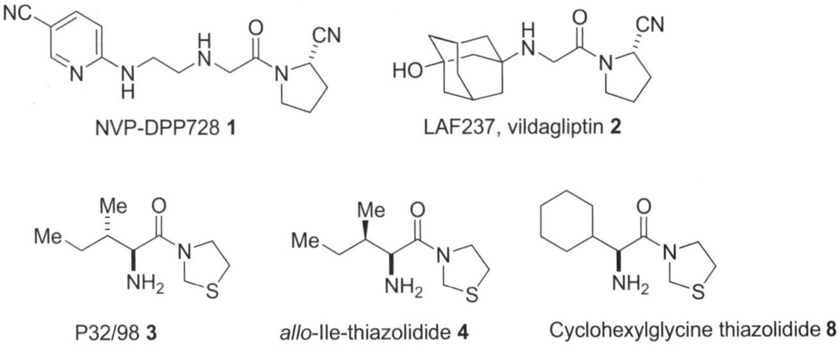

NVP-DPP728 **1** LAF237, vildagliptin **2**

P32/98 **3** *allo*-Ile-thiazolidide **4** Cyclohexylglycine thiazolidide **8**

Figure 2.3 Early reported DPP-4 inhibitors.

While the role of DPP-4 activity in immune function clearly warranted further investigation, the potential of DPP-4 inhibition as a novel oral therapy for T2DM with minimal risk of hypoglycemia and likely beneficial effects on body weight prompted us to initiate a medicinal chemistry effort in 1999. It soon became apparent, however, that others had taken an early lead in this area. In 2002, Novartis reported encouraging 4-week phase II data for its first DPP-4 inhibitor, NVP-728 (**1**) [21], and disclosed development of a second compound, NVP-LAF237 (vildagliptin, **2**) [22,23] (Figure 2.3). The poor pharmacokinetics of NVP-728 necessitated three times daily (TID) administration in T2DM patients. Notwithstanding, significant improvements in fasting, prandial, and 24 h glucose levels were observed without any of the adverse GI events associated with pharmacological activation of the GLP-1 receptor by injectable GLP-1 mimetics. The attractive efficacy/tolerability profile for NVP-728 in the clinic together with the added advantage of oral administration supported positioning small-molecule DPP-4 inhibitors as a viable and earlier alternative to injectable peptides for the treatment of T2DM.

2.2.5 Investigation of DPP-4 Biology: Identification of Candidate Substrates

An important objective of any drug development effort is to predict and evaluate all potential consequences of pharmaceutical intervention, which requires a comprehensive understanding of target biology. DPP-4 had been reported to cleave multiple circulating immunoregulatory, endocrine, and neurological peptides *in vitro* albeit under conditions of nonphysiological substrate concentrations (typically 1–5 μM) and/or excess enzyme [24–28]. Most bioactive peptides and hormones, however, circulate at picomolar concentrations *in vivo*, well below the Michaelis constant (K_M) for protease binding and cleavage, which is typically in the micromolar range. Under these conditions, the efficiency with which a particular peptide undergoes proteolysis is reflected by the apparent second-order rate constant of cleavage (k_{cat}/K_M). We therefore undertook a critical reevaluation of purported DPP-4 substrates in an unbiased screen that measured cleavage kinetics for a library of ~350 mammalian peptides including glucagon superfamily hormones, neuropeptides, chemokines, and other bioactive peptides. Physiologically relevant concentrations of DPP-4 (0.5 nM) and sub-K_M concentrations of each peptide (250 nM) were incubated together and monitored for potential cleavage of the latter using a multiplexed LC/MS assay [29]. Peptides that were efficiently cleaved by DPP-4 *in vitro* ($k_{cat}/K_M > 10^5\ M^{-1}\ s^{-1}$) represented candidate *in vivo* substrates that could be potentially regulated by the enzyme especially if DPP-4 cleavage ablated or altered peptide bioactivity (Table 2.1).

TABLE 2.1 ***In vitro*** **Substrates for DPP-4 that are Efficiently Cleaved by the Enzyme ((K_{cat}/K_M)≥10^5 M^{-1} s^{-1}) in a Multiplexed LC/MS Assay**

Peptide	N-term sequence	$\frac{k_{cat}}{K_M}$, $\times 10^5$ M^{-1} s^{-1}
GHRH	YA↓DA...	30
MCP-4	QP↓DA...	16
LEC	QP↓KV...	16
Endomorphin 2	YP↓FF	14
I-TAC	FP↓MF	13
Substance P	RP↓KP...	13
Neuropeptide Y	YP↓SK...	12
SDF-1β	KP↓VS...	12
GRP	VP↓LP...	10
SDF-1α	KP↓VS...	8.8
PACAP38	HS↓DG...	7.3
Endomorphin 1	YP↓WF	6.3
GH(1–43)	FP↓TI...	6.1
CART(55–102)	VP↓IY...	5.1
GLP-1	HA↓EG...	4.2
BNP	SP↓KM...	3.7
IP-10	VP↓LS...	3.6
MCP-3	QP↓VG...	2.8
PHM	HA↓DG...	2.5
GIP	YA↓EG...	2.3
Ghrelin	GS↓S(oct)F...	2.3
Gro-β	AP↓LA...	2.1
LIX	AP↓SS...	1.7
Pancreatic polypeptide	AP↓LE...	1.6
Oxyntomodulin	HS↓QG...	1.5
Eotaxin	GP↓AS...	1.5
GLP-2	HA↓DG...	0.9
Peptide YY	YP↓IK...	0.6

The associated physiology and pharmacology of these peptides allowed us to identify candidate DPP-4 substrates implicated in metabolic function (in addition to GLP-1 and GIP) and to flag any potential safety issues that could arise from the stabilization of bioactive peptides by a DPP-4 inhibitor.

As summarized in Table 2.1, the best *in vitro* substrates for DPP-4 that were identified contain a penultimate N-terminal Pro or Ala, which is typically required for DPP-4 cleavage. Oxyntomodulin (OXM) and pituitary adenylate cyclase activating polypeptide 38 (PACAP38), however, were identified as novel noncanonical DPP-4 substrates containing a serine residue at this position [29]. DPP-4 cleavage *in vivo* would be anticipated to modulate the activity of most of these peptides since the corresponding N-terminal dipeptides are critical for bioactivity [29,30]. OXM, PACAP38, GH[1–43], CART[55–102], and gastrin-releasing peptide (GRP) are implicated in metabolic function [31–36] and the bioactivity of some of these peptides (administered exogenously) is potentiated by inhibition or genetic ablation of DPP-4 [29,37]. Hence, regulation of substrates other than GLP-1 and GIP may also mediate some of the metabolic effects of DPP-4 inhibitors *in vivo*. Glucose tolerance tests in mice lacking one or both of the GLP-1 and GIP receptors have revealed, however, that the acute glucose lowering effects of DPP-4 inhibitors are mediated solely by these two peptides, at least in rodents [38]. It therefore remains to be determined whether the stabilization of additional *in vivo* DPP-4 substrates contributes to the chronic efficacy of DPP-4 inhibitors in humans.

We next evaluated candidate *in vivo* DPP-4 substrates that could be associated with potential side effects. For most of the *in vitro* substrates (Table 2.1), potential stabilization of the corresponding *endogenous* intact peptides *in vivo* by a DPP-4 inhibitor was anticipated to be well tolerated based on knowledge of corresponding physiology and pharmacology. There was some concern, however, regarding stabilization of growth hormone releasing hormone (GHRH) [39], glucagon-like peptide 2 (GLP-2) [40], substance P [41,42], and various chemokines [25,28], which triggered additional preclinical studies to evaluate the potential regulation of these peptides by DPP-4 *in vivo*. For GHRH and GLP-2, which are growth factors, no significant stabilization of the peptides in the context of DPP-4 inhibition/ablation was observed *in vivo* [43,44]. Furthermore, no adverse events related to elevated levels of substance P (angioedema and pruritus) or altered chemokine tone (increased susceptibility to infection) were observed in DPP-4 deficient mice and in preclinical studies with in-house DPP-4 inhibitors [45,46]. In addition, selective DPP-4 inhibitors had no effect on T-cell proliferation *in vitro* (*vide infra*). Taken together, these preclinical studies increased our confidence in the safety and tolerability of chronic DPP-4 inhibition in T2DM patients, and additional reassurance in this regard was also derived from the published short-term clinical experience with NVP-728 [21].

2.2.6 Preclinical Toxicities of In-Licensed DPP-4 Inhibitors

Given the competitive landscape for DPP-4 inhibitors with at least one company in advanced clinical development [21], we decided to jump-start our nascent drug development program in parallel with ongoing internal lead identification efforts by in-licensing small molecule DPP-4 inhibitors from Probiodrug GmbH in 2000. Specifically, P32/98 (*threo*-isoleucyl-thiazolidide, *threo*-Ile-Thz) **3** [47], and its *allo* diastereomer (*allo*-Ile-Thz) **4** were acquired as potential clinical candidates. Both molecules were equipotent inhibitors of DPP-4 (IC_{50} values of 201 nM and 188 nM, respectively, for soluble human recombinant DPP-4). In addition, P32/98 had an acceptable short-term preclinical safety profile and was well tolerated in a small phase I study conducted by Probiodrug [48]. Unfortunately, the development of P32/98 had to be discontinued at Merck due to serious toxicology findings in chronic studies conducted in rats and dogs [46]. Table 2.2 summarizes the preclinical toxicology profile for P32/98, which included multiorgan pathology in rats, acute GI toxicity in dogs, and mortality upon chronic dosing in both species. Given the potential for multiple peptide substrates in addition to GLP-1 and GIP to be stabilized by a small molecule DPP-4 inhibitor, the initial suspicion was that these adverse effects were mechanism-based (resulting from direct DPP-4 inhibition). This notion was rapidly dispelled, however, by preclinical toxicology studies with the *allo* diastereomer of P32/98. Despite being an equipotent DPP-4 inhibitor and otherwise indistinguishable from P32/98 in terms of metabolism, pharmacokinetics, pharmacodynamics in preclinical species, and selectivity against other target classes as evaluated in an MDS-Pharma PanLabs Screen, *allo*-Ile-Thz reproduced the toxicology signature of P32/98 but was ~10-fold more toxic on a dose or plasma exposure basis in rats and dogs [46] (Table 2.2). The different exposure thresholds for preclinical toxicity with P32/98 and *allo*-Ile-Thz despite comparable (and complete) DPP-4 inhibition *in vivo* by the two compounds strongly suggested that the safety

TABLE 2.2 Comparative Preclinical Toxicities of *threo*- and *allo*-Ile-Thz and Selective DPP Inhibitors in Rats (2 Weeks of Treatment at 10, 30, 100 mg kg^{-1} day^{-1} p.o.) and Dogs (Single Dose, 10 mg kg^{-1}p.o.)

Species	Toxicity	*threo*-Ile-Thz	*allo*-Ile-Thz	DPP-4 selective **5**	QPP-selective **6**	DPP-8/9-selective **7**
Rat	Alopecia		+			+
	Thrombocytopenia	+	+ + +			+ +
	Anemia		+			
	Reticulocytopenia		ND		+	+ +
	Splenomegaly		+ + +			+ + +
	Mortality		+			+
Dog	Bloody diarrhea	+[a]	+			+
	Mortality	+[b]	NT	NT	NT	NT
	CNS toxicity	+[b]	NT	NT	NT	NT

Source: Data summarized from Ref. 46.

For rat data, +, + +, and + + + indicate toxicity observed at high, middle, and low dose, respectively. For dog data, + indicates toxicity was observed. ND = not determined; NT = not tested.

[a]Compound dosed acutely at 225 mg kg^{-1}.

[b]Compound dosed at 75 mg kg^{-1} for >5 weeks.

findings were due to an as yet unidentified off-target activity of these inhibitors. Attention now turned toward confirming this hypothesis.

2.2.7 Correlation of Preclinical Toxicity with Off-Target Inhibition of Pro-Specific Dipeptidase Activity

An early hint of potential off-target activity of the Probiodrug compounds was provided in 2000 in an attempt to catalog other DPP-4 like enzymes. At the time, very little was known about DPP-4 and related peptidases that are able to cleave substrates at a Pro residue and together comprise the "DPP-4 activity and/or structure homologue" (DASH) family [49]. Given the preclinical toxicities of the Probiodrug DPP-4 inhibitors, however, it was important to investigate the consequences of potentially inhibiting these related enzymes. We detected multiple dipeptidases in tissue extracts from *Cd26*$^{-/-}$ mice using a fluorogenic aminomethylcoumarin (AMC)-based P1-positional scanning dipeptide substrate library X-P1-AMC [50] as the probe, where X comprises an isokinetic mixture of norleucine and all coded amino acids except Cys, and the P1 position was scanned across each amino acid. As illustrated in Figure 2.4a, P1-Pro-specific dipeptidase activity in *Cd26*$^{-/-}$ mice was relatively low compared to other dipeptidase activities. When calibrated against recombinant soluble human DPP-4, solubilized P1-Pro-DPP activity from the small intestine of *Cd26*$^{-/-}$ mice was measured to be ~20-fold lower than the corresponding activity in tissue extracts from wild-type mice, where it was completely masked by the relatively high abundance DPP-4. Of note, however, this P1-Pro-DPP activity was potently and selectively inhibited *in vitro* by *allo*-Ile-Thz **4** (IC_{50} = 86 nM), which only modestly inhibited the other dipeptidase activities (<40% inhibition at 100 μM, Figure 2.4b). Our interest was further heightened by the observation that *threo*-Ile-Thz (P32/98) **3** was 8.4-fold less potent in inhibiting this activity (IC_{50} = 726 nM). This differential inhibition of Pro-specific DPP activity was the first significant difference detected between the two compounds *in vitro*, and correlated with the ~10-fold difference in their preclinical toxicities. We therefore refined our hypothesis to postulate that the differential preclinical toxicities of P32/98 and

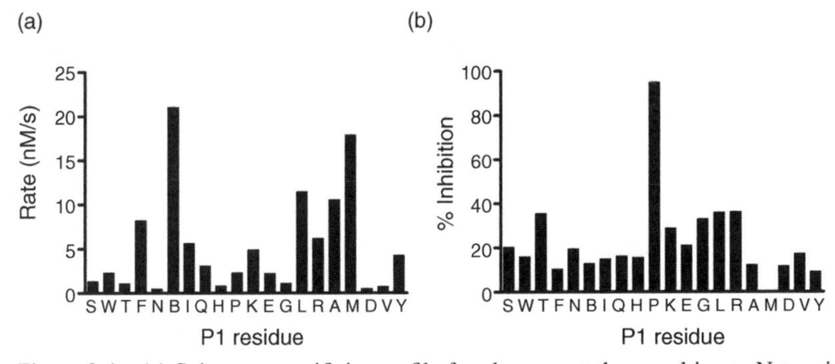

Figure 2.4 (a) Substrate specificity profile for cleavage at the penultimate N-terminal residue (P1 residue) by dipeptidyl peptidase activities present in solubilized tissue extract from the small intestine of *Cd26*$^{-/-}$ mice. P1-Pro-specific DPP activity represents a relatively minor component of DPP activities in tissue. (b) P1-Pro-specific DPP activities in the tissue extract are completely inhibited by addition of 100 μM *allo*-Ile-Thz.

allo-Ile-Thz were not due to inhibition of DPP-4 but due to differential off-target inhibition of one or more related Pro-specific dipeptidases.

2.2.8 Identification of Pro-Specific Dipeptidases Differentially Inhibited by the Probiodrug Compounds

The optimization of a drug that selectively engages its target is an iterative process, facilitated by appropriate *in vitro* counterscreens against related targets, which assess molecular selectivity in medicinal chemistry structure–activity relationship (SAR) studies. A biochemistry effort was initiated to install the appropriate counterscreens for developing a selective and safe DPP-4 inhibitor by characterizing the murine P1-Pro-specific dipeptidases that were differentially inhibited by the Probiodrug inhibitors and by developing the corresponding activity-based assays using recombinant human enzymes. It was anticipated that the latter would also facilitate the development of highly selective inhibitors of the corresponding enzymes for toxicology studies in rats and dogs, which would allow us to unequivocally test the hypothesis of preclinical toxicity arising from off-target inhibition of one or more Pro-specific dipeptidases.

Tissue extracts from the small intestines of DPP-4-deficient mice were fractionated using high-resolution MonoQ anion exchange chromatography. Two P1-Pro-selective dipeptidases were resolved that were each differentially inhibited by the Probiodrug compounds. Although neither of these activities provided useful mass spectrometry data for protein identification, one of the enzymes eluted with the same retention time as that of purified recombinant human DPP-8. In addition, measured IC_{50} values against this Pro-specific DPP activity for a set of structurally diverse DPP-4 inhibitors (including P32/98 and *allo*-Ile-Thz) correlated best with the corresponding IC_{50} values against recombinant human DPP-8 [51] amongst a panel of DPP-4 related enzymes comprising DPP-4, FAP/seprase [52], QPP/DPP-II/DPP-7 [53], DPP-8, prolyl endopeptidase (PEP), aminopeptidase P (APP), and prolidase. Hence, this Pro-specific DPP activity was attributed to be the murine orthologue of DPP-8. A similar analysis of IC_{50} values for the second Pro-specific DPP activity also suggested similarities to DPP-8 but with a few significant outliers (Figure 2.5a). For example, vildagliptin (LAF237, **2**), the second-generation DPP-4 inhibitor from Novartis, was a potent inhibitor of this activity (IC_{50} = 139 nM) but a weak inhibitor of recombinant human DPP-8 (IC_{50} = 5.7 μM). The overall similarity in IC_{50} profiles,

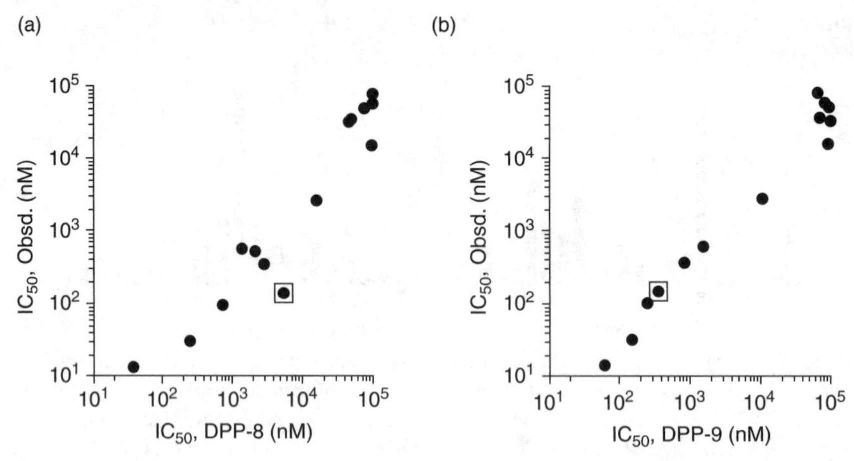

Figure 2.5 Correlation of *in vitro* IC_{50} values measured for a set of structurally diverse DPP-4 inhibitors against an early-eluting Pro-selective dipeptidyl peptidase activity isolated from the small intestine of *Cd26*$^{-/-}$ mice using high-resolution MonoQ anion exchange chromatography and corresponding IC_{50} values against (a) recombinant human DPP-8 and (b) recombinant human DPP-9. The boxed data point corresponds to vildagliptin.

however, suggested that this second P1-Pro-selective dipeptidase was closely related to DPP-8. As illustrated in Figure 2.5b, an excellent linear correlation was subsequently obtained with the IC_{50} values against human DPP-9 [54] (for vildagliptin, $IC_{50} = 363$ nM), when the recombinant enzyme, which exhibits 60% sequence identity to DPP-8, became available in 2002. Hence, the second P1-Pro-DPP activity was identified as the murine orthologue of DPP-9. Although other Pro-selective peptidases (FAP, QPP, PEP, APP, and prolidase) were also detected in solubilized tissue from *Cd26*$^{-/-}$ mice, none of these enzymes (with the possible exception of QPP) were considered relevant to the preclinical toxicities observed with the Probiodrug inhibitors since they are not significantly inhibited by P32/98 and *allo*-Ile-Thz *in vitro* (Table 2.3, entries 1 and 2).

TABLE 2.3 *In vitro* Inhibitory Potencies of *threo*- and *allo*-Ile-Thz and DPP-Selective Inhibitors Against DPP-4 and Related Pro-Specific Peptidases

	IC_{50} (nM)							
Compound	DPP-4	DPP-8	DPP-9	QPP	FAP	PEP	APP	Prolidase
1. *threo*-Ile-Thz **3**	420	2180	1600	14000	$>10^5$	$>10^5$	$>10^5$	$>10^5$
2. *allo*-Ile-Thz **4**	460	220	320	18000	$>10^5$	$>10^5$	$>10^5$	$>10^5$
3. DPP-4-selective **5**	27	69000	$>10^5$	$>10^5$	$>10^5$	$>10^5$	$>10^5$	$>10^5$
4. QPP-selective **6**	1900	22000	11000	19	$>10^5$	63000	$>10^5$	$>10^5$
5. DPP-8,9-selective **7**	30000	38	55	14000	$>10^5$	$>10^5$	$>10^5$	$>10^5$
6. Lys[Z(NO_2)]pyrrolidide	1300	154	165	1210	51000	$>10^5$	$>10^5$	$>10^5$
7. Lys[Z(NO_2)]thiazolidide	410	210	75	210	33000	56000	ND	$>10^5$
8. Lys[Z(NO_2)]piperidide	17000	1100	670	710	$>10^5$	$>10^5$	ND	ND
9. Val-Boro-Pro	<4	4	11	310	560	390	$>10^5$	$>10^5$

ND: not determined.

2.2.9 A Highly Selective DPP-4 Inhibitor is Safe and Well Tolerated in Preclinical Species

The identification of DPP-8 and DPP-9 as Pro-selective-dipeptidyl peptidases (DPP) that are differentially inhibited by the Probiodrug inhibitors (which also modestly inhibit QPP/DPP-II, Table 2.3) underscored the importance of identifying selective inhibitors of DPP-4 and of the other dipeptidases. Our medicinal chemistry team worked to increase the selectivity of a number of structures in order to provide useful tool compounds for biological studies. As summarized in Table 2.3, compounds **5**, **6**, and **7** (Figure 2.6) were highly selective inhibitors of DPP-4, QPP, and DPP-8/9, respectively ($\geq$100-fold selective against other Pro-selective peptidases), with pharmacokinetic properties suitable for chronic dosing in rats and dogs [46]. Each compound was evaluated in a 2-week rat toxicology study at doses of 10, 30, and 100 $mg\,kg^{-1}\,day^{-1}$ and in a single-dose dog tolerability study at 10 $mg\,kg^{-1}$. As summarized in Table 2.2, the QPP-selective inhibitor **6** produced a decrease in reticulocytes in rats at the top dose but no other antemortem or postmortem changes were noticed in either species. In contrast, the DPP-8/9 inhibitor **7** reproduced virtually all the hallmark toxicities of the Probiodrug compounds including multiorgan pathology in rats and acute GI toxicity in dogs (Table 2.2). Of note, the DPP-4-selective inhibitor **5** was completely devoid of any findings in the toxicology studies despite compound exposures that were sufficient for complete plasma DPP-4 inhibition and similar to or greater than the exposures of *allo*-Ile-Thz **4** that had produced toxicity. Hence, we were able to confirm our hypothesis that the preclinical toxicities of the Probiodrug inhibitors were due to off-target inhibition of Pro-specific dipeptidases, specifically DPP-8 and/or DPP-9 [46].

2.2.10 A Highly Selective DPP-4 Inhibitor Does Not Inhibit T-Cell Proliferation *in vitro*

DPP-4/CD26 is a multidomain protein with a classical serine-peptidase fold but with other domains known to mediate intercellular interactions. Considerable evidence suggested that DPP-4 may serve a costimulatory role in T-cell receptor activation [20], but it was unclear as to whether the peptidase activity was involved in this process. While *Cd26*$^{-/-}$ mice exhibited no obvious immune defects, small-molecule DPP-4 inhibitors were reported to suppress CD-4^{+} T-cell proliferation in cell-based assays [55]. We recognized that the DPP-4 inhibitors used in published T-cell proliferation studies were structurally related to the Probiodrug inhibitors and therefore likely to exhibit poor selectivity against other DPP-4 family members. Indeed, as summarized in Table 2.3, entries 6–8, these compounds were revealed to be more potent inhibitors of DPP-8 and DPP-9 than of DPP-4. The availability of selective dipeptidase inhibitors enabled us to now rigorously assess the involvement of DPP-4 activity in T-cell function. Of note, the highly selective and potent DPP-4 inhibitor **5**

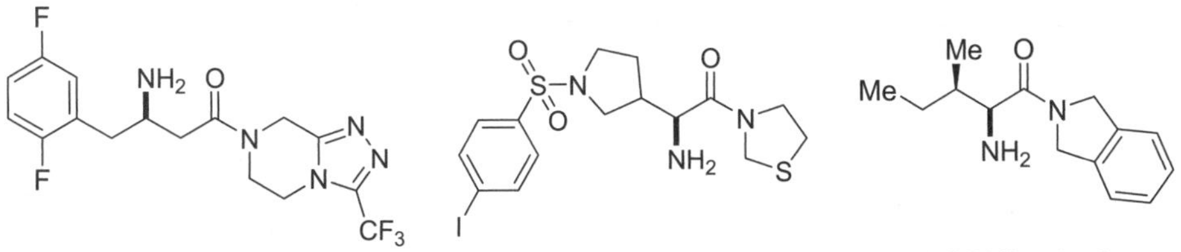

5, DPP-4 selective
DPP-4 IC_{50} = 27 nM

6, QPP selective
QPP IC_{50} = 19 nM

7, DPP8/9 selective
DPP8 IC_{50} = 38 nM
DPP9 IC_{50} = 55 nM

Figure 2.6 DPP-4-, QPP-, and DPP8/9-selective inhibitors used in comparative toxicity studies.

was completely inactive in two cell-based models of T-cell proliferation. In contrast, the DPP-8/9 selective inhibitor **7** potently suppressed T-cell proliferation in these assays, as did the nonselective DPP-4 inhibitor Val-Boro-Pro, Table 2.3, entry 9, which also potently inhibits DPP 8 and DPP-9 [46]. Hence, inhibition of DPP-4 enzyme activity *in vivo* was not anticipated to be a liability for T-cell proliferation and immune function.

2.2.11 DPP-4 Inhibitor Selectivity as a Key Parameter for Drug Development

Our experience with the Probiodrug DPP-4 inhibitors led to an appreciation of the pharmacological consequences of inhibiting other DPP-4-like Pro-selective peptidases as well as to the necessity of developing highly selective inhibitors of these enzymes. We used these tools to demonstrate that *selective* DPP-4 inhibition was safe and well tolerated in preclinical species with no effects on T-cell proliferation *in vitro*. Medicinal chemistry efforts subsequently focused on developing a highly selective (>1000-fold) and potent small-molecule DPP-4 inhibitor suitable for the treatment of T2DM, with excellent selectivity against other related Pro-selective peptidases, especially DPP-8 and DPP-9.

2.3 MEDICINAL CHEMISTRY PROGRAM

2.3.1 Lead Generation Approaches

While there are multiple lead generation strategies available to a nascent drug discovery project, two concurrent approaches were adopted at the onset of our DPP-4 inhibitor program that led to the discovery of sitagliptin phosphate (JANUVIA™). First, a high-throughput screen (HTS) of the Merck sample collection was initiated and this effort yielded two key lead series for the program. Second, a review of publicly disclosed DPP-4 inhibitors was undertaken in order to enable "lead hopping" and initiation of the medicinal chemistry program while the HTS was in progress. This second approach led to the development of a proprietary series of DPP-4 inhibitors with excellent potency and pharmacokinetic properties. An overview of the progression of these three lead series, each structurally distinct from the Probiodrug compounds, is presented. It should be noted that the DPP-4 crystal structure was not available at the time our drug discovery program was initiated. It was, however, employed extensively for structure-based drug design in support of a backup program following publication of the structural information in 2003 [56].

2.3.2 Cyclohexyl Glycine α-Amino Acid Series of DPP-4 Inhibitors

At the time we initiated our medicinal chemistry program, several small-molecule inhibitors of DPP-4 had already been reported in the literature. Of these compounds, **1** and **2** were potent inhibitors of DPP-4 ($IC_{50} = 22$ and 34 nM, respectively), but both contained an electrophilic nitrile group (Figure 2.1 [21,23,47,57]). It had been shown that this nitrile could form a covalent bond with the catalytic serine residue at the DPP-4 active site, and it was also reasoned that this moiety might lead to the poor pharmacokinetic properties observed with some of the known inhibitors [58]. Hence, we made a strategic decision to identify DPP-4 inhibitors that did not possess this electrophilic nitrile moiety. Literature reports indicated that DPP-4 inhibitors lacking the nitrile were more stable but were

TABLE 2.4 4-Substituted Cyclohexylglycine Analogues

Compound	R	X	DPP-4 IC_{50} (nM)
8	H	S	89
9	(3,4-di-F-Ph)CONH-	S	54
10	$PhCH_2OCONH$-	S	25
11	$(4\text{-}CF_3O\text{-}Ph)SO_2NH$-	S	22
12	(3,4-di-F-Ph)CONH-	CH_2	190
13	$PhCH_2OCONH$-	CH_2	94
14	$(4\text{-}CF_3O\text{-}Ph)SO_2NH$-	CH_2	89
15	(3,4-di-F-Ph)CONH-	CF_2	55
16	$PhCH_2OCONH$-	CF_2	27
17	$(4\text{-}CF_3O\text{-}Ph)SO_2NH$-	CF_2	23
18	(3,4-di-F-Ph)CONH-	(*R*)-CHF	110
19	$PhCH_2OCONH$-	(*R*)-CHF	88
20	$(4\text{-}CF_3O\text{-}Ph)SO_2NH$-	(*R*)-CHF	75
21	(3,4-di-F-Ph)CONH-	(*S*)-CHF	54
22	$PhCH_2OCONH$-	(*S*)-CHF	56
23	$(4\text{-}CF_3O\text{-}Ph)SO_2NH$-	(*S*)-CHF	36

generally of modest intrinsic potency. One such example is (*S*)-cyclohexyl glycine thiazolidide **8** ($IC_{50} = 89$ nM) [59], which was only 3- to 4-fold less potent than compounds **1** and **2**. We therefore selected this scaffold as our starting point for modification.

We decided to install an amino group ($R = NH_2$) in the 4-position of the cyclohexyl ring of compound **8** and investigate the effect of diverse nitrogen capping groups on inhibitory activity [60]. This approach yielded a series of highly potent DPP-4 inhibitors, exemplified by analogues **9–11** (IC_{50} values of 22–54 nM, Table 2.4), with excellent pharmacokinetic properties (50–80% oral bioavailability in the rat). This earliest work was performed prior to elucidation of the cause of preclinical toxicity for the Probiodrug inhibitors (*vide supra*); hence, selectivity against DPP-8/9 was not a driver for the SAR of this series. Concerns about potential metabolic issues associated with the thiazolidine ring led us to evaluate alternatives. As anticipated from the parent compounds, replacement of the thiazolidine ring with a pyrrolidine resulted in approximately a 4-fold loss in *in vitro* potency (compounds **12–14**). We therefore evaluated installation of mono- and bis-fluoro substitutions on the pyrrolidine ring [61]. Equivalent activity was observed with 3,3-difluoro-pyrrolidide analogues (compounds **15–17**) as with the thiazolidide ring. The (*R*)-3-fluoro analogues (compounds **18–20**) were less potent, while the (*S*)-3-fluoro substitution (compounds **21–23**) provided the optimal balance between potency and selectivity over QPP (data not shown). This investigation led us to select trifluoromethoxy sulfonamide **23** as a promising lead.

Compound **23** displayed excellent pharmacokinetic properties in preclinical species ($t_{1/2}$ of 4–12 h; 37–90% oral bioavailability). Further evaluation of this compound was

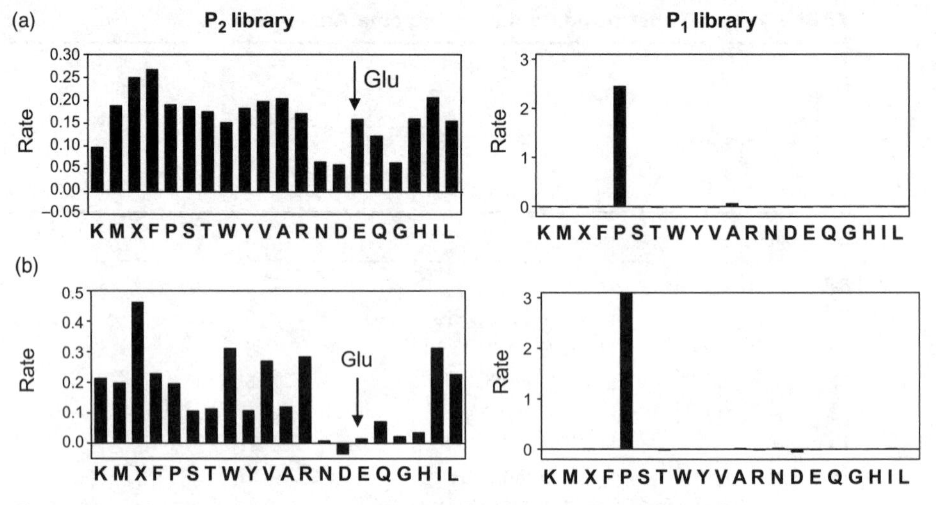

Figure 2.7 Cleavage of peptide scanning libraries by (a) DPP-4 and (b) DPP8.

discontinued, however, upon elucidation of the role of DPP-8/9 in the observed preclinical toxicity of nonselective DPP-4 inhibitors, and in view of the fact that **23** exhibited only modest selectivity against DPP-8 and DPP-9 (IC_{50} values of 1400 and 1700 nM, respectively).

2.3.3 Improving Selectivity of the α-Amino Acid Series

All the α-amino acid analogues that had been prepared thus far in the program were structurally related to compound **23** and showed unacceptable selectivity over DPP-8/9. We therefore focused on improving this profile. From a comparison of substrate P1 and P2 residue selectivities for DPP-4 and DPP-8, using the P1 positional scanning library described earlier and the corresponding P2 library [50], it was evident that while both enzymes showed a strong preference for substrates with a proline at the P1 position (Figure 2.7), DPP-4 was relatively more promiscuous at P2. Notably, dipeptides containing acidic residues such as glutamate were rapidly cleaved by DPP-4 but not by DPP-8. It was hypothesized, therefore, that incorporation of an acidic functionality at sites mapping to the P2 position in our inhibitors could provide analogues with improved selectivity over DPP-8. Similar conclusions were reached by analyzing the substrate selectivity of DPP-9.

Based on the preceding analysis, analogues containing a variety of carboxylic acids and acid bioisosteres were prepared and compounds such as **24** (unpublished results) and **25** [60] were shown to be potent inhibitors of DPP-4 with >100-fold selectivity over DPP-8 (Figure 2.8). Unfortunately, these compounds, as well as other acidic analogues, exhibited extremely poor pharmacokinetic properties in the rat. Hence, work on this series was halted although these issues were ultimately resolved in support of a sitagliptin backup program [62].

2.3.4 Identification and Optimization of the β-Amino Acid Series

High-throughput screening of the Merck sample collection was carried out while SAR studies on the α-amino acid series were underway. Two leads were identified from the screen, from which extensive SAR was developed, and played an integral role in the discovery of sitagliptin. The first lead was the β-amino acid proline amide **26**; this

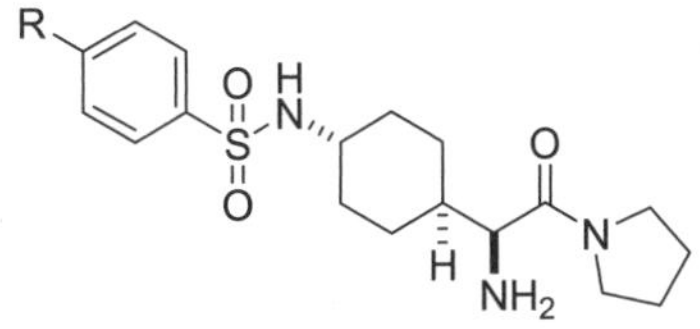

24, R = COOH
DPP-4 IC_{50} = 15 nM
DPP8 IC_{50} = 2800 nM

25, R = $CF_3CH_2SO_2NH$-
DPP-4 IC_{50} = 64 nM
DPP8 IC_{50} = 88,000 nM

Figure 2.8 DPP-4 inhibitors containing acidic functionality.

compound (Figure 2.9) was a moderate inhibitor of DPP-4 ($IC_{50} = 1.9\,\mu M$) and a significantly more potent inhibitor of thrombin ($IC_{50} = 0.052\,\mu M$), the target protease for which it was originally prepared. The second lead was the β-amino piperazine **27**. This compound was originally prepared for an obesity target and was only a weak inhibitor of DPP-4 with an IC_{50} of 11 μM.

Upon inspection of the first lead **26**, it was reasoned that the proline ring might interact with DPP-4 in a manner analogous to that of the pyrrolidide ring in the α-amino acid series. We tested this hypothesis by replacement of the (*R*)-β-amino acid with either isoleucine or cyclohexylglycine, only to find >2-fold loss in potency in each case. More modest changes to the β-phenylalanine side-chain were therefore targeted. For ease of synthesis, these SAR studies were performed in the context of a truncated thiazolidide scaffold **28**, which was only modestly less potent than the original lead (R = H; DPP-4 $IC_{50} = 3\,\mu M$) (Figure 2.10) [63]. Altering the tether length, replacing the phenyl group with heterocyclic or aliphatic moieties, and installing large substituents on the aromatic ring all resulted in a significant loss of activity. The only improvements in potency that could be realized by modifications in this region of the molecule were obtained by installation of fluoro substituents on the aromatic ring. The 2-fluorophenyl analogue **29** exhibited a 3-fold increase in potency, and 3,4-difluoro substitution on the aromatic ring (as in **30**) afforded approximately a 2-fold improvement in activity. These observations prompted a comprehensive evaluation of the positioning of fluorine atoms around the phenyl ring, resulting in identification of the 2,5-difluoro- and 2,4,5-trifluoro analogues (**31** and **32**) as optimal with respect to DPP-4 inhibitory potency (IC_{50} values of 0.27 and 0.12 μM, respectively). At the time the work was performed, this extremely restrictive SAR around the aromatic ring was purely an empirical observation. When the crystal structure of the enzyme was published, the SAR observations were explained, as *in silico* binding studies indicated significant steric constraints within the relevant pocket allowing only the smallest groups (hydrogen and fluorine) to be accommodated [56].

We next turned our attention to optimization of the benzyl amide portion of **26**, and found that cleavage of the cyclopropylamide to the carboxylic acid yielded a modest 2-fold

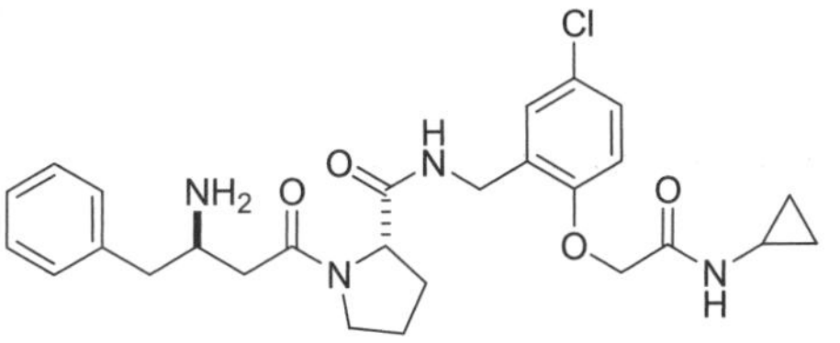

26, IC_{50} = 1900 nM

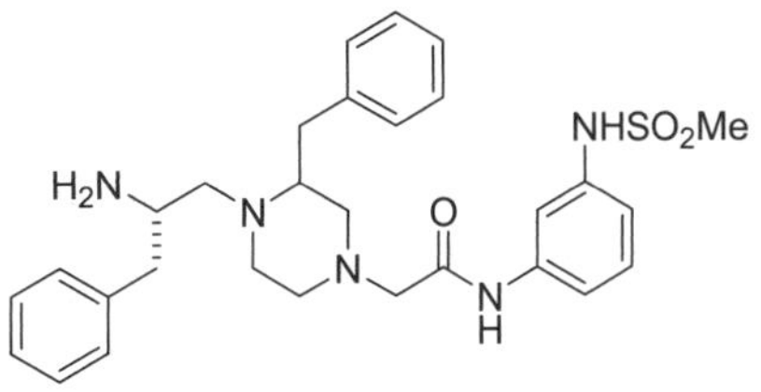

27, IC_{50} = 11, 000 nM

Figure 2.9 DPP-4 inhibitor screening hits.

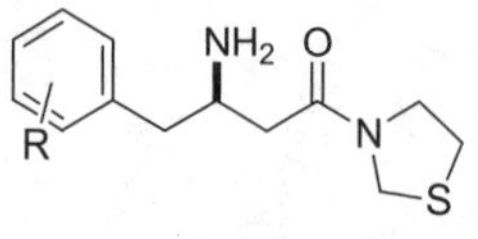

28, R = H, IC_{50} = 3000 nM
29, R = 2-F, IC_{50} = 931 nM
30, R = 3,4diF, IC_{50} = 1700 nM
31, R = 2,5-diF, IC_{50} = 270 nM
32, R = 2,4,5-triF, IC_{50} = 120 nM

Figure 2.10 Optimization of aromatic substitution in the β-amino acid series.

increase in activity (data not shown). Traditional SAR studies in a simpler benzyl acetic acid series revealed that enhanced potency could be obtained by installing the acidic moiety in the *para*-position of the phenyl ring [64]. This yielded a submicromolar inhibitor **33** (DPP-4 $IC_{50} = 0.51\ \mu M$) and, importantly, resulted in a complete ablation of thrombin inhibition (Figure 2.11). Installation of the potency-enhancing 2-fluorophenyl β-amino acid gave an additional 10-fold improvement in potency. Replacement of the right-hand side acetic acid moiety with a substituted glycolic acid further improved DPP-4 inhibitory activity (**34** R = Me, $IC_{50} = 12$ nM; **35** R = ^{i}Pr, $IC_{50} = 1.8$ nM). Finally, installation of a second fluorine in the 5-position of the aromatic ring led to a subnanomolar inhibitor of DPP-4 (**36**, $IC_{50} = 0.48$ nM). Compound **36** was highly selective over related DPPs with no measurable inhibition of QPP, DPP-8, and DPP-9 at concentrations up to 100 μM. This compound was one of the first to demonstrate that exquisitely selective and potent DPP-4 inhibitors were chemically tractable. Compound **36** and a number of related analogues in this series, however, suffered from extremely poor pharmacokinetic properties in the rat, characterized by high plasma clearance ($Cl_p = 150\ mL\ min^{-1}\ kg^{-1}$) and poor oral absorption resulting in unacceptably low oral bioavailability ($F < 1\%$). These issues notwithstanding, the SAR developed here was instrumental to the advancement of the β-amino piperazine series that ultimately led to the discovery of sitagliptin, *vide infra*.

Optimization of the second HTS lead, piperazine **27**, occurred concurrently with that of the β-amino acid proline series but proved challenging since modifications to the right-hand side chain did not result in any substantial improvement in activity. Analogous to SAR in the proline amide series, installation of (*S*)-α-amino amides derived from isoleucine and cyclohexyl glycine on the left-hand side significantly reduced potency [65]. Incorporation of the 3,4-difluorophenyl moiety in compound **37** resulted in a modest 2- to 3-fold increase

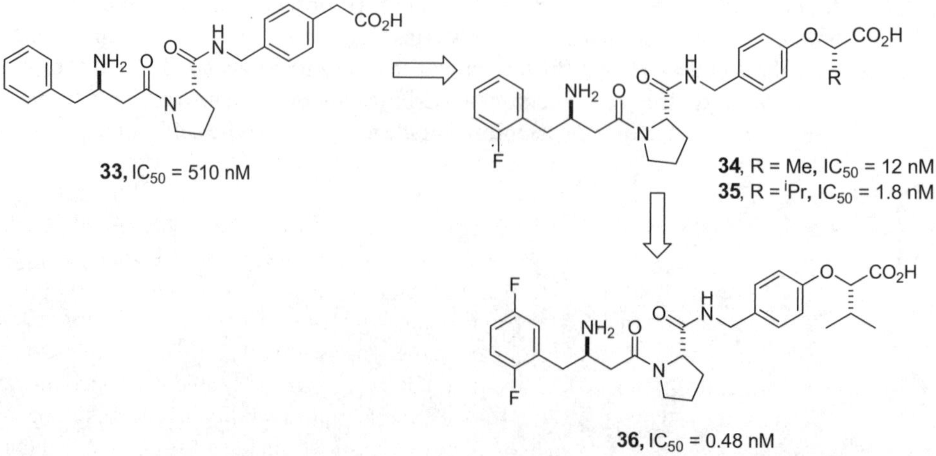

33, IC_{50} = 510 nM

34, R = Me, IC_{50} = 12 nM
35, R = ^{i}Pr, IC_{50} = 1.8 nM

36, IC_{50} = 0.48 nM

Figure 2.11 Optimization of the β-amino acid proline amide series.

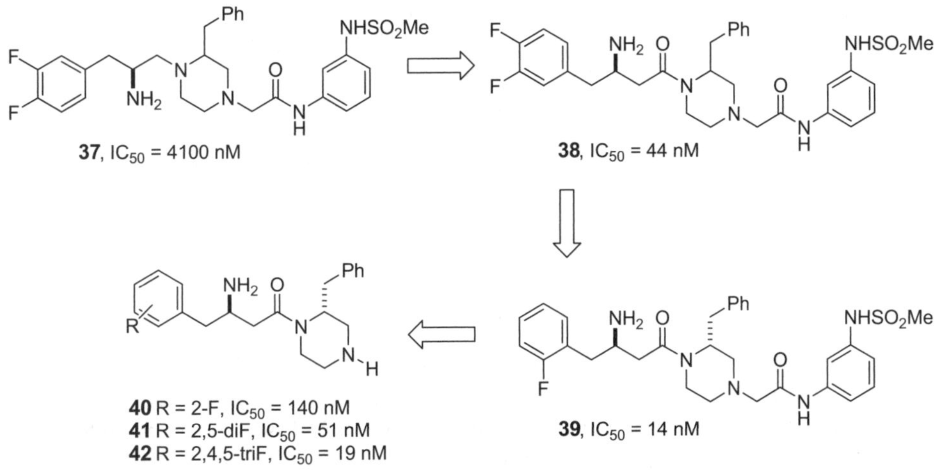

37, IC_{50} = 4100 nM

38, IC_{50} = 44 nM

39, IC_{50} = 14 nM

40 R = 2-F, IC_{50} = 140 nM
41 R = 2,5-diF, IC_{50} = 51 nM
42 R = 2,4,5-triF, IC_{50} = 19 nM

Figure 2.12 Optimization of the piperazine lead series.

in activity as anticipated from SAR of the β-amino acid series (Figure 2.12). Subsequently, the "(*S*)-α-amino amine" moiety was replaced with the left-hand side from the proline amide series (an (*R*)-β-amino amide), to effect a significant 100-fold increase in potency (**38**, DPP-4 $IC_{50} = 44$ nM). Resolution of the corresponding 2-fluorophenyl analogue **39** ($IC_{50} = 14$ nM) revealed that all of the DPP-4 inhibitory activity for the series resided in the (*R,R*)-enantiomers.

In an attempt to reduce the molecular weight of the piperazine leads, the right-hand side was truncated to yield piperazine **40**, a modification that was accompanied by only a 10-fold loss in activity. As anticipated, installation of the optimized 2,5-difluoro- and 2,4,5-trifluoro- substituted phenyl groups (**41** and **42**, respectively) on the left-hand side recovered potency (DPP-4 IC_{50} values of 51 nM and 19 nM, respectively). As with all prior analogues in the β-amino acid series, these compounds had uniformly poor pharmacokinetic properties. This trend was consistent, even for lower molecular weight compounds such as **40–42**. We initially suspected the amino acid portion of the molecule as problematic in this regard. In the piperazine series, however, metabolism studies identified the heterocycle as a site of extensive oxidation, which likely contributed significantly to the poor pharmacokinetic properties.

It was postulated that fusing a five- or six-membered aromatic ring on the right-hand side of the piperazine might result in compounds more resistant to metabolism. A large number of heterocycles were evaluated in a scaffold lacking the 2-benzyl moiety and incorporating the commercially available 3,4-difluorophenyl β-amino acid, yielding compounds that were less potent but more synthetically accessible exemplified by parent **43**. The triazolopiperazine heterocycle proved to be optimal and the discussion that follows will focus on that scaffold alone [66]. An approximately 7-fold increase in potency over the parent analogue **43** ($IC_{50} = 3100$ nM) was obtained when the unsubstituted piperazine was converted to the bicyclic system in compound **44** ($IC_{50} = 460$ nM) (Figure 2.13). An additional increase in DPP-4 inhibitory activity was realized by installing an ethyl substituent on the 3-position of the triazole ring (**45**). This yielded a compound that was completely stable in rat hepatocytes, indicating that oxidation of the piperazine ring had been successfully blocked. Compound **45** still had unacceptable pharmacokinetic properties characterized by very low-to-moderate oral bioavailability in preclinical species (1–2% in rats and monkeys; 33% in dogs). Follow-up studies in the rat suggested that the low oral exposure was likely due to poor and variable absorption. The suboptimal pharmacokinetic

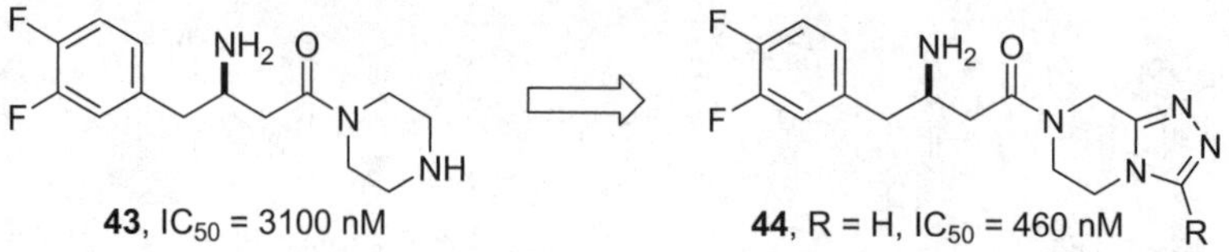

43, IC_{50} = 3100 nM

44, R = H, IC_{50} = 460 nM
45, R = Et, IC_{50} = 230 nM
46, R = CF_3, IC_{50} = 130 nM

Figure 2.13 Optimization of triazolo piperazine replacement.

properties that had plagued the β-amino acid series were ultimately resolved only by exhaustive evaluation of a large number of analogues. Replacement of the ethyl substituent with a trifluoromethyl group resulted in compound **46**, which exhibited a significant improvement in oral absorption in the rat ($F = 44\%$). The success of this semiempirical approach emphasizes the importance of using pharmacokinetics as a screen to identify a compound with optimal properties in a drug discovery program.

The 3,4-difluorophenyl analogue **46** was a 130 nM inhibitor of DPP-4 and, once again, the predictability of the SAR in this series held up as the *in vitro* potency was improved by installation of the 2,5-difluorophenyl (**5**) or the fully optimized 2,4,5-trifluorophenyl (**47**) side chains (IC_{50} values of 27 nM and 18 nM, respectively) (Figure 2.14). The *in vitro* potency was enhanced >25-fold by reinstalling the benzyl substituent on the piperazine ring, thus yielding a subnanomolar DPP-4 inhibitor (**48**, $IC_{50} = 0.66$ nM). This compound, however, was also a submicromolar inhibitor of DPP-8 ($IC_{50} = 620$ nM) and thus did not meet the selectivity criteria for the program [67].

In contrast to benzyl analogue **48,** both the difluoro- and trifluorophenyl analogues (**5** and **47**) had >2500-fold selectivity against DPP-8 and did not inhibit other related enzymes (DPP-9, QPP, PEP, APP, and prolidase) at concentrations up to 100 μM. There were no other significant off-target activities in the MDS-Pharma PanLabs Screen. The pharmacokinetic profiles of both compounds in preclinical species showed short-to-moderate half-lives with good-to-excellent oral bioavailability.

Difluoro analogue **5** was prepared prior to its trifluoro phenyl analogue **47** and so was the first to undergo extensive profiling. The compound was clean in a 2-week toxicological evaluation in the rat dosed up to 100 mg^{-1} kg day^{-1} and showed no acute gastrointestinal toxicity in a dog at 10 mg kg^{-1} day^{-1}. When evaluated intravenously in an anesthetized cardiovascular dog model at doses >1 mg kg^{-1} however, a dose-dependent decrease in blood pressure and increases in heart rate and PR interval were observed (H. Vargas, unpublished results). Evaluation of compound **5** as a preclinical candidate continued, however, as the observed cardiovascular effects were mild and easily monitored in the clinic.

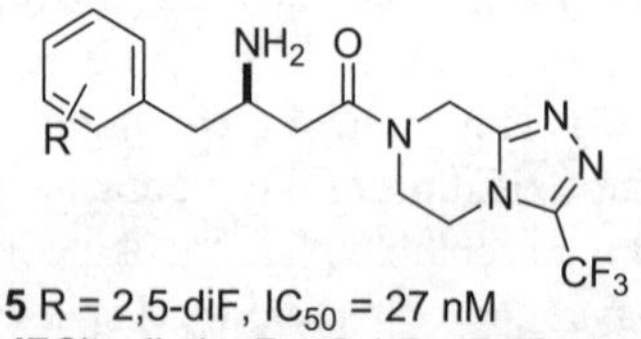

5 R = 2,5-diF, IC_{50} = 27 nM
47 Sitagliptin, R = 2,4,5-triF, IC_{50} = 18 nM

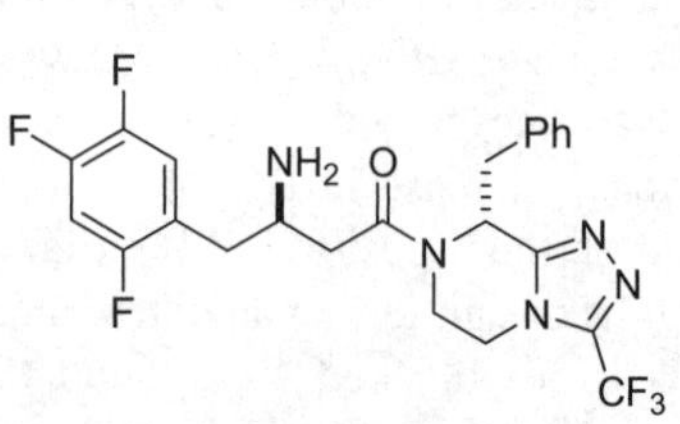

48 DPP-4 IC_{50} = 0.66 nM; DPP-8 IC_{50} = 620 nM

Figure 2.14 JANUVIA™ (sitagliptin, **47**) and related analogues.

Structural similarities between leads **5** and **47** notwithstanding, we continued our evaluation of trifluorophenyl analogue **47** in search of a development candidate lacking any cardiovascular liability. Encouragingly, the extra fluorine atom in compound **47** conferred a significantly improved margin for the observed cardiovascular effects in dog, with a 10-fold higher no-effect level. This molecule therefore replaced the difluoro analogue as our development candidate, and is marketed as JANUVIA™ (sitagliptin phosphate).

2.4 SYNTHETIC AND MANUFACTURING ROUTES TO SITAGLIPTIN

2.4.1 Medicinal Chemistry Route to Sitagliptin and Early Modifications

The original medicinal chemistry synthesis of sitagliptin **47** [63,66] started from chiral template **49** (Scheme 2.1). By applying Schöllkopf's bis-lactim methodology, asymmetric preparation of α-amino acid **50** was realized in two steps. The α-amino acid methyl ester **50** was then transformed into β-amino acid **53** via an Arndt–Eistert homologation through sequential operations: Boc protection, diazo formation, Ag^+-catalyzed Wolff rearrangement, and methyl ester hydrolysis. Coupling β-amino acid **53** and triazole **54** in the presence of EDC afforded the corresponding amide, which was deprotected in HCl/MeOH to give sitagliptin **47**. Triazole **54** was initially prepared according to the method of Potts [68]. Even with modifications [69], however, this synthesis was not suitable for large-scale preparation due to safety hazard issues associated with the use of hydrazine.

Development of an alternative route to triazole **54**, therefore, became an early priority of the Process Research group and is shown in Scheme 2.2 [70]. Selective sequential condensation of 1 equiv of 35% aqueous hydrazine with 1 equiv of ethyl trifluoroacetate followed by 1 equiv of chloroacetyl chloride gave bis-amide **55**. Dehydration of **55** with phosphorus oxychloride afforded the key intermediate chloromethyloxadiazole **56**. The three-step process was efficiently carried out in one pot. In line with the mechanistic understanding about the formation of amidine **58**, the use of methanol was crucial for this transformation. In the presence of nucleophilic methanol, active reaction species **57** was

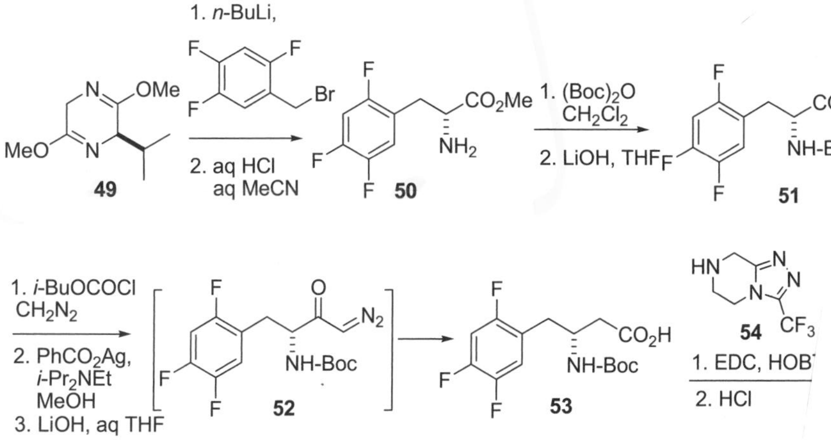

Scheme 2.1 Medicinal chemistry synthesis of sitagliptin.

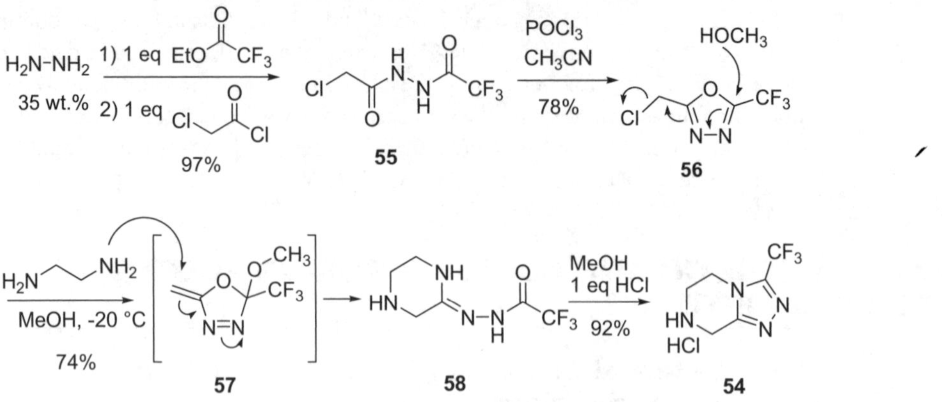

Scheme 2.2 Manufacturing route for the preparation of trizaole **54**.

generated *in situ* and subsequently captured by ethylenediamine to afford amidine **58**. Exposure of **58** to aqueous HCl gave the desired triazole **54**, which was directly isolated as its HCl salt by filtration. The overall yield of this manufacturing process is 52%, nearly double that of the original route. Importantly, the use of 1 equiv of aqueous hydrazine, which is completely consumed in the first step, results in safer operating conditions and cleaner waste streams.

2.4.2 An Asymmetric Hydrogenation Manufacturing Route to Sitagliptin

During the development of sitagliptin, several generations of syntheses suitable for large-scale preparation were developed [69,71,72]. This chapter focuses only on the development of the two manufacturing routes, which addressed the challenges of exercising high standards of "green" chemistry in order to maximize atom-economy and reduce waste burden in an effort to minimize the environmental impact over the lifetime of the commercial product. The initial large-scale syntheses were not considered optimal, mainly due to the number of steps required to set up the stereogenic center of sitagliptin and/or the use of a chiral auxiliary, which generated a by-product that added to the waste burden.

A concise synthesis requires designing a synthetic route with the fewest steps or least functional group manipulations, including minimizing protection-deprotection protocols. Ultimately, an efficient manufacturing route would require moving away from chiral auxiliaries and exploring asymmetric catalysis as the means to install the sitagliptin chiral center. Heavily reliant on efforts to discover new chemistry to realize unprecedented key transformations, the two syntheses discussed below (asymmetric hydrogenation route and enzymatic transamination route) were developed to meet the above criteria.

A concise synthesis of ketoamide **63** and dehydrositagliptin **64** was first developed (Scheme 2.3) [73]. The approach to prepare both compounds capitalized on the ability of Meldrum's acid **60** to act as an acyl anion equivalent. This process involved activation of acid **59** by formation of a mixed anhydride with pivaloyl chloride, in the presence of **60**, *i*-Pr_2NEt, and a catalytic amount of DMAP to form adduct **61**. The formation of β-ketoamide **63** occurred via degradation of **61** to an oxo-ketene intermediate **62** that was trapped with piperazine **54** [73]. Isolation of the ketoamide **63** was important for the enzymatic transamination process and could be achieved directly by addition of water to the reaction mixture. Alternatively, continued processing of the crude reaction stream of **63** by

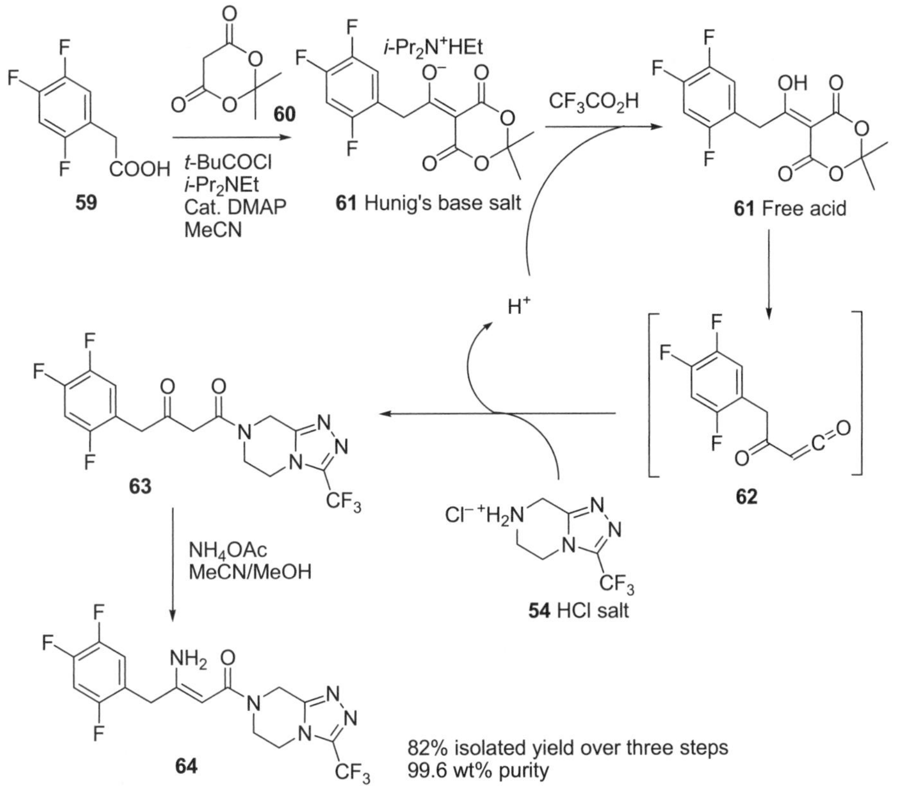

82% isolated yield over three steps
99.6 wt% purity

Scheme 2.3 Synthesis of key intermediates keto amide **63** and enamine amide **64**.

adding NH_4OAc and methanol furnished dehydrositagliptin **64** directly. Importantly, **64** was prepared in an easily operated one-pot process in 82% overall isolated yield with 99.6 wt% purity through a simple filtration, thereby eliminating the need for aqueous workup and minimizing waste generation.

Enamine amide **64** contains the entire structure of sitagliptin **47** save two hydrogen atoms. However, at the time of this work asymmetric hydrogenation of an unprotected enamine was unprecedented. To explore the feasibility of a one-step conversion of **64** to sitagliptin via asymmetric hydrogenation, a focused pilot screen of hydrogenation conditions on substrate **64** with a relatively small set of commercially available chiral bisphosphines in combination with Ir, Ru, and Rh salts was performed (Scheme 2.4) [71,74]. These metal catalysts were selected due to their demonstrated performance in asymmetric hydrogenations. The screening results not only showed the anticipated trend of enantioselectivities but also unexpectedly resulted in the identification of reagents that provided excellent enantiomeric excess. While Ir and Ru catalysts gave poor results, [Rh(COD)$_2$OTf], in particular with ferrocenyl-based JOSIPHOS-type catalysts (e.g., **66**), afforded the desired product with both high conversion and enantioselectivity. Further exhaustive screening for the most suitable hydrogenation catalyst in collaboration with Solvias AG, Switzerland, revealed that other ligands, even those outside the ferrocenyl structural class, could effect this transformation with high enantioselectivity. Using [Rh(COD)Cl]$_2$ as the catalyst, ligands **67–70** provided the highest levels of enantioselectivity for reduction of **64**. In summary, an overall consideration of yield, enantioselectivity, reaction rate, and ligand cost led to a decision to pursue the [Rh(COD)Cl]$_2$-^{t}Bu-JOSIPHOS **66** combination to deliver a viable hydrogenation process for the commercial manufacture of sitagliptin.

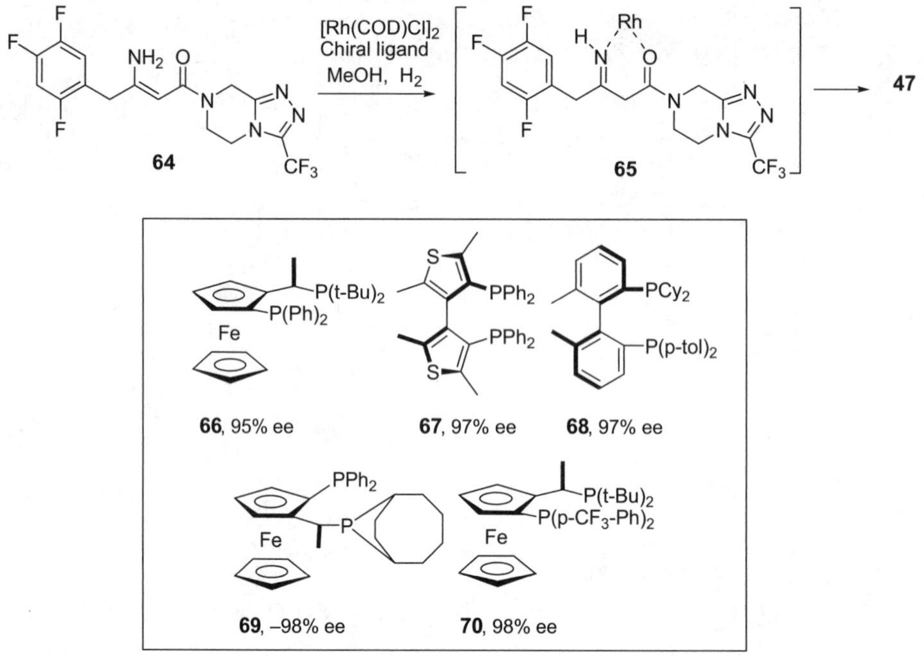

Scheme 2.4 Catalytic hydrogenation optimization of enamine amide **64**.

Further exhaustive optimization showed that hydrogenation of **64** was best performed in methanol. Interestingly, it was found that introducing a small amount of ammonium chloride (0.15–0.3 mol%) was necessary to achieve consistent performance in terms of both enantioselectivity and conversion rate [75]. In addition, by increasing the pressure to 250 psig, catalyst loading was dramatically reduced to 0.15 mol% without sacrificing yield, enantioselectivity, or reaction rate at 50°C. The cost savings achieved by increasing hydrogen pressure and reducing catalyst loading further highlighted the benefits of an asymmetric hydrogenation strategy to set the stereochemistry of **47**.

Mechanistic studies [74] suggest that the hydrogenation of **64** proceeds through the imine tautomer **65**. Under optimal conditions, hydrogenation in the presence of NH_4Cl (0.15 mol%), $[Rh(COD)Cl]_2$ (0.15 mol%), and ^{t}Bu JOSIPHOS **66** (0.155 mol%) in MeOH under 250 psig of hydrogen at 50°C for 16–18 h proved to be extremely robust and afforded sitagliptin **47** in 98% yield and 95% ee, reproducibly. The precious rhodium catalyst was recovered in 90–95% by treating the reaction stream with Ecosorb C-941. The freebase of sitagliptin was then isolated by crystallization in 79% yield with >99% ee and >99% purity, and further converted to the final pharmaceutical form, a monohydrate phosphate salt, in >99.9% purity and >99.9% ee.

The highly efficient asymmetric synthesis of sitagliptin [74] was implemented on an industrial scale. The entire synthesis was carried out with a minimum number of operations: a one-pot preparation of **64** in >99.6 wt% followed by a highly enantioselective hydrogenation. The overall yield of this process is up to 65%. Furthermore, this straightforward approach to **47** reduced significantly the amount of waste produced in the process, in comparison with the early syntheses [69,71,72]. Most strikingly, no aqueous waste was produced in the manufacturing process. This efficient route contained all the elements required for a manufacturing process. However, the quest for an alternative "greener" preparation of sitagliptin continued.

2.4.3 A "Greener" Manufacturing Route to Sitagliptin Employing Biocatalytic Transamination

It was envisioned that the preparation of sitagliptin could be further streamlined and more environment-friendly if the cutting-edge technology of custom-engineering an enzyme to catalyze a reaction [76–78] rather than chemical transformation could be used to enable an enantioselective transamination of ketoamide **63**. As discussed previously, **63** [73] can be intercepted and directly isolated in one-pot from the process developed for the preparation of enamine **64**. Biocatalysis processes can be challenging, however, since they suffer from low turnover numbers, instability toward the demanding conditions of chemical processes, volumetric productivity, and postreaction processing issues. Notwithstanding, a search to identify an unprecedented "parent transamination enzyme" system targeting transformation of substrate **63** to sitagliptin directly was initiated in collaboration with Codexis Inc., USA [79].

Not surprisingly, initial screening with a variety of commercially available transaminases failed to identify an enzyme that could reduce **63** to sitagliptin. In order to induce transaminase activity with ketoamide **63** as a substrate, a "substrate walking" approach [80] was employed. Briefly, this approach applies various standard techniques for forced enzyme evolution. Through successive mutations, an enzyme's binding site is gradually modified by using a series of proxy substrates that eventually link to the desired substrate. Each succeeding proxy substrate more closely resembles the target substrate so that the enzyme gradually "walks" toward the desired activity. Thus, a truncated ketone **71** was prepared, Scheme 2.5, which contained the desired backbone of **63** with the trifluorobenzyl moiety replaced with the less sterically hindering methyl group that is tolerated by several transaminases [81,82].

After screening various transaminases with the "start-up" substrate **71**, it was found that (*R*)-selective transaminase ATA-117, a homologue of an enzyme from *Arthrobacter* spp. [83], effected a modest 4% conversion to the amine **72**. Although the activity of the enzyme was low, this laid the foundation for further evolution and optimization of the enzyme through mutations (Table 2.5). Leveraging recent developments in high-throughput mutagenesis, a combination of *in silico* design and directed evolution was applied to optimize ATA-117. In particular, the S223P mutation, which results in a larger binding pocket, exhibited a 66-fold increase in activity for transamination of **71** to **72** (Table 2.5).

Unfortunately, the S223P variant of ATA-117 exhibited no activity against the desired substrate **63**. However, four residues at the active site (V69, F122, T283, and A284) that

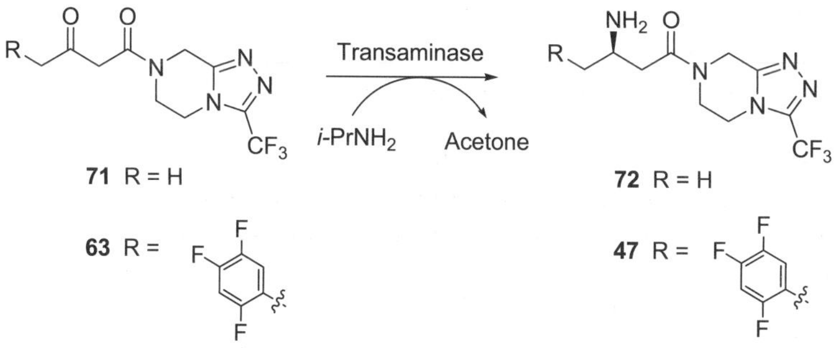

Scheme 2.5 Transaminase optimization of ketoamides **71** and **63**.

TABLE 2.5 Summary of Enzyme Evolution

Substrate	Added mutations[a]	(Substrate) in g L^{-1}	Round identified	Improvement over parent[b]
25	ATA-117	2		N/A
25	S223P	2	1a	66
17	S223P	2	1a	Not active
17	Y26H, V65A, V69G, F122I, A284G	2	1b	1st active
17	H62H, G136Y, E137I, V199I, A209L, T282S	2	2	75
17	S8P, H26Y, G69C, M94I, I137T, G215C, L61Y, C69T, Y136F, T137E, D81G, I94L, I96L, T178S, L269P, T282S, P297S, S321P, Y60F, L94I, A169L, G217N, L273Y, S124H, I122M, H124N, Q329H, N124T, Y150S, V152C, H329Q, S126T	50	11	519

[a]Mutations accumulated in each round of evolution – reference amino acid refers to parent from previous round of evolution.

[b]Fold improvement over parent refers to the parent for that round of evolution.

could potentially interact with the trifluorophenyl group were identified through molecular modeling. Each of these positions was individually subjected to saturation mutagenesis and also included in a combinatorial library that evaluated several substitutions at each position based on structural considerations. Finally, an evolved enzyme incorporating multiple residue changes was identified that exhibited detectable transaminase activity with ketoamide **63**. Although the enzyme activity was extremely low (corresponding to an estimated turnover of 0.1, Table 2.5), this proof-of-concept result triggered additional enzyme optimization and ultimately a mutant with 75-fold increased activity was identified. At this point, methanol and DMSO were also identified as optimal cosolvents in terms of enzyme activity and solubility of the substrate **63**.

Although enzyme activity had been optimized, further mutagenesis of ATA-117 was undertaken to identify an enzyme variant that could survive the reaction conditions. Specifically, since transamination is equilibrium controlled, the enzyme had to tolerate a large excess of isopropylamine and the generation of acetone, which was removed during the reaction. Over the course of 11 rounds of mutation evolution, high-throughput screening ultimately led to an enzyme variant with 27 mutations that was four orders of magnitude more active toward **63** than ATA-117 and produced sitagliptin in >99.9 ee while meeting required process targets (tolerance to DMSO, acetone, and isopropylamine, stability to elevated temperatures, and amenability to expression in an *Eescherichia coli* manufacturing host).

As a consequence of the chemoenzymatic strategy, the preferred manufacturing route to sitagliptin involves treatment of ketoamide **63** (250 g L^{-1}) with isopropylamine in 50% DMSO in the presence of 4.5 wt% of the ATA-117 variant at 50°C, which affords sitagliptin in 92% assay yield with >99.95% ee. The product is then isolated as its final pharmaceutical form, a monohydrate phosphate salt, in 88% yield. In comparison with the asymmetric hydrogenation route, the biocatalytic process afforded sitagliptin with a 10–13% increase in overall yield. In summary, a combination of iterative strategies beginning with asymmetric hydrogenation and culminating in biocatalysis facilitated a safe, efficient and environment-friendly manufacture of sitagliptin without compromising commercial viability.

2.5 DRUG PRODUCT DEVELOPMENT

2.5.1 Overview

In any drug development program, formulation of the drug substance into a tablet for clinical trials and ultimately as a marketed pill is an important process. Sitagliptin was developed as an immediate release tablet for oral administration. Three different doses were developed and commercialized: 25 mg, 50 mg, and 100 mg. The tablet formulation was designed to rapidly release sitagliptin in order to deliver consistent bioavailability and clinical efficacy. When formulated as the monohydrate phosphate salt, sitagliptin is highly soluble ($>40\,mg\,mL^{-1}$) over the entire physiological pH range and thus does not require bioavailability-enhancing excipients. Excipients were chosen to provide a chemically and physically stable formulation and to also ensure a robust tablet manufacturing process. A direct compression (DC) process was selected in which the drug substance and excipients are blended and compressed to form the tablet. The selection of a relatively simple manufacturing process streamlined the process development and helped enable swift technology transfer and launch. A water-soluble polymeric film coat was spray coated onto the compressed tablet to provide a unique and attractive appearance for each dose strength.

2.5.2 Composition Development

A moderately high drug concentration (~32% w/w) was pursued in order to provide a dosage form of acceptably small size for global markets based on the projected maximum efficacious dose (100 mg). The same drug load and excipient concentrations were used to produce tablets for all three dose strengths. Two inactive ingredients were chosen as diluents in order to reduce the concentration of the drug substance into a range where the flow and compaction properties of the powder blend would be optimal for downstream processing. In a DC process, attention must be paid to the selection of excipient physical properties, which can significantly influence final product quality attributes such as dose uniformity and tablet strength. Grades of microcrystalline cellulose (MCC) and dibasic calcium phosphate were selected to provide consistent flow of the powder blend and help minimize segregation propensity of sitagliptin during the compression step, as will be discussed below.

Croscarmellose sodium, a widely used disintegrant [84] was included in the formulation to provide rapid release of sitagliptin from the tablet. Sitagliptin exhibited a propensity to adhere to tablet punch surfaces, and this "sticking" tendency [85] presented a significant challenge in the development of the tablet formulation. Initially, magnesium stearate was selected as the preferred lubricant to minimize defects resulting from transfer of formulation from the tablet surface to the tablet punch surfaces. It was found that the addition of a second lubricant, sodium stearyl fumarate, provided a wider compression process operating window with respect to eliminating the sticking tendency and maximizing tablet hardness. Optimization of the magnesium stearate and sodium stearyl fumarate levels yielded tablets that could be compressed over a wide range of hardness with no significant effect on drug release rate.

2.5.3 Manufacturing Process Development

In order to achieve tablet content uniformity in a DC process, three prerequisites must be met. First, the active ingredient must be evenly distributed throughout the powder mixture at the end of the blending and lubrication steps. Second, segregation of the active ingredient from the blend must be minimized during material transfer and flow through the equipment

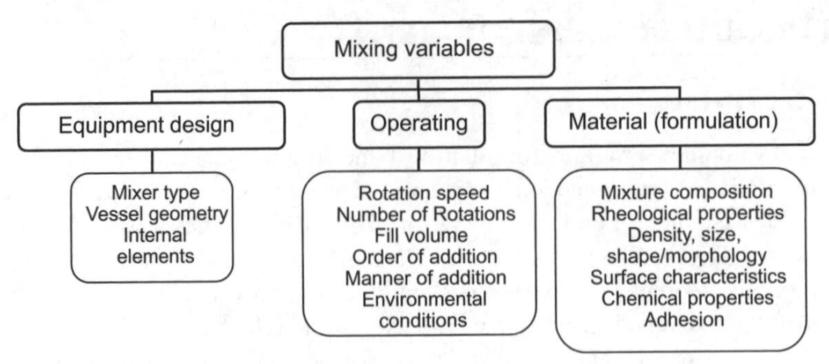

Figure 2.15 Classification of variables in a powder blending process.

during compression. Finally, the tablet weight must be tightly controlled during the compression step to ensure that the desired dose is produced.

The variables that influence blend uniformity in a solid particle mixer can be grouped into three categories—equipment design, operating parameters, and formulation attributes. As shown in Figure 2.15, there are many variables to consider during formulation and process development for products that include a dedicated blending step. The number of these variables and the complexity of their interactions preclude predictive modeling of solid mixing processes based on first principles. From this standpoint, mixing of particulate solids is sharply contrasted with the mixing of fluids [86], which can be simulated computationally based on knowledge of the underlying constitutive equations.

Given the large number of potential variables impacting blending performance, risk-based approaches were taken both to develop sufficient understanding of the key parameters driving product quality attributes and to ensure that appropriate process controls were implemented. The risk analysis indicated that achievement of the initial blend uniformity would be primarily influenced by the number of blending rotations, as well as the blender fill fraction (ratio of the solid's volume to blender volume).

Process Analytical Technology (PAT) was employed during development to provide fundamental insight into the blending kinetics. A near-infrared (NIR) probe installed in the blender was used to monitor the evolution of the blend composition in real time [87]. As illustrated in Figure 2.16, the number of blending rotations required to achieve a uniformity value below 0.01 on the mean spectral standard deviation scale was heavily dependent on the particular batch size ($n = 36$, 42, and 50 rotations for each of the 630 kg, 725 kg, and 820 kg mass of powder fills in the same size blender).

Figure 2.17 shows representative data from two commercial-scale compression runs. The individual tablet assay values were well within the generally accepted limits of 85–115% of the product label claim [88]. These data confirmed that the uniform blend did not undergo significant segregation during the transfer of material from the blender to the tablet press and the subsequent powder feeding into the dies. The absence of any notable degree of segregation of components in the DC formulation was demonstrated in various blender-tablet press equipment trains during product development.

During drug product development, the range of variability in key drug substance properties such as particle size distribution from the future production facility was initially unknown. Risk assessment highlighted both segregation potential and weight control as potentially sensitive to shifts in sitagliptin particle size distribution. Consequently, experiments were designed to elucidate the magnitude of these effects. Coarse and fine fractions of sitagliptin were generated, formulated, processed in compression experiments conducted under controlled conditions. Representative data in Figure 2.18 enabled

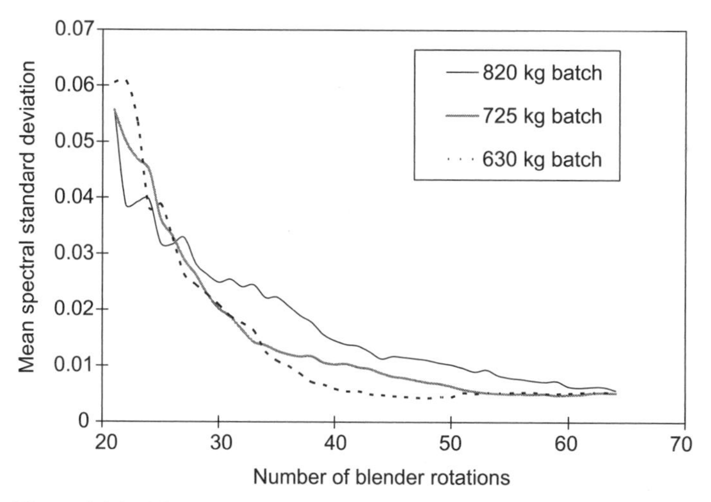

Figure 2.16 Mean spectral standard deviation measured by NIR spectroscopy as a function of number of blender rotations and batch size.

determination of the threshold level for sitagliptin "fines" fraction above which tablet weight uniformity would no longer be acceptable.

Experiments were also conducted whereby the largest particle size batch for sitagliptin was formulated and its segregation tendency (as measured by individual tablet assay values sampled frequently at the very beginning of the compression run) was compared with that of the smallest particle size batch after formulation. As shown in Figure 2.19, the risk of variability in sitagliptin particle size inducing segregation and tablet assay variability was acceptable and within the criteria of the label claim. As sitagliptin particle size was increased, it began to more closely match the size characteristics of the microcrystalline cellulose and the dibasic calcium phosphate excipients. This reduction in the difference between the particle size of the drug substance and the major formulation components was the likely cause of the observed reduction in tablet-to-tablet compositional

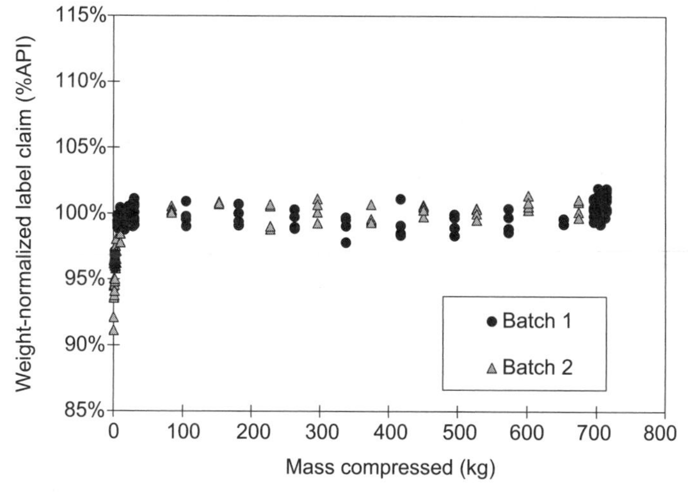

Figure 2.17 Active ingredient uniformity of compressed tablets, expressed as weight-normalized % label claim. Data from two commercial-scale development batches.

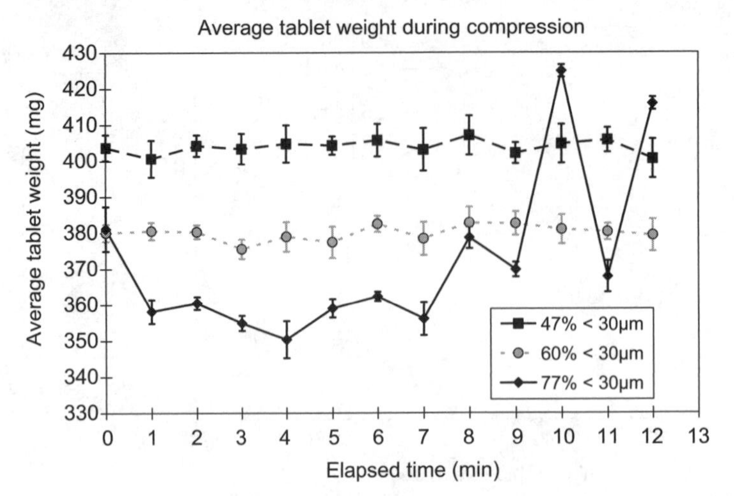

Figure 2.18 Effect of drug substance particle size on tablet weight variability during compression.

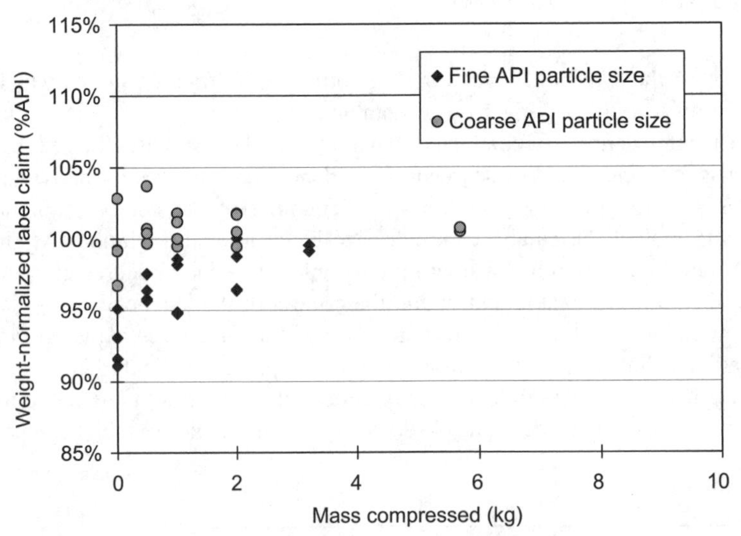

Figure 2.19 Effect of drug substance particle size on drug concentration in tablets at the beginning of the compression run.

variability. These data helped define the target particle size distribution that would provide tablets with the desired critical quality attributes.

2.6 CLINICAL STUDIES

2.6.1 Preclinical PD Studies and Early Clinical Development of Sitagliptin

The clinical development of sitagliptin was facilitated by translational preclinical studies in rodents that established the pharmacokinetic–pharmacodynamic (PK/PD) relationship between circulating inhibitor levels/plasma DPP-4 inhibition and acute glucose lowering efficacy. Phase I clinical trials confirmed this relationship in human subjects [89]. As illustrated in Figure 2.20a, lean mice administered increasing doses of sitagliptin 60 min

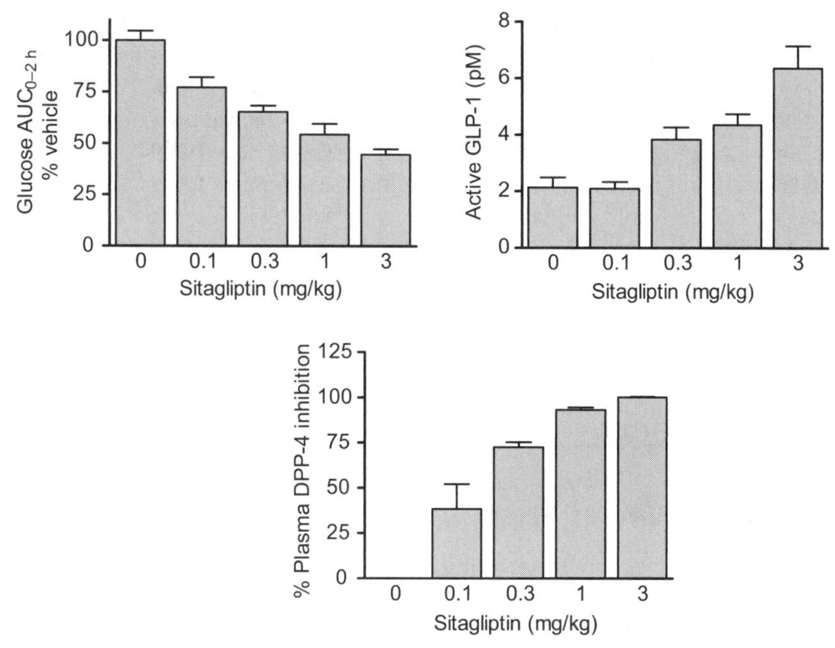

Figure 2.20 Pharmacodynamics of sitagliptin in lean C57/BL6 mice. (a) Blood glucose excursion ($AUC_{0-2\,h}$) in an OGTT initiated 60 min after the sitagliptin dose; (b) plasma levels of active GLP-1 in a matched cohort of animals, measured at 20 min postoral glucose challenge, 80 min postsitagliptin dose; (c) corresponding plasma % DPP-4 inhibition in the same cohort, compared to vehicle-treated animals.

prior to an oral glucose challenge in an "oral glucose tolerance test" (OGTT) exhibited dose-dependent decreases in blood glucose excursions over the 2 h study period. The minimal sitagliptin dose required for maximum glucose lowering efficacy (minimum efficacious dose, MinED) was 1 mg kg^{-1}, corresponding to a reduction in blood glucose $AUC_{0\text{-}2h}$ of 46% relative to vehicle-treated animals. Plasma samples collected from a separate cohort of compound-treated animals at 20 min following oral glucose challenge (80 min post-sitagliptin administration) were analyzed for active GLP-1 levels using a commercial ELISA kit, and for plasma DPP-4 inhibition using the fluorogenic substrate Gly-Pro-AMC [50]. Active GLP-1 levels increased up to 2- to 3-fold in a dose-dependent manner (Figure 2.20b), similar to levels observed in *Cd26*$^{-/-}$ mice following an oral glucose challenge. As illustrated in Figure 2.20c, inhibition of murine DPP-4 by sitagliptin was also dose-dependent, with ~80% enzyme inhibition measured in the plasma DPP-4 activity assay at the MinED of 1 mg kg^{-1}, which corresponds to ~94% plasma DPP-4 inhibition *in vivo* after corrections for assay dilution and presence of fluorogenic substrate [90]. The requirement of ~94% plasma DPP-4 inhibition *in vivo* for maximal acute glucose lowering efficacy in the lean mouse OGTT PD model was confirmed against a panel of 23 structurally diverse DPP-4 inhibitors with varied potencies and pharmacokinetics [91], which reinforced the strategy of using plasma DPP-4 inhibition as a proximal biomarker for target engagement in the clinic.

The clinical development of sitagliptin has been extensively reviewed elsewhere [89,92] and is only briefly summarized herein. A proof-of-concept single rising dose study was conducted in phase I to confirm the relationship between target engagement (plasma DPP-4 inhibition and elevation of postprandial active GLP-1 levels) and disease-related biomarkers (reduction in blood glucose and changes in insulin and glucagon levels) following an OGTT in healthy human subjects [93]. The preclinical pharmacology of DPP-4 inhibition was observed to completely translate to the clinic, with postprandial reductions in circulating glucagon levels and augmented glucose-dependent insulin secretion being observed in addition to blood glucose lowering and endogenous incretin stabilization. The cumulative data from single dose [93,94] and multiple dose studies in phase I [95] facilitated sitagliptin dose-selection for a "direct to phase IIB strategy." A 2- to 3-fold increase in postprandial active GLP-1 levels and >95% plasma DPP-4 inhibition over a 24 h period was observed following administration of a single 100 mg dose of sitagliptin to healthy subjects [93]. The central premise that a PK/PD relationship established with acute dosing would predict glucose lowering efficacy following chronic dosing in T2DM patients was confirmed in 12-week phase IIB studies (*vide infra*), which indicated that 100 mg sitagliptin administered once daily produced near-maximal reductions in plasma HbA1c (an integrated biomarker for long-term glucose control) [96–98].

2.6.2 Summary of Phase II/III Clinical Trials

Once the initial safety and efficacy of a drug have been established in short-term clinical trials with healthy subjects and patients, phase IIB dose-ranging studies are generally conducted in the patient population to select the lowest well-tolerated dose that provides sufficient efficacy for further development. As such, phase IIB studies were conducted with sitagliptin as monotherapy in T2DM patients at 5–50 mg twice daily and at 25–100 mg once daily, or in combination with metformin at 50 mg twice daily [96–98]. Sitagliptin treatment resulted in significant improvement in glycemic control in patients with T2DM as measured by reduced fasting and postprandial glucose levels, and as discussed above, confirmed that optimal glucose lowering efficacy was obtained with a 100 mg once daily administration of the drug (0.79% placebo-subtracted reduction in HbA_{1c} from a baseline HbA_{1c} of 8.0%). These studies also showed that sitagliptin is very well tolerated with an incidence of hypoglycemia and gastrointestinal events similar to that of placebo, and a neutral effect on body weight. A subsequent 12-week study in Japanese patients with a baseline HbA1c of 7.6% showed that a 100 mg dose of sitagliptin resulted in an HbA_{1c} reduction of 1.05% compared to placebo and again the drug was well tolerated [98].

Once a drug dose has been selected for long-term evaluation in patients, large phase III studies, which may be a year or more in duration, are carried out to ensure that the safety and efficacy of the drug are fully characterized. Phase III trials with sitagliptin confirmed that monotherapy with the 100 mg once-daily dose was optimal for chronic glucose lowering in T2DM patients [99]. The efficacy of the drug as an add-on therapy to metformin or pioglitazone was also evaluated in patients inadequately controlled with either drug. The benefits of sitagliptin as an add-on therapy were consistently demonstrated in these phase III studies by incremental and significant decreases in HbA_{1c} compared to the placebo add-on group, and a tolerability profile similar to that of placebo. The glucose-dependent augmentation of insulin secretion by sitagliptin was exemplified in a 52-week phase III study using glipizide (a sulfonylurea) as active comparator in T2DM patients inadequately controlled with metformin [100]. Both add-on groups provided a similar and significant reduction in HbA_{1c} from baseline (0.7%). Sitagliptin therapy, however, was associated with a significantly lower incidence of hypoglycemia (5%) compared to the classical glucose-independent insulin secretagogue glipizide (32%). Furthermore, a 1.5 kg reduction in body weight was obtained with sitagliptin therapy in contrast to a 1.1 kg body weight gain with glipizide. The reduced risk of hypoglycemia and weight neutral profile of sitagliptin are important differentiators in diabetes therapy since many T2DM patients remain poorly controlled and inadequately treated with older agents in part due to concerns of hypoglycemia or excessive weight gain.

2.7 SUMMARY

Several key lessons were learned from the biology, medicinal chemistry, process chemistry, and formulation efforts, which contributed to the discovery and development of JANUVIA™ discussed above. First, licensing and evaluating the Probiodrug compounds gave the program a "jump start" which, although not directly resulting in a drug, afforded early recognition of inhibitor selectivity as being critical for an acceptable safety profile. This realization enabled the medicinal chemistry program to rapidly move away from the early α-amino acid analogues, which did not have the desired selectivity profile, to focus on scaffolds with improved selectivity over other Pro-selective dipeptidases. Second, in the medicinal chemistry effort we saw the importance of pursuing multiple structural classes as a mitigation strategy, should insurmountable issues arise in any one series. We also saw the benefits of a translatable SAR, which allowed us to optimize across chemically tractable leads in a predictable manner. Continual evaluation of pharmacokinetic properties was critical, given the poor oral exposure plaguing all structural classes. Finally, the difference in cardiovascular safety margins observed between sitagliptin and desfluoro sitagliptin (**5**) was a striking example of the importance of comprehensive *in vivo* evaluation of multiple analogues in order to select a development candidate with the optimal profile.

The synthetic route to sitagliptin has been reevaluated and optimized multiple times since the compound entered development. Each successive route has achieved greater efficiency with a reduced environmental impact. The team was not limited by precedented chemistry in their search for an optimal synthesis and, as described above, made several groundbreaking discoveries in the fields of catalytic asymmetric reduction and enzymatic biotransformation. The good physical properties of sitagliptin enabled a relatively straightforward formulation path for the drug substance, while minimizing the risks of variable pharmacokinetics in the clinic and problems in the technology transfer from the development facility to the commercial facility.

The biomarker strategy proved effective in translating from preclinical species to the clinic, hence allowing for accurate dose selection from phase I data. This not only helped drive the clinical program but was also instrumental in reducing the time from introduction into humans to the start of phase III by 1.4 years, compared to the average time for a new chemical entity [101].

Sitagliptin phosphate (JANUVIA™) was approved as the first in class-selective DPP-4 inhibitor for the treatment of type 2 diabetes in October 2006. This drug is the first novel oral therapy for diabetes since the introduction of the thiazolidinediones over a decade ago and is an important addition to the armamentarium available to practitioners in the war against type 2 diabetes.

REFERENCES

1. WHO. World Health Organization Global Strategy on Diet, Physical Activity and Health. World Health Organization, 2010.
2. Wright, A., Burden, A. C. F., Paisey, R. B., Cull, C. A., and Holman, R. R. Sulfonylurea inadequacy: efficacy of addition of insulin over 6 years in patients with type 2 diabetes in the UK Prospective Diabetes Study (UKPDS 57). *Diabetes Care* **2002**, *25*(2), 330–336.
3. Aaboe, K., Krarup, T., Madsbad, S., and Holst, J. J. GLP-1: physiological effects and potential therapeutic

applications. *Diabetes Obes. Metabol.* **2008**, *10*(11), 994–1003.

4. Irwin, N. and Flatt, P. R. Therapeutic potential for GIP receptor agonists and antagonists. *Best Pract. Res. Clin. Endocrinol. Metab.* **2009**, *23*(4), 499–512.
5. Roges, O. A., Baron, M., and Philis-Tsimikas, A. The incretin effect and its potentiation by glucagon-like peptide 1-based therapies: a revolution in diabetes management. *Expert Opin. Investig. Drugs* **2005**, *14* (6), 705–727.
6. Baggio, L. L. and Drucker, D. J. Biology of incretins: GLP-1 and GIP. *Gastroenterology* **2007**, *132*(6), 2131–2157.
7. Zander, M., Madsbad, S., Madsen, J. L., and Holst, J. J. Effect of 6-week course of glucagon-like peptide 1 on glycaemic control, insulin sensitivity, and beta-cell function in type 2 diabetes: a parallel-group study. *Lancet* **2002**, *359*(9309), 824–830.
8. Gault, V. A., O'Harte, F. P. M., and Flatt, P. R. Glucose-dependent insulinotropic polypeptide (GIP): anti-diabetic and anti-obesity potential? *Neuropeptides* **2003**, *37*(5), 253–263.
9. Nauck, M. A., Heimesaat, M. M., Orskov, C., Holst, J. J., Ebert, R., and Creutzfeldt, W. Preserved incretin activity of glucagon-like peptide-1 [7–36 amide] but not of synthetic human gastric-inhibitory polypeptide in patients with type-2 diabetes-mellitus. *J. Clin. Invest.* **1993**, *91*(1), 301–307.
10. Kieffer, T. J., McIntosh, C. H. S., and Pederson, R. A. Degradation of Glucose-dependent insulinotropic polypeptide and truncated glucagon-like peptide-1 *in-vitro* and *in-vivo* by dipeptidyl peptidase-IV. *Endocrinology* **1995**, *136*(8), 3585–3596.
11. Mentlein, R., Gallwitz, B., and Schmidt, W. E. Dipeptidyl-peptidase-IV hydrolyzes gastric-inhibitory polypeptide, glucagon-like peptide-1(7-36)amide, peptide histidine methionine and is responsible for their degradation in human serum. *Eur. J. Biochem.* **1993**, *214*(3), 829–835.
12. Deacon, C. F., Nauck, M. A., Toftnielsen, M., Pridal, L., Willms, B., and Holst, J. J. Both subcutaneously and intravenously administered glucagon-like peptide-I are rapidly degraded from the amino-terminus in type-II diabetic-patients and in healthy-subjects. *Diabetes* **1995**, *44*(9), 1126–1131.
13. Deacon, C. F., Pridal, L., Klarskov, L., Olesen, M., and Holst, J. J. Glucagon-like peptide 1 undergoes differential tissue-specific metabolism in the anesthetized pig. *Am. J. Physiol. Endocrinol. Metab.* **1996**, *34*(3), E458–E464.
14. Gentilella, R., Bianchi, C., Rossi, A., and Rotella, C. M. Exenatide: a review from pharmacology to clinical practice. *Diabetes Obes. Metab.* **2009**, *11*(6), 544–556.
15. Montanya, E. and Sesti, G. A. Review of efficacy and safety data regarding the use of liraglutide, a once-daily human glucagon-like peptide 1 analogue, in the treatment of type 2 diabetes mellitus. *Clin. Ther.* **2009**, *31*(11), 2472–2488.
16. Astrup, A., Rossner, S., Van Goal, L., Rissanen, A., Niskanen, L., Al Hakim, M., Madsen, J., Rasmussen, M. F., and Lean, M. E. J. Effects of liraglutide in the treatment of obesity: a randomised, double-blind, placebo-controlled study. *Lancet* **2009**, *374*(9701), 1606–1616.
17. Garber, A., Henry, R., Ratner, R., Garcia-Hernandez, P. A., Rodriguez-Pattzi, H., Olvera-Alvarez, I., Hale, P. M., Zdravkovic, M., and Bode, B. Liraglutide versus glimepiride monotherapy for type 2 diabetes (LEAD-3 Mono): a randomised, 52-week, phase III, double-blind, parallel-treatment trial. *Lancet* **2009**, *373*(9662), 473–481.
18. Kendall, D. M., Cuddihy, R. M., and Bergenstal, R. M. Clinical application of incretin-based therapy: therapeutic potential, patient selection and clinical use. *Eur. J. Intern. Med.* **2009**, *20*, S329–S339.
19. Marguet, D., Baggio, L., Kobayashi, T., Bernard, A. M., Pierres, M., Nielsen, P. F., Ribel, U., Watanabe, T., Drucker, D. J., and Wagtmann, N. Enhanced insulin secretion and improved glucose tolerance in mice lacking CD26. *Proc. Natl. Acad. Sci. USA* **2000**, *97* (12), 6874–6879.
20. Morimoto, C. and Schlossman, S. F. The structure and function of CD26 in the T-cell immune response. *Immunol. Rev.* **1998**, *161*, 55–70.
21. Ahren, B., Simonsson, E., Larsson, H., Landin-Olsson, M., Torgeirsson, H., Jansson, P. A., Sandqvist, M., Bavenholm, P., Efendic, S., Eriksson, J. W., Dickinson, S., and Holmes, D. Inhibition of dipeptidyl peptidase IV improves metabolic control over a 4-week study period in type 2 diabetes. *Diabetes Care* **2002**, *25*(5), 869–875.
22. Hughes, T. E., Russell, M. E., Bolognese, L., Li, X., Burkey, B. F., Wang, P. R., and Villhauer, E. B. NVP-LAF237, a highly selective and long-acting dipeptidyl peptidase IV inhibitor. *Diabetes* **2002**, *51*, A67.
23. Villhauer, E. B., Brinkman, J. A., Naderi, G. B., Burkey, B. F., Dunning, B. E., Prasad, K., Mangold, B. L., Russell, M. E., and Hughes, T. E. 1-[[(3-hydroxy-1-adamantyl)amino]acetyl]-2-cyano-(*S*)-pyrrolidine: a potent, selective, and orally bioavailable dipeptidyl peptidase IV inhibitor with antihyperglycemic properties. *J. Med. Chem.* **2003**, *46*(13), 2774–2789.
24. Lambeir, A. M., Durinx, C., Proost, P., Van Damme, J., Scharpe, S., and De Meester, I. Kinetic study of the processing by dipeptidyl-peptidase IV/CD26 of neuropeptides involved in pancreatic insulin secretion. *FEBS Lett.* **2001**, *507*(3), 327–330.
25. Lambeir, A. M., Proost, P., Durinx, C., Bal, G., Senten, K., Augustyns, K., Scharpe, S., Van Damme, J., and De Meester, I. Kinetic investigation of chemokine truncation by CD26/dipeptidyl peptidase IV reveals a striking selectivity within the chemokine family. *J. Biol. Chem.* **2001**, *276*(32), 29839–29845.
26. De Meester, I., Durinx, C., Bal, G., Proost, P., Struyf, S., Goossens, F., Augustyns, K., and Scharpe, S. Natural substrates of dipeptidyl peptidase IV. In: *Cellular Peptidases in Immune Functions and*

Diseases 2 (eds J. Langner and S. Ansorge), Plenum, pp. 67–87.

27. Mentlein, R. Dipeptidyl-peptidase IV (CD26)-role in the inactivation of regulatory peptides. *Regul. Pept.* **1999**, *85*(1), 9–24.
28. Van Damme, J., Struyf, S., Wuyts, A., Van Coillie, E., Menten, P., Schols, D., Sozzani, S., De Meester, I., Proost, P., and Mantovani, A. The role of CD26/DPP IV in chemokine processing. In *Chemical Immunology: Chemokines* (ed Alberto Mantovani), vol. **72**, S Karger Pub., **1999**, pp. 42–56.
29. Zhu, L., Tamvakopoulos, C., Xie, D., Dragovic, J., Shen, X. L., Fenyk-Melody, J. E., Schmidt, K., Bagchi, A., Griffin, P. R., Thornberry, N. A., and Sinha Roy, R. The role of dipeptidyl peptidase IV in the cleavage of glucagon family peptides: *in vivo* metabolism of pituitary adenylate cyclase-activating polypeptide-(1-38). *J. Biol. Chem.* **2003**, *278*(25), 22418–22423.
30. Robberecht, P., Gourlet, P., Deneef, P., Woussencolle, M. C., Vandermeerspiret, M. C., Vandermeers, A., and Christophe, J. Receptor occupancy and adenylate-cyclase activation in Ar-4-2J rat pancreatic acinar cell-membranes by analogs of pituitary adenylate cyclase-activating peptides amino-terminally shortened or modified at position 1, 2, 3, 20, or 21. *Mol. Pharmacol.* **1992**, *42*(2), 347–355.
31. Wynne, K. and Bloom, S. R. The role of oxyntomodulin and peptide tyrosine-tyrosine (PYY) in appetite control. *Nat. Clin. Pract. Endocrinol. Metab.* **2006**, *2*(11), 612–620.
32. Salem, M. A. M., Lewis, U. J., Haro, L. S., Kishi, K., McAllister, D. L., Seavey, B. K., Bee, G., and Wolff, G. L. Effects of hypophysectomy and the insulin-like and anti-insulin pituitary peptides on carbohydrate-metabolism in yellow Avy/A (Balb/C x Vy)F1 hybrid mice. *Proc. Soc. Exp. Biol. Med.* **1989**, *191*(4), 408–419.
33. Salem, M. A. M. Effects of the amino-terminal portion of human growth-hormone on glucose clearance and metabolism in normal, diabetic, hypophysectomized, and diabetic-hypophysectomized rats. *Endocrinology* **1988**, *123*(3), 1565–1576.
34. Rohner-Jeanrenaud, F., Craft, L. S., Bridwell, J., Suter, T. M., Tinsley, F. C., Smiley, D. L., Burkhart, D. R., Statnick, M. A., Heiman, M. L., Ravussin, E., and Caro, J. F. Chronic central infusion of cocaine- and amphetamine-regulated transcript (CART 55-102): effects on body weight homeostasis in lean and high-fat-fed obese rats. *Int. J. Obes.* **2002**, *26*(2), 143–149.
35. Abiko, T. and Ogawa, R. Chemical syntheses of CART (human, 55-102) analogues and their anorectic effect on food intake in rats induced by neuropeptide Y. *Protein Pept. Lett.* **2001**, *8*(4), 289–295.
36. Yamada, K., Wada, E., and Wada, K. Bombesin-like peptides: studies on food intake and social behaviour with receptor knock-out mice. *Ann. Med.* **2000**, *32*(8), 519–529.
37. Ahren, B. and Hughes, T. E. Inhibition of dipeptidyl peptidase-4 augments insulin secretion in response to exogenously administered glucagon-like peptide-1, glucose-dependent insulinotropic polypeptide, pituitary adenylate cyclase-activating polypeptide, and gastrin-releasing peptide in mice. *Endocrinology* **2005**, *146*(4), 2055–2059.
38. Hansotia, T., Baggio, L. L., Delmeire, D., Hinke, S. A., Yamada, Y., Tsukiyama, K., Seino, Y., Holst, J. J., Schuit, F., and Drucker, D. J. Double incretin receptor knockout (DIRKO) mice reveal an essential role for the enteroinsular axis in transducing the glucoregulatory actions of DPP-IV inhibitors. *Diabetes* **2004**, *53*(5), 1326–1335.
39. Bongers, J., Lambros, T., Ahmad, M., and Heimer, E. P. Kinetics of dipeptidyl peptidase-IV proteolysis of growth hormone-releasing factor and analogs. *Biochim. Biophys. Acta* **1992**, *1122*(2), 147–153.
40. Drucker, D. J., Shi, Q., Crivici, A., SumnerSmith, M., Tavares, W., Hill, M., DeForest, L., Cooper, S., and Brubaker, P. L. Regulation of the biological activity of glucagon-like peptide 2 *in vivo* by dipeptidyl peptidase IV. *Nat. Biotechnol.* **1997**, *15*(7), 673–677.
41. Ahmad, S., Wang, L. H., and Ward, P. E. Dipeptidyl (amino)peptidase-IV and aminopeptidase-M metabolize circulating substance-P *in vivo*. *J. Pharmacol. Exp. Ther.* **1992**, *260*(3), 1257–1261.
42. Heymann, E. and Mentlein, R. Liver dipeptidyl aminopeptidase-IV hydrolyzes substance-P. *FEBS Lett.* **1978**, *91*(2), 360–364.
43. Faidley, T. D., Leiting, B., Pryor, K. D., Lyons, K., Hickey, G. J., and Thompson, D. R. Inhibition of dipeptidyl-peptidase IV does not increase circulating IGF-1 concentrations in growing pigs. *Exp. Biol. Med.* **2006**, *231*(8), 1373–1378.
44. L'Heureux, M. C. and Brubaker, P. L. Therapeutic potential of the intestinotropic hormone, glucagon-like peptide-2. *Ann. Med.* **2001**, *33*(4), 229–235.
45. Vora, K. A., Porter, G., Peng, R. C., Cui, Y., Pryor, K., Eiermann, G., and Zaller, D. M. Genetic ablation or pharmacological blockade of dipeptidyl peptidase IV does not impact T cell-dependent immune responses. *BMC Immunol.* **2009**, *10*, 19.
46. Lankas, G. R., Leiting, B., Sinha Roy, R., Eiermann, G. J., Beconi, M. G., Biftu, T., Chan, C. C., Edmondson, S., Feeney, W. P., He, H. B., Ippolito, D. E., Kim, D., Lyons, K. A., Ok, H. O., Patel, R. A., Petrov, A. N., Pryor, K. A., Qian, X. X., Reigle, L., Woods, A., Wu, J. K., Zaller, D., Zhang, X. P., Zhu, L., Weber, A. E., and Thornberry, N. A. Dipeptidyl peptidase IV inhibition for the treatment of type 2 diabetes: potential importance of selectivity over dipeptidyl peptidases 8 and 9. *Diabetes* **2005**, *54*(10), 2988–2994.
47. Sorbera, L. A., Revel, L., and Castaner, J. P32/98. Antidiabetic, dipeptidyl-peptidase IV inhibitor. *Drugs Future* **2001**, *26*(9), 859–864.
48. Demuth, H. U., Hoffmann, T., Glund, K., McIntosh, C. H. S., Pederson, R. A., Fuecker, K., Fischer, S., and Hanefeld, M. Single dose treatment of diabetic patients by the DP IV inhibitor p32/98. *Diabetes* **2000**, *49*, 413.

49. Sedo, A. and Malik, R. Dipeptidyl peptidase IV-like molecules: homologous proteins or homologous activities? *Biochim. Biophys. Acta Protein Struct. Mol. Enzymol.* **2001**, *1550*(2), 107–116.
50. Leiting, B., Pryor, K. D., Wu, J. K., Marsilio, F., Patel, R. A., Craik, C. S., Ellman, J. A., Cummings, R. T., and Thornberry, N. A. Catalytic properties and inhibition of proline-specific dipeptidyl peptidases II, IV and VII. *Biochem. J.* **2003**, *371*, 525–532.
51. Abbott, C. A., Yu, D. M. T., Woollatt, E., Sutherland, G. R., McCaughan, G. W., and Gorrell, M. D. Cloning, expression and chromosomal localization of a novel human dipeptidyl peptidase (DPP) IV homolog, DPP8. *Eur. J. Biochem.* **2000**, *267*(20), 6140–6150.
52. Goldstein, L. A., Ghersi, G., PineiroSanchez, M. L., Salamone, M., Yeh, Y. Y., Flessate, D., and Chen, W. T. Molecular cloning of seprase: a serine integral membrane protease from human melanoma. *Biochimi. Biophys. Acta Mol. Basis Disease* **1997**, *1361*(1), 11–19.
53. Underwood, R., Chiravuri, M., Lee, H., Schmitz, T., Kabcenell, A. K., Yardley, K., and Huber, B. T. Sequence, purification, and cloning of an intracellular serine protease, quiescent cell proline dipeptidase. *J. Biol. Chem.* **1999**, *274*(48), 34053–34058.
54. Ajami, K., Abbott, C. A., McCaughan, G. W., Gorrell, M. D. Dipeptidyl peptidase 9 has two forms, a broad tissue distribution, cytoplasmic localization and DPIV-like peptidase activity. *Biochim. Biophys. Acta Gene Struct. Expression* **2004**, *1679*(1), 18–28.
55. Reinhold, D., Hemmer, B., Gran, B., Born, I., Faust, J., Neubert, K., McFarland, H. F., Martin, R., and Ansorge, S. Inhibitors of dipeptidyl peptidase IV/CD26 suppress activation of human MBP-specific CD4+T cell clones. *J. Neuroimmunol.* **1998**, *87* (1–2), 203–209.
56. Rasmussen, H. B., Branner, S., Wiberg, F. C., and Wagtmann, N. Crystal structure of human dipeptidyl peptidase IV/CD26 in complex with a substrate analog. *Nat. Struct. Biol.* **2003**, *10*(1), 19–25.
57. Ahren, B., Landin-Olsson, M., Jansson, P. A., Eriksson, J., Pacini, G., Thomaseth, K., and Schweizer, A. The DPPIV inhibitor, LAF237, reduces fasting and postprandial glucose in subjects with type 2 diabetes over a 4 week period by increasing active GLP-1, sustaining insulin and reducing glucagon. *Diabetes* **2003**, *52*, A15.
58. Oefner, C., D'Arcy, A., Mac Sweeney, A., Pierau, S., Gardiner, R., and Dale, G. E. High-resolution structure of human apo dipeptidyl peptidase IV/CD26 and its complex with 1-[({2-[(5-iodopyridin-2-yl)amino]-ethyl}amino)-acetyl]-2-cyano-(*S*)-pyrrolidine. *Acta Crystallogr. D Biol. Crystallogr.* **2003**, *59*, 1206–1212.
59. Ashworth, D. M., Atrash, B., Baker, G. R., Baxter, A. J., Jenkins, P. D., Jones, D. M., and Szelke, M. 2-Cyanopyrrolidides as potent, stable inhibitors of dipeptidyl peptidase IV. *Bioorg. Med. Chem. Lett.* **1996**, *6*(10), 1163–1166.
60. Parmee, E. R., He, J. F., Mastracchio, A., Edmondson, S. D., Colwell, L., Eiermann, G., Feeney, W. P., Habulihaz, B., He, H. B., Kilburn, R., Leiting, B., Lyons, K., Marsilio, F., Patel, R. A., Petrov, A., Di Salvo, J., Wu, J. K., Thornberry, N. A., and Weber, A. E. 4-Amino cyclohexylglycine analogues as potent dipeptidyl peptidase IV inhibitors. *Bioorg. Med. Chem. Lett.* **2004**, *14*(1), 43–46.
61. Caldwell, C. G., Chen, P., He, J. F., Parmee, E. R., Leiting, B., Marsilio, F., Patel, R. A., Wu, J. K., Eiermann, G. J., Petrov, A., He, H. B., Lyons, K. A., Thornberry, N. A., and Weber, A. E. Fluoropyrrolidine amides as dipeptidyl peptidase IV inhibitors. *Bioorg. Med. Chem. Lett.* **2004**, *14*(5), 1265–1268.
62. Edmondson, S. D., Mastracchio, A., Mathvink, R. J., He, J. F., Harper, B., Park, Y. J., Beconi, M., Di Salvo, J., Eiermann, G. J., He, H. B., Leiting, B., Leone, J. F., Levorse, D. A., Lyons, K., Patel, R. A., Patel, S. B., Petrov, A., Scapin, G., Shang, J., Sinha Roy, R., Smith, A., Wu, J. K., Xu, S. Y., Zhu, B., Thornberry, N. A., and Weber, A. E. (2S, 3S)-3-Amino-4-(3,3-difluoro-pyrrolidin-1-yl)-*N,N*-dimethyl4-oxo-2-(4-[1,2, 4]tria-zolo [1,5-a]pyridin-6-ylphenyl)butanamide: a selective alpha-amino amide dipeptidyl peptidase IV inhibitor for the treatment of type 2 diabetes. *J. Med. Chem.* **2006**, *49* (12), 3614–3627.
63. Xu, J. Y., Ok, H. O., Gonzalez, E. J., Colwell, L. F., Habulihaz, B., He, H. B., Leiting, B., Lyons, K. A., Marsilio, F., Patel, R. A., Wu, J. K., Thornberry, N. A., Weber, A. E., and Parmee, E. R. Discovery of potent and selective beta-homophenylalanine based dipeptidyl peptidase IV inhibitors. *Bioorg. Med. Chem. Lett.* **2004**, *14*(18), 4759–4762.
64. Edmondson, S. D., Mastracchio, A., Beconi, M., Colwell, L. F., Habulihaz, B., He, H. B., Kumar, S. J., Leiting, B., Lyons, K. A., Mao, A., Marsilio, F., Patel, R. A., Wu, J. K., Zhu, L., Thornberry, N. A., Weber, A. E., and Parmee, E. R. Potent and selective proline derived dipeptidyl peptidase IV inhibitors. *Bioorg. Med. Chem. Lett.* **2004**, *14*(20), 5151–5155.
65. Brockunier, L. L., He, J. F., Colwell, L. F., Habulihaz, B., He, H. B., Leiting, B., Lyons, K. A., Marsilio, F., Patel, R. A., Teffera, Y., Wu, J. K., Thornberry, N. A., Ann, A. E., and Parmee, E. R. Substituted piperazines as novel dipeptidyl peptidase IV inhibitors. *Bioorg. Med. Chem. Lett.* **2004**, *14*(18), 4763–4766.
66. Kim, D., Wang, L. P., Beconi, M., Eiermann, G. J., Fisher, M. H., He, H. B., Hickey, G. J., Kowalchick, J. E., Leiting, B., Lyons, K., Marsilio, F., Mccann, M. E., Patel, R. A., Petrov, A., Scapin, G., Patel, S. B., Sinha Roy, R., Wu, J. K., Wyvratt, M. J., Zhang, B. B., Zhu, L., Thornberry, N. A., and Weber, A. E. (2R)-4-Oxo-4-[3-(trifluoromethyl)-5,6-dihydro[1,2,4]triazolo[4,3-alpha]p yrazin-7(8*H*)-yl]-1-(2,4,5-trifluorophenyl)butan-2-amine: a potent, orally active dipeptidyl peptidase IV inhibitor for the treatment of type 2 diabetes. *J. Med. Chem.* **2005**, *48*(1), 141–151.

67. Kim, D., Kowalchick, J. E., Brockunier, L. L., Parmee, E. R., Eiermann, G. J., Fisher, M. H., He, H. B., Leiting, B., Lyons, K., Scapin, G., Patel, S. B., Petrov, A., Pryor, K. D., Sinha Roy, R., Wu, J. K., Zhang, X., Wyvratt, M. J., Zhang, B. B., Zhu, L., Thornberry, N. A., and Weber, A. E. Discovery of potent and selective dipeptidyl peptidase IV inhibitors derived from beta-aminoamides bearing substituted triazo-lopiperazines. *J. Med. Chem.* **2008**, *51*(3), 589–602.
68. Nelson, P. J. and Potts, K. T. 1,2,4-Triazoles. VI.1 The synthesis of some s-triazolo[4,3-a]pyrazines. *J. Org. Chem.* **1962**, *27*(9), 3243–3248.
69. Hansen, K. B., Balsells, J., Dreher, S., Hsiao, Y., Kubryk, M., Palucki, M., Rivera, N., Steinhuebel, D., Armstrong, J. D., Askin, D., and Grabowski, E. J. J. First generation process for the preparation of the DPP-IV inhibitor sitagliptin. *Org. Process Res. Dev.* **2005**, *9*(5), 634–639.
70. Balsells, J., DiMichele, L., Liu, J. C., Kubryk, M., Hansen, K., and Armstrong, J. D. Synthesis of [1,2,4] triazolo[4,3-alpha,]piperazines via highly reactive chloromethyloxadiazoles. *Org. Lett.* **2005**, *7*(6), 1039–1042.
71. Hsiao, Y., Rivera, N. R., Rosner, T., Krska, S. W., Njolito, E., Wang, F., Sun, Y. K., Armstrong, J. D., Grabowski, E. J. J., Tillyer, R. D., Spindler, F., and Malan, C. Highly efficient synthesis of beta-amino acid derivatives via asymmetric hydrogenation of unprotected enamines. *J. Am. Chem. Soc.* **2004**, *126* (32), 9918–9919.
72. Ikemoto, N., Tellers, D. M., Dreher, S. D., Liu, J. C., Huang, A., Rivera, N. R., Njolito, E., Hsiao, Y., McWilliams, J. C., Williams, J. M., Armstrong, J. D., Sun, Y. K., Mathre, D. J., Grabowski, E. J. J., and Tillyer, R. D. Highly diastereoselective heterogeneously catalyzed hydrogenation of enamines for the synthesis of chiral beta-amino acid derivatives. *J. Am. Chem. Soc.* **2004**, *126*(10), 3048–3049.
73. Xu, F., Armstrong, J. D., Zhou, G. X., Simmons, B., Hughes, D., Ge, Z. H., and Grabowski, E. J. J. Mechanistic evidence for an alpha-oxoketene pathway in the formation of beta-ketoamides/esters via Meldrum's acid adducts. *J. Am. Chem. Soc.* **2004**, *126*(40), 13002–13009.
74. Hansen, K. B., Yi, H., Xu, F., Rivera, N., Clausen, A., Kubryk, M., Krska, S., Rosner, T., Simmons, B., Balsells, J., Ikemoto, N., Sun, Y., Spindler, F., Malan, C., Grabowski, E. J. J., and Armstrong, J. D. Highly efficient asymmetric synthesis of sitagliptin. *J. Am. Chem. Soc.* **2009**, *131*(25), 8798–8804.
75. Clausen, A. M., Dziadul, B., Cappuccio, K. L., Kaba, M., Starbuck, C., Hsiao, Y., and Dowling, T. M. Identification of ammonium chloride as an effective promoter of the asymmetric hydrogenation of a beta-enamine amide. *Org. Process Res. Dev.* **2006**, *10*(4), 723–726.
76. Shin, J. S. and Kim, B. G. Exploring the active site of amine:pyruvate aminotransferase on the basis of the substrate structure–reactivity relationship: how the enzyme controls substrate specificity and stereo selectivity. *J. Org. Chem.* **2002**, *67*(9), 2848–2853.
77. Cho, B. K., Park, H. Y., Seo, J. H., Kim, J. H., Kang, T. J., Lee, B. S., and Kim, B. G. Redesigning the substrate specificity of omega-aminotransferase for the kinetic resolution of aliphatic chiral arnines. *Biotechnol. Bioeng.* **2008**, *99*(2), 275–284.
78. Crump, S. P. and Rozzell, J. D. *Biocatalytic Production of Amino Acids and Derivatives*, Wiley, New York, 1993.
79. Savile, C. K., Janey, J. M., Mundorff, E. C., Moore, J. C., Tam, S., Jarvis, W. R., Colbeck, J. C., Krebber, A., Fleitz, F. J., Brands, J., Devine, P. N., Huisman, G. W., and Hughes, G. J. Biocatalytic asymmetric synthesis of chiral amines from ketones applied to sitagliptin manufacture. *Science* **2010**, *329*(5989), 305–309.
80. Chen, Z. L. and Zhao, H. M. Rapid creation of a novel protein function by *in vitro* coevolution. *J. Mol. Biol.* **2005**, *348*(5), 1273–1282.
81. Koszelewski, D., Clay, D., Rozzell, D., and Kroutil, W. Deracemisation of alpha-chiral primary amines by a one-pot, two-step cascade reaction catalysed by omega-transaminases. *Eur. J. Org. Chem.* **2009**, *14*, 2289–2292.
82. Truppo, M. D., Turner, N. J., and Rozzell, J. D. Efficient kinetic resolution of racemic amines using a transaminase in combination with an amino acid oxidase. *Chem. Commun.* **2009**, 2127–2129.
83. Iwasaki, A., Yamada, Y., Kizaki, N., Ikenaka, Y., and Hasegawa, J. Microbial synthesis of chiral amines by (*R*)-specific transamination with *Arthrobacter* sp KNK168. *Appl. Microbiol. Biotechnol.* **2006**, *69*(5), 499–505.
84. Rowe, R. C., Sheskey, P. J., and Quinn, M. E. *Handbook of Pharmaceutical Excipients*, 6th ed., Pharmaceutical Press, London, 2009.
85. Lachman, L., Lieberman, J. L., and Kanig, J. L. *The Theory and Practice of Industrial Pharmacy*, 2nd ed., Lea & Febiger, Philadelphia, **1976**. pp. 321–358.
86. Jaeger, H. M. and Nagel, S. R. Physics of the granular state. *Science* **1992**, *255*(5051), 1523–1531.
87. Sekulic, S. S., Ward, H. W., Brannegan, D. R., Stanley, E. D., Evans, C. L., Sciavolino, S. T., Hailey, P. A., and Aldridge, P. K. On-line monitoring of powder blend homogeneity by near-infrared spectroscopy. *Anal. Chem.* **1996**, *68*(3), 509–513.
88. Council of, Europe., *European Pharmacopoeia*, Chapter 2.9.6, 5th ed., Council of Europe, Strasbourg, 2004.
89. Krishna, R., Herman, G., and Wagner, J. A. Accelerating drug development using biomarkers: a case study with sitagliptin, a novel DPP4 inhibitor for type 2 diabetes. *AAPS J.* **2008**, *10*(2), 401–409.
90. Alba, M., Sheng, D., Guan, Y., Williams-Herman, D., Larson, P., Sachs, J. R., Thornberry, N., Herman, G., Kaufman, K. D., and Goldstein, B. J. Sitagliptin 100 mg daily effect on DPP-4 inhibition and compound-specific

glycemic improvement. *Curr. Med. Res. Opin.* **2009**, *25*(10), 2507–2514.

91. Sinha Roy, R., Wu, J., Eiermann, G., Lyons, K., He, H. B., Weber, A., and Thornberry, N. Plasma DPP-4 inhibition by sitagliptin and other DPP-4 inhibitors correlates with and predicts glucose lowering efficacy. *Diabetes* **2009**, *58*, A612.
92. Karasik, A., Aschner, P., Katzeff, H., Davies, M. J., and Stein, P. P. Sitagliptin, a DPP-4 inhibitor for the treatment of patients with type 2 diabetes: a review of recent clinical trials. *Curr. Med. Res. Opin.* **2008**, *24* (2), 489–496.
93. Herman, G. A., Stevens, C., Van Dyck, K., Bergman, A., Yi, B. M., De Smet, M., Snyder, E., Hilliard, D., Tanen, M., Tanaka, W., Wang, A. Q., Zeng, W., Musson, D., Winchell, G., Davies, M. J., Ramael, S., Gottesdiener, K. M., and Wagner, J. A. Pharmacokinetics and pharmacodynamics of sitagliptin, an inhibitor of dipeptidyl peptidase IV, in healthy subjects: results from two randomized, double-blind, placebo-controlled studies with single oral doses. *Clin. Pharmacol. Ther.* **2005**, *78*(6), 675–688.
94. Herman, G. A., Bergman, A., Stevens, C., Kotey, P., Yi, B. M., Zhao, P., Dietrich, B., Golor, G., Schrodter, A., Keymeulen, B., Lasseter, K. C., Kipnes, M. S., Snyder, K., Hilliard, D., Tanen, M., Cilissen, C., De Smet, M., Lepeleire, I., Van Dyck, K., Wang, A. Q., Zeng, W., Davies, M. J., Tanaka, W., Holst, J. J., Deacon, C. F., Gottesdiener, K. M., and Wagner, J. A. Effect of single oral doses of sitagliptin, a dipeptidyl peptidase-4 inhibitor, on incretin and plasma glucose levels after an oral glucose tolerance test in patients with type 2 diabetes. *J. Clin. Endocrinol. Metab.* **2006**, *91*(11), 4612–4619.
95. Bergman, A. J., Stevens, C., Zhou, Y. Y., Yi, B. M., Laethem, M., De Smet, M., Snyder, K., Hilliard, D., Tanaka, W., Zeng, W., Tanen, M., Wang, A. Q., Chen, L., Winchell, G., Davies, M. J., Ramael, S., Wagner, J. A., and Herman, G. A. Pharmacokinetic and pharmacodynamic properties of multiple oral doses of sitagliptin, a dipeptidyl peptidase-IV inhibitor: a double-blind, randomized, placebo-controlled study in healthy male volunteers. *Clin. Ther.* **2006**, *28*(1), 55–72.
96. Scott, R., Wu, M., Sanchez, M., and Stein, P. Efficacy and tolerability of the dipeptidyl peptidase-4 inhibitor sitagliptin as monotherapy over 12 weeks in patients with type 2 diabetes. *Int. J. Clin. Pract.* **2007**, *61*(1), 171–180.
97. Hanefeld, M., Herman, G. A., Wu, M., Mickel, C., Sanchez, M., Stein, P. P., and Sitagliptin, S. O. Once-daily sitagliptin, a dipeptidyl peptidase-4 inhibitor, for the treatment of patients with type 2 diabetes. *Curr. Med. Res. Opin.* **2007**, *23*(6), 1329–1339.
98. Nonaka, K., Kakikawa, T., Sato, A., Okuyama, K., Fujimoto, G., Kato, N., Suzuki, H., Hirayama, Y., Ahmed, T., Davies, M. J., and Stein, P. P. Efficacy and safety of sitagliptin monotherapy in Japanese patients with type 2 diabetes. *Diabetes Res. Clin. Pract.* **2008**, *79*(2), 291–298.
99. Herman, G. A., Stein, P. P., Thornberry, N. A., Wagner, J. A. Dipeptidyl peptidase-4 inhibitors for the treatment of type 2 diabetes: focus on sitagliptin. *Clin. Pharmacol. Ther.* **2007**, *81*(5), 761–767.
100. Nauck, M. A., Meininger, G., Sheng, D., Terranella, L., and Stein, P. P., Sitagliptin Study 024 Group. Efficacy and safety of the dipeptidyl peptidase-4 inhibitor, sitagliptin, compared with the sulfonylurea, glipizide, in patients with type 2 diabetes inadequately controlled on metformin alone: a randomized, double-blind, non-inferiority trial. *Diabetes Obes. Metab.* **2007**, *9*(2), 194–205.
101. Kaitin, K. I. Deconstructing the drug development process: the new face of innovation. *Clin Pharmacol. Ther.* **2010**, *87*(3), 356–361.

CHAPTER 3

OLMESARTAN MEDOXOMIL: AN ANGIOTENSIN II RECEPTOR BLOCKER

Hiroaki Yanagisawa, Hiroyuki Koike, and Shin-ichiro Miura

3.1 BACKGROUND

3.1.1 Introduction

Hypertension is often called a silent killer because its symptoms do not manifest themselves until the late stage of the disease. The number of hypertensive patients worldwide is estimated to be one billion and one quarter of all adults are afflicted with hypertension [1]. As hypertension is an independent risk factor for cardiovascular events, control of hypertension is of great concern not only in advanced countries, but also in developing ones.

The sphygmomanometric method for determining systolic and diastolic blood pressure was established by Korotkoff in 1905, but it was not until the 1950s that high blood pressure was recognized as a disease. The term "essential hypertension" was introduced in the late 1920s, but it was misunderstood as an important compensatory mechanism to provide adequate blood flow to vital organs. This misconception persisted for decades and many physicians, until as late as the 1940s, believed that high blood pressure was not a disease and should "be left alone." In a leading textbook at the time, *Practice of Medicine* (ed. Tice, 1946), R. D. Scott wrote: "Many cases of essential hypertension not only do not need any treatment but are better off without it. Generally the less said about the blood pressure in such people, the better" [2]. The conception that control of high blood pressure could prevent cardiovascular complications was established after large-scale clinical studies were conducted in the 1960–1980s.

Many types of antihypertensive drugs were developed since the 1950s: diuretics, α-blockers, β-blockers, and calcium channel blockers. However, these drugs were not well tolerated because they had adverse effects on glucose and lipid metabolism and the cardiovascular system. Inhibition of the renin angiotensin system (RAS, Figure 3.1) made it possible to develop antihypertensives that are free from these adverse effects. The RAS dates from 1889 when Tigerstedt and Bergman demonstrated that saline extracts of the kidney elevated blood pressure. An active principle in the crude extract was designated renin, which was later shown to be an enzyme that liberates a decapeptide, angiotensin I (Ang I), from angiotensinogen in the α_2-globlin fraction. Biologically inactive Ang I is further converted to a biologically active octapeptide, angiotensin II (Ang II), by the action of angiotensin converting enzyme (ACE). The basic function of the RAS was elucidated in the late 1960s. However, the system was not acknowledged to be a contributing factor to the development and maintenance of high blood pressure until the late 1970s when captopril, the first ACE inhibitor, [3] proved effective in lowering blood pressure in patients with

Case Studies in Modern Drug Discovery and Development, Edited by Xianhai Huang and Robert G. Aslanian.

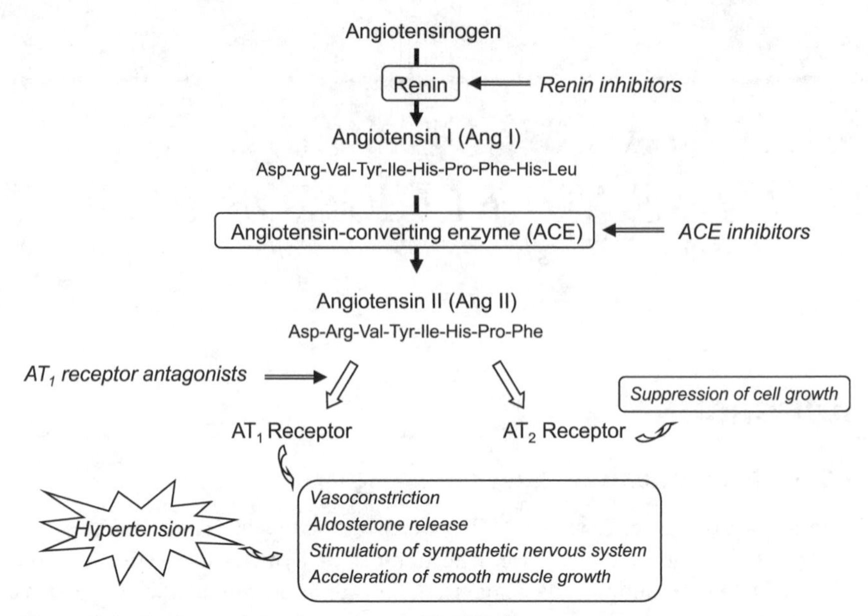

Figure 3.1 Renin–angiotensin system and its blockers.

essential hypertension. Effective blood pressure control with captopril and other ACE inhibitors that followed eventually established the importance of the RAS in the pathogenesis of hypertension.

ACE inhibitors were devoid of the adverse effects associated with previous antihypertensive drugs but had peculiar side effects: dry cough and angioedema, which were postulated to be due to the inhibition of ACE that is identical to kininase II, and a subsequent increase of plasma concentrations of kinins and substance P. This speculation prompted the development of angiotensin receptor blockers (ARBs), which were anticipated not to cause dry cough and angioedema. ARBs developed from the late 1980s to the 1990s proved to be highly effective in controlling blood pressure with safety profiles similar to those of a placebo. They are considered one of the first-line antihypertensive drugs, particularly in patients with type 2 diabetes millitus.

The development of ARBs has led not only to enormous progress in the drug therapy of hypertension, but also to great progress in the physiology of Ang II and its receptors. Two types of Ang II receptor antagonists developed simultaneously and independently in the 1980s at two different laboratories, DuP 753 (losartan) and PD-123177, made clear the existence of the two types of Ang II receptors that had been postulated for decades. The receptors that interact with losartan and PD 123177 were designated as AT_1 and AT_2, respectively [4]. Both receptors are the members of the G-protein-coupled receptors (GPCRs) and have seven transmembrane α-helical segments. AT_1 and AT_2 receptors have only 37% similarity in their amino acid sequence. Known actions of Ang II are mostly mediated through the AT_1 receptor, and are therefore blocked by ARBs.

3.1.2 Prototype of Orally Active ARBs

Peptide-type ARBs, created by modifying the Ang II molecule, were studied in the 1960s and, as a result, saralasin was developed in 1971. These ARBs in general showed a partial antagonist activity and were not effective upon oral administration. The practical study of the orally active nonpeptide ARB started when the prototype of the nonpeptide ARBs was

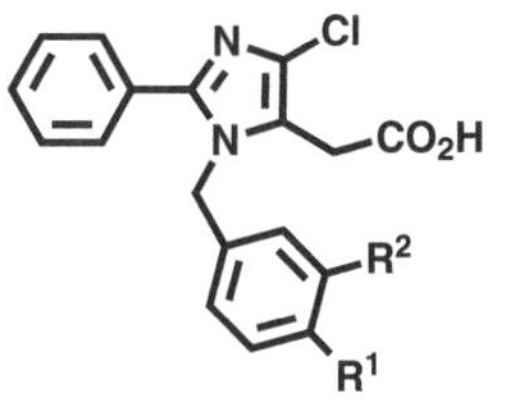

CV-2198 (1): R^1, R^2 = H

CV-2973 (2): R^1 = OMe, R^2 =Me

Figure 3.2 Prototype of an orally active ARB.

discovered by the Takeda Research Group [5]. They found that the benzyl-imidazole acetic acid CV-2198 (**1**) had diuretic activity during the diuretic and antihypertensive screening of heterocyclic compounds (Figure 3.2). Compound **1** exhibited antihypertensive activity at a dose that showed no diuretic activity. The Takeda Research Group proved that the blood pressure-lowering activity of **1** was caused by the selective inhibition of the Ang II-induced pressor response. Takeda conducted a clinical trial of CV-2973 (**2**) in 1981, which had both antihypertensive and potent diuretic activities, but unfortunately they gave up its further development due to poor results. They filed applications for the patents of these prototype compounds [6] and suspended the research and development of ARBs.

3.2 THE DISCOVERY OF OLMESARTAN MEDOXOMIL (BENICAR)

3.2.1 Lead Generation

3.2.1.1 Birth of Losartsan, the First ARB The DuPont Research Group, which had been interested in orally active ARBs, paid attention to the Takeda patents and chose the sodium salt CV-2961, S-8308 (**3**), which is the most potent compound in the Takeda patents, as the lead compound for developing clinically useful ARBs [7]. They overlapped the chemical structure of **1** with Ang II by using Dreiding models and computer modeling, and supposed that the carboxyl group of **1** played a similar role to that of the carboxyl group of Phe^8 in Ang II, which interacted with the positive charge in the receptor. The imidazole group of **1** corresponded with the imidazole ring of His^6 in Ang II, and the benzyl group of **1** pointed toward the N-terminus of Ang II. Introduction of the carboxyl group at the 4-position of the benzyl group of **1** gave EXP6155 (**4**), which had a 12-fold more potent binding affinity than **3**. The carboxyl group was proposed to correspond to the phenolic hydroxyl group of Tyr^4 or the carboxyl group of Asp^1 of Ang II. The next step in the drug design was the addition of the phthalamic acid moiety at the 4-position of the benzyl group in order to increase the molecular size to give a 10-fold increase in the binding affinity [EXP6803 (**5**)]. The carboxyl group of **5** is located at the same position as in **4**. Compound **5** demonstrated antihypertensive activity in renal hypertensive rats upon intravenous administration, but not upon oral administration. Replacement of the methoxycarbonylmethyl and the aromatic groups of **5** with the hydroxymethyl and biphenyl groups, respectively, gave orally active EXP7711 (**6**). Finally, the carboxyl group of **6** was replaced with a bioisostere, tetrazole, to give DuP 753 (later designated as losartan) (**7**), in which the binding affinity was increased more than 10-fold and the oral activity improved. DuPont applied for the patent of DuP 753 in 1986 and losartan was launched by Merck in 1995 as the first orally active ARB. After the successful development of losartan, many pharmaceutical companies initiated studies in the development of more effective ARBs (Figure 3.3).

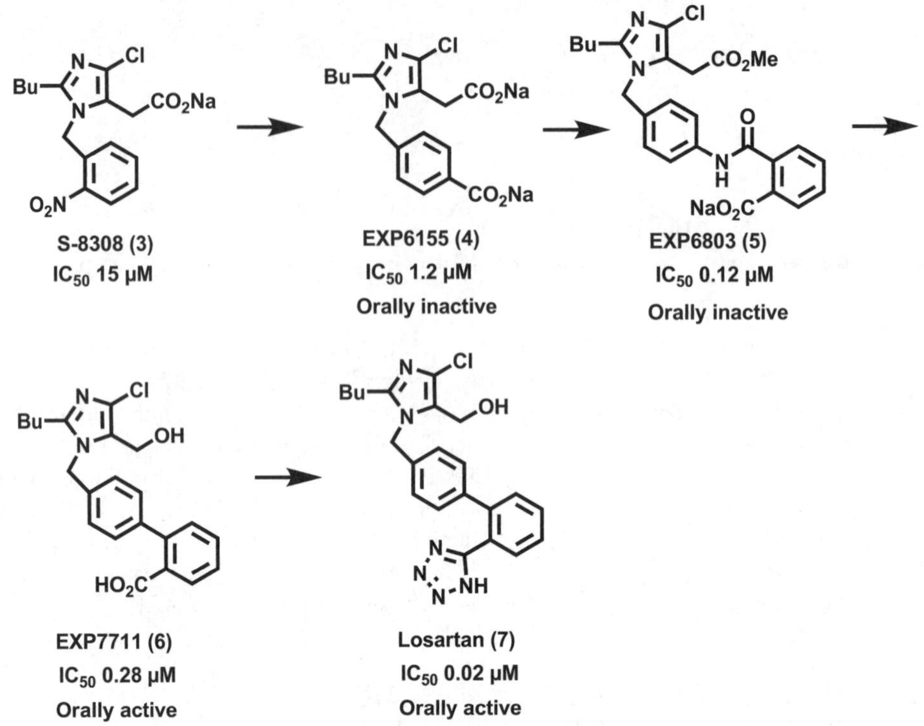

S-8308 (3)
IC_{50} 15 μM

EXP6155 (4)
IC_{50} 1.2 μM
Orally inactive

EXP6803 (5)
IC_{50} 0.12 μM
Orally inactive

EXP7711 (6)
IC_{50} 0.28 μM
Orally active

Losartan (7)
IC_{50} 0.02 μM
Orally active

Figure 3.3 Discovery of losartan (**7**) from the lead compound (**3**).

3.2.1.2 Information on ARBs in the Spring of 1990 DuPont disclosed the pharmacological activities of losartan in experimental animals at the 43rd Annual Meeting of the Council for High Blood Pressure Research of the American Heart Association in Cleveland in September 1989. This information was encouraging since Daiichi Sankyo had developed its own ACE inhibitor, temocapril, and had long been interested in the other means to interrupt the RAS.

In the spring of 1990, two papers [8,9] were published by DuPont in the *Journal of Medicinal Chemistry*, in which the structure–activity relationships (SAR) of the lead **3** were presented. They suggested that the addition of the phenyl group to the benzyl group of the lead, the carboxyl group at the *ortho*-position of the terminal phenyl group in **6**, three to five carbon atoms at the 2-position in the imidazole ring and the group capable of making a hydrogen bond at the 5-position of the imidazole ring were recommended for the potent activity. Furthermore, the 4-chloro regioisomers had a stronger binding affinity than the 5-chloro isomers. All of the compounds discussed in the papers reduced blood pressure only slightly or not at all upon oral administration.

3.2.1.3 Strategies for the Development of Novel ARBs The goal was to discover compounds that had at least 10 times more potent activity than losartan with a long-lasting effect suitable for once-a-day dosing. Due to the limited information available at the time, effort was made to search for in-house lead compounds by synthesizing heterocyclic compounds that had various types of substituents in the heterocyclic ring.

In order to quickly achieve the goal, the first screening of the synthesized compounds was done by an *in vivo* method, not by an *in vitro* assay. This method makes it possible to evaluate various aspects of the compounds, such as the antagonistic potency and duration of action, whereas *in vitro* assay only gives information about the binding affinity to the

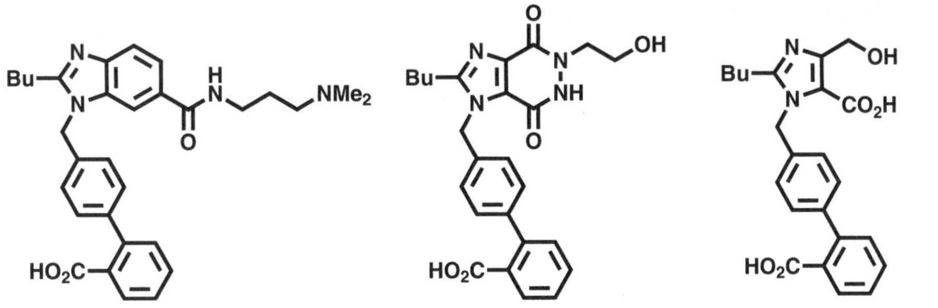

8 9 10

Figure 3.4 Benzimidazole (**8**), imidazopyridazine (**9**), and imidazole (**10**) having potent Ang II antagonist activity upon intravenous administration.

receptor. The compounds were intravenously administered to rats, and the inhibition of the pressor response induced by Ang II was determined. Compounds that showed a favorable profile in the first screening were then evaluated in rats after oral administration, and the time course of the inhibitory effect on Ang II-induced pressor response was examined.

3.2.1.4 Lead Compound Three potent compounds (**8**, **9**, and **10**) were identified in the first screening, chemical structures of which are shown in Figure 3.4. Benzimidazole (**8**) and imidazopyridazine (**9**) had six to ten times more potent antagonist activity than losartan after intravenous administration, but showed poor results when orally administered to rats. On the other hand, imidazole (**10**) which has the hydroxymethyl and carboxyl groups at the 4- and 5-positions in the imidazole ring, respectively, not only had two times more potent activity than losartan after intravenous administration, but also showed a favorable profile after oral administration. This result contradicted the prevailing conception that the hydrophobic group, such as the chlorine atom, be favored at the 4-position in the imidazole ring. In 1991, DuPont researchers stated in their paper [10] that the large lipophilic and electron-withdrawing substituents were preferred at the 4-position in imidazoles and developed the potent ARB, DuP 532, which has the large lipophilic CF_3CF_2 group at the 4-position [11]. Contrary to their preferences, however, the hydrophilic hydroxymethyl group in **10** seemed to have an important role in the potent antagonist activity. Compound **10** was selected as the lead compound for the lead optimization.

3.2.2 Lead Optimization

3.2.2.1 SAR Studies to the Discovery of Olmesartan

1-(2′-Carboxybiphenylyl)imidazole Series Derivatives of the lead **10** were synthesized to study the SAR [12]. The results are shown in Table 3.1. The table contains the binding affinity (*in vitro*) and the inhibitory activity against Ang II-induced pressor response (*in vivo*) of our compounds, EXP7711 (**6**) and **28**, an active metabolite of **6**.

The *in vitro* and *in vivo* activities increased with the size of the 4-hydroxyalkyl groups, as shown in CH_2OH (**11**), CHMeOH (**12**), and CMe_2OH (**13**), but the bulkier groups, CMeEtOH (**14**) and CEt_2OH (**15**), reduced the activity. These compounds were more potent than references **6** and **28**.

Removal of the hydroxyl group from the 4-hydroxyalkyl group diminished the activity. The 4-hydroxyalkyl compounds (**11–13**) were 1.9- to 13-fold more potent in the binding affinity and 1.4- to 4.3-fold more potent in the antagonist activity *in vivo* than the

TABLE 3.1 Biological Activities of 2′-Carboxybiphenylylmethylimidazoles

Compound	R^1	R^2	R^3	*In vitro* IC_{50}[a] (nM)	*In vivo* ID_{50}[b] ($mg\ kg^{-1}$)
11	Pr	CH_2OH	CO_2H	58	0.069
12	Pr	CHMeOH	CO_2H	28	0.062
13	Pr	CMe_2OH	CO_2H	28	0.056
14	Pr	CMeEtOH	CO_2H	51	0.074
15	Pr	CEt_2OH	CO_2H	110	0.11
16	Pr	H	CO_2H	60	0.22
17	Pr	Me	CO_2H	110	0.096
18	Pr	Et	CO_2H	100	0.27
19	Pr	$CHMe_2$	CO_2H	360	0.14
20	Pr	CH_2OH	CO_2Et	840	1.5
21	Pr	CMe_2OH	CO_2Et	600	1.2
21	Pr	CH_2OH	CH_2OH	2700	2.1
23	Pr	CO_2H	CH_2OH	20000	8.8
24	Pr	CO_2H	H	45000	8.2
25	Pr	CO_2H	CO_2H	320	0.67
26	Et	CMe_2OH	CO_2H	37	0.3
27	Bu	CMe_2OH	CO_2H	30	0.066
6[c]	Bu	Cl	CH_2OH	490	2.3
28[d]	Bu	Cl	CO_2H	130	0.21

[a]Determined by radioligand-binding assay using [125I]Ang II (0.1 nM) and bovine adrenal cortex.

[b]Determined by inhibitory activity to the Ang II-induced pressor response in rats. The compounds were intravenously administered and then Ang II (50 ng kg^{-1}) was injected 2 min later.

[c]EXP7711.

[d]Active metabolite of **6**.

corresponding 4-alkyl compounds (**17–19**). The activities of **17–19** were comparable to those of **28**. The compound (**16**), having no substituent at the 4-position, had the same binding affinity as that of **11** but its antagonist activity was less.

Ethyl esters (**20**, **21**) of the 5-carboxyl group in **11** and **13** reduced both the *in vitro* and *in vivo* activities to less than one tenth. Their activities were equivalent to **6**. Replacement (**22**) of the chlorine atom of **6** with the hydroxymethyl group reduced the binding affinity. These results suggest that the carboxyl group at the 5-position is capable of forming not only a hydrogen bonding but also an electrostatic interaction with the receptor, and thus contributes to the potent activity. The position of the carboxyl group is favorable at the 5-position, and **16** was markedly more potent than **24**. The potent activity of **11–13** is derived from the combination of the 4-hydroxyalkyl group and the 5-carboxyl group. The regioisomer (**23**) of **11** was substantially less active than **11**, which means that the positions of their groups are essential for the activity. The 4,5-dicarboxylic acid (**25**) demonstrated activity similar to **28** but less than that of **11–13**. The propyl group (**13**) at the 2-position achieved better results than the ethyl (**26**) and the butyl (**27**) groups.

The best compound in this series was **13**, as it has the propyl, hydroxyisopropyl, and carboxyl groups at the 2-, 4-, and 5-positions, respectively, and was more potent than losaratan (**7**).

1-(2′-Tetrazolylbiphenylyl)imidazole Series Table 3.2 shows the activities of the tetrazole derivatives of the compounds in Table 3.1 in comparison with **7** and the active metabolite of **7**, EXP3174 (**42**) [13]. Replacement of the carboxyl group with the tetrazolyl group enhanced the *in vitro* and *in vivo* activities. The SAR of this series had little difference from that of the 2′-carboxybiphenylyl series. The 4-hydroxyalkyl compounds (**29–31**) were more potent than the 4-alkyl compounds (**33–35**) in the *in vitro* and *in vivo* activities. The 4-alkyl compounds (**33–35**) showed binding affinities comparable to **42**, and the *in vivo* activities were less than **42**. Ethyl ester (**36**) was less active than the carboxylic acid (**31**) in both *in vitro* and *in vivo* assays. Replacement (**37**) of the carboxyl group at the 5-position of **39** with the hydroxymethyl group markedly reduced the *in vitro* and *in vivo* activities. The 2-ethyl compound (**40**) had a more potent binding affinity (*in vitro*) but less antagonist activity (*in vivo*) than **31**.

The 4-hydroxyisopropyl compound (**31**) was slightly less active than the other 4-hydroxyalkyl compounds (**29**, **30**), although the 4-hydroxyisopropyl group was the best in the 2-carboxybiphenylyl series. In order to evaluate these compounds as an oral drug, **29–31** were orally administered to rats. All of these compounds had potent and long-lasting antagonist activity, as seen in Figure 3.5. The hydroxyisopropyl compound (**31**) showed the most potent and longest-lasting activity among them, and was 30 times more active than losartan. Compound **31** was temporarily chosen as a clinical candidate and designated it later as olmesartan. However, **31** had room for improvement in terms of oral absorption because the bioavailability of **31** was estimated to be only 4.1% in rats in a pharmacokinetic study.

TABLE 3.2 Biological Activities of 2′-Tetrazolylbiphenylylmethylimidazoles

Compound	R^1	R^2	R^3	*In vitro* IC_{50}[a] (nM)	*In vivo* ID_{50}[b] (mg kg^{-1})
29	Pr	CH_2OH	CO_2H	6.9	0.0062
30	Pr	CHMeOH	CO_2H	4.9	0.0063
31[c]	Pr	CMe_2OH	CO_2H	8.1	0.0079
32	Pr	H	CO_2H	9.1	0.018
33	Pr	Me	CO_2H	11	0.028
34	Pr	Et	CO_2H	12	0.019
35	Pr	$CHMe_2$	CO_2H	46	0.014
36	Pr	CMe_2OH	CO_2Et	200	0.32
37	Pr	CO_2H	CH_2OH	4600	1.7
38	Pr	CO_2H	H	14000	2.4
39	Pr	CO_2H	CO_2H	100	0.031
40	Et	CMe_2OH	CO_2H	5.3	0.019
41	Bu	CMe_2OH	CO_2H	9.5	0.017
7	Bu	Cl	CH_2OH	120	0.3
42[d]	Bu	Cl	CO_2H	22	0.1
52	Pr	CMe_2OH	$CONH_2$		

[a]Determined by radioligand-binding assay using [125I]Ang II (0.1 nM) and bovine adrenal cortex.

[b]Determined by inhibitory activity to the Ang II-induced pressor response in rats. The compounds were intravenously administered and then Ang II (50 ng kg^{-1}) was injected 2 min later.

[c]Olmesartan.

[d]EXP3174, active metabolite of **7**.

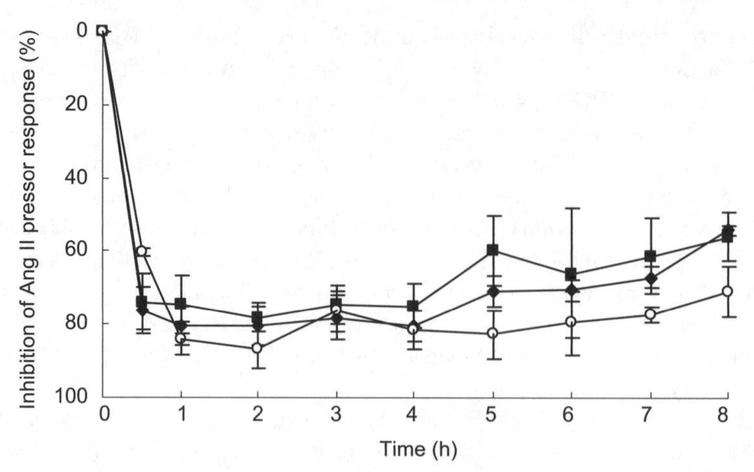

Figure 3.5 Time courses of **29** (■), **30** (◆) and olmesartan **31** (○) for inhibition of Ang II (50 ng/kg, i.v.)-induced pressor response in conscious normotensive rats ($n = 3$–5). The compounds were administered orally at a dose of 0.3 mg/kg.

3.2.2.2 Prodrug of Olmesartan: The Way to Olmesartan Medoxomil

Improving the oral activity of **13,** the most potent compound in the carboxybiphenylyl series, was attempted. There are several means to improve oral absorption: alteration of the physicochemical property by modifying the chemical structure, replacement of a functional group with its bioisostere, the preparation of prodrugs or employing different formulation formulas. There are many types of prodrugs but the desirable prodrug type is dependent upon the target molecule [14]. Effort was attempted to produce prodrugs of **13** by esterification [12]. The prodrug ester would readily cross the intestinal wall and enter the blood stream due to the increased lipophilicity of the molecule, and it would liberate the parent compound by the action of esterase in the body. Compound **13** has the two carboxyl groups, one at the 5-position of the imidazole ring and the other in the terminal phenyl group. The ethyl ester (**21**) of the carboxyl group in the imidazole ring was less active than **13**. The esters of (5-methyl-2-oxo-1,3-dioxol-4-yl)methyl (DMDO, **43**), pivaloyloxymethyl (POM, **44**), [(isopropoxycarbonyl)oxy]methyl (IPM, **45**), and phthalidyl (PHT, **46**), which are useful pro-moieties of orally active β-lactam antibiotics, showed two to three times more potent and long-lasting antagonist activity than **13** (see Figure 3.6 for their chemical structures). On the other hand, the POM ester (**47**) of the carboxyl group at the terminal phenyl group decreased the potency of **13**. These results demonstrated that prodrugs at the 5-position in the imidazole ring with the specific pro-moieties improved oral absorption.

The same results were obtained from the prodrugs of olmesartan (**31**), except for the PHT ester (**51**). The DMDO (**48**), POM (**49**), and IPM (**50**) esters were three times more potent than olmesartan and had longer lasting activity, but the PHT ester (**51**) was less active. Compound **48** was obtained as crystals having a melting point of 180–182 °C, whereas **49** and **50** were amorphous solids. It was finally decided to develop **48** for the clinical study and designated it as olmesartan medoxomil. Crystallization is an important factor in drug development. The bioavailability of **48** was 21.5% in rats, which meant a fivefold improvement by prodrug formation. Figure 3.7 shows the time courses of **31**, **48**, and losartan (**7**) for the inhibition of Ang II induced-pressor response after oral administration in rats. Olmesartan medoxomil (**48**) had 100 times more potent activity than losartan (**7**) and was three times more potent than olmesartan (**31**).

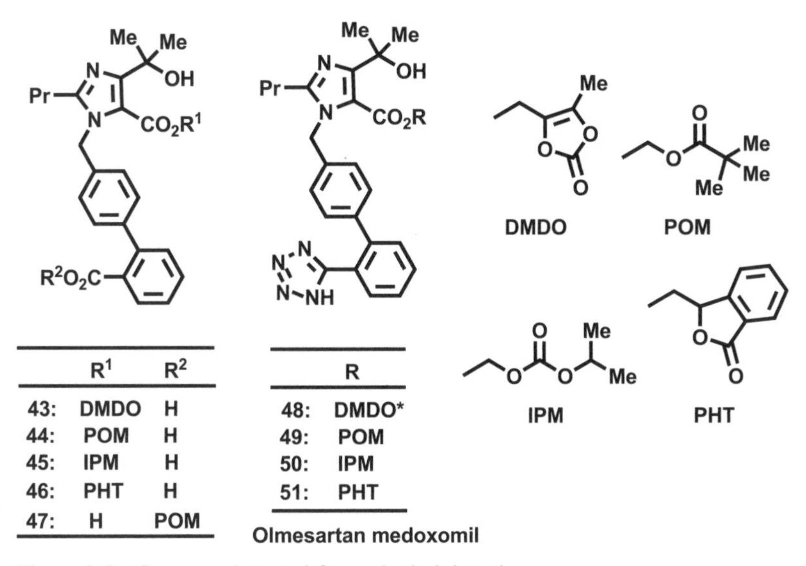

Figure 3.6 Compounds tested for oral administration.

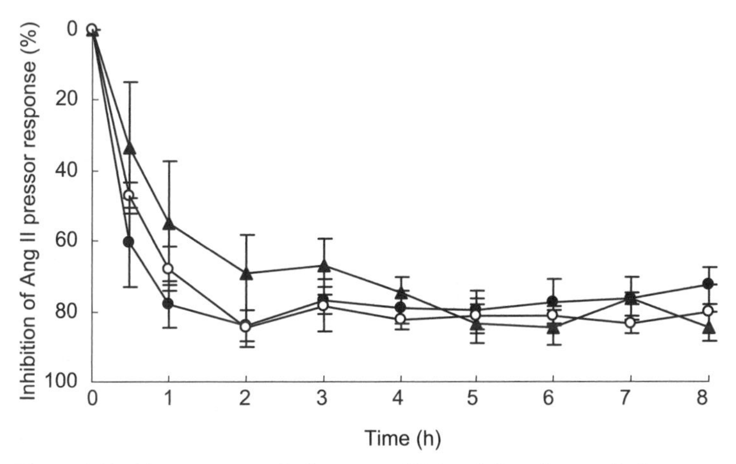

Figure 3.7 Time courses of olmesartan **31** (●, 0.3 mg/kg, p.o.),olmesartan medoxomil **48** (○, 0.1 mg/kg, p.o.) and losartan **7** (▲, 10 mg/kg, p.o.) for inhibition of Ang II (50 ng/kg, i.v.)-induced pressor response in conscious normotensive rats ($n = 3$–5).

3.3 CHARACTERISTICS OF OLMESARTAN

After the development of losartan by DuPont, a large number of ARBs were announced by pharmaceutical companies, but only seven ARBs, shown in Figure 3.8, have been successfully launched. The patent applications for these compounds were filed between 1989 and 1991, except for losartan, which was filed in 1986. All ARBs except eprosartan have the tetrazolylbiphenylyl or carboxybiphenylyl groups. The substituents corresponding to the butyl group of losartan are straight chains with a C3 to C4 length: propyl, butyl, or ethoxy groups. Olmesartan medoxomil and candesartan cilexetil are the prodrugs derived from the modification of the carboxyl group.

These ARBs have the same mechanism of antihypertensive activity and block the Ang II action by binding to the AT_1 receptor, but their pharmacological features such as potency,

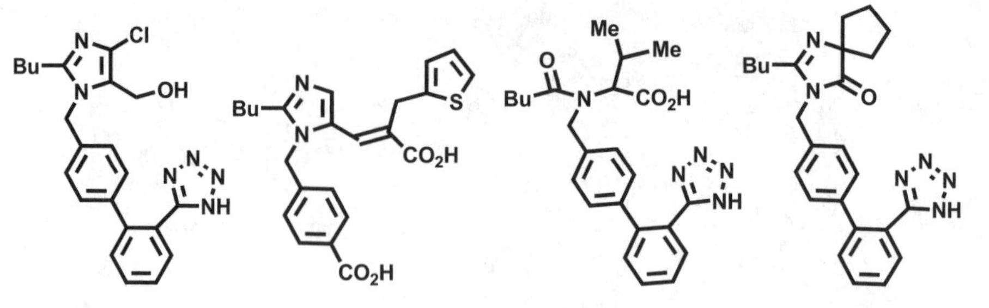

Losartan Eprosartan Valsartan Irbesartan

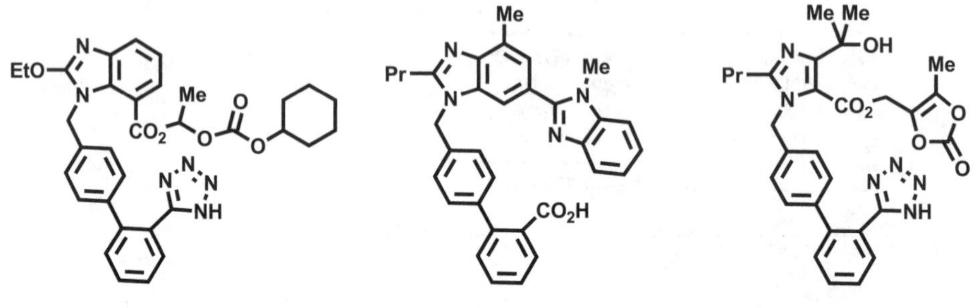

Candesartan cilexetil Telmisartan Olmesartan medoxomil

Figure 3.8 Seven ARBs launched in the world.

PK/PD profiles and the type of the antagonist activity differ with their chemical structures. The pharmacological feature characteristics of olmesartan discussed here are assumed to be the result of hydrophilic 4-hydroxyisopropyl and 5-carboxyl groups in the imidazole ring.

The biological feature of olmesartan is characterized by potent AT_1 receptor blockade, insurmountable antagonist activity, inverse agonist activity, and metabolic stability. These characteristics are accounted for at least partly by unique chemical structures as described in this section.

(i) *Strong antagonist activity*. As mentioned in the previous sections, the hydroxyisopropyl and carboxyl groups at the 4- and 5-positions in olmesartan contribute to its strong antagonist activity. Also, olmesartan had the most potent antagonist activity in the study of the contractile response to Ang II in rabbit aortas. Details are described in Section 3.6.2.

(ii) *Insurmountable antagonist activity*. Olmesartan is a potent insurmountable antagonist. Olmesartan does not easily dissociate from the receptor and is not easily replaced by Ang II after binding to the receptor. Pretreatment of rabbit aortas with a very low concentration of olmesartan markedly reduced the maximal contraction induced by a high concentration of Ang II. On the other hand, the compounds that had the hydroxymethyl (**29**) and isopropyl (**35**) groups at the 4-position and the carbamoyl group (**52**; shown in Table 3.2) at the 5-position did not show potent insurmountable antagonist activity. These data suggest that the 4-hydroxyisopropyl and 5-carboxyl groups are essential for the insurmountable antagonism. Details are discussed in Section 3.6.2.

Similar results were obtained in a study with HEK 293 cells expressing the AT_1 receptor. In these cells olmesartan decreased the maximum response of AngII-induced ERK activation, whereas the compound that has the isopropyl group at the 4-position (36) or the carbamoyl group at the 5-posion (52) produced a right-wards shift of the concentration-response curve for AngII induced ERK activation (15).

Le et al. reported that olmesartan has a higher degree of insurmountability, slower dissociation and higher affinity to the receptor than telmisartan, as demonstrated in the experiments of radioligand binding and the inhibition of Ang II-induced inositol phosphate accumulation in CHO-K1 cells expressing the human AT_1 receptor [16]. These results were assumed to be due to the 5-carboxyl group and possibly other substituents in the imidazole ring of olmesartan.

(iii) *Inverse agonist activity*. GPCRs, including the AT_1 receptor, have spontaneous activity in the absence of agonists, which would cause organ damage over time. This activity is suppressed by an inverse agonist, which stabilizes the receptor in the inactive conformation. Olmesartan was examined to check its inverse agonist activity using COS1 cells expressing the AT_1 receptor or the mutated receptor, and the result demonstrated that the drug does have strong inverse agonist activity due to the combination of the hydroxyisopropyl and carboxyl groups in the imidazole ring (see Section 3.4 for detailed discussion) [17].

A similar result was reported by Qin et al. [15]. The basal c-fos promoter activity in HEK293 cells expressing the N111G mutated AT_1 receptor was suppressed by olmesartan, but not by **36** and **52**. Also, ERK activation by stretching cardiomyocytes isolated and cultured from neonatal rats was suppressed by olmesartan in the absence of Ang II and not by **36** and **52**. These results show that the combination of the hydroxyisopropyl group with the carboxyl group is essential for the potent inverse agonist activity of olmesartan. The inverse agonist activity of olmesartan was also observed in mesangial cells isolated from rat kidney [18]. Olmesartan attenuated the activation of ERK and NADPH oxidase by mechanical strain in mesangial cells in the absence of Ang II.

(iv) *Metabolic stability*. As most hypertensive patients take multiple drugs, hypertensive agents are expected not to have a drug–drug interaction due to cytochrome P450. Kamiyama et al. examined the effect on the hydroxylation of *(S)*-warfarin by CYP2C9, which is the major enzyme involved in the metabolization of ARBs [19]. Olmesartan did not inhibit the hydroxylation of warfarin (Figure 3.9a). On the other hand, other ARBs inhibited hydroxylation

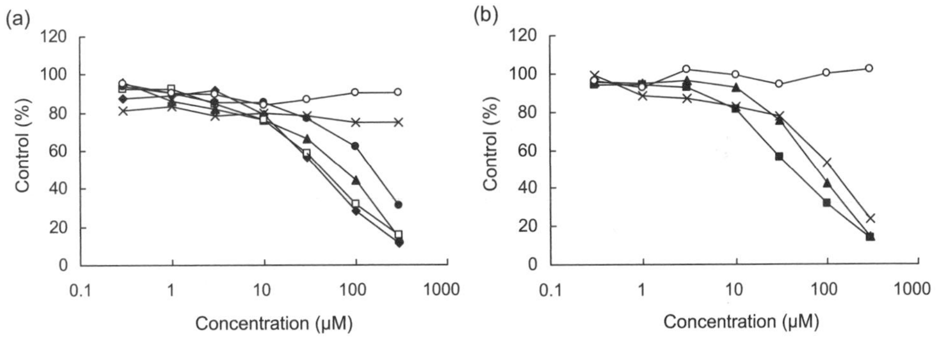

Figure 3.9 Inhibitory effects of ARBs on 7-hydroxylation of (*S*)-warfarin (final concentration, 5 μM) with CYP2C in human liver microsomes. The reaction mixture was incubated at 37°C for 40 min. Each symbol represents the mean of quadruplicate determinations. (a) Olmesartan (○), valsartan (×), irbesartan (●), candesartan (▲), telmisartan (□) and losartan (○). (b) Olmesartan (○), **33** (×), **34** (▲) and **35** (■).

except valsartan which does not have an imidazole ring. Also, the compounds which have the alkyl groups (**33–35**) instead of the hydroxyalkyl groups at the 4-position of the imidazole ring inhibited CYP2C9 (Figure 3.9b). This is due to the hydrophilic property of olmesartan, which is the highest among ARBs, and also to the inept interaction of the 4-hydroxyisopropyl group in olmesartan with the hydrophobic pocket of CYP2C9.

3.4 BINDING SITES OF OMLERSARTAN TO THE AT_1 RECEPTOR AND ITS INVERSE AGONOIST ACTIVITY

3.4.1 Binding Sites of Olmesartan to the AT_1 Receptor

The octapeptide Ang II binds to the AT_1 receptor by four main interactions. First two interactions may be important for docking the receptor, one between the guanidino group of Arg^2 of Ang II and Asp^{281} of the AT_1 receptor and the other between the α-carboxyl group of Phe^8 of Ang II and Lys^{199} of the AT_1 receptor [20,21]. In addition, it has been shown that the second two important interactions are necessary to activate the receptor, one between Phe^8 of Ang II and His^{256} of the AT_1 receptor [21] and the other between Tyr^4 of Ang II and Asn^{111} [22]. Since part of the structures of peptide-type ARBs is similar to that of Ang II, it is possible that ARBs may interact with these binding sites. On the other hand, non-peptide-type ARBs have been reported to interact with the binding sites differently from those for Ang II [23].

Most nonpeptide ARBs have a common chemical structure that includes a biphenyl-tetrazole group substituted imidazole core. Olmesartan however has a hydroxyisopropyl group and a carboxyl group at the 4- and 5-positions, respectively, in addition to these shared chemical features. These small, but significant, differences in the chemical structure lead to unique binding behaviors. The binding sites of the AT_1 receptor to these functional groups of olmesartan was studied [17]. In order to clarify the specific amino acid residues of the AT_1 receptor that interact with olmesartan, binding affinities of olmesartan and its related compounds, **29**, **35**, and **52**, which differ at the 4- or 5-positions from olmesartan, as shown in Table 3.2, to the wild-type (WT) and mutant AT_1 receptors were examined. A large reduction of binding affinity in the mutant AT_1 receptor compared to the WT receptor would suggest that the mutated amino acid in the mutant receptor should be a candidate for a binding interaction with the AT_1 receptor with olmesartan. The results demonstrated that residues Tyr^{113}, Lys^{199}, His^{256}, Gln^{257}, Thr^{260}, Thr^{287}, and Tyr^{295} in the AT_1 receptor were considered to interact with olmesartan. Among them, Tyr^{113}, Lys^{199}, and Gln^{257} were essential for binding to the AT_1 receptor. It was speculated that these amino acids interacted with olmesartan as follows: Tyr^{113} binds to the hydroxyl group at the 4-position of olmesartan, Lys^{199} exhibits electrostratic interaction with the carboxyl group at the 5-position, and the carbamoyl group of Gln^{257} interacts with the tetrazolyl group of olmesartan.

3.4.2 Inverse Agonist Activity of Olmesartan

Although no naturally occurring mutant AT_1 receptor that has constitutive activity has been found, a recombinant WT AT_1 receptor expressed at a high density showed constitutive activity. As the WT AT_1 receptor has some constitutive activity, it can be used to analyze the molecular mechanism that underlies the inverse agonist activity [24]. Inverse agonist activity was estimated by suppression of the basal inositol phosphate (IP) production. Olmesartan significantly suppressed basal IP production whereas **29**, **35**, and **52** did not. In order to study more details, the AT_1-N111G mutant and F77A/N111A double mutant receptors were used instead of the WT AT_1 receptor. Their constitutive activities were increased due to a conformational change of the receptor. The results suggested that the coexistence of both the carboxyl and hydroxyisopropyl groups of olmesartan was required for the potent inverse agonist activity.

Next, effort was made to investigate which binding sites between olmesartan and the AT_1 receptor were critical for the inverse agonist activity of olmesartan. The inhibitory effects on IP production were evaluated in the receptors mutated at Tyr^{113}, Lys^{199}, His^{256}, and Gln^{257} in the N111G and F77A/N111G. It turned out that cooperative interactions between the hydroxyl group of olmesartan and Tyr^{113} [transmembrane (TM) III] and between the carboxyl group and His^{256} (TM VI) are crucial for the potent inverse agonist activity. These specific interactions would stabilize the AT_1 receptor in an inactive conformation, which does not allow G protein coupling. Interaction between the tetrazolyl group and Gln^{257} was only a little involved in the inverse agonist activity, while this interaction was important for binding to the AT_1 receptor.

3.4.3 Molecular Model of the Interaction between Olmesartan and the AT_1 Receptor

Computer modeling of the interaction of the AT_1 receptor with olmesartan was performed by the use of Glide program. The structure of the AT_1 receptor was based on the X-ray crystal structure of bovine rhodopsin. Based on the mutation data, olmesartan was docked to the receptor utilizing three critical interactions: between Tyr^{113} and the hydroxyl group of olmesartan, between Lys^{199} and the carboxyl group, and between Gln^{257} and the tetrazolyl group as shown in Figure 3.10.

The distances between Tyr^{113} and the hydroxyl group, Lys^{199} and the carboxyl group, and Gln^{257} and the tetrazolyl group are 2.7, 2.8, and 3.1 Å, respectively, which are

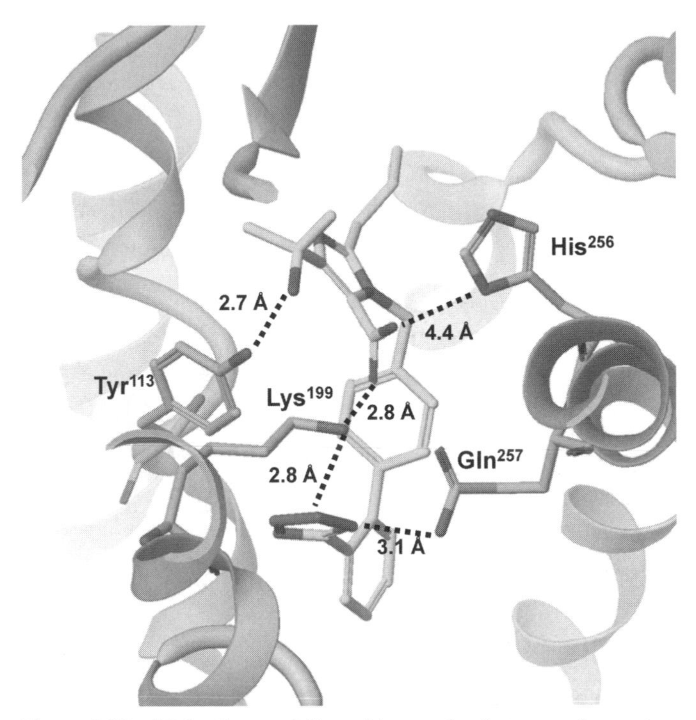

Figure 3.10 Molecular modeling of interaction between olmesartan and the AT_1 recep

reasonable distances for contributing to electrostatic and/or hydrogen bond interactions. Lys^{199} is also close to the tetrazolyl group, that is, the distance between them is 2.8 Å, suggesting the electrostatic interaction between them. The other amino acid, His^{256}, which is critical for the inverse agonist activity, is located 4.4 Å from the carboxyl group, a distance at which interaction between them is possible.

The amino acid residues, Lys^{199}, His^{256}, and Gln^{257} also interact with losartan (**7**) [25]. According to the molecular modeling, olmesartan binds to amino acid residues located deeper in the TM domains of the receptor than those to which losartan binds. More importantly, the hydroxyl and carboxyl groups of olmesartan, which are not shared by losartan, interact with the AT_1 receptor. This mode of olmesartan binding, which is distinct from that of losartan, underlies potent inverse agonism of olmesartan.

3.5 PRACTICAL PREPARATION OF OLMESARTAN MEDOXOMIL

The practical route for scale up production of olmesartan medoxomil (**48**) is shown in Scheme 3.1. The starting compound, 2-propylimidazole-4,5-dicarbonitrile (**53**), was quantitatively prepared by the condensation of diaminomaleonitrile with trimethyl orthobutyrate. After the conversion of **53** to the diester (**54**), **54** was treated with excess MeMgCl (>3 eq.) to give 4-hydroxyisopropylimidazole (**55**) in a high yield . Benzylation of **55** with bromide (**56**) afforded exclusively **57**, without the formation of the regioisomer due to the bulky hydroxyisopropyl group. After the conversion of **57** to olmesartan (**32**), protection of the tetrazolyl group with the trityl group, esterification with **58**, and finally, removal of the trityl group gave olmesartan medoxomil (**48**).

Preparation of olmesartan medoxomil. i. 6N HCl; ii. HCl/EtOH; iii. >3 eq. MeMgCl; . NaOH; vii. Ph_3CCl/DBU; vii. **58**/DBU; viii. aq. AcOH.

. STUDIES

eceptor Blocking Action

or. xomil is a prodrug that liberates the active metabolite olmesartan after ydrolysis of olmesartan medoxomil occurs readily by the action of esterases, which are present abundantly in the gastro-intestinal tract, liver, and plasma. Olmesartan selectively binds to the AT_1 receptor. The IC_{50} values for the inhibition of ^{125}I-Ang II binding to the human AT_1 and AT_2 receptors were 1.3 and 20000 nM, respectively. Other ARBs also have AT_1/AT_2 selectivity similar to that of olmesartan. In other studies with bovine adrenal cortex preparation, the specific binding of ^{125}I-Ang II was displaced by ARBs. The concentration of olmesartan producing a 50% inhibition of Ang II binding (IC_{50}) to the AT_1 receptor was 7.7 ± 1.0 nM, which was twelve and two times lower than losartan (92 ± 5 nM) and EXP3174 (16 ± 1 nM), respectively. The Scatchard, Hill, and Lineweaver–Burk analysis of the effects of ARBs on Ang II binding to the AT_1 receptor revealed that olmesartan, as well as losartan, interacts with the receptor in a reversible and competitive manner [26].

3.6.2 Inhibition of Ang II-Induced Vascular Contraction

The effects of olmesartan and other ARBs on Ang II-induced vascular contraction were examined in isolated rabbit aortas. A concentration–response curve was constructed by increasing Ang II concentration in the bathing solution (Figure 3.11) [27]. Drug concentrations at which the contractile response to Ang II (10 nM) was inhibited by 50% (IC_{50}) were calculated for different ARBs, and the results are listed in Table 3.3. The potency of olmesartan was slightly higher than or almost the same as that of candesartan and considerably higher than other ARBs. Losartan (Figure 3.11b) and irbesartan (data not

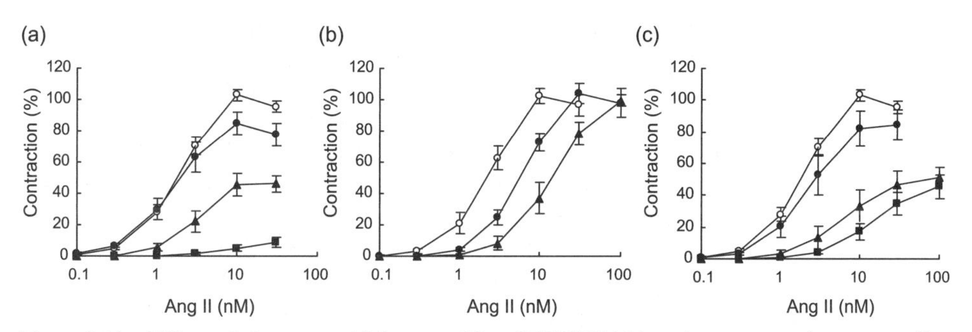

Figure 3.11 Effects of olmesartan (a), losartan (b) and EXP3174 (c) on the concentration-contractile response curves for Ang II in rabbits aortas. (a) ○ Vehicle ($n = 12$), ● 0.03 nM ($n = 6$), ▲ 0.1 nM ($n = 6$), ■ 0.3 nM ($n = 6$). (b) ○ vehicle ($n = 6$), ● 10 nM ($n = 6$), ▲ 30 nM ($n = 6$). (c) ○ vehicle ($n = 12$), ● 0.1 nM ($n = 6$), ▲ 0.3 nM ($n = 6$), ■ 1 nM ($n = 6$).

TABLE 3.3 Inhibitory Action of ARBs on Ang II-Induced Contraction in Isolated Rabbit Aorta

Compound	IC_{50} (nM)
Olmesartan	0.083
Losartan	19
EXP3174	0.20
Candesartan	0.09
Valsartan	0.59
Irbesartan	1.3
Telmisartan	1.8

shown) caused a parallel rightward shift of the concentration-response curve for Ang II, indicating a "surmountable" antagonism. On the other hand, olmesartan (Figure 3.11a) and candesartan (data not shown) produced a marked reduction in the maximal response to Ang II with a little right-ward shift of the concentration-response curves, indicating that the antagonistic mode of these ARBs is "insurmountable." EXP3174 (Figure 3.11c), valsartan (data not shown) and telmisartan (data not shown) caused a nonparallel rightward shift with a moderate reduction in the maximal response, indicating a mixed mode of action.

In general, an irreversible receptor blocker such as phenoxibenzamine, an α-adrenergic blocker, reduces the maximal response to the ligand. However, olmesartan has been proved to be a reversible AT_1 receptor blocker, as described in Section 3.6.1. The insurmountable blockade of the AT_1 receptor with olmesartan is attributed to a slow dissociation characteristic of olmesartan in interaction with the AT_1 receptor [16].

3.6.3 Inhibition of the Pressor Response to Ang II

Inhibition of the pressor response to Ang II was examined in conscious rats. Ang II (50 ng kg^{-1}) was intravenously administered before and after a single oral administration of olmesartan medoxomil or losartan. Figure 3.7 shows the time course for the inhibition of Ang II-induced pressor response. Olmesartan medoxomil at 0.1 mg kg^{-1} produced a maximal inhibition of the pressor response 2 h after administration, whereas losartan at 10 mg kg^{-1} produced a gradual inhibition with a maximal inhibition 5 h after administration. Both drugs inhibited the Ang II-pressor response for more than 8 h after a single oral administration.

Losartan has an oxidized metabolite, EXP3174 [13], that is more potent than the parent compound in blocking the AT_1 receptor. An intravenous administration of losartan (1 mg kg^{-1}) or olmesartan medoxomil (0.01 mg kg^{-1}) inhibited the pressor response to Ang II (50 ng kg^{-1}, i.v.) in anesthetized rats (Figure 3.12). The maximal inhibition was achieved within 1 h after olmesartan medoxomil administration, and the inhibition gradually decreased thereafter (Figure 3.12a). Losartan exhibited a biphasic inhibitory effect (Figure 3.12b). The first maximal inhibition was achieved immediately after administration, and then the inhibition rapidly decreased. The inhibitory effect of losartan increased again 1 h after administration. Pretreatment with a CYP inhibitor, SKF-525A (50 mg kg^{-1}, i.p.), abolished the second phase of inhibition by losartan but did not affect the inhibition by olmesartan medoxomil. These results suggest that the inhibition of the pressor response to Ang II by losartan is partly attributed to its metabolite, EXP3174.

3.6.4 Blood Pressure Lowering Effects

The antihypertensive effects after a single oral administration of olmesartan medoxomil were evaluated in different models of hypertension in rats. Olmesartan medoxomil was the most effective in lowering blood pressure in renal hypertensive rats (RHR), followed by spontaneously hypertensive rats (SHR), normotensive rats (NTR), and DOCA-salt hypertensive rats (DOCA). In DOCA rats olmesartan medoxomil was totally ineffective in lowering blood pressure at doses up to 30 mg kg^{-1}. This order of potency among different types of hypertension is similar to that of ACE inhibitors and suggests that the antihypertensive effects of olmesartan medoxomil depend on plasma renin activity [28].

The effects of olmesartan (0.01 or 0.1 mg kg^{-1}, i.v.) on central and peripheral hemodynamics were examined by the tracer microsphere method in anesthetized SHR [28]. Olmesartan lowered blood pressure without affecting heart rate. In higher doses, olmesartan increased cardiac output. The total peripheral resistance was decreased in a dose-related

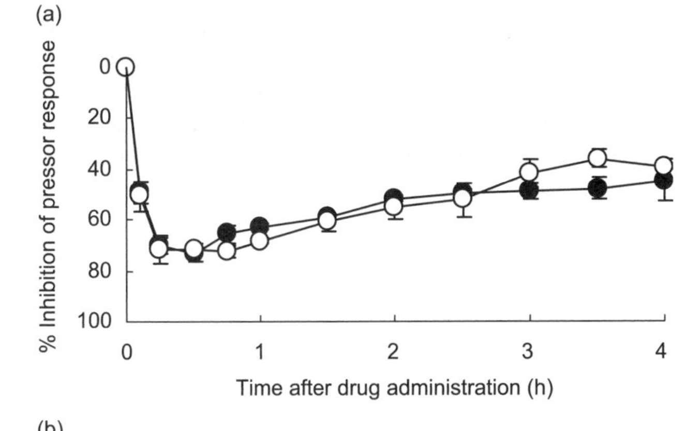

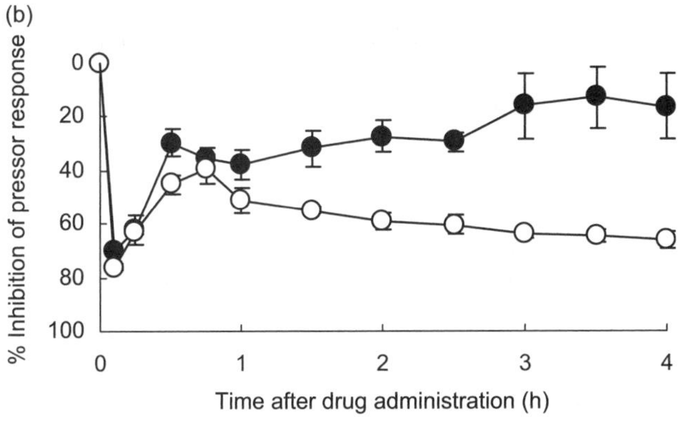

Figure 3.12 Inhibitory effects of (a) olmesartan medoxomil (0.01 mg/kg, i.v.) or (b) losartan (1 mg/kg, i.v.) on the Ang II-pressor response with or without SK&F-525A in anaesthetized rats. Values are means ±S.E.M. (a) ○ Vehicle ($n = 5$), ● SK&F-525A ($n = 4$). (b) ○ vehicle ($n = 5$), ● SK&F-525A ($n = 4$).

manner. Blood flow in the kidneys was increased markedly, while blood flow in other organs was not changed. The results suggest that vasodilatation in the kidneys, among other organs, is a major factor in the decrease of total peripheral resistance, which leads to blood pressure reduction (data not shown) [28].

3.6.5 Organ Protection

Besides classical actions such as vasoconstriction and sodium retention, the following actions have been known for Ang II: the stimulation of cell growth and fibrosis, and increased production of reactive oxygen species and inflammatory cytokines [29,30]. These new actions are unrelated to blood pressure control. As most of the harmful actions of Ang II are mediated through the AT_1 receptor, ARBs confer beneficial effects beyond the lowering of blood pressure. Organ protections produced by olmesartan medoxomil are at least partly attributed to the inverse agonist activity. However, the extent to which this activity is involved remains to be determined.

Sustained exposure to Ang II leads to cardiovascular remodeling due to stimulation of cell growth and the increased formation of matrix protein and fibroblast. Long-term treatment with olmesartan medoxomil reduced cardiac hypertrophy in SHR and increased the survival rate in a rat model of myocardial infarction [28]. The drug has also been demonstrated to improve the endothelial function in different models of vascular dysfunction [31–33] and to reduce fatty streaks in animal models of atherosclerosis [34–36]. The protective effects on the kidney have been shown in early and late phase nephropathy in ZDF, a type 2 diabetes model rat [37,38] and SHR/ND mc-cp rats [39]. These effects are most probably shared by other ARBs.

Several types of beneficial effects have been reported for olmesartan medoxomil in disease models that are unrelated to the cardiovascular system. These effects include the improvement of insulin resistance in fructose-fed rats [40], suppression of liver fibrosis formation in a liver cirrhosis model rat [41], the prevention of oxygen-induced retinopathy in mice and VEGF-induced corneal neovasculization in rabbits [42], and the suppression of collagen-induced arthritis in mice [43].

3.7 CLINICAL STUDIES

Clinical development of olmesartan medoxomil started at the same time in Japan, the United States, and Europe in the mid-1990s. More than 50 clinical reports were published by the time olmesartan medoxomil was approved in the United States in 2002. These studies of over 4000 patients revealed the pharmacokinetics, safety profiles and efficacy of olmesartan medoxomil. Olmesartan medoxomil is a prodrug that readily liberates the parent compound, olmesartan after ingestion. Olmesartan is excreted through the kidneys and liver without being further metabolized: only olmesartan is detected in the plasma and urine after oral dosing in humans. This is in contrast to other ARBs, from which metabolites of the active drugs have been found in human urine [44]. The metabolic stability of olmesartan is attributed to its higher hydrophilicity than other ARBs (see Sections 3.3 and 3.6.3). In clinical pharmacological studies, olmesartan was proven not to interact with antiacid, warfarin, and digoxin [27].

3.7.1 Antihypertensive Efficacy and Safety

Antihypertensive efficacy and safety was assessed on the basis of data from seven randomized, double-blind, placebo-controlled, parallel group studies in patients with essential hypertension [45]. In a total of 2693 patients, 2145 patients were treated with olmesartan medoxomil (daily dose of 2.5–80 mg) and 548 patients were with placebo. The degree of blood pressure reduction at 8–12 weeks increased in a dose-related manner. The incidence of adverse events did not increase with the dose of olmesartan medoxomil and remained similar to that of the placebo group. From these dose-finding studies, the daily olmesartan medoxomil dose has been set at 5, 10, 20, or 40 mg worldwide.

Head-to-head comparison studies were conducted in the United States and Europe. A study in the United States compared the effects of olmesartan medoxomil (20 mg) and other ARBs at the starting doses (losartan 50 mg, valsartan 80 mg, and irbsartan 150 mg) [46]. Another study evaluated the achievement of the blood pressure guideline goal at higher doses of different ARBs (olmesartan medoxomil 40 mg, losartan 100 mg, and valsartan 320 mg) [47]. A study in Europe compared olmesartan medoxomil (20 mg) and candesartan cilexetil (8 mg) [48]. These early studies demonstrated that olmesartan medoxomil offered better blood pressure control than ARBs comparators. For a more comprehensive evaluation of different ARBs, see a recent review [49].

A double blind, head-to-head comparison with amlodipine was conducted in the United States [50]. A total of 440 patients with essential hypertension received olmesartan medoxomil 20 mg, amlodipine 5 mg or placebo for 8 weeks. The results showed that olmesartan medoxomil and amlodipine produced identical reductions in blood pressure. However, olmesartan medoxomil was significantly more effective than amlodipine at reaching the blood pressure goals set for this study. The percentage of patients who achieved the systolic blood pressure goal of 130 mmHg was 33.9% for olmesartan medoxomil and 17.4% for amlodipine. The percentage attainment of the diastolic pressure goal of 85 mmHg was 48.0% for olmesartan medoxomil and 34.3% for amlodipine. These findings suggest that olmesartan medoxomil offers stricter blood pressure control than amlodipine.

3.7.2 Organ Protection

As shown in animal studies, olmesartan medoxomil exhibits beneficial effects on the cardiovascular and renal systems in humans as well. These effects are not necessarily accounted for by blood pressure reduction and are thus referred to as "beyond blood pressure-lowering" effects. Treatment with olmesartan medoxomil for 6–12 weeks reduced the biochemical markers of vascular inflammation, including a highly sensitive C-reactive protein (hsCRP), TNF-α, IL-6, and monocyte chymoattractant protein 1 (MCP-1) in patients with essential hypertension [51].

A study in the United States examined the effects of olmesartan medoxomil on the morphology of small, resistant arteries isolated from subcutaneous gluteal fat [52]. Biopsies were conducted before and after 1 year treatment with olmesartan medoxomil in patients with essential hypertension. Olmesartan medoxomil reduced the wall-to-lumen ratio to the levels of normotensive subjects. In hypertensive patients with high cardiovascular risk, the effects of olmesartan medoxomil on atherosclerotic plaque volume in the carotid artery were examined [53]. The plaque volume, measured by means of a 3D ultrasound method decreased after 2-year treatment with olmesartan medoxomil.

Regarding renal protection, the following two studies are completed but not yet published. One is the ROADMAP study, which addresses the question of whether an ARB prevents or delays the onset of microalbuminuria in diabetic patients, and whether this translates into protection against cardiovascular and renal disease [54]. This European study has enrolled a total of 4400 type 2 diabetes patients with normoalbuminuria who were randomly assigned to 40 mg of olmesartan medoxomil or a placebo. The primary end point of the study is the occurrence of microalbuminuria, and the secondary end points include fatal and nonfatal cardiovascular events. The study is event-driven and will be discontinued when 328 patients reach the end point. The second study is the ORIENT study, which is being conducted in Japan and Hong Kong, to evaluate the renal preventive effects of olmesartan medoxomil in type 2 diabetic patients with overt proteinuria [55]. The primary outcome is the composite endpoint of time to the first occurrence of serum creatinin doubling, and end stage renal disease or death. The average follow-up period is 4 years.

3.8 CONCLUSION

Olmesartan medoxomil was launched in the United States and Europe in 2002 under the trade names of Benicar® and Olmetec®, respectively. The drug has been marketed in 58 countries. The crucial proposition in the development of olmesartan medoxomil was the introduction of a hydrophilic group at the 4-position in the imidazole ring instead of a hydrophobic one, which was believed to be favorable at the time. The lead compound has the hydroxymethyl and carboxyl groups at the 4- and 5-positions in the imidazole ring, respectively, which characterizes the biological profile of olmesartan as described in Sections 3.4 and 3.6. The important point at issue for any improved drug is to have a specific profile that differentiates the new drug from the preceding drugs. This was achieved by the discovery of olmesartan. Another important point was the development of the prodrug of olmesartan by the medoxomil pro-moiety, affording olmesartan medoxomil, which was improved in bioavailability and the physicochemical property.

After the launch of losartan, ARBs have been steadily replacing ACE inhibitors, which had a large share of the hypertensive market in the 1980s, and in addition, ARBs have created their own market. Olmesartan medoxomil is the latest ARB. Nevertheless, it has been well accepted by physicians specialized in cardiovascular disease as well as by general practitioners because of excellent efficacy and safety profile.

REFERENCES

1. The Scientific Meeting of the 21st International Society of Hypertension, October 15–19 2006, at Hukuoka, Japan.
2. Moser, M. *The Treatment of Hypertension*, 2nd ed., Le Jacq Communications, Inc., Darien, CT, **2002**, pp. 1–10.
3. Ondetti, M. A., Rubin, B., and Cushman, D. W. Design of specific inhibitor of angiotensin converting enzyme. *A new class of orally active antihypertensive agents. Science* **1977**, *196*, 441–444.
4. Bumpus, F. M., Catt, K. J., Chiu, A. T., De Casparo, M., Goodfriend, T., Husain, A., Peach, M. J., Taylor, D. J., and Timmermans, P. B. M. W. M. Nomenclature for angiotensin receptors. A report of the Nomenclature Committee of the Council for High Blood Pressure Research. *Hypertension* **1991**, *17*, 720–721.
5. Naka, T., Kubo, K., Nishikawa, K., Inada, Y., and Furukawa, Y. Angiotensin II receptor antagonists: candesartan cilexetil. *Yakugaku Zasshi* **2000**, *120*, 1261–1275.
6. (a) Furukawa, Y., Kishimoto, S., and Nishikawa, K. Imidazole derivatives, their production and use. *EP Patent 0028833*, **1981**. (b) Furukawa, Y., Kishimoto, S., and Nishikawa, K. Imidazole-5-acetic acid derivatives, their production and use. *EP Patent 0028834*, 1981.
7. Johnson, A. L., Carini, D. J., Chiu, A. T., Duncia, J. V., Price, W. A., Jr., Wells, G. J., Wexler, R. R., Wong, P. C., and Timmermans, P. B. M. W. M. Nonpeptide angiotensin II receptor antagonists. *Drug NewsPerspects* **1990**, *3*, 337–351.
8. Dancia, J. V., Chiu, A. T., Carini, D. J., Gregory, G. B., Johnson, A. L., Price, W. A., Wells, G. J., Wong, P. C., Calabrese, J. C., and Timmermans, P. B. M. W. M. The discovery of potent nonpeptide angiotensin II receptor antagonists: a new class of potent antihypertensives. *J. Med. Chem.* **1990**, *33*, 1312–1329.
9. Carini, D. J., Dancia, J. V., Johnson, A. L., Chiu, A. T., Price, W. A., Wong, P. C., and Timmermans, P. B. M. W. M. Nonpeptide angiotensin II receptor antagonists: N-[(benzyloxy)benzyl]imidazoles and related compounds as potent antihypertensives. *J. Med. Chem.* **1990**, *33*, 1330–1336.
10. Carini, D. J., Dancia, J. V., Aldrich, P. E., Chiu, A. T., Johnson, A. L., Pierce, M. E., Price, W. A., SantellaIII, J. B., Wells, G. J., Wexler, R. R., Wong, P. C., Yoo, S.-E., and Timmermans, P. B. M. W. M. Nonpeptide angiotensin II receptor antagonists: the discovery of a series of N-(biphenylmethyl)imidazoles as potent, orally active antihypertensives. *J. Med. Chem*, **1991**, *34*, 2525–2547.
11. Carini, D. J., Chiu, A. T., Wong, P. C., Johnson, A. L., Wexler, R. R., and Timmermans, P. B. M. W. M. The preparation of (perfluoroalkyl)imidazoles as nonpeptide angiotensin II receptor antagonists. *Bioor. Med. Chem. Lett.* **1993**, *13*, 895–898.
12. Yanagisawa, H., Amemiya, Y., Kanazaki, T., Shimoji, Y., Fujimoto, K., Kitahara, Y., Sada, T., Mizuno, M., Ikeda, M., Miyamoto, S., Furukawa, Y., and Koike, H. Nonpeptide angiotensin II receptor antagonists: synthesis, biological activities, and structure-activity relationships of imidazole-5-carboxylic acids bearing alkyl, alkenyl, and hydroxyalkyl substituents at the 4-position and their related compounds. *J. Med. Chem.* **1996**, *39*, 323–338.
13. Wong, P. C., Price, W. A., Chiu, A. T., Duncia, J. V., Carini, D. J., Wexler, R. R., Johnson, A. L., and Timmermans, P. B. M. W. M. Nonpeptide angiotensin II receptor antagonists. XI. Pharmacology of EXP3174: an active metabolite of Dup 753, an orally active antihypertensive agent. *J. Pharmacol. Exp. Ther.*, **1990**, *255*, 211–217.
14. Cho, A. Recent advances in oral prodrug discovery. *Annu. Rep. Med. Chem.*, **2006**, *41*, 395–407.
15. Qin, Y., Yasuda, N., Akazawa, H., Ito, K., Kudo, Y., Liao, C., Yamamoto, R., Miura, S., Saku, K., and Komuro, I. Multivalent ligand–receptor interactions elicit inverse agonist activity of AT_1 receptor blockers against stretch-induced AT_1 receptor activation. *Hypertens. Res.*, **2009**, *32*, 875–883.
16. Le, M. T., Pugsley, M. K., Vauquelin, G., and Liefde, I. V. Molecular characterization of the interactions between olmesartan and telmisartan and the human angiotensin II AT_1 receptor. *Br. J. Pharmacol.* **2007**, *151*, 952–962.
17. Miura, S., Fujino, M., Hanzawa, H., Kiya, Y., Imaizumi, S., Matsuo, Y., Tomita, S., Uehara, Y., Karnik, S.S., Yanagisawa, H., Koike, H., Komuro, I., and Saku, K. Molecular mechanism underlying inverse agonist of angiotensin II type receptor. *J. Biol. Chem.*, **2006**, *281*, 19288–19295.
18. Yatabe, J., Sanada, H., Sasaki Yatabe, M., Hashimoto, S., Yoneda, M., Felder, R. A., Jose, P. A., and Watanabe, T. Angiotensin II type 1 receptor blocker attenuates the activation of ERK and NADPH oxidase by mechanical strain in mesangial cells in the absence of angiotensin II. *Am. J. Renal Physiol.*, **2009**, *296*, F1052–F1060.

19. Kamiyama, E., Yoshigae, Y., Kasuya, A., Takei, M., Kurihara, A., and Ikeda, T. Inhibitory effects of angiotensin receptor blockers on CYP2C9 activity in human liver microsomes. *Drug Metab. Pharmacokinet.*, **2007**, *22*, 267–275.
20. Feng, Y. -H., Noda, K., Saad, Y., Liu, X-p., Husain, A., and Karnik, S.S. The docking of Arg^2 of angiotensin II with Asp^{281} of AT_1 receptor is essential for full agonism. *J. Biol. Chem.*, **1995**, *270*, 12846–12850.
21. Noda, K., Saad, Y., and Karnik, S. S. Interaction of Phe^8 of angiotensin II with Lys^{199} and His^{256} of AT_1 receptor in agonist activation. *J. Biol. Chem.*, **1995**, *270*, 28511–28514.
22. Miura, S., Feng, Y. -H., Husain, A., Karnik, S. S. Role of aromaticity of agonist switches of angiotensin II in the activation of the AT_1 receptor. *J. Biol. Chem.*, **1999**, *274*, 7103–7110.
23. Shabmbye, H. T., Hjorth, S. A., Bergsma, D. J., Sathe, G., and Schwartz, T. W. Differentiation between binding sites for angiotensin II and nonpeptide antagonists on the angiotensin II type 1 receptors. *Proc. Natl. Acad. Sci. USA*, **1994**, *91*, 7046–7050.
24. Miura, S., Kiya, Y., Kanazawa, T., Imaizumi, S., Fujino, M., Matsuo, Y., Karnik S. S., and Saku, K. Differential bonding interactions of inverse agonists of angiotensin II type 1 receptor in stabilizing the inactive state. *Mol. Endocrinol.*, **2008**, *22*, 139–146.
25. Baleanu-Gogonea, C., and Karnik, S. Model of the whole rat AT_1 receptor and the ligand-binding site. *J. Mol. Model.*, **2006**, *12*, 325–337.
26. Mizuno, M., Sada, T., Ikeda, M., Fukuda, N., Miyamoto, M., Yanagisawa, H., and Koike, H. Pharmacology of CS-866, a novel nonpeptide angiotensin II receptor antagonist. *Eur. J. Pharmacol.*, **1995**, *285*, 181–188.
27. Koike, H., Konse, T., Sada, T., Ikeda, T., Hyogo, A., Hinman, D., Saito, H., and Yanagisawa, H. Olmesartan medoxomil, a novel potent angiotensin II blocker. *Annu. Rep. Sankyo Res. Lab.*, **2003**, *55*, 1–99.
28. Koike, H., Sada, T., and Mizuno, M. *In vitro* and *in vivo* pharmacology of olmesartan medoxomil, an angiotensin II type AT_1 receptor antagonist. *J. Hypertens.*, **2001**, *19* (suppl 1), S3–S14.
29. Goodfriend, TL. Angiotensins: actions and receptors. In *Hypertension Primer*, 4th ed. (eds J.L. Izzo, Jr., H.R. Black), Lippincott Wilkins, New York, **2008**, pp. 54–58.
30. Shao, J., Nangaku, M., Miyata, T., Inagi, R., Yamada, K., Kurokawa, K., and Fujita, T. Imbalance of T-cell subsets in angiotensin II-infused hypertensive rats with kidney injury. *Hypertension*, **2003**, *42*, 31–38.
31. Kim, S., Izumi, Y., Izumiya, Y., Zhan, Y., Taniguchi, M., and Iwao, H. Beneficial effects of combined blockade of ACE and AT_1 receptor on intimal hyperplasia in balloon-injured rat artery. *Arterioscler. Thromb. Vasc. Biol.*, **2002**, *22*, 1299–1304.
32. Mukai, Y., Shimokawa, H., Higashi, M., Morikawa, K., Matoba, T., Hiroki, J., Kunihiro, I., Talkder, H. M. A., and Takeshita, A. Inhibition of renin-angiotensin system ameliorates endothelial dysfunction associated with aging in rats. *Arteriosclerosis, Thrombosis, and Vascular Biology*, **2002**, *22*, 1445–1450.
33. Kato, T., Nasu, T., Sonoda, H., Ito, K. M., Ikeda, M., and Ito K., Evaluation of olmesartan medoxomil in the rat monocrotaline model of pulmonary hypertension. *J. Cardiovasc. Pharmacol.*, **2008**, *51*, 18–23.
34. Kato, M., Sada, T., Mizuno, M., Kitayama, K., Inaba, T., and Koike, H. Effect of combined treatment with an angiotensin II receptor antagonist and an HMG-CoA reductase inhibitor on atherosclerosis in genetically hyperlipidemic rabbits. *J. Cardiovasc. Pharmacol.*, **2005**, *46*, 556–562.
35. Kato, M., Sada, T., Chuma, H., Mizuno, M., Terashima, H., Fukushima, Y., and Koike, H. Severity of hyperlipidemia does not affect antiatherosclerotic effect of an angiotensin II receptor blocker in apolipoprotein E-deficient mice. *J. Cardiovasc. Pharmacol.*, **2006**, *47*, 764–769.
36. Takai, S., Jin, D., Sakaguchi, M., Muramatsu, M., and Miyazaki, M. The regressive effect of an angiotensin receptor blocker on formed fatty streaks in monkeys fed a high-cholesterol diet. *J. Hypertens.*, **2005**, *23*, 1879–1886.
37. Mizuno, M., Sada, T., Kato, M., and Koike, H. Renoprotective effects of blockade of angiotensin II AT_1 receptors in an animal model of type 2 diabetes. *Hypertens. Res.*, **2002**, *25*, 271–278.
38. Mizuno, M., Sada, T., Kato, M. Fukushima, Y., Terashima, H., and Koike, H. The effect of angiotensin II receptor blockade on an end-stage renal failure model of type 2 diabetes. *J. Cardiovasc. Pharmacol.*, **2006**, *48*, 135–142.
39. Nangaku, M., Miyata, T., Sada, T., Mizuno, M., Inagi, R., Ueda, Y., Ishikawa, N., Yuzawa, H., Koike, H., van Ypersele de Strihou, C., and Kurokawa, K. Antihypertensive agents inhibit in vivo the formation of advanced glycation end product and improve renal damage in a type 2 diabetic nephropathy rat model. *J. Am. Soc. Nephrol.*, **2003**, *14*, 1212–1222.
40. Higashiura, K., Ura, N., Takada, T., Li, Y., Torii, T., Togashi, N., Takada, M., Takizawa, H., and Shimamoto, K. The effect of an angiotensin converting enzyme and an angiotensin II receptor antagonist on insulin resistance in fructose-fed rats. *Am. J. Hypertens.*, **2000**, *13*, 290–297.
41. Kurikawa, N., Suga, M., Kuroda, S., Yamada, K., and Ishikawa, H. An angiotensin II type 1 receptor antagonist, olmesartan medoxomil, improves experimental liver fibrosis by suppression of proliferation and collagen synthesis in activated hepatic stellate cells. *Br. J. Pharmacol.*, **2003**, *139*, 1085–1094.
42. Nakamura, H., Inoue, T., Arakawa, N., Shimizu, Y., Yoshigae, Y., Fujimori, I., Shimakawa, E., Toyoshi, T., and Yokoyama, T. Pharmacological and pharmacokinetic study of olmesartan medoxomil in animal diabetic retinopathy models. *Eur. J. Pharmacol.*, **2005**, *512*, 239–246.
43. Sagawa, K., Nagatani, K., Komagata, Y., and Yamamoto, K. Angiotensin receptor blockers suppress

antigen-specific T cell response and ameliorate collagen-induced arthritis in mice. *Arthritis Rheum.*, **2005**, *52*, 1920–1928.

44. Schmidt, B., and Scieffer, B. Angiotensin AT_1 receptor antagonists. Clinical implications of active metabolites. *J. Med. Chem.*, **2003**, *46*, 2261–2270.
45. Neutel, J. M. Clinical studies of CS-866, the newest angiotensin II receptor antagonist. *Am. J. Cardiol.*, **2001**, *87*, 37c–43c.
46. Oparil, S., Williams, D., Crysant, S.G., Marbury, T.C., and Neutel, J. M. Comparative efficacy of olmesartan, losartan, valsartan and irbsartan. *J. Clin. Hypertens.*, **2001**, *3*, 283–291.
47. Giles, T. D., Oparil, S., Silfani, T. N., Wang, A., and Walker, J. F. Comparison of increasing doses of olmesartan medoxomil, losartan potassium and valsartan in patients with essential hypertension. *J. Clin. Hypertens.*, **2007**, *9*, 187–195.
48. Brunner, H. R., Stumpe, K. O., and Januszewicz, A. Antihypertension efficacy of olmesartan medoxomil and candesartan cilexedil assessed by 24-hr ambulatory blood pressure monitoring in patients with essential hypertension. *Clin. Drug Investig.*, **2003**, *23*, 419–430.
49. Smith, D. H. G. Comparison of angiotensin II type 1 receptor antagonists in the treatment of essential hypertension. *Drugs*, **2008**, *68*, 1207–1225.
50. Chrysant, S. G., Marbury, T. C., and Robinson, T. D. Antihypertensive efficacy and safety of olmesartan medoxomil compared with amlodipine for mild-to-moderate hypertension. *J. Hum. Hypertens*, **2003**, *17*, 425–432.
51. Fliser, D., Buchholz, K., and Haller, H. Anti-inflammatory effects of angiotensin II subtype 1 receptor blockade in hypertensive patients with microinflammation. *Circulation*, **2004**, *110*, 1103–1107.
52. Smith, R. D., Yokoyama, H., Averill, D. B., Schiffrin, E. L., and Ferrario, C. M. Reversal of vascular hypertrophy in hypertensive patients through blockade of angiotensin II receptors. *J. Am. Soc. Hypertens.*, **2008**, *2*, 165–172.
53. Stumpe, K. O., Agabiti-Rosei, E., Zielinski, T., Schremmer, D., Scholze, J., Laeis, P., Schwandt, P., and Ludwig, M. Carotid intima-media thickness and plaque volume changes following 2-year angiotensin II-receptor blockade. The multicentre olmesartan atherosclerosis regression evaluation (MORE) study. *Ther. Adv. Cardiovasc. Dis.*, **2007**, *1*, 97–106.
54. Ritz, E., Viberti, G. C., Ruilope, L. M., Rabelink, A. J., Izzo, J. L., Katayama, S., Ito, S., Mimram, A., Menne, J., Rum, L. C., Januszewicz, A., and Haller, H. Determinants of urinary albumin excretion within the normal range in patients with type 2 diabetes: the randomized olmesartan and diabetes microalbuminuria prevention (ROADMAP) study. *Diabetologia*, **2010**, *53*, 49–57.
55. Imai, E., Ito, S., Haneda, M., Chang, J. C. N., Makino, H., for the ORIENT investigators. Olmesartan reducing incidence of endstage renal disease in diabetic nephropathy trial (ORIENT): rationale and study design. *Hypertens. Res.*, **2006**, *29*, 703–709.

CHAPTER 4

DISCOVERY OF HETEROCYCLIC PHOSPHONIC ACIDS AS NOVEL AMP MIMICS THAT ARE POTENT AND SELECTIVE FRUCTOSE-1, 6-BISPHOSPHATASE INHIBITORS AND ELICIT POTENT GLUCOSE-LOWERING EFFECTS IN DIABETIC ANIMALS AND HUMANS

Qun Dang and Mark D. Erion

4.1 INTRODUCTION

Type 2 diabetes (T2DM) is a prevalent disease with an increasing patient population worldwide. Hyperglycemia is one of many hallmarks for T2DM, which has been linked to serious diabetic complications such as nephropathy, vision loss, and heart diseases [1]. It is well established that increased endogenous glucose production is a major contributor to the abnormally high blood glucose levels in T2DM patients [2–4], and hepatic gluconeogenesis (GNG, by which 3-carbon precursors are converted enzymatically to glucose) was further identified as the major culprit for hepatic glucose overproduction in T2DM patients [5].

Several classes of oral hypoglycemic agents are on the market to treat T2DM, such as sulfonylureas (e.g., glimepiride [6]), PPAR-γ agonists (e.g., pioglitazone [7]), biguanides (e.g., metformin [8]), and the recently approved DPP4 inhibitor Januvia [9], Figure 4.1. However, none of these agents directly inhibit the GNG pathway to reduce hepatic glucose output in T2DM.

It is logical to hypothesize that the combination of a direct GNG inhibitor (that will reduce excess hepatic glucose production) with an existing agent (that will improve either glucose utilization or clearance) might lead to significantly higher clinical efficacy in T2DM.

Fructose-1,6-bisphosphatase (FBPase), as the second-to-last enzyme in GNG (Figure 4.2), controls the incorporation of all 3-carbon substrates into glucose [10]. Furthermore, the FBPase step is not involved in the breakdown of glycogen and is well

Case Studies in Modern Drug Discovery and Development, Edited by Xianhai Huang and Robert G. Aslanian.

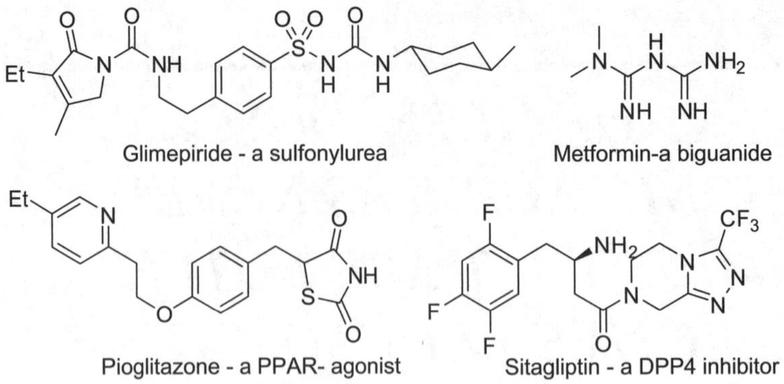

Glimepiride - a sulfonylurea

Metformin-a biguanide

Pioglitazone - a PPAR- agonist

Sitagliptin - a DPP4 inhibitor

Figure 4.1 Oral hypoglycemic agents on the market.

removed from the mitochondrial steps of the pathway, theoretically reducing risk of hypoglycemia and other mechanistic toxicities. The potential of an FBPase inhibitor to exhibit an adequate safety margin was supported by the clinical profiles of humans genetically deficient in FBPase, and their propensity to exhibit episodes of hypoglycemia, increased lactate levels and increased circulating triglycerides [11]. These individuals have near normal biochemical and clinical parameters provided they maintain an appropriate diet and avoid prolonged fasting.

Human liver FBPase is a cytosolic enzyme that consists of four identical 36.7 kD subunits each containing a substrate site and an allosteric site [10]. The intracellular activity of FBPase is regulated synergistically by fructose-2,6-bisphosphate (F2,6BP), an inhibitor that binds to the substrate site, and adenosine-5′-monophosphate (AMP), an inhibitor that binds to the allosteric site [12,13]. Both the substrate site and the AMP site of FBPase have been the target of drug discovery efforts; however, efforts to identify noncompetitive AMP site inhibitors have not led to FBPase inhibitors entering human clinical trials [14–26]. Recently, a structure-guided approach using AMP as a medicinal chemistry lead yielded the first oral FBPase inhibitor, MB06322 (also known as CS-917) [27,28], advancing to phase 2 human clinical trials as a potential treatment for T2DM [29]. Herein, the discovery efforts leading to MB06322 are presented with a focus on medicinal chemistry aspects.

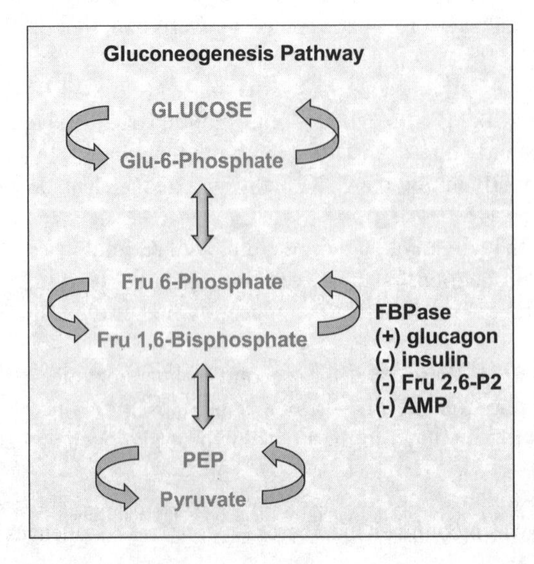

Figure 4.2 Major substrate cycles of the GNG pathway (+ sign denotes stimulation; – sign denotes inhibition).

4.2 THE DISCOVERY OF MB06322

4.2.1 Research Operation Plan

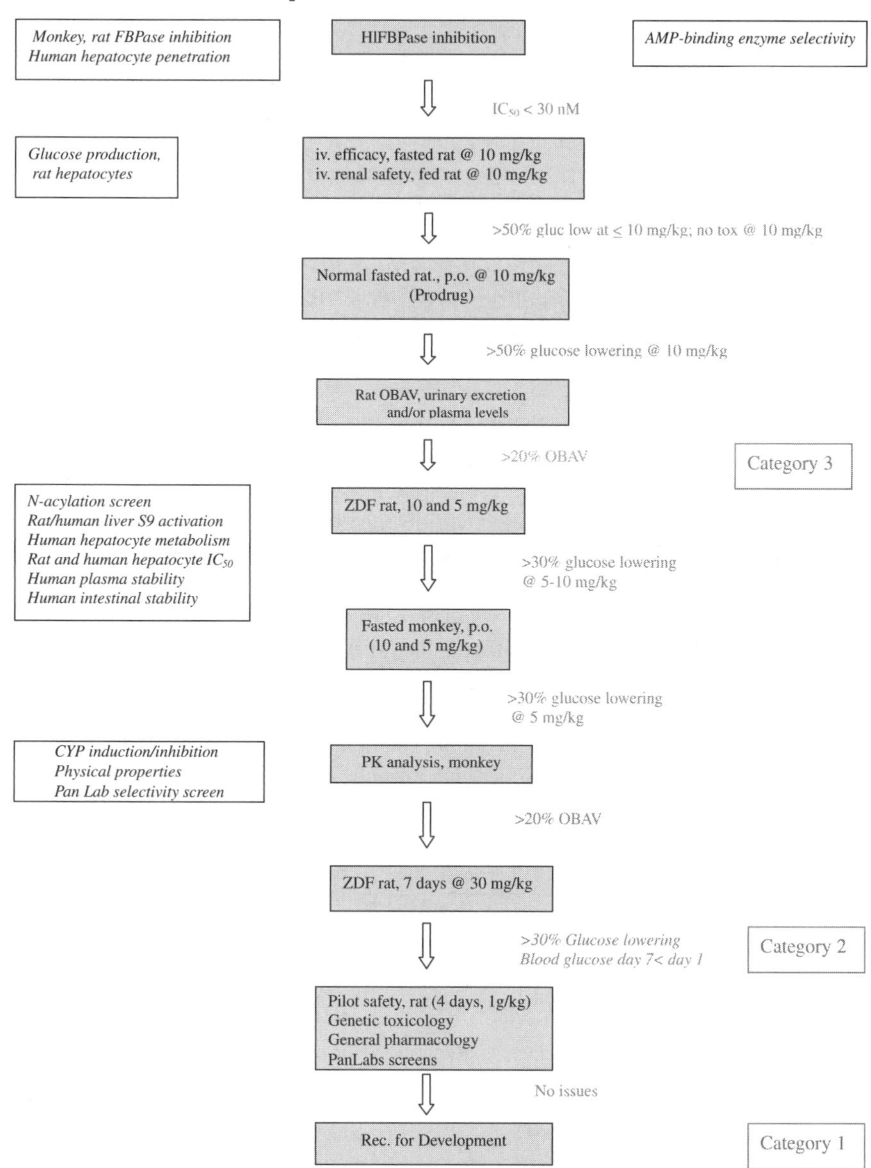

4.2.2 Discovery of Nonnucleotide AMP Mimics as FBPase Inhibitors [30]

4.2.2.1 Rational Design of Novel AMP Mimics as FBPase Inhibitors

The program was initiated in 1992 targeting the AMP binding site of FBPase. Since there was no known allosteric FBPase inhibitor targeting the AMP site, we used AMP as our lead. X-ray crystallographic studies of human FBPase complexed with AMP [31] indicated that the phosphate group forms a constellation of hydrogen bond interactions that are essential for binding affinity. Therefore, it was recognized that there are significant challenges using

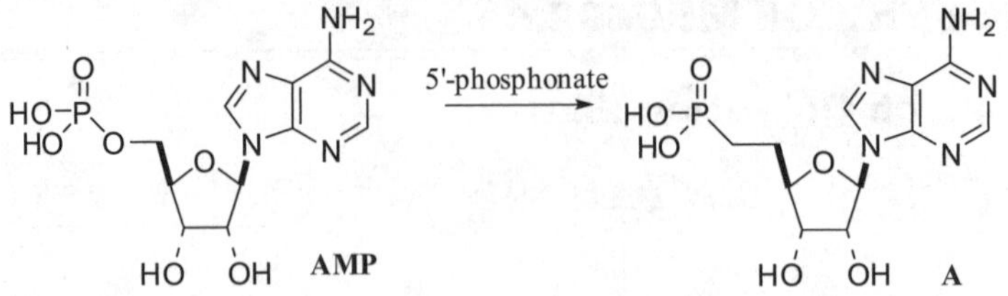

Scheme 4.1 5′-Phosphonate analog as a potential AMP mimic.

AMP as a medicinal chemistry drug discovery lead: poor stability of the 5′-phosphate group in biological fluids; removal of the phosphate group will likely lead to significant loss in binding affinity; selectivity toward other AMP-binding enzymes and receptors is a must-have. Consequently, our initial efforts to design FBPase-specific AMP mimics focused on the 5′-phosphate group. The first challenge was the identification of a phosphate surrogate that retained most of the associated binding affinity while exhibiting good stability in biological fluids.

Phosphonates are structurally and electronically very similar to phosphates, and have been successfully applied as phosphate mimics [32]. Therefore, the first logical phosphonate analog of AMP is the direct 5′-phosphonate AMP analog **A** (Scheme 4.1); however, compound **A** surprisingly exhibited >2000-fold loss in inhibitory potency compared to AMP, suggesting that the discovery of a suitable phosphate mimic would be challenging and might require novel design approaches [33].

Supported by crystallography and computational chemistry, a structure-guided drug design approach was utilized to identify novel AMP mimics as FBPase inhibitors [34].

Careful examination of the FBPase–AMP complex (Figure 4.3) revealed that the phosphate binding site might be accessed from the 8-position of the purine base. Accordingly, we sought a suitable linker to connect a phosphonic acid group to the 8-position of the purine nucleus (compound B, Scheme 4.2).

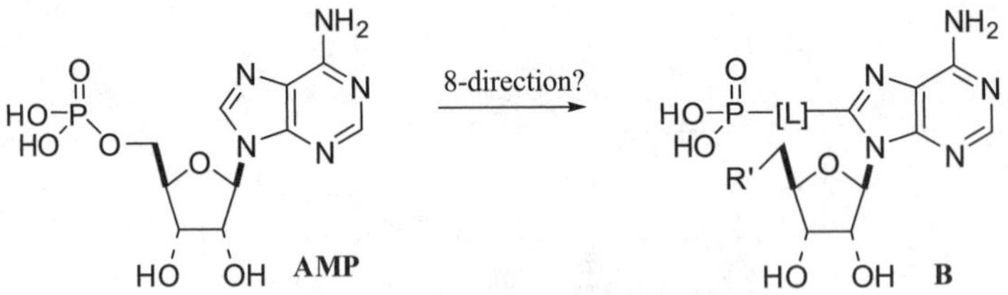

Scheme 4.2 8-Purine-phosphonates as potential AMP mimics.

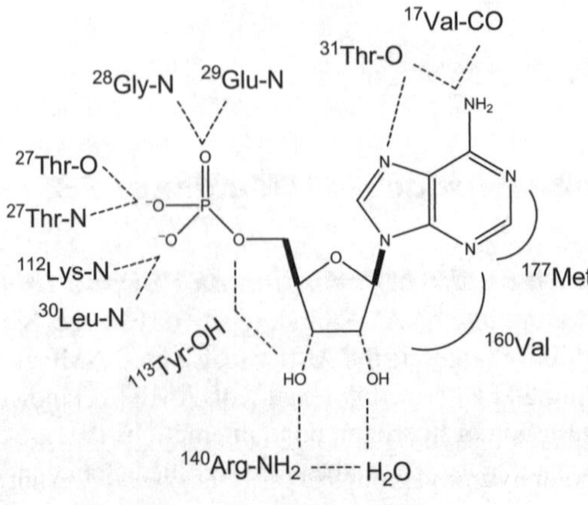

Figure 4.3 AMP key interactions with human FBPase.

TABLE 4.1 SAR of Adenosine C8-Analogs (1.1–1.9)

Compound	R^8	R'	IC_{50} (μM)[a]
AMP			1
1.1	-CH=CHCO$_2$H	OH	≫100[b]
1.2	-(CH$_2$)$_2$CO$_2$H	OH	≫100[b]
1.3	-NHCH$_2$CO$_2$H	OH	≫100[b]
1.4	-NH(CH$_2$)$_2$CO$_2$H	OH	≫100[b]
1.5	-NHCH$_2$PO$_3$H$_2$	OH	≫100[b]
1.6	-NH(CH$_2$)$_2$PO$_3$H$_2$	OH	100
1.7	-NH(CH$_2$)$_3$PO$_3$H$_2$	OH	≫100[b]
1.8	-NH(CH$_2$)$_2$OPO$_3$H$_2$	OH	140
1.9	-NH(CH$_2$)$_2$PO$_3$H$_2$	H	100

[a]Inhibition of human liver FBPase is reported as IC_{50} values, and represent an average of three runs;

[b]<25% inhibition at 100 μM.

4.2.2.2 Lead Generation and Optimization Working under the assumption that the phosphate and the ribosyl groups are important for AMP to function as an FBPase inhibitor, adenosine was selected as the initial scaffold for lead generation, and various acidic groups were linked to the 8-position of the purine base in order to find a suitable phosphate mimic (Table 4.1).

Initially, carboxylic acids with various 2- to 4-atom linkers were explored. Analogs **1.1**–**1.4** showed little inhibition of FBPase (Table 4.1), which may be due to the poor mimicry of AMP by these carboxylate analogs, both electronically and geometrically. Next we examined phosphonic acids since they more closely resemble a phosphate. The 2- and 4-atom linked analogs **1.5** and **1.7** (Table 4.1) were inactive, but the 3-atom linked analog **1.6** showed moderate inhibition of FBPase with an IC_{50} of 100 μM. This represented a significant observation given that the AMP analog wherein the phosphate was replaced with $CH_2PO_3^{2-}$ (compound **A**, Scheme 4.1) showed an IC_{50} of 2000 μM. The 20-fold enhancement in potency suggested that the 8-position enabled better alignment of the phosphonic acid in the phosphate-binding pocket of the AMP site compared to the 5′-position. The 4-atom linked phosphate analog **1.8** showed FBPase inhibition comparable to the 3-atom linked phosphonate analog **1.6**. This observation suggests that electronic effects are also important, since computer modeling studies indicate a 3-atom linker provides the optimum distance. Removing the 5′-hydroxyl group of analog **1.6** gave analog **1.9**, which retained similar potency, suggesting that this hydroxyl group is not critically involved in binding to FBPase. Although the inhibitory activity of analog **1.6** was still weak, this discovery provided encouragement to further pursue this scaffold using our structure-guided drug discovery approach. Thus, an X-ray crystal structure of compound **1.6** bound to FBPase was obtained (Figure 4.4). Detailed analysis of the interactions between compound **1.6** and FBPase provided key insights into the binding mode of this compound.

A crystallographic study confirmed that compound **1.6** does indeed bind to the AMP site of FBPase. Analysis of the structural information showed that the adenine base formed three hydrogen bonds in the same manner as AMP. More importantly, the phosphonate group linked via the 8-position of the adenine serves as an excellent mimic of the binding interactions between the phosphate of AMP and FBPase. Six strong hydrogen bonds are formed between the phosphonate group and the enzyme just as with the phosphate group of AMP. An important finding was the lack of hydrogen bond interactions between the ribose moiety and the enzyme. Since the polar hydroxyl groups of the ribose moiety do not enhance

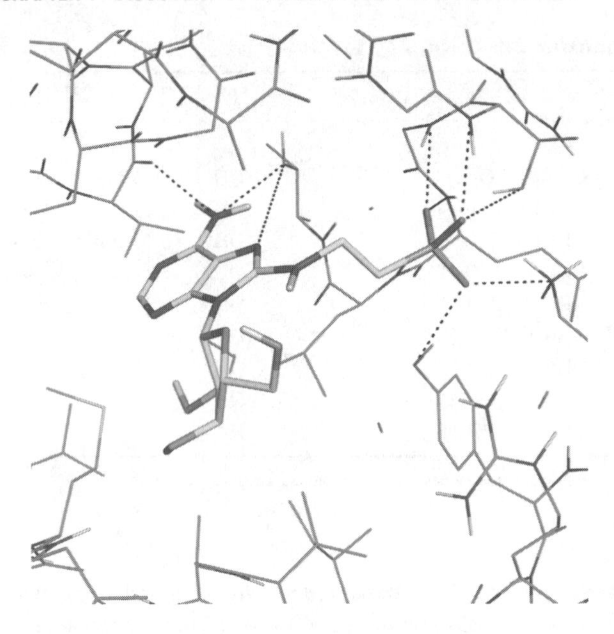

Figure 4.4 X-ray structural analysis of **1.6** bound to FBPase. (See color version of the figure in Color Plate section)

binding affinity but require higher desolvation energy, the presence of the ribosyl group likely contributed to the moderate activity of compound **1.6**. It was therefore logical to replace the ribosyl group with a simple hydrophobic group, which would simplify the scaffold and facilitate rapid exploration of SAR. Further optimization of compound **1.6** was carried out and results are summarized in Table 4.2.

Replacing the ribosyl group in compound **1.6** with a phenethyl group gave compound **2.1**, which showed no loss in FBPase inhibition confirming our hypothesis that the ribosyl group is not contributing to bind affinity for compound **1.6**. Given that the

TABLE 4.2 SAR of Phosphonic Acid-Containing Purine Analogs

Compound	R^2	R^9	Linker	IC_{50} (μM)[a]
1.6	H	Ribosyl	$-NHCH_2CH_2-$	100
2.1	H	$-CH_2CH_2Ph$	$-NHCH_2CH_2-$	100
2.2	H	$-CH_2CH_2Ph$	$-CH_2OCH_2-$	23
2.3	H	$-CH_2CH_2Ph$	2,5-Furanyl	5
2.4	H	$-CH_2CH_2Ph$	2,5-Thienyl	48
2.5	H	Cyclopropyl	2,5-Furanyl	1.5
2.6	H	-Et	2,5-Furanyl	1.8
2.7	H	Isobutyl	2,5-Furanyl	1.5
2.8	H	Neopentyl	2,5-Furanyl	0.8
2.9	H	Adamantyl	2,5-Furanyl	>10[b]
2.10	-SMe	Isobutyl	2,5-Furanyl	0.7
2.11	$-SO_2Me$	Isobutyl	2,5-Furanyl	28
2.12	$-NH_2$	Neopentyl	2,5-Furanyl	5.5
2.13	-SMe	Neopentyl	2,5-Furanyl	1.1

[a]Inhibition of human liver FBPase is reported as IC_{50} values and represents an average of three runs;
[b]<25% inhibition at 10 μM.

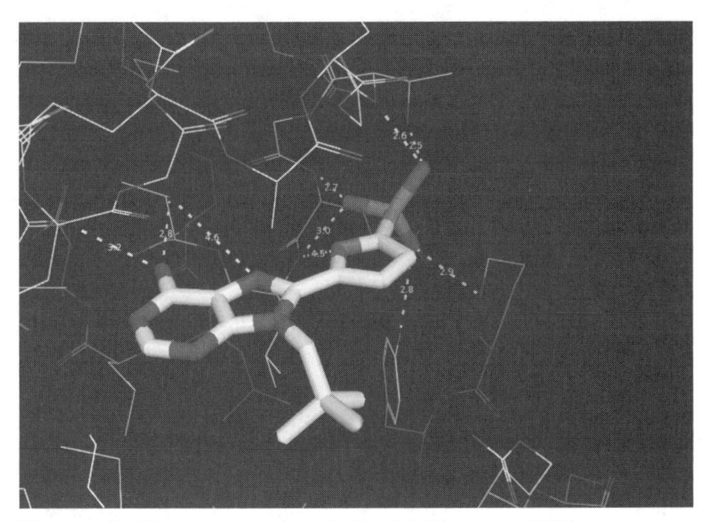

Figure 4.5 X-ray structural analysis of **2.8** bound to FBPase.

amino moiety of the linker in compound **2.1** is not picking up hydrogen-bonding interaction, our lead optimization (LO) efforts were focused on optimizing the linker group with a focus on various 3-atom linkers, which was suggested by modeling efforts to have the optimal distance between the C8 of purine and the phosphonic acid group. Significant potency improvement was obtained through the optimization of the linker group: compounds **2.2** and **2.3** are 4- and 20-fold more potent than compound **2.1**, respectively. Compound **2.3** can be viewed as a conformationally restricted linker analog of compound **2.2**, which is likely the reason for the observed >4-fold improvement in potency. On the other hand, the thienyl analog (compound **2.4**) of compound **2.3** is approximately 10-fold weaker, suggesting that the oxygen atom of the furan linker may be involved in either electrostatic or hydrogen-bonding interactions with the enzyme. Optimization of the R^9 group (compounds **2.5–2.9**) led to compound **2.8** with fivefold improvement over compound **2.3**, while limited SAR exploration at the 2-position of the purine nucleus (compounds **2.10–2.13**) did not lead to further enhancement in potency. To understand the binding mode for these novel purine FBPase inhibitors, an X-ray structure of purine **2.8** was obtained as shown in Figure 4.5.

Analysis of the structural information showed that purine **2.8** binds to FBPase in a similar fashion to AMP and purine **1.6**: the adenine base formed three hydrogen bonds; the phosphonate group formed six strong hydrogen bonds just as with the phosphate group of AMP. Two important findings were noted, the furan linker picks up a strong electrostatic interaction with ^{31}Thr, and the neopentyl group occupies the same place as the ribose moiety of purine **1.6**. Both factors likely contribute to the significant potency improvement for purine **2.8** compared to purine **1.6**.

4.2.2.3 Selectivity Toward Enzymes with an AMP Site To determine the selectivity of the purine series of novel AMP mimics, effects of FBPase inhibitors **2.3** and **2.8** on five key AMP binding enzymes were measured [35]. The results are summarized in Table 4.3.

Compound **2.3** is a relatively weak inhibitor of FBPase. However, it displays excellent selectivity against most of these AMP-binding enzymes except for AMP deaminase (AMPDA), which it inhibits with an IC_{50} of 6.7 μM. It was envisioned that further improving

TABLE 4.3 Selectivity of Compounds 2.3 and 2.8[a]

Enzymes	Compound 2.3	Compound **2.8**
FBPase	$IC_{50} = 5.0\,\mu M$	$IC_{50} = 0.8\,\mu M$
Adenosine kinase	$IC_{50} \gg 100\,\mu M$	$IC_{50} \gg 100\,\mu M$
Adenylate kinase	$IC_{50} \gg 500\,\mu M$	$IC_{50} \gg 500\,\mu M$
AMP deaminase	$IC_{50} = 6.7\,\mu M$	$IC_{50} = 390\,\mu M$
Glycogen phosphorylase	$EC_{50} \gg 250\,\mu M$	$EC_{50} \gg 100\,\mu M$
Phosphofructokinase	$EC_{50} \gg 200\,\mu M$	$EC_{50} \gg 100\,\mu M$

[a]Inhibition of enzymes is reported as IC_{50}, while activation of enzymes is reported as EC_{50}.

the FBPase inhibitory potency for compounds in this series would likely increase selectivity against AMPDA as well. Indeed, the more potent compound **2.8** (hlFBPase $IC_{50} = 0.8\,\mu M$) maintained excellent selectivity toward most AMP-binding enzymes and exhibited >480-fold selectivity against AMPDA ($IC_{50} = 390\,\mu M$).

Thus, a series of purine analogs were designed as AMP mimics using a structural-guided drug design approach. Through this approach, a series of purine phosphonic acids, which mimic AMP and its effects on FBPase activity following binding to the FBPase allosteric binding site, were discovered. Further lead optimization produced purine analogs such as compounds **2.8** and **2.10,** which are essentially equipotent with AMP with regard to inhibition of human liver FBPase. This represents a significant advance in the field: these compounds are non-nucleotides since they lack a phosphate group and a ribosyl moiety, yet they inhibit FBPase in the same manner as AMP. Evaluation of these compounds further demonstrated that they are capable of inhibiting glucose production in hepatocytes and lowering blood glucose levels in fasted rats. The lead compound discovered, purine **2.8**, is a potent inhibitor of both human and rat liver FBPase, and has excellent selectivity toward five other AMP-binding enzymes. Moreover, compound **2.8** elicited profound glucose lowering (65%) in fasted SD rats after intraperitoneal administration at a dose of $20\,mg\,kg^{-1}$, validating the approach of FBPase inhibition to lower blood glucose levels. The structure–activity relationships established with these purine analogs became the basis for the discovery of other series of heterocyclic phosphonic acids as highly potent and selective FBPase inhibitors.

4.2.3 Discovery of Benzimidazole Phosphonic Acids as FBPase Inhibitors [36]

Although compound **2.8** inhibits human liver FBPase at the same level as AMP, it still contains a purine base which might lead to potential selectivity issues. To enhance the potency and possibly the specificity of the purine series of FBPase inhibitors, we focused our attention on the N^1 and N^3 atoms of the purine ring. Crystallographic data suggest that neither N^1 nor N^3 appeared to form a hydrogen bond with the FBPase binding site (Figure 4.3). Consequently, removal of one or both of the nitrogens was considered unlikely to result in a loss of binding affinity and more likely to improve inhibitor potency by minimizing any losses due to desolvation. Moreover, since many purine-containing nucleotides form hydrogen bonds to one or both nitrogens, their removal could enhance specificity for the AMP binding site of FBPase over other AMP binding sites. The resulting benzimidazoles could be further optimized by attaching lipophilic groups to the core to pick up favorable van der Waals interactions with residues such as ^{177}Met and ^{160}Val in the vicinity of N^1 and N^3 atoms.

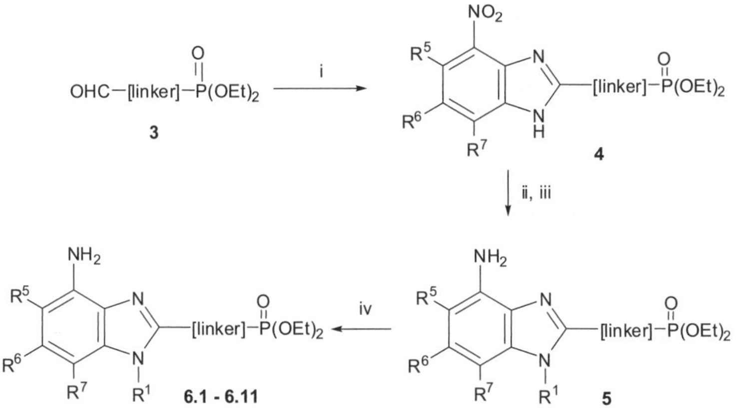

Scheme 4.3 Synthesis of benzimidazole analogs. Conditions and reagents: (i) 3-nitro-benzene-1,2-diamine, $FeCl_3$-SiO_2, DMSO, 80°C, 2 h; (ii) (a) R^1-OH, PPh_3, DEAD or (b) R^1Br, NaH, DMF; (iii) H_2, Pd-C, EtOH; (iv) TMSBr, CH_2Cl_2.

4.2.3.1 Synthesis of Benzimidazole Analogs The N^1-substituted 4-aminobenzimidazole phosphonate analogs were prepared from 5-diethylphosphono-2-furaldehyde (**3**) via a four-step procedure as shown in Scheme 4.3. The cyclization of aldehyde **3** with 3-nitro-benzene-1,2-diamine using the $FeCl_3$-promoted cyclization reaction developed for purine synthesis gave benzimidazole **4** in 81% yield. The R^1 group was introduced via either Mitsunobu reactions with alcohols or alkylation reactions with alkyl bromides using sodium hydride as the base. The nitro group was subsequently reduced to its corresponding amino group under hydrogenation conditions to give compounds **5**, and the phosphonate diethyl esters were cleaved using TMSBr to yield compounds **6.1–6.11**.

4.2.3.2 Evaluations of Benzimidazole Phosphonate Analogs Replacing the N^1 and N^3 nitrogen atoms in compound **2.7** with CH generates the benzimidazole analog **6.1**, which exhibited identical FBPase inhibitory potency as **2.7**, Table 4.4. This

TABLE 4.4 SAR of Benzimidazole Analogs[a]

	R^1	R^5	R^7	HL IC_{50} (μM)	RL IC_{50} (μM)	EC_{50} (μM)
2.7				1.5		
6.1	Isobutyl	H	H	1.5	4	20
6.2	Isobutyl	Cl	H	0.2	2	15
6.3	Isobutyl	Br	H	0.4	2	14
6.4	Isobutyl	F	H	0.1	2	2.4
6.5	cPr-CH_2-[b]	F	H	0.055	2	3.3
6.6	Isobutyl	F	Cl	0.1	1.6	3.6
6.7	Isobutyl	F	Br	0.1	2	5
6.8	Isobutyl	F	Vinyl	0.28	0.9	25
6.9	Isobutyl	F	cPr-	0.055	0.4	1.5
6.10	Isobutyl	F	Ph	0.09	0.9	18
6.11	Isobutyl	F	Et	0.055	0.55	3.5

[a]HL, human liver FBPase; RL, rat liver FBPase; IC_{50} is an average of three runs; EC_{50}, inhibition of glucose production in primary rat hepatocytes;
[b]cPr, cyclopropyl.

observation validated our hypothesis that neither N^1 nor N^3 of our initial purine series of FBPase inhibitors are required for binding affinity. Next, the SAR of the benzimidazole scaffold were carefully investigated with > 1000 analogs; some key compounds, which were important to establish important SAR for the benzimidazole scaffold, are summarized in Table 4.4. An amino group at the 4-position is important for binding affinity, while small branched alkyl groups such as isobutyl and cyclopropylmethyl groups are preferred at the N^1-position. Introduction of halo groups at the 5-position led to significant potency boost (compounds **6.1–6.4**) and a fluoro group gave the highest degree of potency enhancement. Fine tuning of compound **6.4** by varying substituents at 1-, 5-, 6-, and 7-position led to compound **6.11**, which showed twofold better potency than compound **6.4**. Consistent with previous reports, rat FBPase inhibitory potency was 2- to 25-fold less than human FBPase potency. In general, the rat liver FBPase potency for these compounds correlates well with the relative inhibitory potency measured in the primary rat hepatocyte assay; however, some compounds appear to be outliers. For example, compound **6.10** is slightly more potent (about 2-fold) against rat liver FBPase compared to compound **6.4**, but it is almost 10-fold less potent in the cellular assay. It is likely that these phosphonic acids penetrate cells via organic anion transporters (OATPs) [37]. Therefore, both rat liver FBPase IC_{50} and OATP substrate specificity may be determinants of potency at the cellular level.

The *in vitro* efficacy observed by benzimidazole FBPase inhibitors such as compounds **6.9** and **6.11** was also translated into *in vivo* glucose-lowering effects in a normal rat assay: intravenous dosing of compounds **6.9** and **6.11** at doses of 10 mg kg^{-1} led to 64% reduction of blood glucose levels in over night fasted normal rats. Since compounds **6.9** and **6.11** have very similar profiles, compound **6.11** was selected for further evaluations based on ease of chemical synthesis. A dose response and time course study of compound **6.11** was carried in Zucker diabetic fatty (ZDF) rats, a rodent model of T2DM. Compound **6.11** was administered to 5 h-fasted ZDF rats (12 weeks of age, tail vein infusion) at doses of 1, 3, and 10 mg kg^{-1} h^{-1}, and blood glucose levels were measured hourly up to 6 h; results are summarized in Figure 4.6.

The 10 mg kg^{-1} h^{-1} dose of compound **6.11** produced rapid and profound glucose lowering and by 5th and 6th hour time points almost normalized glucose levels; the study

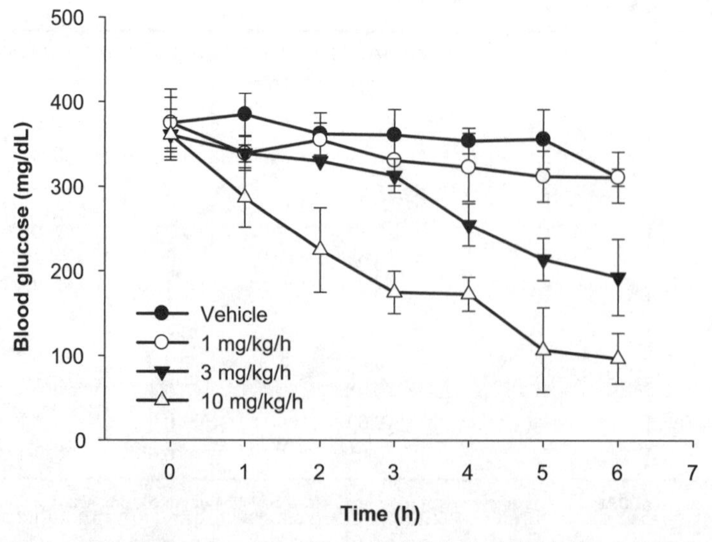

Figure 4.6 Glucose-lowering effects of **6.11** in male ZDF rats ($n = 8$/group).

revealed the minimum efficacious dose is 3 mg kg^{-1} h^{-1}. Therefore, the *in vivo* efficacy of compound **6.11** in ZDF rats demonstrated proof of concept (POC) for FBPase inhibitors as hypoglycemic agents with the potential to lower glucose levels in T2DM.

LO efforts of the initial purine series of FBPase inhibitors were aided by a structure-guided drug design approach, which led to improvements in the potency and selectivity profiles for the early purine phosphonate series of FBPase inhibitors. Replacements of both N^1 and N^3 atoms in the purine scaffold with carbon atoms produced new benzimidazole analogs with similar FBPase inhibitory activity relative to analogs of the purine series. Further optimization of the new benzimidazole scaffold led to the discovery of several analogs with IC_{50} values < 100 nM, which represents a significant improvement over the early purine series of FBPase inhibitors (e.g., purine **2.8**, $IC_{50} = 0.8$ μM). Compound **6.11** emerged as a lead inhibitor based on its potent inhibition of human liver FBPase ($IC_{50} = 55$ nM), enzyme specificity, potent cellular activity ($EC_{50} = 3.5$ μM) and significant glucose-lowering (64%) in normal fasted rats. Evaluation of **6.11** in the ZDF rat demonstrated for the first time that FBPase inhibitors could significantly reduce glucose levels in an animal model of T2DM.

4.2.4 Discovery of Thiazole Phosphonic Acids as Potent and Selective FBPase Inhibitors [38]

Even though the purine and benzimidazole FBPase inhibitor series (e.g., purine **2.8** and benzimidazole **6.11**) demonstrated potent *in vivo* glucose-lowering effects after parenteral administration, their high molecular weight (MW) was deemed as a potential structural limitation for achieving acceptable oral bioavailability (OBAV), which likely contributed to the inability of using prodrug approaches to deliver these two series of FBPase inhibitors orally. Therefore, we focused our redesign efforts on reducing the number of atoms. The strategy to trim the purine and benzimidazole scaffolds was guided by both existing SAR and the X-ray crystal structures of FBPase–inhibitor complexes (e.g. AMP–FBPase complex, Figure 4.3). Since the six-membered ring portion of the purine/benzimidazole forms few direct interactions with the binding site, efforts focused on five-membered heterocycles that could be substituted in a manner that retained the two hydrogen bond interactions with ^{31}Thr and ^{17}Val gained by the amino substituent on the six-membered ring. Following extensive evaluation of compounds containing various five-membered heterocycles and substituents by molecular modeling and *in vitro* testing, the thiazole scaffold was selected for further investigation.

4.2.4.1 *Synthesis of Thiazoles* Phosphonate-containing ketones **7** were readily converted to 2-aminothiazoles: bromination of ketones **7** with copper(II) bromide followed by cyclization reactions with thiourea gave aminothiazoles **8**, whereas cyclization with thioamides gave C2-substituted thiazole analogs **9** (Scheme 4.4). Final thiazole phosphonic acids (Table 4.5) were readily obtained via TMSBr-mediated removal of the phosphonate diethyl esters from thiazoles **10** (Scheme 4.5).

4.2.4.2 *Evaluations of Thiazole Phosphonic Acids* To test the thiazole concept, thiazole **11.1** was first prepared and interesting, the C2-methyl thiazole **11.1** potently inhibited human liver FBPase ($IC_{50} = 100$ nM). Moreover, after intravenous (i.v.) administration to fasted normal rats at a dose of 10 mg kg^{-1}, thiazole **11.1** lowered blood glucose (C_{max}) by 55% compared to vehicle-treated animals, indicating that thiazole **11.1** was also able to inhibit GNG *in vivo*. The initial encouraging activity exhibited by thiazole

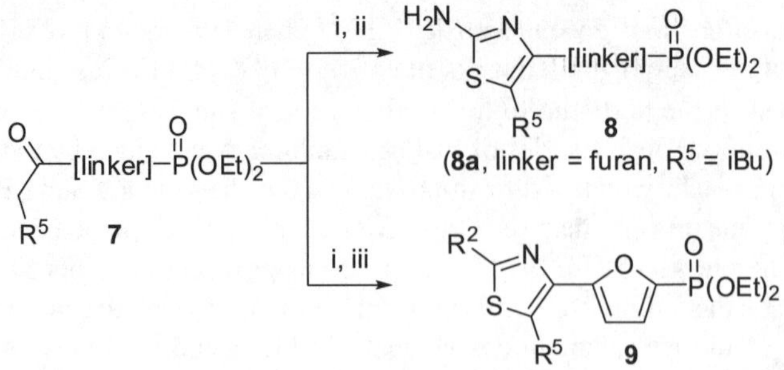

Scheme 4.4 Synthesis of thiazole phosphonates. Conditions: (i) $CuBr_2$, EtOAc-$CHCl_3$; (ii) thiourea, EtOH; (iii) R^2CSNH_2, EtOH.

TABLE 4.5 SAR of Thiazole Analogs[a]

	R^2	R^5	[linker]	HL IC_{50} (μM)	G-LOW (%)
11.1	Me	IBu	2,5-Furan	0.1	55
11.2	Et	IBu	2,5-Furan	0.4	ND[b]
11.3	H	IBu	2,5-Furan	0.5	ND
11.4	NH_2	IBu	2,5-Furan	0.025	65
11.5	NHMe	IBu	2,5-Furan	1	ND
11.6	NHAc	IBu	2,5-Furan	10	ND
11.7	NH_2	H	2,5-Furan	0.45	ND
11.8	NH_2	Me	2,5-Furan	0.12	7
11.9	NH_2	n-Pr	2,5-Furan	0.03	64
11.10	NH_2	Neopentyl	2,5-Furan	0.012	80
11.11	NH_2	Cyclobutyl	2,5-Furan	0.019	24
11.12	NH_2	Cl	2,5-Furan	0.07	17
11.13	NH_2	Br	2,5-Furan	0.05	20
11.14	NH_2	I	2,5-Furan	0.1	0
11.15	NH_2	n-PrS	2,5-Furan	0.016	82
11.16	NH_2	$CONMe_2$	2,5-Furan	1.7	ND
11.17	NH_2	CO_2Et	2,5-Furan	0.014	76
11.18	NH_2	Ph	2,5-Furan	0.014	76
11.19	NH_2	n-Pr	2,5-Thienyl	>10	ND
11.20	NH_2	n-Pr	CO_2CH_2	0.05	63
11.21	NH_2	2-thienyl	$CONHCH_2$	0.95	ND
11.22	NH_2	H	2,6-Pyridyl	2	ND
11.23	NH_2	H	1,3-Phenyl	1.3	ND
11.24	NH_2	n-Pr	1,3-Phenyl	0.25	0

[a]HL, human liver FBPase; G-LOW, glucose lowering (C_{max}) in fasted normal rats after i.v. administration at doses of 10 mg kg^{-1}; [b]ND, not determined.

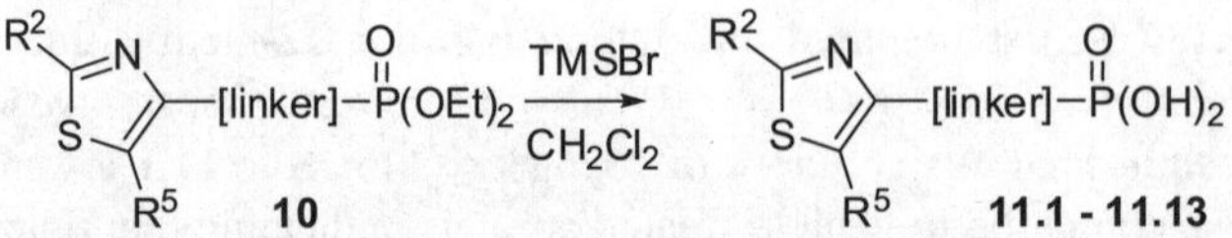

Scheme 4.5 Synthesis of thiazole phosphonic acids.

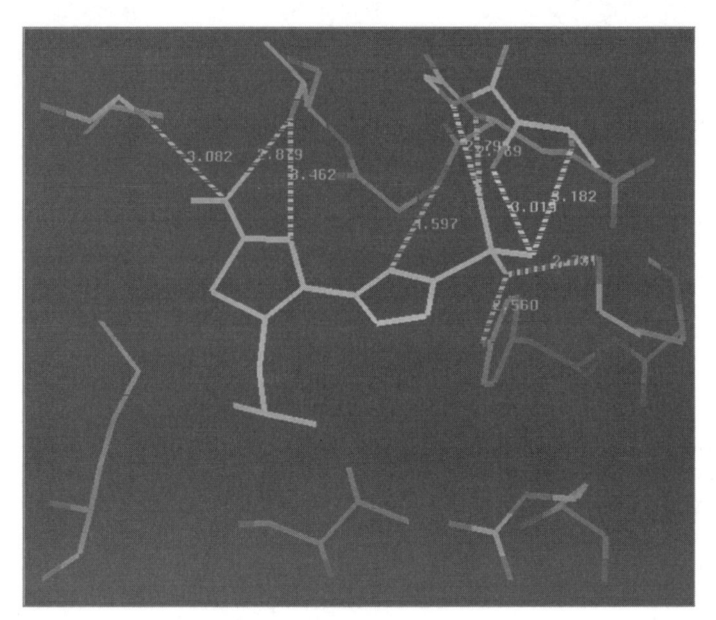

Figure 4.7 X-ray structural analysis of **11.4** (in yellow) bound to FBPase.

11.1 prompted us to explore the full SAR of the thiazole scaffold at C2-, C5-positions, and various linker groups; representative results are summarized in Table 4.5.

Increase or decrease the size of the C2-group in thiazole **11.1** (thiazoles **11.2** and **11.3**) resulted in loss of potency, indicating that the C2-region has very sensitive SAR. Replacement of the C2-methyl group with an amino group gave analog **11.4**, which is 4-fold more potent than **11.1** and more importantly it elicits potent glucose lowering in fasted normal rats (65%). *N*-Methylation and acetylation of the 2-amino group of **11.4** are detrimental for potency (thiazoles **11.5** and **11.6**). Therefore, the C2-SAR indicates the binding pocket around the C2-position prefers a small hydrogen bond donating group. Having identified that an amino group is optimal at the C2-position, 2-aminothiazoles with various groups at the C5-position were explored next (thiazoles **11.7–11.18**). Diverse groups are tolerated at the C5-position with medium sized alkyl groups (such as isobutyl, neopentyl, and cyclobutyl), halo, alkylthio, aryl, and ester groups all leading to potent FBPase inhibitors with $IC_{50} < 100$ nM. On the other hand, the linker SAR is very tight with only the ester linker analog **11.20** showing comparable potency as the furan linker analog **11.4**. All other attempts to replace the 2,5-furan linker (thiazoles **11.19**, **11.21–11.24**) resulted in significant loss in enzyme inhibition potency compared to compound **11.4**. To better understand the binding of thiazole FBPase inhibitors, an X-ray structure of thiazole **11.4** was obtained, Figure 4.7.

Analysis of the **11.4** FBPase-bound X-ray structure revealed that the phosphonic acid group is an excellent mimic of the phosphate group of AMP since it picks up all six hydrogen bonds formed by AMP. The 2-amino group of thiazole **11.4** forms two hydrogen bonds just like the 6-amino group of AMP, while the 3-nitrogen of thiazole **11.4** picks up a hydrogen bond in a similar manner as the N^7 of AMP. The oxygen of the important furan linker is 4.6 Å away from ^{29}Glu, indicating an electrostatic interaction with the enzyme, which explains why most other linkers resulted in a loss in potency. Thus, results from the crystallographic study of **11.4** and human liver FBPase are consistent with the SAR observed experimentally.

4.2.5 The Discovery of MB06322 Through Prodrug Strategy

Phosphonic acids are often reported to have very limited oral bioavailability; thus, prodrug approaches are widely explored in order to achieve acceptable oral delivery [39,40]. A prodrug is a pharmacological substance (drug) administered in an inactive (or significantly less active) form. Once administered, the prodrug is metabolized *in vivo* into an active metabolite, a process termed bioactivation. The rationale behind the use of a prodrug is generally for absorption, distribution, metabolism, and excretion (ADME) optimization. Prodrugs are usually designed to improve oral bioavailability, with poor absorption from the gastrointestinal tract usually being the limiting factor.

4.2.5.1 An Introduction to Phosphonate Prodrugs At physiological pH, phosphonic acids are ionized and exist as highly charged species, which prevent cell penetration via passive diffusion. Consequently, oral delivery of phosphonic acids are often attempted via their neutral prodrugs, which are prepared to mask the charges in order to enhance oral absorption via passive diffusion [39,40]. Successful development of prodrug strategies will expand the chemical space for drug discovery programs, which lessens the concerns of poor ADME properties for highly polar compounds such as phosphonic acids. Incorporation of prodrug strategies to a drug discovery project does increase additional complexity and requires diligent planning by both chemistry and biology teams.

4.2.5.2 Synthesis of FBPase Inhibitor Prodrugs [41] To deliver thiazole phosphonate FBPase inhibitors orally, various prodrugs were prepared to mask the double negative charge. The classic acyloxyalkyl ester prodrugs (**35a–35e**) were obtained via direct alkylation reactions, while other prodrug esters (**35f–35i**) were prepared via the phosphonic dichloride coupling method as depicted in Scheme 4.6.

4.2.5.3 The Discovery of MB06322 Thiazole **11.4** possesses all the desired attributes of a clinical candidate except for the very low OBAV (F% = 2, Table 4.6); therefore, it was selected for prodrug syntheses in order to achieve oral delivery [41]. The SAR of thiazole **11.4** prodrugs is summarized in Table 4.6.

Acyloxyalkyl phosphonate esters are a proven approach to improve OBAV for some phosphonic acids [40]; however, this type of prodrug (prodrugs **12.1** and **12.2**) only

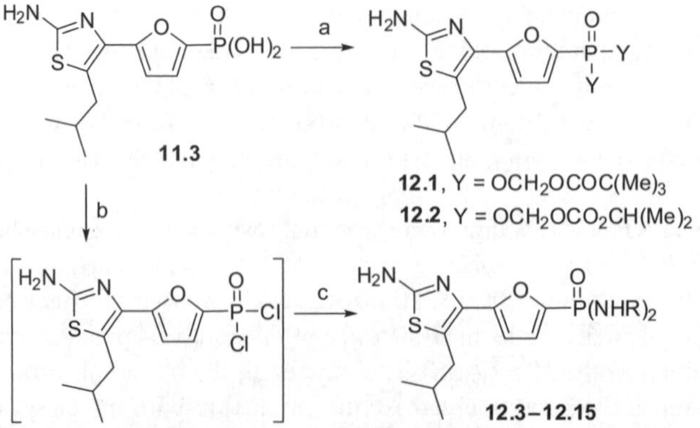

11.3

12.1, Y = $OCH_2OCOC(Me)_3$

12.2, Y = $OCH_2OCO_2CH(Me)_2$

12.3–12.15

Scheme 4.6 Synthesis of the prodrugs. Conditions and reagents: (a) $ICH_2OCOC(Me)_3$ or $ICH_2OCO_2CH(Me)_2$, DCMC, DMF; (b) thionyl chloride, pyridine, $(CH_2Cl)_2$; (c) RNH_2, Hunig's base, CH_2Cl_2.

TABLE 4.6 OBAV SAR of Thiazole 11.4 and Its Prodrugs (12.1–12.13)[a]

Compound	X	OBAV (%)	G-Low (%)
11.4	OH	2	0
12.1	$OCH_2OCOC(Me)_3$	11	0
12.2	$OCH_2OCO_2CH(Me)_2$	13	0
12.3	$NHCH_2CO_2Et$	26	51
12.4	$NHCH_2CO_2Bn$	17	ND[b]
12.5	$NHCH_2CO_2Bu$-*t*	9	ND
12.6	(*S*)-NHCH(Me)CO_2Et	22	59
12.7	(*S*)-NHCH(Me)CO_2Bn	11	ND
12.9	(*R*,*S*)-NHCH(Me)CO_2Et	28	52
12.10	(*S*)-NHCH(Me)CO_2Pr-*i*	31	63
12.12	(*S*)-NHCH(Me)CO_2Bu-*i*	10	ND
12.13	(*R*)-NHCH(Me)CO_2Me	22	26
12.15	(*S*)-NHCH(CH_2Pr-i)CO_2Et	3	ND
12.16	(*S*)-NHCH(Pr-i)CO_2Et	7	ND
12.17	(*S*)-NHCH(Bn)CO_2Et	3	ND
12.19	NHC$(Me)_2CO_2Et$	47	45

[a]OBAV, determined by measuring urinary excretion of **11.4** following oral administration of the prodrug versus i.v. administration of **11.4**; G-LOW, glucose lowering (C_{max}) in normal fasted rats after oral administration of a 10 mg kg^{-1} dose;

[b]ND, not determined.

produced marginal improvement in OBAV (<15%) for thiazole **11.4**. On the other hand, our recently discovered phosphonic diamide prodrugs [41] proved to be amendable to deliver thiazole **11.4** orally with many prodrugs achieving OBAV in the range of 20–47%. Phosphonic diamides derived from simple alkyl (methyl, ethyl, propyl) esters of alanine tend to give consistently good OBAV (20–30%). It is also noteworthy that the stereochemistry of the amino acids had no effect on OBAV, as diamides derived from L-, D- and D,L-alanine all gave similar OBAV results. This observation is in stark contrast to other phosphoramidate prodrugs of antiviral compounds. McGuigan et al. reported that the phosphoramidate prodrugs of [(1*R*)-4-[2-amino-6-(cyclopropylamino)purin-9-yl]-1-cyclopent-2-enyl]methanol (abacavir) showed a clear preference for L-amino acids: the abacavir prodrug from L-alanine methyl ester is 50-fold more potent than the corresponding prodrug from D-alanine methyl ester in a cellular anti-HIV assay [42]. Substitution on the α-methyl group of alanine was also explored, but led to a significant decrease in OBAV, which may be attributed to either decreased oral absorption or being poor substrates of the enzyme that is responsible for cleavage of the final P–N bond. The phosphonic diamides derived from 2-methylalanine ethyl ester (**12.19**) gave higher OBAV (30–50%) than diamides derived from either glycine or alanine ethyl esters.

OBAV determination by measuring the urinary recovery of the parent phosphonic acid was a useful tool in rapidly assessing a composite of oral absorption and *in vivo* prodrug conversion. However, an assay with a pharmacological endpoint is needed to assess whether drug levels achieved by these diamide prodrugs were sufficient for efficacy. In addition to inhibiting human FBPase, thiazole **11.4** is also a potent inhibitor of the rat FBPase, and when administered intravenously, thiazole **11.4** lowered plasma glucose levels in 18 h fasted normal Sprague Dawley (SD) rats (>50% at doses $\leq$ 10 mg kg^{-1}) [27]. This efficacy assay was selected based on the fact that glycogen storage should be largely depleted following an 18 h fast in a normal rat, and therefore the majority of endogenous glucose production is the result of gluconeogenesis, providing maximum sensitivity to the effects of a gluconeogenesis inhibitor. Therefore, compounds that passed the urinary OBAV screen (>20%) were evaluated for their ability to reduce plasma glucose levels following oral dosing in SD rats; the results are also shown in Table 4.6. Most of the diamides with >20% OBAV elicited a significant decrease (>40%) in fasting plasma glucose levels in this model at a dose of 30 mg kg^{-1}. On the other hand, some diamides (e.g., **12.13**) displayed weak efficacy (<30%) despite good OBAV (22–30%) demonstrated in the urinary excretion assay.

Several diamides (**12.3**, **12.6**, **12.9**, **12.10**, and **12.19**) showed >20% OBAV and produced significant glucose lowering in our normal fasted rat assay; however, further confirmatory studies (such as full pharmacokinetic studies, and efficacy in animal models of T2DM) led us to select thiazole **12.6** for characterization as a preclinical development candidate.

4.3 PHARMACOKINETIC STUDIES OF MB06322

Full pharmacokinetic (PK) studies of thiazole **12.6** were carried out in three species and the results are summarized in Table 4.7.

TABLE 4.7 Pharmacokinetic Profiles of Thiazole 12.6 in Three Species[a]

	Rat		Dog		Monkey		
Compound	$T_{1/2}$	OBAV	$T_{1/2}$	OBAV	$T_{1/2}$	OBAV	Protein binding, %
11.4	0.6 h	2 %	2.4 h	ND	0.4 h	ND	99, rat; 96, human
12.6	2.7 h	21 %	2.4 h	20 %	2.4 h	24%	90, rat; 93, human

[a]Fed male Sprague Dawley rats, bengle Dogs, cynomolgus monkeys were used; protein binding determined using heparinized rat and human plasma.

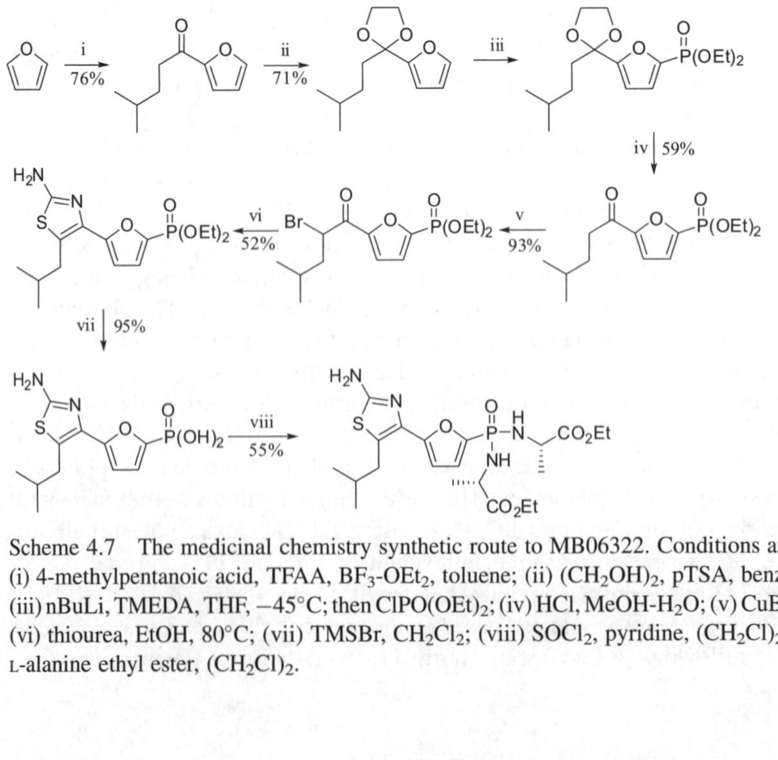

Scheme 4.7 The medicinal chemistry synthetic route to MB06322. Conditions and reagents: (i) 4-methylpentanoic acid, TFAA, BF_3-OEt_2, toluene; (ii) $(CH_2OH)_2$, pTSA, benzene, 80°C; (iii) nBuLi, TMEDA, THF, −45°C; then $ClPO(OEt)_2$; (iv) HCl, MeOH-H_2O; (v) $CuBr_2$, EtOH, 80°C; (vi) thiourea, EtOH, 80°C; (vii) TMSBr, CH_2Cl_2; (viii) $SOCl_2$, pyridine, $(CH_2Cl)_2$, 105°C; then L-alanine ethyl ester, $(CH_2Cl)_2$.

Exploratory toxicology studies of thiazole **12.6** were also conducted: in rats, no significant toxicity was observed at doses up to 300 mg kg^{-1}, qd p.o. dosing for 14 days; in monkeys, only hypoglycia was observed at > 300 mg kg^{-1} (mechanistic pharmacology); no other significant toxicity was observed up to 2000 mg kg^{-1}, p.o. qd dosing for 14 days; negative in Ames test at 5000 μg $plate^{-1}$ with (generation of thiazole **11.4**) or without S9.

4.4 SYNTHETIC ROUTES TO MB06322

The medicinal chemistry synthetic route to MB06322 consisted of eight steps starting from furan with an overall yield of 8.0%, as shown in Scheme 4.7.

Friedel-Crafts acylation of furan with 4-methylpentanoic acid gave the 2-ketofuran, and the resulting ketone was protected as a cyclic ketal. Lithiation of the 5-position of the furan followed by reaction with diethyl chlorophosphate, and removal of the cyclic ketal gave the key 2-keto-furan-5-phosphonate diethyl ester (59% yield over two steps). Bromination of the ketone followed by thiazole formation and final TMSBr-mediated removal of the phosphonate diethyl ester gave the desired FBPase inhibitor. The phosphonic acid FBPase inhibitor was converted to its corresponding phosphorus dichloridate and subsequent coupling with L-alanine ethyl ester gave the diamide prodrug MB06322.

4.5 CLINICAL STUDIES OF MB06322

4.5.1 Efficacy Study of Thiazole 12.6 in Rodent Models of T2DM

Compound **12.6** inhibits glucose production in both human and rat primary hepatocytes in a concentration-dependent manner [43]. The inhibitory potency of compound **12.6** was independent of substrates used for the hepatocyte assay (i.e., lactate or glycerol), which is consistent with the expected mechanism of action, that is, blocking of GNG via FBPase inhibition. Moreover, compound **12.6** demonstrated oral glucose-lowering effects in several rodent models of T2DM (e.g., STZ, ZDF and GK rats, and db/db mice), establishing it as the first FBPase inhibitor with reported oral activity in animal models [44,45].

One study was carried out in 6-week-old male ZDF rats in both prevention and intervention modes to evaluate compound **12.6** as a potential treatment for T2DM [46]. Compound **12.6** was studied using three cohorts of rats: one group of control animals treated with vehicle, a second group in which drug treatment was initiated at 6 weeks of age (prevention mode) and a third group in which drug treatment was initiated at 10 weeks of age (intervention mode). Compound **12.6** was administered as a food admixture in these studies (0.4%). In the prevention mode, drug treatment delayed the development of T2DM as indicated by the slow progression of hyperglycemia compared to vehicle-treated animals (Figure 4.8). In the intervention mode, treatment with **12.6** resulted in a marked correction of established hyperglycemia relative to the control group. Therefore, the study results suggest that compound **12.6** might be useful to treat both the early and late stages of T2DM.

Compound **12.6** was administered as a food admixture (0.4%, w/w) to 6-week-old (prevention) or 10-week-old (intervention) rats. $n = 8$/group. $^{*}p < 0.05$ compared to controls (ANOVA).

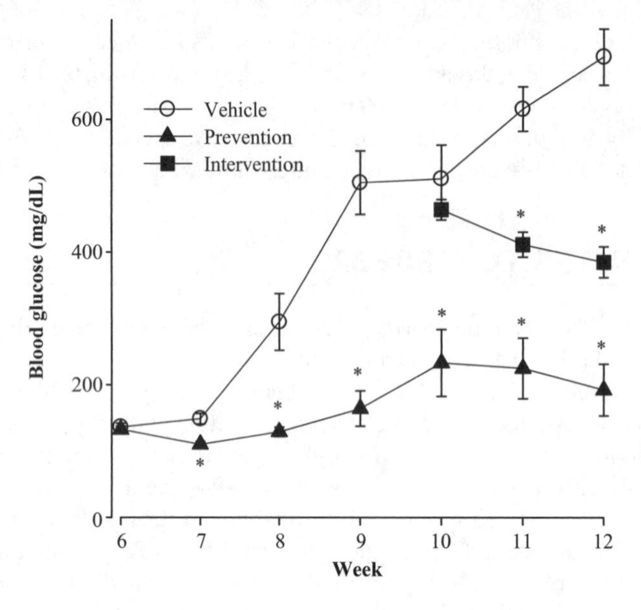

Figure 4.8 Effects of **12.6** prevention and intervention therapy in male ZDF rats.

4.5.2 Phase I/II Clinical Studies

In phase 2 randomized, double-blind, placebo-controlled 14-day studies, MB06322 was safe and well tolerated significant. Moreover, all of the doses (ranging 50 to 400 mg) with the exception of 100-mg dose produced statistically significant plasma glucose-lowering effects compared to placebo. All MB06322-treated patients maintained plasma lactate levels in the normal range. MN06322 was rapidly absorbed and efficiently converted to MB05032, and showed linear pharmacokinetics for the 50- to 200-mg dose range. Therefore, these results suggest that MB0633 has the potential as a therapy for type 2 diabetes.

4.6 SUMMARY

Having a drug-like lead molecule is key for a high probability of success for a medicinal chemistry program; however, sometimes a program is forced to start with a non-drug-like lead such as AMP. Using a structure-guided drug-design approach we were able to take AMP as our lead molecule and discover multiple series of potent and selective FBPase inhibitors, Figure 4.9. The program overcame many significant medicinal chemistry challenges. Our first goal was to discover a novel non-nucleotide AMP mimic, which was met by the discovery of phosphonic acid-containing purines and benzimidazoles; these phosphonic acids function as FBPase inhibitors *in vivo* and elicit profound glucose-lowering activity in animal models of T2DM. However, extensive prodrug efforts to deliver these phosphonic acids orally were not successful. Thus, our second challenge was to search for a new scaffold that is suitable for oral delivery via prodrugs. A redesign of the 5,6-fused heterocyclic nucleus in purine and benzimidazole was once again guided by X-ray crystallography studies, which led to the discovery of phosphonic acid-containing thiazoles as potent and selective FBPase inhibitors. The final hurdle was the oral delivery of phosphonic acid-containing thiazoles. Modification of thiazole FBPase inhibitors using commonly used phosphonate prodrugs did not produce oral efficacy, thus a new phosphonate prodrug approach had to be developed. To this end, a phosphonic diamide prodrug

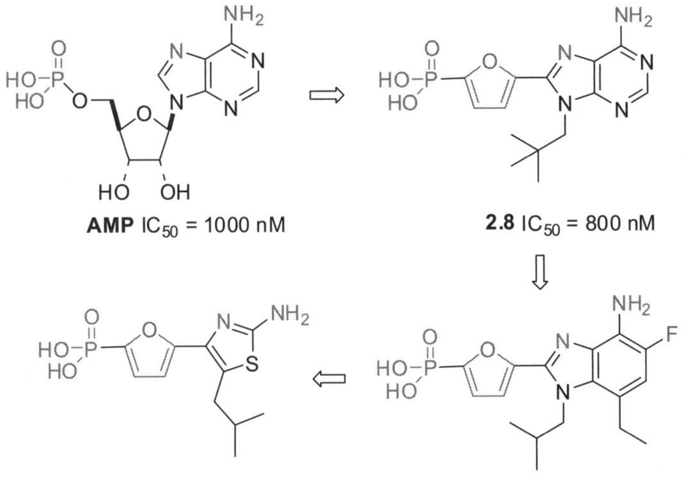

Figure 4.9 Evolution of novel AMP mimics as FBPase inhibitors.

approach was discovered, which successfully delivered our phosphonic acid-containing thiazoles orally with OBAV of 20–40% and potent oral glucose-lowering effects in animal models of T2DM. Years of collaborative team effort culminated in the discovery of compound **12.6** (MB06322) as the first oral FBPase inhibitor to advance to human clinical trials in patients with T2DM [22]. Significant lowering of plasma glucose levels in T2DM patients was demonstrated during the clinical studies of MB06322. A second generation FBPase inhibitor, MB07803, was discovered by Metabasis Therapeutics, and demonstrated improved PK profiles in both preclinical species and phase 1 clinical trials. MB07803 advanced to a phase 2A study and demonstrated statistical significant glucose-lowering in T2DM patients.

REFERENCES

1. Smushkin, G. and Vella, A. What is type 2 diabetes? *Medicine (Baltimore)*, **2010**, *38*, 597–601.
2. DeFronzo, R. A., Ferrannini, E., and Simonson, D. C. Type 2 diabetes mellitus: epidemiology. *Metabolism* **1989**, *38*, 387–395.
3. Jeng, C. Y., Sheu, W. H., Fuh, M. M., Chen, Y. D., and Reaven, G. M. Relationship between hepatic glucose production and fasting plasma glucose concentration in patients with NIDDM. *Diabetes* **1994**, *43*, 1440–1444.
4. Perriello, G., Pampanelli, S., Del Sindaco, P., Lalli, C., Ciofetta, M., Volpi, E., Santeusanio, F., Brunetti, P., and Bolli, G. B. Evidence of increased systemic glucose production and gluconeogenesis in an early stage of NIDDM. *Diabetes* **1997**, *46*, 1010–1016.
5. Magnusson, I., Rothman, D. L., Katz, L. D., Shulman, R. G., and Shulman, G. I. increased rate of gluconeogenesis in type 11 diabetes mellitus. A 13C nuclear magnetic resonance study. *J. Clin. Invest.* **1992**, *90*, 1323–1327.
6. Davis, S. N. The role of glimepiride in the effective management of type 2 diabetes. *J. Diabetes Complications* **2004**, *18*, 367–376.
7. Gillies, P. S. and Dunn, C. J. Pioglitazone. *Drugs* **2000**, *60*, 333-343;discussion 344–345.
8. Hundal, R. S., Krssak, M., Dufour, S., Laurent, D., Lebon, V., Chandramouli, V., Inzucchi, S. E., Schumann, W. C., Petersen, K. F., Landau, B. R., and Shulman, G. I. Mechanism by which metformin reduces glucose production in type 2 diabetes. *Diabetes* **2000**, *49*, 2063–2069.
9. Thornberry, N. A. and Weber, A. E. Discovery of JANUVIA (Sitagliptin), a selective dipeptidyl peptidase IV inhibitor for the treatment of type 2 diabetes. *Curr. Top. Med. Chem.* **2007**, *7*, 557–568.
10. el-Maghrabi, M. R., Gidh-Jain, M., Austin, L. R., and Pilkis, S. J. Isolation of a human fructose-1, 6-bisphosphatase cDNA and expression of the protein in Escherichia coli. *J. Biol. Chem.* **1993**, *268*, 9466–9472.

11. Steinmann, B., van den Bergh, S. G., Gitzelmann, R. Disorders of fructose metabolism. *The Metabolic and Molecular Bases of Inherited Disease, seventh edition*, Vol 1 (eds C. R. Scriver, A. L. Beaudet, W. S. Sly, and D. Valle), McGraw-Hill, New York, **1995**, p. 905.
12. Pilkis, S. J. and Claus, T. H. Hepatic gluconeogenesis/glycolysis: regulation and structure/function relationships of substrate cycle enzymes. *Annu. Rev. Nutr.* **1991**, *11*, 465–515.
13. Ke, H. M., Liang, J. Y., Zhang, Y. P., and Lipscomb, W. N. Conformational transition of fructose-1, 6-bisphosphatase: structure comparison between the AMP complex (T form) and the fructose 6-phosphate complex (R form). *Biochemistry* **1991**, *30*, 4412–4420.
14. Maryanoff, B. E., Reitz, A. B., Tutwiler, G. F., Benkovic, S. J., Benkovic, P. A., and Pilkis, S. J. Stereoselective synthesis and biological activity of beta- and alpha-D-arabinose 1, 5-diphosphate: analogs of a potent metabolic regulator. *J. Am. Chem. Soc.* **1984**, *106*, 7851–7853.
15. Wright, S. W., Carlo, A. A., Carty, M. D., Danley, D. E., Hageman, D. L., Karam, G. A., Levy, C. B., Mansour, M. N., Mathiowetz, A. M., McClure, L. D., Nestor, N. B., McPherson, R. K., Pandit, J., Pustilnik, L. R., Schulte, G. K., Soeller, W. C., Treadway, J. L., Wang, I. K., and Bauer, P. H. Anilinoquinazoline inhibitors of fructose 1,6-bisphosphatase bind at a novel allosteric site: synthesis, *in vitro* characterization, and X-ray crystallography. *J. Med. Chem.* **2002**, *45*, 3865–3877.
16. Wright, S. W., Carlo, A. A., Danley, D. E., Hageman, D. L., Karam, G. A., Mansour, M. N., McClure, L. D., Pandit, J., Schulte, G. K., Treadway, J. L., Wang, I. K., and Bauer, P. H. 3-(2-carboxyethyl)-4,6-dichloro-1H-indole-2-carboxylic acid: an allosteric inhibitor of fructose-1, 6-bisphosphatase at the AMP site. *Bioorg. Med. Chem. Lett.* **2003**, *13*, 2055–2058.
17. Choe, J. Y., Nelson, S. W., Arienti, K. L., Axe, F. U., Collins, T. L., Jones, T. K., Kimmich, R. D., Newman, M. J., Norvell, K., Ripka, W. C., Romano, S. J., Short, K. M., Slee, D. H., Fromm, H. J., and Honzatko, R. B. Inhibition of fructose-1, 6-bisphosphatase by a new class of allosteric effectors. *J. Biol. Chem.* **2003**, *278*, 51176–51183.
18. Lai, C., Gum, R. J., Daly, M., Fry, E. H., Hutchins, C., Abad-Zapatero, C., and von Geldern, T. W. Benzoxazole benzenesulfonamides as allosteric inhibitors of fructose-1, 6-bisphosphatase. Bioorg. *Med. Chem. Lett.* **2006**, *16*, 1807–1810.
19. von Geldern, T. W., Lai, C., Gum, R. J., Daly, M., Sun, C., Fry, E. H., and Abad-Zapatero, C. Benzoxazole benzenesulfonamides are novel allosteric inhibitors of fructose-1, 6-bisphosphatase with a distinct binding mode. *Bioorg. Med. Chem. Lett.* **2006**, *16*, 1811–1815.
20. Shaikh, M. S., Mittal, A., and Bharatam, P. V. Design of fructose-2, 6-bisphosphatase inhibitors: a novel virtual screening approach. *J. Mol. Graph. Model* **2008**, *26*, 900–906.
21. Tsukada, T., Kanno, O., Yamane, T., Tanaka, J., Yoshida, T., Okuno, A., Shiiki, T., Takahashi, M., and Nishi, T. Discovery of potent and orally active tricyclic-based FBPase inhibitors. *Bioorg. Med. Chem.* **2008**, *18*, 5346–5351.
22. Heng, S., Gryncel, K. R., and Kantrowitz, E. R. A library of novel allosteric inhibitors against fructose 1, 6-bisphosphatase. *Bioorg. Med. Chem*, **2009**, *17*, 3916–3922.
23. Rudnitskaya, A., Huynh, K., Torok, B., and Stieglitz, K. Novel heteroaromatic organofluorine inhibitors of fructose-1, 6-bisphosphatase. *J. Med. Chem.* **2009**, *52*, 878–882.
24. Heng, S., Harris, K. M., and Kantrowitz, E. R. Designing inhibitors against fructose 1,6-bisphosphatase: exploring natural products for novel inhibitor scaffolds. *Eur, J. Med. Chem.* **2010**, *45*, 1478–1484.
25. Kitas, E., Mohr, P., Kuhn, B., Hebeisen, P., Wessel, H. P., Haap, W., Ruf, A., Benz, J., Joseph, C., Huber, W., Sanchez, R. A., Paehler, A., Benardeau, A., Gubler, M., Schott, B., and Tozzo, E. Sulfonylureido thiazoles as fructose-1, 6-bisphosphatase inhibitors for the treatment of type-2 diabetes. *Bioorg. Med. Chem. Lett.* **2010**, *20*, 594–599.
26. Rudnitskaya, A., Borkin, D. A., Huynh, K., Torok, B., and Stieglitz, K. Rational design, synthesis, and potency of *N*-substituted indoles, pyrroles, and triarylpyrazoles as potential fructose 1, 6-bisphosphatase inhibitors. *Chem. Med. Chem.* **2010**, *5*, 384–389.
27. Erion, M. D., van Poelje, P. D., Dang, Q., Kasibhatla, S. R., Potter, S. C., Reddy, M. R., Reddy, K. R., Jiang, T., and Lipscomb, W. N. MB06322 (CS-917): a potent and selective inhibitor of fructose 1, 6-bisphosphatase for controlling gluconeogenesis in type 2 diabetes. *Proc. Natl. Acad. Sci. USA* **2005**, *102*, 7970–7975.
28. Wang, Y., and Tomlinson, B. Managlinat dialanetil, a fructose-1, 6-bisphosphatase inhibitor for the treatment of type 2 diabetes. *Curr. Opin. Investig. Drugs* **2007**, *8*, 849–858.
29. Triscari, J., Walker, J., Feins, K., Tao, B., and Bruce, S. R. A novel fructose-1, 6-bisphosphatase (FBPase) inhibitor. *Subjects with Type 2 Diabetes Treated for 14 Days*. The American Diabetes Association 66th Scientific Session, Washington, DC, **2006**.
30. Dang, Q., Brown, B. S., Liu, Y., Rydzewski, R. M., Robinson, E. D., van Poelje, P. D., Reddy, M. R., and Erion, M. D. Fructose-1, 6-bisphosphatase inhibitors: 1. Purine phosphonic acids as novel AMP mimics. *J. Med. Chem.* **2009**, *52*, 2880–2898.
31. Gidh-Jain, M., Zhang, Y., van Poelje, P. D., Liang, J. Y., Huang, S., Kim, J., Elliott, J. T., Erion, M. D., Pilkis, S. J., and Raafat el-Maghrabi, M. The allosteric site of human liver fructose-1, 6-bisphosphatase. Analysis of six AMP site mutants based on the crystal structure. *J. Biol. Chem.* **1994**, *269*, 27732–27738.
32. Dang, Q. Organophosphonic acids as drug candidates. *Exp. Opin. Therapeutic Patents* **2006**, *16*, 343.

33. Reddy, M. R.; Erion, M. D. *J. Am. Chem. Soc.* **2007**, *129*, 9296–9297.
34. Erion, M. D.; Dang, Q.; Reddy, M. R.; Kasibhatla, S. R.; Huang, J.; Lipscomb, W. N.; van Poelje, P. D. Structure-Guided Design of AMP Mimics that Inhibit Fructose 1,6-Bisphosphatase with High Affinity and Specificity. *J. Am. Chem. Soc.* **2007**, *129*, 15480–15490.
35. Erion, M. D.; Srinivas, R. K.; Bookser, B. C.; van Poelje, P. D.; Reddy, M. R.; Gruber, H. E.; Appleman, J. R. *J. Am. Chem. Soc.* **1999**, *121*, 308–319.
36. Dang, Q., Kasibhatla, S. R., Xiao, W., Liu, Y., Dare, J., Taplin, F., Reddy, K. R., Scarlato, G. R., Gibson, T., van Poelje, P. D., Potter, S. C., and Erion, M. D. Fructose-1,6-bisphosphatase inhibitors: 2. Design, synthesis, and structure–activity relationship of a series of phosphonic acid containing benzimidazoles that function as 50-adenosinemonophosphate (AMP) mimics. *J. Med. Chem.* **2010**, *53*, 441–451.
37. Sun, W., Wu, R. R., van Poelje, P. D., and Erion, M. D. Isolation of a family of organic anion transporters from human liver and kidney. *Biochem. Biophys. Res. Commun.* **2001**, *283*, 417–422.
38. Dang, Q., Liu, Y., Cashion, D. K., Kasibhatla, S. R., Jiang, T., Taplin, F., Jacintho, J. D., Li, H., Sun, Z., Fan, Y., Dare, J., Tian, F., Li, W., Gibson, T., Lemus, R., van Poelje, P. D., Potter, S. C., and Erion, M. D. Discovery of a series of phosphonic acid-containing thiazoles and orally bioavailable diamide prodrugs that lower glucose in diabetic animals through inhibition of fructose-1, 6-bisphosphatase. *J. Med. Chem.* **2011**, *54*, 153–165.
39. Krise, J. P. and Stella, V. J. Prodrugs of phosphates, phosphonates, and phosphinate. *Adv. Drug Deliv. Rev.* **1996**, *19*, 287–310.
40. Hecker, S. J. and Erion, M. D. Prodrugs of phosphates and phosphonates. *J. Med. Chem.* **2008**, *51*, 2328–2345.
41. Dang, Q., Kasibhatla, S. R., Jiang, T., Fan, K., Liu, Y., Taplin, F., Schulz, W., Cashion, D. K., Reddy, K. R., van Poelje, P. D., Fujitaki, J. M., Potter, S. C., and Erion, M. D. Discovery of phosphonic diamide prodrugs and their use for the oral delivery of a series of fructose 1, 6-bisphosphatase inhibitors. *J. Med. Chem.* **2008**, *51*, 4331–4339.
42. McGuigan, C. M., Harris, S. A., Daluge, S. M., Gudmundsson, K. S., McLean, E. W., Burnette, T. C., Marr, H., Hazen, R., Condreay, L. D., Johnson, L., De Clercq, E., and Balzarini, J. Application of Phosphoramidate Pronucleotide Technology to Abacavir Leads to a Significant Enhancement of Antiviral Potency. *J. Med. Chem.* **2005**, *48*, 3504–3515.
43. Dang, Q., Kasibhatla, S. R., Reddy, K. R., Jiang, T., Reddy, M. R., Potter, S. C., Fujitaki, J. M., van Poelje, P. D., Huang, J., Lipscomb, W. N., and Erion, M. D. Discovery of potent and specific fructose-1, 6-bisphosphatase inhibitors and a series of orally-bioavailable phosphoramidase-sensitive prodrugs for the treatment of type 2 diabetes. *J. Am. Chem. Soc.* **2007**, *129*, 15491–15502.
44. Van Poelje, P. D.; Dang, Q.; Erion, M. D. Fructose 1,6-bisphosphatase as a therapeutic target for type 2 diabetes. *Drug Discovery Today: Ther. Strategies* **2007**, *4*, 103–109.
45. Van Poelje, P. D.; Dang, Q.; Erion, M. D. Discovery of fructose 1,6-bisphosphatase inhibitors for the treatment of type 2 diabetes. *Curr. Opin. Drug Discovery Dev.* **2007**, *10*, 430–437.
46. Van Poelje, P. D.; Potter, S. C.; Chandramouli, V. C.; Landau, B. R.; Dang, Q.; Erion, M. D. Inhibition of fructose 1,6-bisphosphatase reduces excessive endogenous glucose production and attenuates hyperglycemia in zucker diabetic Fatty rats. *Diabetes* **2006**, *55*, 1747–1754.

CHAPTER 5

SETTING THE PARADIGM OF TARGETED DRUGS FOR THE TREATMENT OF CANCER: IMATINIB AND NILOTINIB, THERAPIES FOR CHRONIC MYELOGENOUS LEUKEMIA

Paul W. Manley and Jürg Zimmermann

5.1 INTRODUCTION

Cancer comprises over 200 different malignancies, driven by genetic damage which results in a large variety of tumors having quite different pathophysiologies. The cancer cell phenotype initially arises through the stepwise acquisition of mutations in genes that reactivate and modify processes to provide a growth advantage. The nascent tumor then continues to malignantly evolve in a Darwinian fashion, incorporating random mutations and epigenetic changes that prove to be beneficial, to acquire the key hallmarks of cancer: self-sufficiency in growth signaling, evading apoptosis, limited replicative potential, sustained angiogenesis, tissue invasion and metastasis, and insensitivity to antigrowth signals [1]. The gene mutations which can drive this process result in gain-of-function, amplification, and/or overexpression of oncogenes, together with loss-of-function, deletion, and/or epigenetic silencing of key tumor suppressor genes [2].

Many current cancer therapeutics continue to be general cytotoxic agents that impact tumor cells as well as other rapidly dividing cells, such that in a large patient population they frequently achieve little patient benefit at the price of high toxicity. However, since the year 2000, targeted drugs have been devised which are aimed at pathways central to tumor cell survival, and as such are intended to achieve high patient benefit in relatively smaller patient populations that are homogenous with regard to expressing the molecular target of the drug and, in the absence of off-target liabilities, should be better tolerated. Imatinib (Glivec®) was the first targeted cancer therapy, and by virtue of its dramatic success in improving the outcomes of patients with a particular type of leukemia, this drug has set a new paradigm for the treatment of cancer.

Case Studies in Modern Drug Discovery and Development, Edited by Xianhai Huang and Robert G. Aslanian.

5.2 CHRONIC MYELOGENOUS LEUKEMIA (CML) AND EARLY TREATMENT OF THE DISEASE

In his treatise on medical microscopy published in 1844, Alfred Donné provided an early description of leukemic cells and this paved the way for Bennett, Neumann, and Virchow to characterize leukemia as a disease of the bone marrow [3]. Building upon this foundation, it was recognized that CML progressed in three clinical phases, exemplifying the malignant evolution of tumors, beginning with a relatively asymptomatic chronic phase (CP), marked by greatly increased numbers of mature granulocytes in the peripheral blood and committed myeloid progenitors (myeloblasts) in the bone marrow, together with the enlargement of the spleen. In the absence of effective treatment, after a medium of 3.5 years patients advance to a transient accelerated phase (AP), when the myeloblasts lose their ability to differentiate and start to appear in the circulation, after which they progress into the terminal blast phase (BP), where blasts constitute >30% of cells in the circulation and bone marrow, leading to breakdown of the immune system, hemorrhage, and inevitably death [4]. It is now estimated that at diagnosis, CP CML patients can typically have a disease burden of 1×10^{13} leukemic cells in their bone marrow, blood, and other organs, and responses to therapy are now quantified as partial hematological response (PHR; peripheral blood leukocytes $<1 \times 10^{8}\,L^{-1}$), complete hematological response (CHR; as for PHR, but with no splenomegaly and no immature cells in peripheral blood), major cytogenetic response (MCyR; <34% of dividing cells from bone marrow carrying the Ph chromosome), complete cytogenetic response (CCyR; none of 20 dividing cells from bone marrow carrying the Ph chromosome), and major molecular response (MMR; a 1000-fold reduction in *BCR-ABL1* mRNA from cells in peripheral blood by reverse-transcription PCR) [5].

Following the early descriptions of CML and the possibility for diagnosis, in 1865, Heinrich Lissauer reported the first successful treatment of the symptoms of the disease, after administering Fowler's solution, which is comprised of arsenic trioxide dissolved in potassium bicarbonate [6]. Arsenic then became established as a treatment for leukemia until 1903, when splenic irradiation with X-rays demonstrated a similar control of symptoms, but with less toxicity [3]. Interestingly, arsenic continues to be a successful therapy for acute promyelocytic leukemia (APL), where it binds to cysteine residues within the oncogenic fusion protein PML-RARa, which results from a t(15;17) chromosome translocation and causes the disease, to induce oligomerization and sumoylation thereby promoting protein degradation [7]. Studies on the effects of mustard gas on victims from the First World War revealed an effect on hematopoiesis and studies in the 1940s with bis-(β-chloroethyl)methylamine confirmed some efficacy in leukemia, particularly in patients resistant to radiotherapy [8]. In medicinal chemistry, the approach to enhance the therapeutic efficiency of nitrogen mustards as alkylating agents, Geoffrey Timmis, working at the Chester Beatty Research Institute in London, synthesized the orally bioavailable 1,4-bis (methanesulfonoxy)butane (busulphan, Myleran®; Table 5.1) [9]. The mechanism of action of busulphan involved the cross-linking of DNA and the drug showed superiority to radiotherapy in achieving PHR in most patients at tolerated doses, with lung, marrow, and heart fibrosis being the main side effects. Subsequently, *N*-hydroxyurea (Hydrea®; Table 5.1), a drug originally developed by Bristol-Myers Squibb and the University of Chicago, largely replaced busulphan as the standard cytotoxic drug for CML patients. Hydroxyurea arrests DNA replication, probably by inhibiting ribonucleotide reductase by free radical mechanism [10], and was the first drug to prolong survival in CML patients (Table 5.1) [11]. Being relatively well tolerated, this drug continues to have some use today. The next advance in treating CML started with the use of alpha-interferon (IFN-α) in

TABLE 5.1 Evolution of Treatments for Chronic Phase Chronic Myelogenous Leukemia

Therapy	Structure	Introduction	Response Assessments from Initiation of Treatment
Arsenic	As_2O_3	ca. 1865	Data unavailable
Radiotherapy	X-Rays	1903	Median survival 28 months[15]
Busulphan	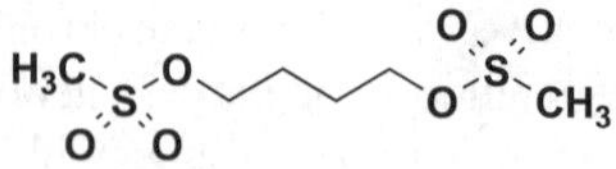	1959	Median survival 35–48 months[15]
Hydroxyurea	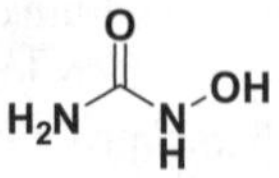	1968	Median survival 48–56 months[15]
Interferon-α	Glycosylated Protein	1994	Median survival 98, 65 & 42 months for low, medium & high risk patients[13]
Imatinib	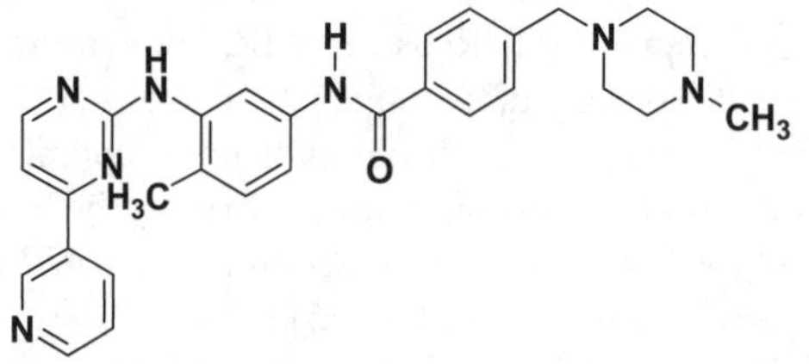	2001	Estimated survival rates in newly diagnosed CP CML at 36 months[38]: 92% in imatinib (400 mg q24h) treated patients 84% in interferon-α plus cytarabine treated patients
Nilotinib	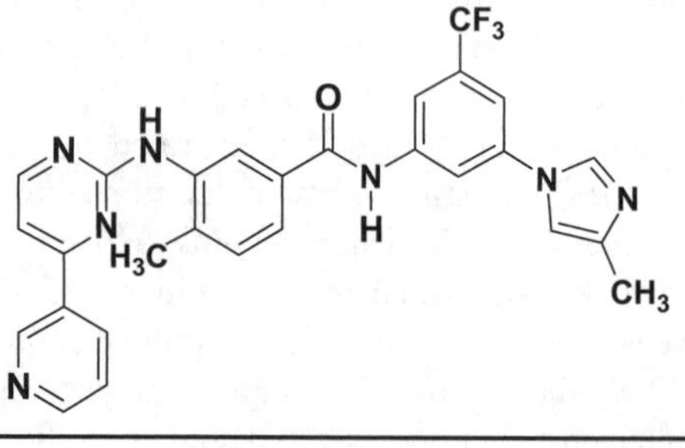	2010	Response rates in newly diagnosed CP CML at 12 months[56]: 80% CCyR & 44% MMR in nilotinib (300 mg q12h) treated patients 65% CCyR & 22% MMR in imatinib (400 mg q24h) treated patients

1983 [12]. Interferons are glycoproteins produced by lymphocytes in response to pathogens, which interact with receptors on cells to activate transcription factors that modulate immune responses, although they can also have a direct antitumor effect. IFN-α became standard therapy either as a single agent or in combination with cytotic agents, giving stable and durable CCyR in up to 33% of patients with overall survival at 9–10 years in the range of 27–53% [13,14]. However prior to the year 2000, despite improvements over the arsenic treatment of the mid-nineteenth century, most patients had a life expectancy of just 6–7 years following a diagnosis of CML (Table 5.1) [15].

The paradigm shift toward targeted therapy for this disease was based upon an understanding of CML on a molecular level and started in 1960, when Nowell and Hungerford discovered that a truncated version of chromosome 22, termed the Philadelphia (Ph) chromosome, was diagnostic of CML [16]. Some 13 years later, Janet Rowley showed that the Ph chromosome was the product of a t(9;22)(q34,q11) reciprocal chromosome translocation, where the ends of the long arms of chromosomes 9 (q34-ter) and 22 (q11-ter) break off and become fused to their opposite members [17]. In studies unknown to be related to CML, in 1970, Abelson and Rabstein [18] isolated the Abelson retrovirus that triggered leukemia in mice, which was subsequently shown to incorporate a fragment of a normal mouse gene (*ABL1*) into its own DNA leading to a protein that overstimulated cell growth [19]. These studies converged [20] when it was recognized that in the Ph chromosome translocation a fragment of the Abelson gene (*ABL1*), situated at the breakpoint on chromosome 9, becomes attached to a fragment of the breakpoint cluster region (*BCR*) gene on chromosome 22 [21]. The resulting *BCR-ABL1* fusion gene encodes a 210 kDa protein (BCR-ABL1), having tyrosine kinase domain corresponding to that of the viral Abelson oncoprotein [22].

In humans, 518 genes encode protein kinases and these play a central role in signal transduction pathways in all cells. These enzymes catalyze the transfer of a phosphate group from intracellular adenosine triphopshate (ATP) onto particular sidechain hydroxyl groups of serine, threonine, or tyrosine amino acid residues of their client proteins, thus enabling the phosphorylated residues to provide docking sites for other proteins and thereby allow signal transmission. Because of their critical role in signal transduction, the tight regulation of kinase activity is crucial and deregulation, by various mechanisms, has been observed for many of kinases in association with a number of human diseases. Thus gain- or loss–of-function mutations in kinases are frequently the cause of the deregulated signal transduction in cells that leads to the cancer phenotype, and by inhibiting the mutated kinase in tumor cells, it is possible to impede cell proliferation and restore apoptosis. Because the ATP-binding sites of kinases are often druggable, these enzymes are particularly attractive targets for cancer therapy. However, the ATP-binding site, which is located between two lobes of the kinase catalytic domain (SH1), is highly conserved across the kinome, and in the preimatinib era there was much scepticism as to whether the discovery of potent and selective kinase inhibitors, suitable for clinical efficacy and safety, would ever be achievable.

Whereas ABL1 is ubiquitously expressed in cells and is normally tightly regulated, the chimeric oncoprotein lacks an *N*-terminal ABL1 regulatory domain and, via the BCR domain, forms a tetrameric complex [23,24] which undergoes autophosphorylation, leading to self-activation and imparting constitutive activity to the tyrosine kinase domain. In the transformed haematopoietic cells, this deregulated phosphorylation of protein tyrosine residues induces growth factor-independent proliferation and neoplastic transformation, through the activation of Janus kinase, PI3 kinase, the RAS GTPase, and STAT5 (a Signal Transducer and Activator of Transcription). The expression of BCR-ABL1 is sufficient for the transformation of hematopoietic cells *in vitro* and *in vivo*, where it leads to a CML-like myeloproliferative disorder in mice [25] and this supports the belief that the aberrant tyrosine kinase activity alone is able to account for the pathophysiology of CP CML.

This understanding of CML helped to make ABL1 an attractive drug target, and from a pharmacological point of view, this was further supported by the knowledge that ABL1 knock-out mice exhibited a viable phenotype, demonstrating that the enzyme was not absolutely essential for survival [26]. However, prior to the development of imatinib, protein kinases were generally considered to be poor drug targets because all members of the serine–threonine and tyrosine kinase families, encoded by 518 genes [27], bound their substrate adenosine triphosphate (ATP) in a very similar manner to catalyze the transfer of the terminal phosphate group onto protein serine, threonine, or tyrosine residues in a highly homologous fashion. At the time this belief was further supported by kinetic arguments, such as the weak binding of ATP, coupled to millimolar intracellular ATP concentrations [28]. Researchers at Ciba-Geigy in Basel, Switzerland, under the leadership of Alex Matter were not so pessimistic, and in the late 1980s, several drug discovery programs were being pursued that targeted protein kinases. One of these was directed against the serine–threonine specific, protein kinase C (PKC), and it was this research that provided the lead compound for a medicinal chemistry effort directed toward inhibitors of BCR-ABL1.

5.3 IMATINIB: A TREATMENT FOR CHRONIC MYELOGENOUS LEUKEMIA (CML)

A key aspect of any new drug discovery program is the identification of tractable, drug-like lead compounds which hold promise for medicinal chemistry optimization. Strategies for lead finding range from high-throughput screening of compound libraries, to more rational methods, such as *de novo* design with insight from liganded or unliganded protein structures, database mining employing pharmacophore models derived from known compounds, or upon mechanistic insight. It was the latter method that led to the breakthrough compound, imatinib. Following a hypothesis that compounds displaying activity in animal models of inflammation might in part be acting through protein kinase C inhibition, in an effort to find new lead structures as kinase inhibitors, compounds reported to have anti-inflammatory properties as a result of unknown mechanisms were evaluated for their effects on kinase activity. One such class of compounds that inhibited histamine release from basophils was disclosed in a patent by researchers at American Cyanamid as having anti-asthmatic activity [29,30]. One of the three most active compounds disclosed (Example 231; **1** in Figure 5.1) was synthesized and found to inhibit several protein kinases and in particular the tyrosine phosphorylation of the Asp–Arg–Val–Tyr–Val–His–Pro–Phe substrate by a bacterial construct ABL1 [31]. Table 5.2 illustrates the selectivity of **1**, where it inhibits the tyrosine phosphorylation of the PolyAEKY substrate, catalyzed by several recombinant kinase domains, with IC_{50} values in the range of 90–3300 nM and a rank order of potency of CDK1 > PDGFRβ > KIT > SRC > PKCα/β1 > ABL1. This new kinase inhibitor chemotype was optimized for activity against ABL1 using an empirical approach, firstly based upon structure–activity relationships (SAR) for potency and selectivity, and latter to improve solubility and pharmacokinetic properties (Figure 5.1) [32,33]. Initial SAR studies employed a modular approach to vary the structure and utilized various substituted 3-nitroanilines and acetylheterocycles as building blocks to prepare compounds prepared via Brederick's keto-enamine primidine synthesis (Figure 5.2) [34]. Important observations were that the activity against the SRC kinase was greatly reduced by replacing the imidazole group in **1**, by amides in particular, and that the introduction of a methyl group *ortho* to the aminopyrimidine substituent abrogated activity against the PKC and improved potency against ABL1. Thus compound **2a** (Figure 5.1) inhibited ABL1, PKCα, and SRC with IC_{50} values of 430 nM, 72 μM, and 100 μM, respectively. However, aryl amides such as **2a**, despite being quite potent inhibitors of ABL1, failed to demonstrate activity either in cellular assays or in a murine model of CML. This was attributable to the high lipophilicity of the molecules and their poor water solubility (e.g., compound **2a**, Figure 5.1, has a $\log P_{\mathrm{Oct/Water}}$ value of 4.2 and aqueous solubility at pH 4 of 2 mg L^{-1}, compared to values of 3.1 and >200 mg L^{-1} for imatinib), and consequently in an attempt to improve oral bioavailability the effect of incorporating polar groups, such as the ionizable *N*-methylpiperazine moiety, was investigated. Based upon the SAR for ABL1 inhibition, the *N*-methylpiperazine group was attached to the *para*-position of the benzamide ring in compound **2a**, via a methylene-linker in order to avoid the introduction of a further aromatic amino group, in the belief that this would not interfere with binding to the protein. The resulting compound **3** (CGP057148) potently inhibited ABL1, PDGFRβ, and KIT in biochemical assays, with IC_{50} values in the sub-micromolar range (Table 5.2). The importance of introducing the solubilizing *N*-methylpiperazine group was immediately

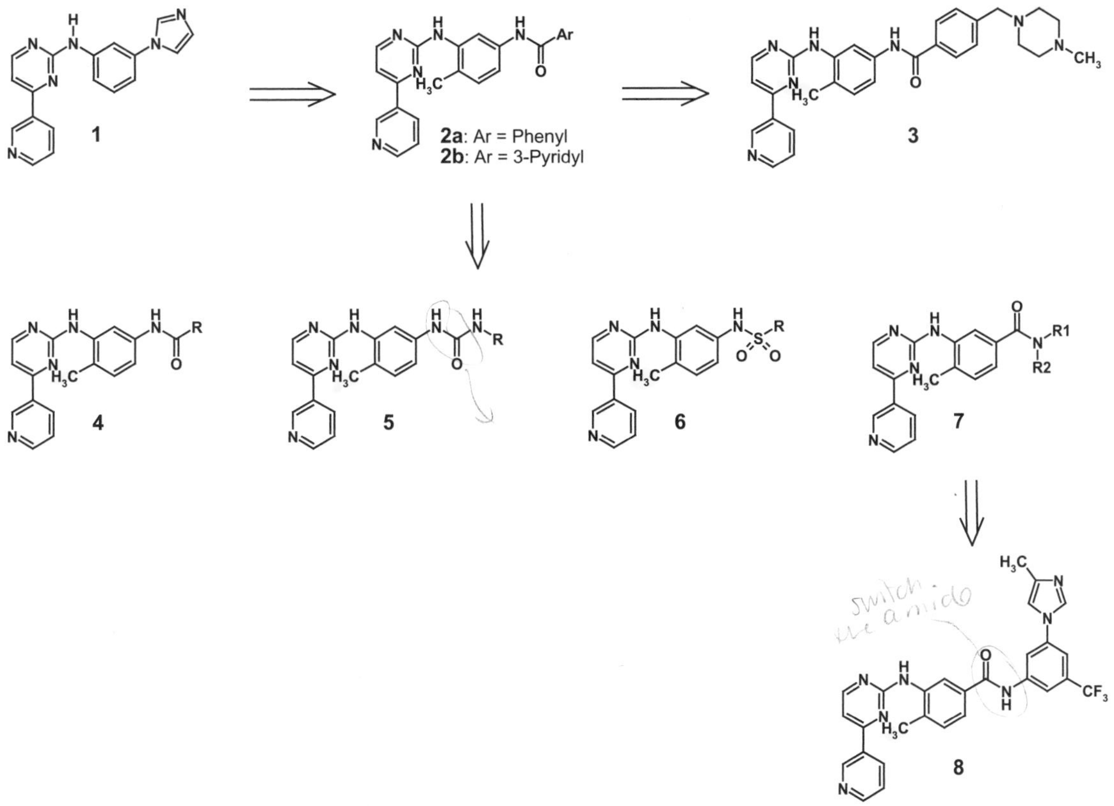

Figure 5.1 Genesis of imatinib (**3**) and nilotinib (**8**). The anti-inflammatory lead phenylaminopyrimidine **1** was optimized for ABL1 kinase inhibition, leading to a series of amides, typified by **2a**, which was further elaborated to optimize drug-like properties to culminate in imatinib **3**. With structural biology insight, the structure–activity relationships for BCR-ABL1 inhibition of the phenylaminopyrimidines **4–7** were investigated and the benzamide **7** was further optimized to afford nilotinib, **8**.

apparent from the activity of **3** in cell-based assays, where it dose-dependently inhibited ABL1 tyrosine autophosphorylation in transfected PB-3c mast cells and full-length BCR-ABL1 kinase in transfected murine 32D hematopoietic cells, but had no effect on SRC tyrosine kinase activity in 32D SRC cells. This *in vitro* activity translated into *in vivo* activity in a tumor xenograft model, where **3** dose-dependently inhibited the growth of

TABLE 5.2 Comparison of Effects of Lead Compound and Imatinib on Kinase Transphosphorylation

Kinase	Lead Compound (1)	Imatinib (3)
	Inhibition of transphosphorylation, IC_{50} (nM)	
PKC-α	1,000	>10,000
PKC-β1	2,500	>10,000
ABL1	3,300 ± 1,100	188 ± 13
KIT	1,100 ± 200	413 ± 23
PDGFR-β	390 ± 58	386 ± 111
c-SRC	1,700	100,000
VEGFR-2	1,400	10,000
FGFR-1	2,500	>10,000
CDK1/cycB	92 ± 4	>10,000

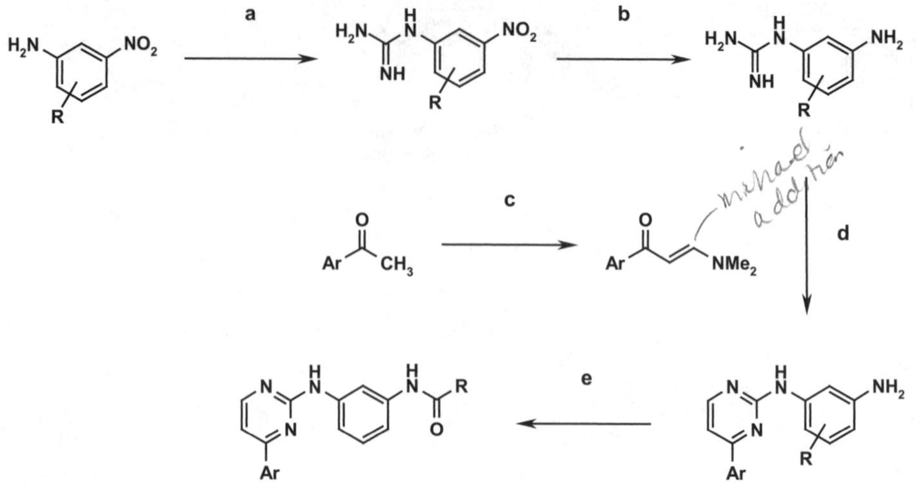

Figure 5.2 Synthesis scheme employed for the preparation of imatinib analogs. Acid-catalyzed addition of commercially available 3-nitroanilines with cyanamide afforded the corresponding 3-nitrophenylguanidines, which were subjected to palladium-catalyzed hydrogenation to reduce the nitro-group. The resulting aminophenylguanidines were then reacted with diverse enaminones, derived from commercially available acetophenones by condensation with dimethylformamide dimethylacetal, to give diverse pyrimidin-2-ylamino-anilines. These anilines were then converted to a wide range of amides using a variety of standard methods. Reagents and conditions: (a) H_2NCN, c. HCl, *n*-butanol, 90°C; (b) H_2, Pd/C, *n*-butanol; (c) $Me_2NCH(OMe)_2$, xylene, 140°C; (d) NaOH, *i*-PrOH, 95°C; (e) amide formation.

32D-p210-BCR-ABL1 tumor xenografts in mice following intraperitoneal administration, but was inactive against 32D-SRC tumors [35].

The compound advanced through extensive preclinical testing and entered clinical trials as the beta-crystal form of the methanesulphonate salt in 1998, with once daily oral dosing at up to 1000 mg day in CML patients who had failed interferon therapy [36]. The drug was well absorbed to give dose-proportional exposure with a plasma half-life of between 13 and 16 hours and, with the most common adverse events being nausea, myalgias, edema, and diarrhea, the maximum tolerated dose was not reached. Hematological responses were seen in all patients receiving doses ≥140 mg day, and 53 of 54 patients who received doses of ≥300 mg day, for a period of at least 4 weeks, showed a CHR. Of these 54 patients, 54% showed cytogenic responses, with 13% having a CCyR. These early results were substantiated in larger Phase II studies [37], and following accelerated review the drug (imatinib: Gleevec®) was approved by the US Food and Drugs Administration (FDA), in May 2001 for the treatment of CML refractory to treatment with interferon. A Phase III open-label International Randomized Study of Interferon versus STI571 (IRIS) trial that compared imatinib to the previous standard of care showed greatly improved survival over interferon plus the cytotoxic agent cytarabine (Table 5.1) [38] and confirmed the long-term safety and durability of response [39].

5.4 THE NEED FOR NEW INHIBITORTS OF BCR-ABL1 AND DEVELOPMENT OF NILOTINIB

In contrast to CP CML patients, CHR and CCyR remissions were less frequently achieved in patients who had progressed to AP or to BC prior to starting imatinib therapy, and the responses were less durable with many patients relapsing within a short period due to the

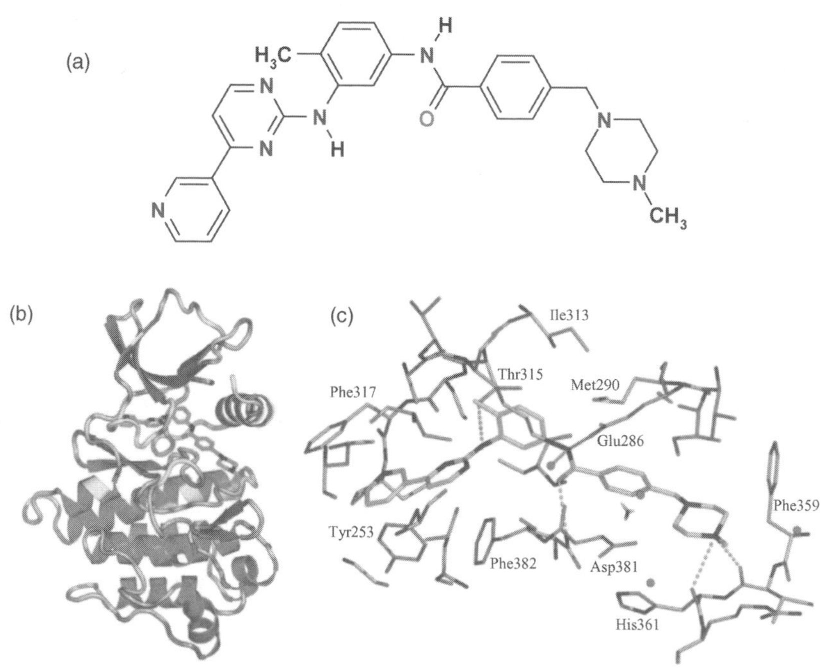

Figure 5.3 (a) Chemical structure of imatinib in pose similar to that in 3b and 3c. (b) Ribbon diagram showing the binding of imatinib (green C atoms, blue N atoms and red O atom) within the ATP-binding cleft between the two lobes of the ABL kinase SH1 domain (helices in red, strands in blue, loops and turns in gray), with the locations of mutants isolated from imatinib-resistant patients shown in yellow. (c) Details of the binding of imatinib (color-coded as in 3b) to ABL kinase (gray C atoms, blue N atoms and red O atoms; conserved water molecules shown as red spheres) showing potential hydrogen bonds as orange dotted lines and, clearly showing the hydrogen bond between the imatinib-NH and the oxygen atom of the threonine315 CH(Me)OH sidechain, that is not possible for the $CH(Me)CH_2CH_3$ isoleucine sidechain of the T315I mutant enzyme. (Adapted from [49] with permission from Elsevier.) (See color version of the figure in Color Plate section)

development of imatinib resistance [37]. Thus in interferon-resistant and interferon-intolerant CP patients, the rates of resistance and relapse to imatinib at 24 months were 4% and 13% respectively, whereas in AP these rates were 24% and 51%, and for BC 66% and 88%, respectively. Imatinib resistance could be recapitulated *in vitro*, by culturing either Ph-positive human K562 cells or BCR-ABL1-transformed murine haematopoietic cells in the presence of sublethal concentrations of drug to generate resistant cell lines. The mechanisms for both *in vitro* and patient resistance are multifactorial, with increased expression of BCR-ABL1 and upregulation of drug-efflux transporters being involved. However, although to some extent anticipated in *in vitro* studies by Brian Druker [40], the most frequent cause of resistance was revealed by Charles Sawyers and co-workers when they detected mutant forms of BCR-ABL1 in CML cells from imatinib-resistant patients [41]. In this study, sequencing the RNA of the *ABL1* kinase domain from leukemic cells revealed a cytosine to thymine nucleotide substitution in six of nine patients who had developed resistance to imatinib. This nucleotide substitution changed the adenine–thymine–cytosine nucleotide triad into adenine–thymine–thymine and thus encoded a single amino acid substitution of the threonine315 residue with isoleucine in the kinase domain of BCR-ABL1. This point mutation (T315I) rendered the tyrosine kinase activity of the protein insensitive to imatinib and this could be explained on a structural basis following a publication by John Kuriyan's group of an X-ray crystal structure of an analog of imatinib bound to the ABL1 kinase domain [42]. This pyridyl analog, which lacked the *N*-methylpiperazine group (**2b**; Figure 5.1), was believed (and subsequently confirmed) to bind in a similar fashion to that of imatinib (Figure 5.3), with the aniline-NH of the inhibitor donating a hydrogen bond to the sidechain hydroxyl group of the Thr315 residue and the methyl group of the same residue in van der Waal's contact with the aniline ring. In the case of the isoleucine mutant form of the enzyme, the replacement of the sidechain hydroxyl group with an ethyl group, the absence of the hydrogen bond and steric hindrance from the ethyl group precluded imatinib from binding to the catalytic site and rendered it insensitive to the drug (see Figure 5.3). Since the discovery of T315I BCR-ABL1, over 100 different mutant forms of the enzyme have been detected in imatinib-resistant leukemia patients having varying degrees of drug insensitivity [43], which impede the binding of the drug and this mechanism is the most common cause of patient relapse in CP (42%) and AP (57%) [44,45]. In general, imatinib binding is impeded by two mechanisms, which can operate either independently or in concert. The most obvious mechanism is where the mutation alters the binding surface between imatinib and the protein, leading to steric clashes and/or the loss of hydrogen-bond interactions (e.g. T315I), but a second mechanism involves the destabilization of the imatinib-binding conformation (discussed in more detail below), such that the active, DFG-in conformation becomes thermodynamically preferred, as in the case of the substitution of Glutamate255 (e.g., E255V, where loss of hydrogen-bond interactions between the sidechain of Glu255 and the sidechain of Tyr257 and Lys247 in the protein destabilize the DFG-out conformation) [46].

With this understanding that imatinib resistance and relapse in CML patients resulted from the emergence and expansion of leukemic clones resistant to the inhibitor, as a consequence of exposing BCR-ABL1-dependent cells to sub-lethal imatinib concentrations, it was reasoned that a more potent BCR-ABL1 kinase inhibitor would reduce the reservoir of leukemic cells in patients and thereby reduce, or at least substantially slow, the emergence of drug resistance. With this hypothesis a new program was initiated with the goal to find a BCR-ABL1 kinase inhibitor to combat imatinib resistance.

The medicinal chemistry direction for this new endeavor was steered by the detailed knowledge of how imatinib bound within the ATP-binding pocket of the ABL1 kinase domain (Figure 5.3) [47–49]. Although imatinib binds in the cleft between the N- and C-terminal lobes as originally postulated based upon homology modeling, a crucial difference revealed by the crystal structure was that it did not bind to the catalytically active conformation of the kinase domain, but to a conformation where the Asp381–Phe382–Gly383 triad flips out (DFG-out or inactive conformation) to open access to a pocket beyond the Thr315 residue for the benzamide and *N*-methylpiperazine groups to bind (Figure 5.4). Rather than sitting at the protein–water interphase, the protonated *N*-methylpiperazine group makes strong hydrogen bonds with the backbone-CO groups of Ile360 and His361 within the binding pocket. Other hydrogen-bond interactions involve the pyridine-N and the backbone-NH of Met318, the aniline-NH and the sidechain hydroxyl of residue Thr315, the amide-NH and the sidechain carboxylate of Glu286 from helix C, and the amide-CO and the backbone-NH of Ala380, which just precedes the highly conserved DFG motif. This assembly of hydrogen bonds is complemented by extensive hydrophobic interactions over the whole length of the inhibitor. This DFG-out conformation is incapable of binding ATP and is catalytically inactive, so that imatinib inhibits the kinase by stabilizing this conformation, rather than by directly competing with ATP-binding to the active conformation. The new medicinal chemistry effort therefore focused on optimizing the binding of the phenylpyrimidine scaffold to this conformation. This approach was thought to be feasible, since imatinib only showed an IC_{50} value in the range of 250–800 nM against BCR-ABL1 in cellular assays, which was considerably higher than what might be

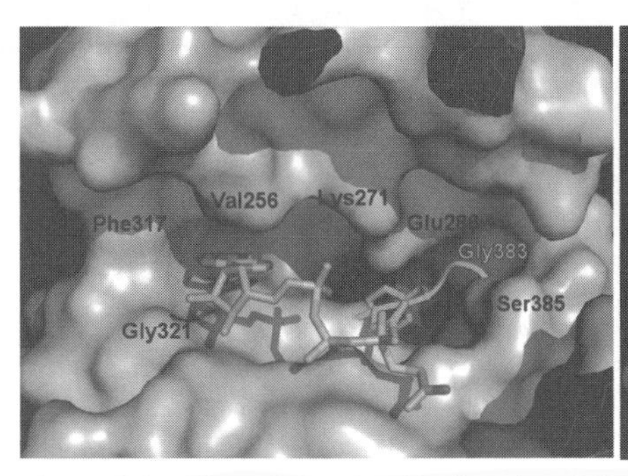

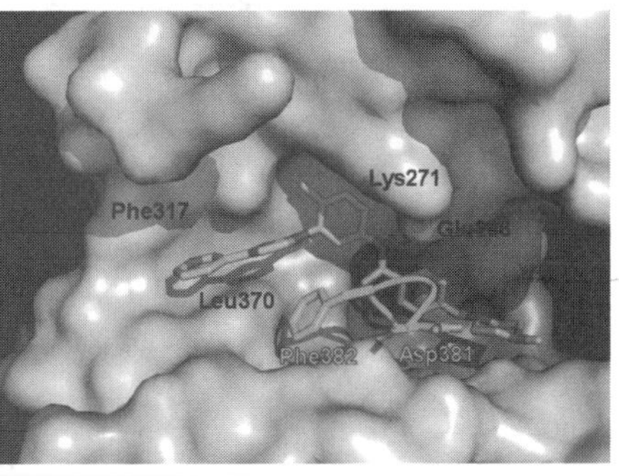

Figure 5.4 View of the ATP-binding site of ABL kinase with ATP bound (left-hand panel) and with imatinib bound (right-hand panel), with the locations of several residues lining the binding labeled. In both panels the solvent accessible surface of ABL is shown in gray, with the activation loop beyond the DFG motif (green) and the P-loop removed for clarity, as these loops cover the binding site. The DFG motif is buried in the active conformation (left) and it is flipped out in the inactive conformation required for binding imatinib (right, with Phe382 labeled), thus lengthening the channel within which inhibitors can bind. The locations of several residues important for inhibitor binding are indicated with labels. (Adapted from [52] with permission from Elsevier.)

predicted based upon the seven hydrogen-bond and lipophilic interactions observed in the crystal structure [50]. The first step in this approach was to keep the 3-pyridyl-4-anilino-pyrimidine half of the imatinib structure constant, and to prepare small focused libraries of compounds to probe the binding pocket opened up in the DFG-out conformation. Four such libraries were prepared (Figure 5.1) based upon anilide (**4**), urea (**5**), sulphonamide (**6**), and benzamide (**7**) linker groups [51]. From this study the most promising lead compounds for BCR-ABL1 inhibition were from the anilide and benzamide chemotypes, bearing a meta-trifluoromethyl substituted phenyl group. Further studies to optimize the binding interactions, with emphasis on improving the topological fit as supported by X-ray crystallography, revealed that this phenyl group could be further substituted,10x(8) both to increase potency and selectivity toward BCR-ABL1 inhibition, and to optimize the drug-like properties (e.g., lipophilicity, oral bioavailability in rodents, cytochrome P450 inhibition) of the molecule. Thus iterative optimization eventually resulted in the identification of AMN107 (**8**; nilotinib; Tasigna®), which showed up to 30-fold greater potency than imatinib as an inhibitor of BCR-ABL1 [50] (with a selectivity profile toward protein kinases of DDR-1/-2 > BCR-ABL1 > PDGFR > KIT > EPHB4 > CSF-1R, compared to that of imatinib of DDR-1/-2 > PDGFR > KIT > BCR-ABL1 > CSF-1R ≫ EPHB4 (Table 5.3))[52]. The enhanced potency over imatinib was consistent with the X-ray structure of nilotinib in complex with ABL (Figure 5.5). This *in vitro* activity translated into good oral efficacy in murine models of CML [50,53]. For example, following inoculation of 32D-p210-Luc cells, vehicle-treated mice develop a rapidly fatal, myeloproliferative disease, characterized by leukocytosis and splenomegaly, whereas treatment with nilotinib dose-dependently reduced disease burden, as assessed by light emission, with tumor stasis observed at 45 mg kg^{-1} q24h or 30 mg kg^{-1} q12h and higher doses giving regressions.

The greater binding affinity of nilotinib to the DFG-out, ABL1 kinase domain enabled it to inhibit the majority (31/32 tested) of imatinib-resistant mutant forms of BCR-ABL1, with only the T315I mutant being unaffected by non-physiologically-relevant drug concentrations [54]. Furthermore, *in vitro* mutagenesis studies showed that in comparison to imatinib, nilotinib had a much lower potential for the emergence of drug-resistant mutations, with the only commonly selected mutations occurring in residues G250, Y253, E255, T315, and F359 [55–57].

TABLE 5.3 Comparison of Effects of Imatinib and Nilotinib on Intracellular Kinase Autophosphorylation[a]

		Imatinib (3)	Nilotinib (8)
Kinase	Cell line	Inhibition of autophosphorylation, IC_{50} (nM)	
BCR-ABL1	Transfected Ba/F3	221 ± 31	20 ± 2
BCR-ABL1	K562	473 ± 60	42 ± 8
PDGFR-α & -β	A31	72 ± 10	71 ± 5
KIT (K642E)	GIST882	97 ± 12	217 ± 8
DDR-1	Transfected HEK393	43 ± 2.4	3.7 ± 1.2
DDR-2	Transfected HEK393	141 ± 33	5.2 ± 3.3
CSF-1R	Transfected HEK393	291 ± 54	677 ± 437

[a]As a consequence of binding to catalytically inactive conformations of their kinase targets, imatinib and nilotinib exhibit time-dependent kinase inhibition in in enzymatic assays, and consequently their effects on kinase activity is best assessed following incubation of cells with drug and measuring kinase autophosphorylation using capture enzyme linked immunosorbant assays (ELISA) in cell lysates [52].

With this preclinical profile, coupled with a satisfactory preclinical safety assessment, nilotinib as the hydrochloride salt progressed into Phase I clinical trials in May 2004 in patients with imatinib-resistant or imatinib-intolerant CML or Ph+ acute lymphoblastic leukemia. Solubility-limited drug absorption resulted in twice-daily administration

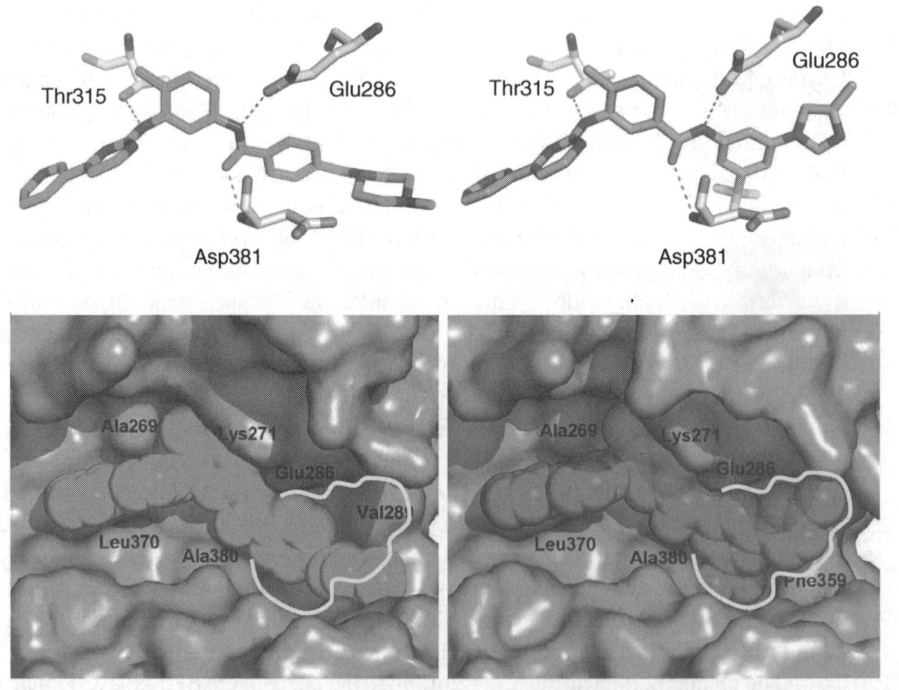

Figure 5.5 Cartoon illustrating the differences in how imatinib and nilotinib bind to ABL as determined by X-ray crystallography [49]. The upper panel illustrates how the amide groups of imatinib (green) and nilotinib (gold) differ in their hydrogen-bond interactions with Glu286 and Asp381 of the ABL protein. The lower panel illustrates how nilotinib (red) has a better topological fit, mediated primarily via van der Waal's interactions, than that of imatinib (green) to the pocket opened up by flipping-out of the DFG motif in the inactive conformation (see Figure 5.4) of the ABL protein (solvent accessible surface shown in gray). (Adapted from [52] with permission from Elsevier.)

affording optimum drug exposure with nilotinib at 400 mg bid delivering steady-state plasma trough levels of 1.95 μM and regimen was adopted for single-arm Phase II efficacy studies [58]. Nilotinib proved to be efficacious in imatinib-resistant or imatinib-intolerant patients with CML in chronic, accelerated, and blastic phases, and the drug produced sustained cytogenetic and hematological responses, particularly in chronic- and accelerated-phase patients [45,59]. (The differences in the structure and target selectivity between nilotinib and imatinib are reflected in the drugs having substantially different preclinical pharmacology and a lack of cross-intolerance in patients, which translates into nilotinib being an efficacious treatment for CML, with a favorable side-effect profile [52].

Based upon the Phase 2 studies, nilotinib gained health authority approved throughout the world for the treatment of patients with CML in CP and AP following imatinib failure, and Phase 3 trials then commenced to comparing the efficacy and safety of nilotinib with imatinib, as first-line treatment of newly diagnosed CP CML [60]. Reflecting the advances in the control of CML seen with imatinib, the primary endpoint in this study was the rate of MMR at 12 months, which was superior for nilotinib 300 mg q12h compared with imatinib (44% versus 22%) and nilotinib 400 mg q12h compared with imatinib (43% versus 22%). Furthermore, by the cutoff date, fewer patients had progressed to AP or BC in either nilotinib arm (0.7% at 300 mg and 0.4% at 400 mg) in comparison to the imatinib arm (3.9%), indicating that the greater potency, leading to greater reduction in tumor burden, indeed leads to an improvement in the survival rate of CML patients. A New Drug Application for nilotinib in newly diagnosed CML was approved by the FDA in June 2010.

5.5 CONCLUSION

The unprecedented efficacy of imatinib in CML, coupled with the duration of responses and long-term tolerability of the drug, which reflects its selectivity profile as an ABL kinase inhibitor, set a new paradigm of molecularly targeted agents for the treatment of cancer. Building upon an in-depth understanding of the efficacy of imatinib as an inhibitor of BCR-ABL1 and how it bound to ABL at a molecular level, nilotinib was designed as a new, improved drug and the improved preclinical features of the drug have been borne out in patients. The speed with which nilotinib was discovered and developed to Health Authority approval for use in CML (6.5 years from programme start) also reflects the value of having a clearly validated disease target, therapeutically relevant *in vitro* assays to develop SAR, and efficient clinical development. This success of the targeted drug paradigm has been translated into treatments for other malignancies with highly selective kinase inhibitors, such as non-small-cell lung cancer where erlotinib (Tarceva®; OSI Pharmaceuticals and Roche) and gefitinib (Iressa®; AstraZeneca) target the epidermal growth factor receptor (EGFR), metastatic breast cancer where lapatinib (Tykerb®; GlaxoSmithKline) is a dual inhibitor of EGFR and the estrogen receptor kinase (ERBB2), and gastrointestinal stromal tumors where imatinib also targets the stem cell factor receptor kinase, KIT. With respect to CML, it is hoped that the next therapeutic advance will be to effect a cure for this malignancy, such that patients can cease CML therapy without the re-emergence of the disease. One approach toward this goal is to selectively target the CML stem cells, which remain resistant and invulnerable to current therapies because of their quiescent state, either directly through an Achilles heel in their defence, or through driving them out of the quiescent state to render them sensitive towards BCR-ABL1 inhibitors. Thus in the search for cures for cancers in general, it is hoped that CML will provide a platform of success, that is translatable to other malignancies.

REFERENCES

1. Hanahan, D. and Weinberg, R. A. The Hallmarks of Cancer. *Cell* **2000**, *100*, 57–70.
2. Hahn, W. C. and Weinberg, R. A. Modelling the molecular circuitry of cancer. *Nat. Rev. Cancer* **2002**, *2*, 331–341.
3. Piller, G. J. Leukaemia—a brief historical review from ancient times to 1950. *Br. J. Haematol.* **2001**, *112*, 282–292.
4. Melo, J. V. and Barnes, D. J. Chronic myeloid leukaemia as a model of disease evolution in human cancer. *Nat. Rev. Cancer* **2007**, *7*, 441–453.
5. Baccarani, M., Cortes, C., Pane, F., Niederwieser, D., Saglio, G., Apperley, J., Cervantes, F., Deininger, M., Gratwohl, A., Guilhot, F., Hochhaus, A., Horowitz, M., Hughes, T., Kantarjian, H., Larson, R., Radich, J., Simonsson, B., Silver, R. T., Goldman, J., and Hehlmann, R. Chronic myeloid leukemia: an update of concepts and management recommendations of European leukemia Net. *J. Clin. Oncol.* **2009**, *27*, 6041–6051.
6. Lissauer, H. Zwei Falle von Leukamie. *Berliner Klinische Wochenschrift* **1865**, *2*, 403–404.
7. Zhang, X., Yan, X., Zhou, Z., Yang, F., Wu, Z., Sun, H., Liang, W., Song, A., Lallemand-Breitenbach, V., Jeanne, M., Zhang, Q., Yang, H., Huang, Q., Zhou, G., Tong, J., Zhang, Y., Wu, J., Hu, H., de Thé, H., Chen, S., and Chen, Z. Arsenic trioxide controls the fate of the PML-RARa oncoprotein by directly binding PML. *Science* **2010**, *328*, 240–243.
8. Gilman, A., and Philips, F. S. The biological actions and therapeutic applications of the b chloroethyl amines and sulfides. *Science* **1946**, *103*, 409–415.
9. Haddow, A. and Timmis, G. M. Myleran in chronic myeloid leukaemia chemical constitution and biological action. *Lancet* **1953**, *261*, 207–208.
10. Jiang, W., Xie, J., Varano, P. T., Krebs, C., and Bollinger, J. M., Jr., Two distinct mechanisms of inactivation of the class Ic ribonucleotide reductase from Chlamydia trachomatis by hydroxyurea: implications for the protein gating of intersubunit electron transfer. *Biochemistry* **2010**, *49*, 5340–5349.
11. Hehlmann, R., Berger, U., Pfirrmann, M., Hochhaus, A., Metzgeroth, G., Maywald, O., Hasford, J., Reiter, A., Hossfeld, D. K., Kolb, H.-J., Loeffler, H., Pralle, H., Queisser, W., Griesshammer, M., Nerl, C., Kuse, R., Tobler, A., Eimermacher, H., Tichelli, A., Aul, C., Wilhelm, M., Fischer, J. T., Perker, M., Scheid, C., Schenk, M., Weiss, J., Meier, C. R., Kremers, S., Labedzki, L., Schmeiser, T., Lohrmann, H.-P., and Heimpel, H. Randomized comparison of interferon-alpha and hydroxyurea with hydroxyurea monotherapy in chronic myeloid leukemia (CML-study II): prolongation of survival by the combination of interferon-alpha and hydroxyurea. *Leukemia* **2003**, *17*, 1529–1537.
12. Griesshammer, M., Hehlmann, R., Hochhaus, A., Talpaz, M., Tura, S., Stryckmans, P., Allan, N. C., Tanzer, J., Kolb, H. J., and Heimpel, H. Interferon in chronic myeloid leukemia: a workshop report. *Ann. Hematol.* **1993**, *67*, 101–106.
13. Hasford, J., Pfirrmann, M., Hehlmann, R., Allan, N. C., Baccarani, M., Kluin-Nelemans, J. C., Alimena, G., Steegmann, J. L., and Ansari, H. A new prognostic score for survival of patients with chronic myeloid leukemia treated with interferon alfa. Writing Committee for the Collaborative CML Prognostic Factors Project Group. *J. Natl. Cancer Inst.* **1998**, *90*, 850–858.
14. Baccarani, M., Russo, D., Rosti, G., and Martinelli, G. Interferon-alfa for chronic myeloid leukemia. *Semin. Hematol.* **2003**, *40*, 22–33.
15. Griffin, J. D. Management of chronic myelogenous leukemia. *Semin. Hematol.* **1986**, *23*, 20–26.
16. Nowell, P. C. Discovery of the Philadelphia chromosome: a personal perspective. *J. Clin. Invest.* **2007**, *117*, 2033–2035.
17. Rowley, J. D. Letter: a new consistent chromosomal abnormality in chronic myelogenous leukaemia identified by quinacrine fluorescence and Giemsa staining. *Nature* **1973**, *243*, 290–293.
18. Abelson, H. T., and Rabstein, L. S. Lymphosarcoma: virus-induced thymic-independent disease in mice. *Cancer Res.* **1970**, *30*, 2213–2222.
19. Witte, O. N., Rosenberg, N., Paskind, M., Shields, A., and Baltimore, D. Identification of an Abelson murine leukemia virus-encoded protein present in transformed fibroblast and lymphoid cells. *Proc. Natl. Acad. Sci. USA.* **1978**, *75*, 2488–2492.
20. Hunter, T. Treatment for chronic myelogenous leukemia: the long road to imatinib. *J. Clin. Invest.* **2007**, *117*, 2036–2043.
21. Heisterkamp, N., Stephensen, J. R., Groffen, J., Hansen, P. F., De Klein, A., Bartram, C. R., and Grosveld, G. Localization of the c-abl oncogene adjacent to a translocation break point in chronic myelocytic leukaemia. *Nature* **1983**, *306*, 239–242.
22. Kurzrock, R., Gutterman, J. U., and Talpaz, M. The molecular genetics of Philadelphia chromosome-positive leukemias. *New Engl. J. Med.* **1988**, *319*, 990–998.
23. Beissert T., Puccetti E., Bianchini A., Guller S., Boehrer S., and Hoelzer D. Targeting of the N-terminal coiled coil oligomerization interface of BCR interferes with the transformation potential of BCR-ABL and increases sensitivity to STI571. *Blood* **2003** *102*, 2985–2993.
24. Brehme, M., Hantschel, O., Colinge, J., Kaupe, I., Planyavsky, M., Kocher, T., Mechtler, K., Bennett, K. L., and Superti-Furga, G. Charting the molecular network of the drug target Bcr-Abl. *Proc. Natl. Acad. Sci. USA* **2009**, *106*, 7414–7419.
25. Daley, G. Q., Van Etten, R. A., and Baltimore, D. Induction of chronic myelogenous leukemia in mice by the P210bcr/abl gene of the Philadelphia chromosome. *Science* **1990**, *247*, 824–830.

26. Schwartzberg, P. L., Stall, A. M., Hardin, J. D., Bowdish, K. S., Humaran, T., Boast, S., Harbison, M. L., Robertson, E. J., and Goff, S. P. Mice homozygous for the ablm1 mutation show poor viability and depletion of selected B and T cell populations. *Cell* **1991**, *65*, 1165–1175.
27. Manning, G., Whyte, D. B., Martinez, R., Hunter, T., and Sudarsanam, S. The protein kinase complement of the human genome. *Science* **2002**, *298*, 1912–1934.
28. Rüegg, U. T. and Burgess, G. M. Staurosporine, K-252 and UCN-01: potent but nonspecific inhibitors of protein kinases. *Trends Pharm. Sci.* **1989**, *10*, 218–220.
29. Torley, L. W., Johnson, B. D., and Dusza, J. P.4,5,6-Substituted pyridinamines. *European Patent Application* 233461, August 26, 1987.
30. Paul, R., Hallett, W. A., Hanifin, J. W., Reich, M. F., Johnson, B. D., Lenhard, R. H., Dusza, J. P., Kerwar, S. S., Lin, Y., Pickett, W. C., Seifert, C. M., Torley, L. W., Tarrant, M. E., and Wrenn, S. Preparation of substituted *N*-phenyl-4-aryl-2-pyrimidinamines as mediator release inhibitors. *J. Med. Chem.* **1993**, *36*, 2716–2725.
31. Lydon, N. B., Adams, B., Poschet, J. F., Gutzwiller, A., and Matter, A. An *E. coli* expression system for the rapid purification and expression of a v-abl tyrosine protein kinase. *Oncogene Res.* **1990**, *5*, 161–173.
32. Zimmermann, J., Buchdunger, E., Mett, H., Meyer, T., Lydon, N. B., and Traxler, P. (Phenylamino)pyrimidine (PAP) derivatives: a new class of potent and highly selective PDGF-receptor autophosphorylation inhibitors. *Bioorg. Med. Chem. Lett.* **1996**, *6*, 1221–1226.
33. Zimmermann J., Buchdunger, E., Mett, H., Meyer, T., and Lydon, N. B. Potent and selective inhibitors of the ABL-kinase: phenylaminopyrimidine (PAP) derivatives. *Bioorg. Med. Chem. Lett.* **1997**, *7*, 187–192.
34. Bredereck, H., Effenberger, F., and Botsch, H. Untersuchungen über die reaktionsfähigkeit von formamidinen, dimethylformamid-diäthylacetal (Amidacetal) und bis-dimethylamino-methoxy-methan (Aminalester). *Chem. Ber.* **1964**, *97*, 3397–3406.
35. Druker, B. J., Tamura, S., Buchdunger, E., Ohno, S., Segal, G. M., Fanning, S., Zimmermann, J., and Lydon, N. B. Effects of a selective inhibitor of the Abl tyrosine kinase on the growth of Bcr-Abl positive cells. *Nat. Med.* **1996**, *2*, 561–566.
36. Druker, B. J., Talpaz, M., Resta, D. J., Peng, B., Buchdunger, E., Ford, J. M., Lydon, N. B., Kantarjian, H., Capdeville, R., Ohno-Jones, S., and Sawyers, C. L. Efficacy and safety of a specific inhibitor of the BCR-ABL tyrosine kinase in chronic myeloid leukemia. *N. Engl. J. Med.* **2001**, *344*, 1031–1037.
37. Guilhot, F. Indications for imatinib mesylate therapy and clinical management. *Oncologist* **2004**, *9*, 271–281.
38. Roy, L., Guilhot, J., Krahnke, T., Guerci-Bresler, A., Druker, B. J., Larson, R. A., O'Brien, S., So, C., Massimini, G., and Guilhot, F. Survival advantage from imatinib compared with the combination interferon-α plus cytarabine in chronic-phase chronic myelogenous leukemia: historical comparison between two phase 3 trials. *Blood* **2006**, *108*, 1478–1484.
39. Hochhaus, A., O'Brien, S. G., Guilhot, F., Druker, B. J., Branford, S., Foroni, L., Goldman, J. M., Müller, M.C., Radich, J. P., Rudoltz, M., Mone, M., Gathmann, I., Hughes, T. P., and Larson, R. A. Six-year follow-up of patients receiving imatinib for the first-line treatment of chronic myeloid leukemia. *Leukemia* **2009**, *23*, 1054–1061.
40. Corbin, A. S., Toledo, L. M., Lydon, N. B., Buchdunger, E., Kuriyan, J., and Druker, B. J. Analysis of the structural basis of specificity of inhibition of the Abl kinase by STI571. *Blood* **2000**, *96*, 470a.
41. Gorre, M. E., Mohammed, M., Ellwood, K., Hsu, N., Paquette, R., Rao, P. N., and Sawyers, C. L. Clinical resistance to STI-571 cancer therapy caused by BCR-ABL gene mutation or amplification. *Science* **2001**, *293*, 876–880.
42. Schindler, T., Bornmann, W., Pellicena, P., Miller, W. T., Clarkson, B., and Kuriyan, J. Structural mechanism for STI-571 inhibition of Abelson tyrosine kinase. *Science* **2000**, *289*, 1938–1942.
43. Apperley, J. F. Part I: mechanisms of resistance to imatinib in chronic myeloid leukemia. *Lancet Oncol.* **2007**, *8*, 1018–1029.
44. Kantarjian, H. M., Giles, F., Gattermann, N., Bhalla, K., Alimena, G., Palandri, F., Ossenkoppele, G. J., Nicolini, F.-E., O'Brien, S. G., Litzow, M., Bhatia, R., Cervantes, F., Haque, A., Shou, Y., Resta, D. J., Weitzman, A., Hochhaus, A., and Le Coutre, P. Nilotinib (formerly AMN107), a highly selective BCR-ABL tyrosine kinase inhibitor, is effective in patients with Philadelphia chromosome-positive chronic myelogenous leukemia in chronic phase following imatinib resistance and intolerance. *Blood* **2007**, *110*, 3540–3546.
45. Le Coutre, P., Ottmann, O. G., Giles, F., Kim, D.-W., Cortes, J., Gattermann, N., Apperley, J. F., Larson, R. A., Abruzzese, E., O'Brien, S. G., Kuliczkowski, K., Hochhaus, A., Mahon, F.-X., Saglio, G., Gobbi, M., Kwong, Y.-L., Baccarani, M., Hughes, T., Martinelli, G., Radich, J. P., Zheng, M., Shou, Y., and Kantarjian, H. Nilotinib (formerly AMN107), a highly selective BCR-ABL tyrosine kinase inhibitor, is active in patients with imatinib-resistant or -intolerant accelerated-phase chronic myelogenous leukemia. *Blood* **2008**, *111*, 1834–1839.
46. Cowan-Jacob, S. W., Guez, V., Fendrich, G., Griffin, J. D., Fabbro, D., Furet, P., Liebetanz, J., Mestan, J., and Manley, P. W. Imatinib (STI571) resistance in chronic myelogenous leukemia: molecular basis of the underlying mechanisms and potential strategies for treatment. *Mini-Rev. Med. Chem.* **2004**, *4*, 285–299.
47. Nagar, B., Bornmann, W. G., Pellicena, P., Schindler, T., Veach, D. R., Miller, W. T.RRCR.R. Clarkson, B., and Kuriyan, J. Crystal structures of the kinase domain of c-Abl in complex with the small molecule inhibitors PD173955 and imatinib (STI-571). *Cancer Res.* **2002**, *62*, 4236–4243.

48. Manley, P. W., Cowan-Jacob, S. W., Buchdunger, E., Fabbro, D., Fendrich, G., Furet, P., Meyer, T., and Zimmermann, J. Imatinib: a selective tyrosine kinase inhibitor. *Eur. J. Cancer* **2002**, *38*, S19–S27.
49. Cowan-Jacob, S. W., Fendrich, G., Floersheimer, A., Furet, P., Liebetanz, J., Rummel, G., Rheinberger, P., Centeleghe, M., Fabbro, D., and Manley, P. W. Structural biology contributions to the discovery of drugs to treat chronic myelogenous leukaemia. *Acta Crystallogr. D Biol. Crystallogr.* **2007**, *D63*, 80–93.
50. Weisberg, E., Manley, P. W., Breitenstein, W., Brüggen, J., Cowan-Jacob, S.W., Ray, A., Huntly, B., Fabbro, D., Fendrich, G., Hall-Meyers, E., Kung, A. L., Mestan, J., Daley, G. Q., Callahan, L., Catley, L., Cavazza, C., Azam, M., Neuberg, D., Wright, R. D., Gilliland, D. G., and Griffin, J. D. Characterization of AMN107, a selective inhibitor of native and mutant Bcr-Abl. *Cancer Cell* **2005**, *7*, 129–141.
51. Manley, P. W., Breitenstein, W., Brüggen, J., Cowan-Jacob, S. W., Furet, P., Mestan, J., and Meyer, T. Urea-derivatives of STI571 as inhibitors of Bcr-Abl and PDGFR kinases. *Bioorg. Med. Chem. Lett.* **2004**, *14*, 5793–5797.
52. Manley, P. W., Stiefl, N., Cowan-Jacob, S. W., Kaufman, S., Mestan, J., Wartmann, M., Wiesmann, M., Woodman, R., and Gallagher, N. Structural resemblances and comparisons of the relative pharmacological properties of imatinib and nilotinib. *Bioorg. Med. Chem.* **2010**, *18*, 6977–6986.
53. Jensen, M. R., Brüggen, J., DiLea, C., Mestan, J., and Manley, P. W. AMN107: efficacy of the selective Bcr-Abl tyrosine kinase inhibitor in a murine model of chronic myelogenous leukemia. *Proc. Am. Assoc. Cancer Res.* **2006**, *47*, 61–62.
54. Weisberg, E., Manley, P. W., Mestan, J., Cowan-Jacob, S., Ray, A., and Griffin, J. D. AMN107 (nilotinib): a novel and selective inhibitor of BCR-ABL. *Br. J. Cancer.* **2006**, *94*, 1765–1769.
55. von Bubnoff N., Manley P. W., Mestan J., Sanger J., Peschel C., and Duyster J. Bcr-Abl resistance screening predicts a limited spectrum of point mutations to be associated with clinical resistance to the Abl kinase inhibitor nilotinib (AMN107). *Blood* **2006**, *108*, 1328–1333.
56. Bradeen H. A., Eide C. A., O'Hare T., Johnson K. J., Willis S.G., Lee F. Y., Druker B. J., and Deininger M. W. Comparison of imatinib mesylate, dasatinib (BMS-354825), and nilotinib (AMN107) in an *N*-ethyl-*N*-nitrosourea (ENU)-based mutagenesis screen: high efficacy of drug combinations. *Blood* **2006**, *108*, 2332–2338.
57. Ray A., Cowan-Jacob S. W., Manley P. W., Mestan J., and Griffin J. D. Identification of Bcr/Abl point mutations conferring resistance to the Abl kinase inhibitor AMN107 (Nilotinib) by a random mutagenesis study. *Blood* **2007**, *109*, 5011–5015.
58. Tanaka, C., Yin, O., Sethuraman, V., Smith, T., Wang, X. F., Grouss, K., Kantarjian, H., Giles, F., Ottmann, O. G., Galitz, L., and Schran, H. Clinical pharmacokinetics of the BCR-ABL tyrosine kinase inhibitor nilotinib. *Clin. Pharmacol. Ther.* **2010**, *87*, 197–203.
59. Kantarjian, H., Giles, F., Wunderle, L., Bhalla, K., O'Brien, S., Wassmann, B., Tanaka, C., Manley, P., Rae, P., Mietlowski, W., Bochinski, K., Hochhaus, A., Griffin, J. D., Hoelzer, D., Albitar, M., Dugan, M., Cortes, J., Alland, L., and Ottmann, O. G. Nilotinib in imatinib-resistant CML and Philadelphia chromosome-positive ALL. *New Engl. J. Med.* **2006**, *354*, 2542–2551.
60. Saglio, G., Kim, D.-W., Issaragrisil, S., Le Coutre, P., Etienne, G., Lobo, C., Pasquini, R., Clark, R. E., Hochhaus, A., Hughes, T. P., Gallagher, N., Hoenekopp, A., Dong, M., Haque, A., Larson, R. A., and Kantarjian, H. M. Nilotinib is superior to imatinib in patients with newly diagnosed chronic myeloid leukemia in chronic phase: results from ENESTnd. *New Engl. J. Med.* **2010**, *362*, 2251–2259.

CHAPTER 6

AMRUBICIN, A COMPLETELY SYNTHETIC 9-AMINOANTHRACYCLINE FOR EXTENSIVE-DISEASE SMALL-CELL LUNG CANCER

Mitsuharu Hanada

6.1 INTRODUCTION

Lung cancer is the most common cancer in the world [1], and small-cell lung cancer (SCLC) accounts for approximately 15% to 20% of all cases of lung cancer. Although SCLC is highly responsive to initial chemotherapy or radiotherapy, complete responses (CRs) are seen in a minority of patients, response durations are short, and overall survival (OS) is still dismal [2]. Non-small-cell lung cancer (NSCLC) comprises approximately 80% to 90% of lung cancer, and the majority of patients have locally advanced stage III or metastatic stage IV at diagnosis. Combination chemotherapy has an overall response rate (ORR) of 25% to 50% against NSCLC; however, NSCLC remains generally refractory to systemic chemotherapy when compared to SCLC.

The currently accepted global standard for previously untreated SCLC patients is combination chemotherapy including cisplatin (CDDP) and etoposide. Since a phase III trial in patients with extensive disease -SCLC (ED-SCLC) demonstrated that a combination of CDDP and irinotecan yielded a highly significant improvement in survival over a standard regimen consisting of CDDP and etoposide, the former combination is now regarded as the standard treatment for ED-SCLC in Japan [3]. New active agents, including irinotecan, paclitaxel, docetaxel, gemcitabine, and vinorelbine (Figure 6.1), were introduced for the treatment of naïve SCLC patients around 1990; however, there has been no significant improvement in the survival of patients with SCLC [4]. After completion of the first-line treatment, approximately 80% of limited-disease patients and almost all patients with extensive disease will develop disease relapse or progression. There is evidence that response to second-line chemotherapy is influenced by the treatment-free interval after first-line therapy. Patients with "refractory" SCLC who relapse less than 3 months after first-line therapy are less likely to show an objective response than patients with "sensitive" SCLC who relapse more than 3 months after therapy. Topotecan has been recognized as a key drug in the second-line treatment of SCLC and is the only agent approved for this condition in the United States and Europe, primarily based on data from three phase III trials (Figure 6.1) [5,6]. One demonstrated that topotecan as a single agent was at least as effective as the combination of cyclophosphamide, doxorubicin (adriamycin), and vincristine (CAV)

Case Studies in Modern Drug Discovery and Development, Edited by Xianhai Huang and Robert G. Aslanian.

in patients with sensitive SCLC (Figure 6.1) [5]. Greater symptom improvement and less toxicity were associated with topotecan treatment than CAV treatment although there was no significant difference in the response rate (RR) and median survival. However, the prognosis for patients who receive second-line chemotherapy after relapse remains extremely poor; therefore, there is a clear need for novel and effective agents and/or combinations to treat patients with SCLC.

Anthracycline derivatives are among the most widely used antitumor agents in clinical oncology today. Approximately 60% to 80% of patients with acute myeloid leukemia achieve complete remission with a standard induction regimen including cytarabine and daunorubicin (DNR) (Figure 6.1) [7]. Anthracyclines, such as doxorubicin (DXR) and epirubicin (Figure 6.1), have been used for over 30 years and are widely considered as the standard first-line chemotherapy for metastatic breast cancer. Anthracycline-based

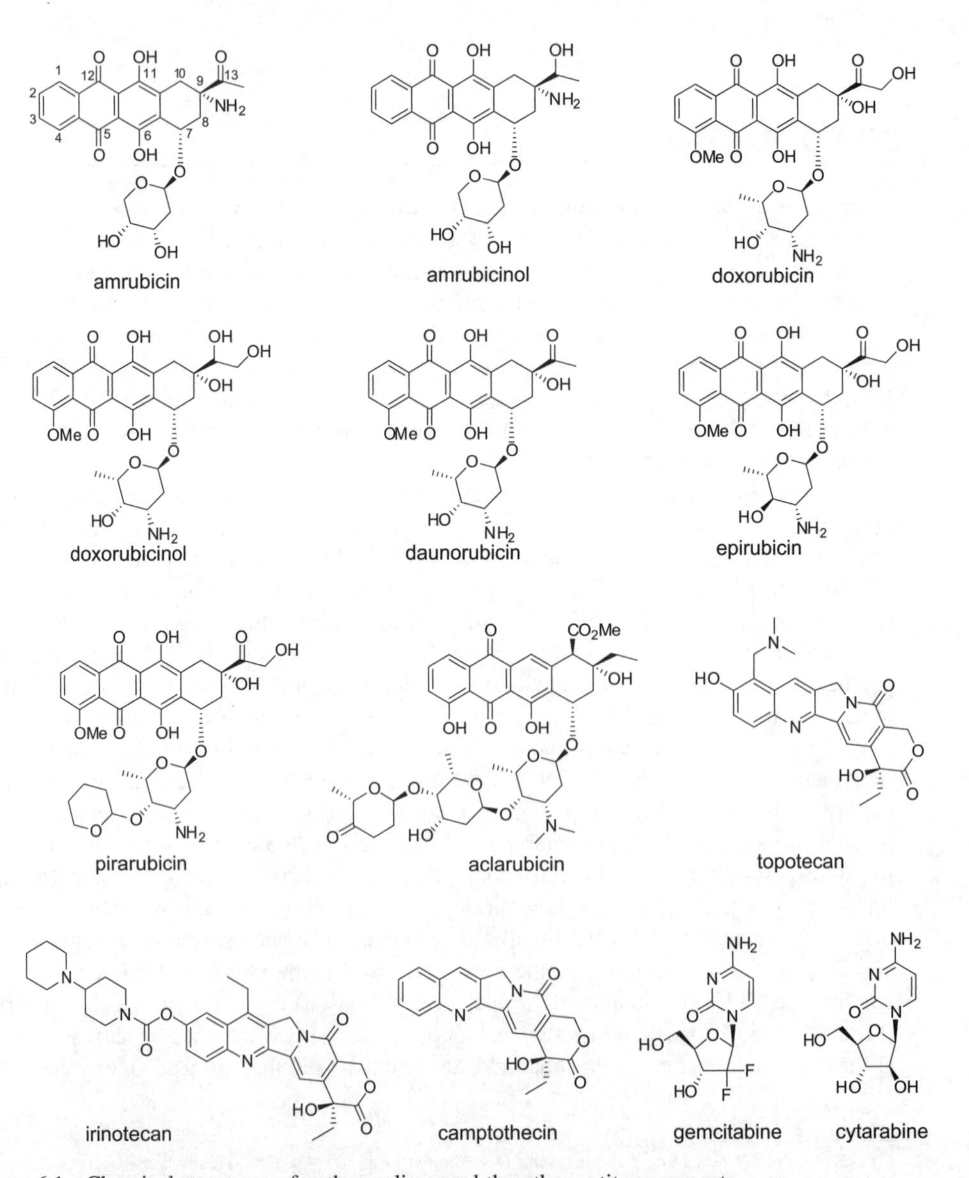

Figure 6.1 Chemical structures of anthracyclines and the other antitumor agents.

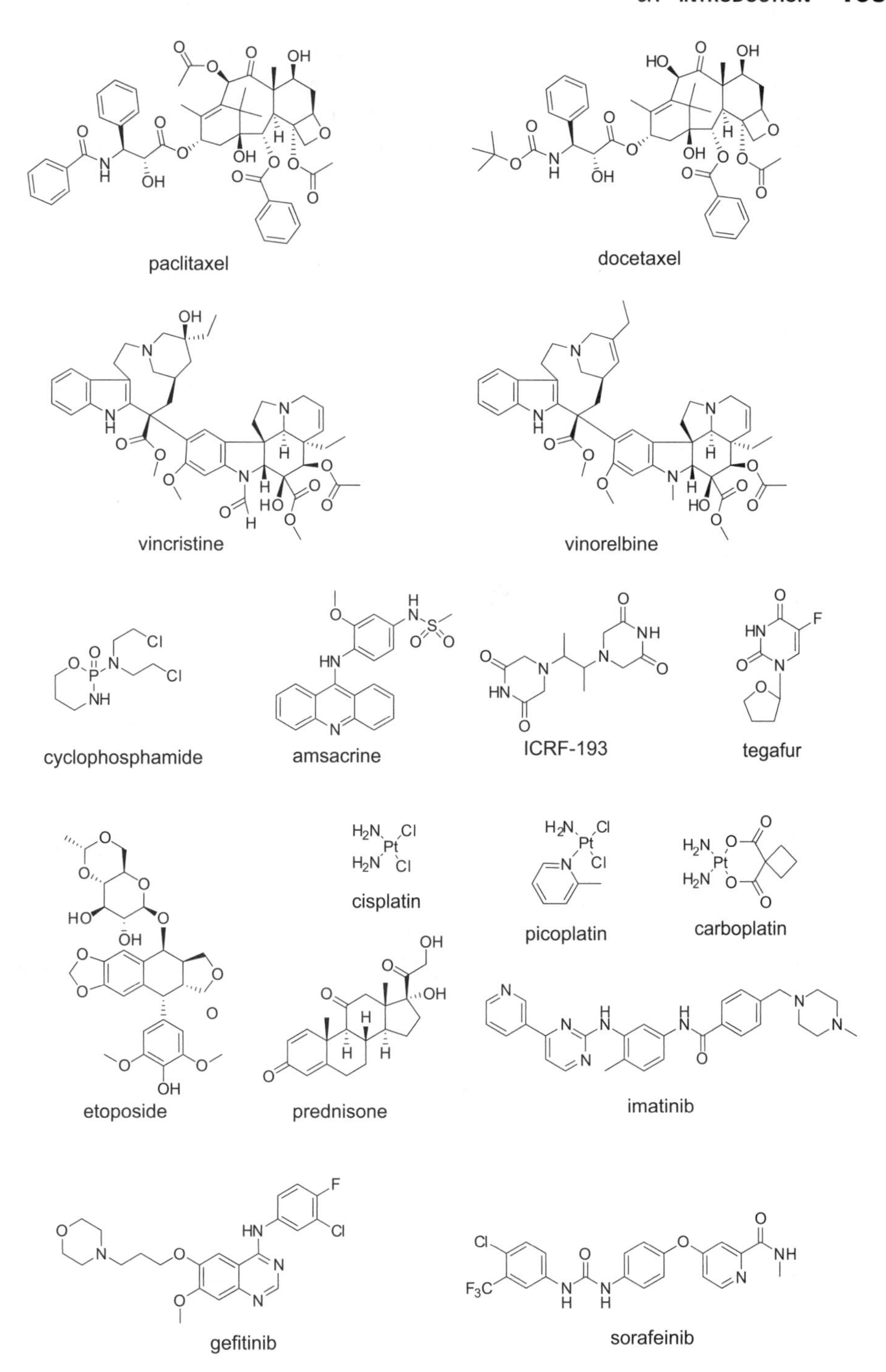
paclitaxel
docetaxel
vincristine
vinorelbine
cyclophosphamide
amsacrine
ICRF-193
tegafur
cisplatin
picoplatin
carboplatin
etoposide
prednisone
imatinib
gefitinib
sorafeinib

Figure 6.1 (*Continued*)

regimens with cyclophosphamide, DXR, and docetaxel are often associated with improved RR and time to progression [8]. In the past, combination chemotherapy, consisting of cyclophosphamide, DXR (hydroxydaunorubicin), vincristine (Oncovin ®), and prednisone (CHOP), was considered the gold-standard treatment for aggressive non-Hodgkin's lymphoma (NHL). The addition of rituximab to CHOP is now considered the standard of care for the treatment of diffuse large B-cell lymphoma, the most common form of NHL, because it has been associated with improvements in OS and progression-free survival (PFS) without increased toxicity [9].

Anthracyclines rank among the most effective antitumor agents ever developed; however, their clinical use is hampered by such serious problems as the development of resistance by tumor cells or toxicity in healthy tissues, most notably in the form of chronic cardiomyopathy and congestive heart failure (CHF) [10]. Anthracycline-induced cardiomyopathy and CHF are dose-dependent, and their incidence increases sharply when the cumulative dose of anthracycline exceeds 500 mg m^{-2}; therefore, the maximum recommended cumulative dose of DXR has been tentatively set at 450–600 mg m^{-2}.

6.2 THE DISCOVERY OF AMRUBICIN: THE FIRST COMPLETELY SYNTHETIC ANTHRACYCLINE

Since DNR and DXR produced by *Streptomyces* were isolated early in the 1960s, a great effort has been made to identify superior novel anthracyclines in terms of activity and/or cardiac tolerability. Although various chemical modifications, substitutions, and conjugations have been introduced in the tetracyclic ring, the side chain, or amino sugar, only a few derivatives have obtained clinical approval. These include epirubicin, idarubicin, pirarubicin, and aclarubicin (Figure 6.1). Most clinically available anthracycline derivatives have been produced by fermentation or semisynthesis, which might make it difficult to markedly improve the chemical structure of anthracycline derivatives without limit. All clinically available anthracyclines have a hydroxyl group at the 9-position and an amino sugar moiety at the 7-position. To discover novel anthracycline derivatives, a different approach was adopted using total synthesis. After establishing a synthetic route for 9-amino-9-deoxydaunomycin [11], we investigated whether various 9-aminoanthracycline derivatives could show a clear advantage over DXR in terms of antitumor activity and safety *in vivo*. Our primary screening assay evaluated the increase in lifespan of mice implanted with the mouse leukemia cell line P388 intraperitoneally, and active derivatives were secondarily tested in human tumor xenografts to compare with DXR. Among these derivatives, amrubicin hydrochloride (formerly SM-5887, Calsed®) was almost equipotent to DXR against the murine experimental tumors and exhibited greater efficacy in human tumor xenografts [12]. All nine human tumors tested showed apparent responses to intravenously administered amrubicin, and the growth of seven was suppressed by amrubicin 25 mg kg^{-1} with minimum T/C values of 50% or less (Table 6.1). T/C values were calculated by comparing the tumor volume of the treated group with those of the control group. Compared with DXR, amrubicin was significantly more effective in several tumors, including the breast cancer cell line MX-1 and the SCLC cell line LX-1.

Amrubicin, the first completely synthetic anthracycline derivative in the world, is characterized by a 9-amino group and a simple sugar moiety at the 7-position (Figure 6.1). Many modifications were needed to establish a synthetic method for the commercial production of amrubicin hydrochloride based on the original synthetic route (Figure 6.2) [13]. Due to the low solubility in organic solvents of the intermediates with an anthracycline structure, solvents choices were very limited. Most of the reaction

TABLE 6.1 Antitumor Effects of Amrubicin and Doxorubicin on the Growth of Human Tumor Xenograft Models[a]

		Minimum *T/C* (%)	
	Cell lines	Amrubicin	Doxorubicin
Breast	MX-1	13	30
Lung	LX-1	25	44
	QG-56	53	28
Stomach	SC-6	12	38
	SC-7	51	52
	SC-9	27	45
	St-4	23	16
	St-15	45	40
	4-1ST	4	26

[a]Female athymic nude mice, BALB/c nu/nu, were injected subcutaneously with tumor fragments in the flank. A few weeks after this inoculation, mice bearing a tumor approximately 100–300 mm^3 in volume were randomly allocated into different treatment groups and a control group, each of which consisted of 6 mice. Amrubicin and doxorubicin were administered intravenously at doses of 25 and 12.5 mg/kg, respectively. *T/C* values were calculated by comparing the tumor volume of the treated group with those of the control group. Minimum *T/C* was the lowest value of *T/C* for each day that the tumors were measured.

intermediates were chemically unstable because of the unique structure of the labile amino group on the quaternary carbon center, which required strict control of pH and temperature. The main changes in the synthesis were as follows. To introduce the methylketone safely, the solvent was changed to methyl phenyl sulfone from dimethyl sulfoxide. The protecting group for the 9-amino moiety was changed from an acetyl group to a trifluoroacetyl group. Instead of ethylene glycol and *p*-toluenesulfonic acid, neopentyl glycol and Amberlyst 15 resin were used to protect the 13-keto group. Keeping the water content in the range of 3–8%, more preferably 4–7%, was important not only for the storage of amrubicin hydrochloride but also during its drying in order to control the final content of aglycon and deamination by-products in the final manufacturing step.

6.3 TOXICOLOGICAL PROFILE OF AMRUBICIN

Although amrubicin is distinctly different in chemical structure from existing anthracyclines, including DXR, this does not necessarily indicate that amrubicin shows any clinical benefit superior to DXR. In order to confirm that amrubicin is a suitable candidate worthy of clinical trials, its pharmacological and toxicological profile was examined, focusing on the difference between amrubicin and DXR.

The major long-term side effect of anthracyclines is cardiotoxicity. It has been shown that amrubicin has less cardiotoxicity than DXR in beagle and rabbit models [14,15]. Morphological changes in myocardial tissue and electrocardiogram (ECG) changes in rabbits administered DXR (0.8 mg kg^{-1}, three times a week for 8 weeks) were remarkable; marked vacuolation due to enlargement of the sarcoplasmic reticulum, lysis of myofibrils, bradycardia, prolongation of QTc interval, and S–T changes were observed. Histopathological findings of myocardial tissue in the amrubicin group (0.8 or 1.6 mg kg^{-1}) were quantitatively comparable to those in the negative control group. ECG changes such as prolongation of QRS interval and ST–T changes were observed, but these changes were transient and reversible in amrubicin groups. Dogs receiving DXR (1.5 mg kg^{-1}, every

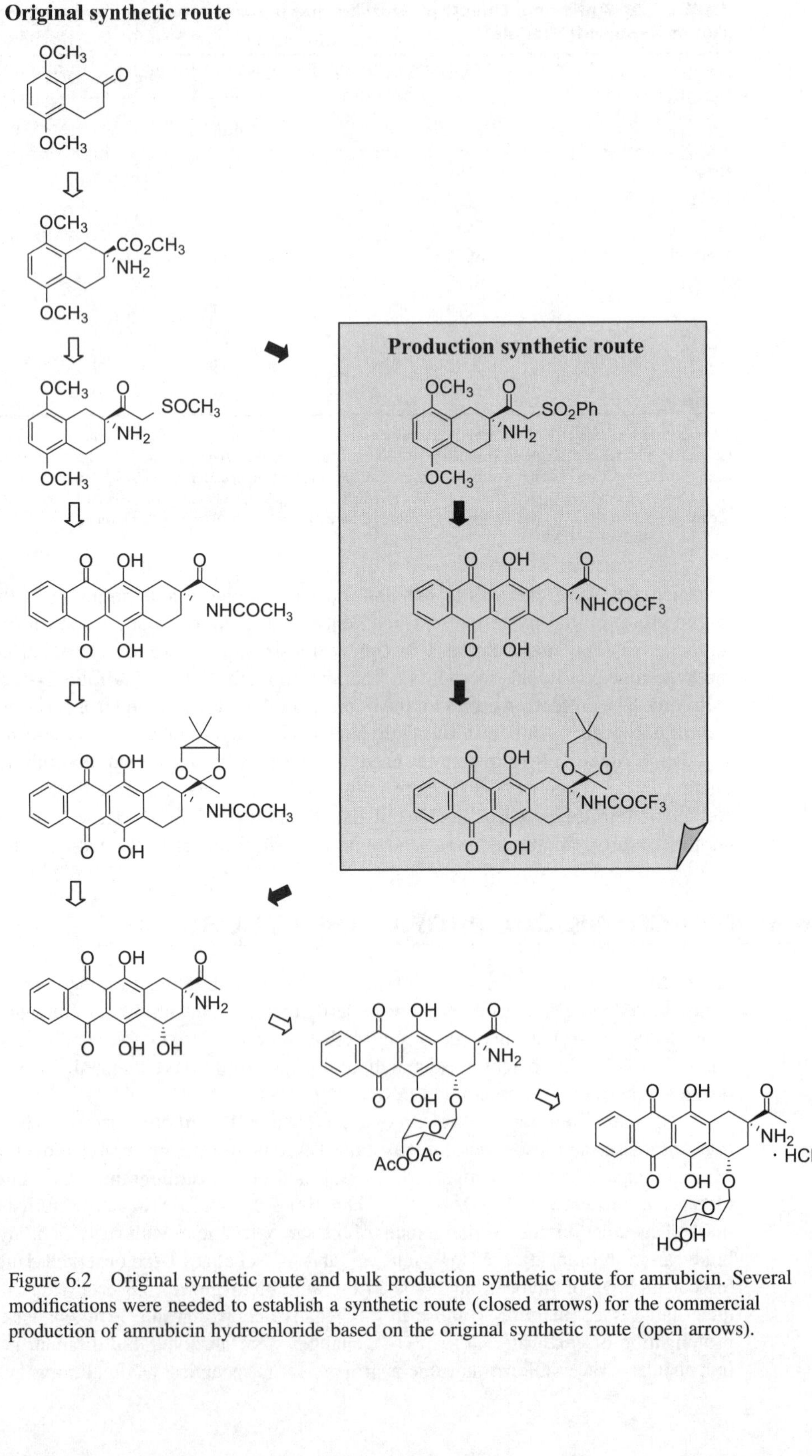

Original synthetic route

Production synthetic route

Figure 6.2 Original synthetic route and bulk production synthetic route for amrubicin. Several modifications were needed to establish a synthetic route (closed arrows) for the commercial production of amrubicin hydrochloride based on the original synthetic route (open arrows).

3 weeks for 6 months) demonstrated ECG changes, low blood pressure, and high-grade cardiomyopathy, while those administered amrubicin (1.5 or 2.5 mg kg^{-1}) did not show any changes in ECG, blood pressure, and histopathological examinations. In addition, amrubicin did not progress the grade of cardiomyopathy induced in dogs by DXR. The cardiac safety profile of amrubicin was confirmed by data from a pooled study of two phase II studies in ED-SCLC [16]. The study demonstrated a minimal change in the left ventricular ejection fraction (LEVF) percentage from the baseline in 115 patients treated with amrubicin, even at a cumulative dose exceeding 1000 mg m^{-2}. The C-13 hydroxyl metabolite of anthracyclines, especially doxorubicinol, influences the risk of anthracycline-related cardiotoxicity. Cardiomyopathy correlates with the accumulation of doxorubicinol in the heart, and anthracyclines that form less C-13 hydroxyl metabolite are less cardiotoxic. Despite the importance of DXR reduction, the underlying enzymes and their tissue distribution are poorly characterized. Thus far, DXR reduction has been shown for carbonyl reductase 1 (CBR1), aldo-keto reductase (AKR) 1A1, and AKR 1B1. Transgenic mice that overexpress human CBR1 in the heart show increased heart damage followed by decreased survival after DXR treatment [17], while knockouts heterozygous for *Cbr1* are less sensitive to DXR [18]. These data implicate CBR as a potent contributor to DXR-induced cardiotoxicity. It has been shown that CBR was one of the enzymes mediating the metabolism of amrubicin to amrubicinol [19], suggesting that CBR-mediated reduction of amrubicin might potentially influence cardiotoxicity.

Besides cardiotoxicity at a high cumulative dose of DXR, various side effects, such as myelosuppression, mucositis, alopecia, and gastrointestinal toxicity, restrict its clinical use. In general, preclinical data obtained from mice suggested that toxic effects of amrubicin were more reversible and controllable than those of DXR. The acute toxicities of amrubicin and DXR in mice, such as body weight decrease, ataxia, hair loss, and myelosuppression, were qualitatively similar [20]. The maximum tolerated doses (MTD) following a single intravenous administration in mice were estimated to be 25 mg kg^{-1} for amrubicin and 12.5 mg kg^{-1} for DXR, with no toxic death or body weight loss of more than 3 g. The tissue distribution of amrubicin at this dose was 3.2 L kg^{-1}, and the half-life was 1.6 h [21], revealing that amrubicin had a smaller distribution volume and a shorter half-life than DXR. DXR caused frequent and dose-dependent delayed-type lethal toxicity at doses of more than 10 mg kg^{-1}, while amrubicin had little effect. When agents were administered into the mouse tail vain, DXR induced a dose-dependent and long-lasting severe local inflammatory response, whereas this response due to amrubicin was much milder, even at a four-fold higher dose than DXR. On the other hand, amrubicin caused more severe myelosuppression than DXR although there was faster recovery from myelosuppression induced by amrubicin than by DXR. The early myelosuppression and its rapid recovery observed in mice treated with amrubicin might depend on colony-forming units of granulocytes and monocytes [22]. These phenomenon might depend upon differences of absorption, half-life in blood, metabolism, or affinity for stem cells between amrubicin and DXR. This seemed to be reflected in the clinical outcome that amrubicin's major toxicity was myelosuppression, especially neutropenia, as described later. A recent report by Kassner *et al.* showed that CBR1 is the predominant DXR reductase in the human liver; in contrast, DXR reduction in the heart is mediated most likely by AKR 1A1, using purified reductases and a panel of normal human tissues [23]. Gonzalez-Covarrubias *et al.* observed that CBR1 1096G>A polymorphism was significantly associated with lower hepatic CBR1 expression and lower CBR activity [24]. Pharmacokinetic study of amrubicin and amrubicinol revealed that the areas under curves (AUCs) seemed to be associated with the severity of hematologic toxicity [25]. Significant relationships were apparent between the AUC of amrubicinol and leucopenia. These findings suggest that the pharmacological modulation of reductases metabolizing amrubicin might be explored as an alternative strategy to improve the safety of amrubicin. Pretreatment with a CBR1 inhibitor, like hydroxyl-PP [26], might prevent or reduce the severe neutropenia caused by amrubicin. Compared with free DXR, pegylated liposomal DXR is characterized by dose-limiting mucosal and cutaneous toxicities, milder myelosuppression, reduced alopecia, and reduced cardiotoxicity [27,28]. The extended circulation time of liposomal antitumor agents results in changes in the distribution, elimination, and toxicological profile, and sometimes in enhanced efficacy due to their ability to extravasate through the leaky vasculature of tumors. Thus, a pegylated liposomal formulation of amrubicin might be another strategy to reduce or prevent neutropenia.

6.4 DNA TOPOISOMERASE II INHIBITION AND APOPTOSIS INDUCTION BY AMRUBICIN

Mammalian DNA topoisomerase (topo) II is a nuclear enzyme regulating DNA topology through strand breakage, strand passage, and ligation. Thus, topo II is extensively involved in DNA metabolism, including replication, transcription, recombination, and sister chromatid segregation (Figure 6.3). The enzyme is also the primary cellular target of a number of antitumor agents, such as DXR, DNR, amsacrine, and etoposide [29]. These agents interfere

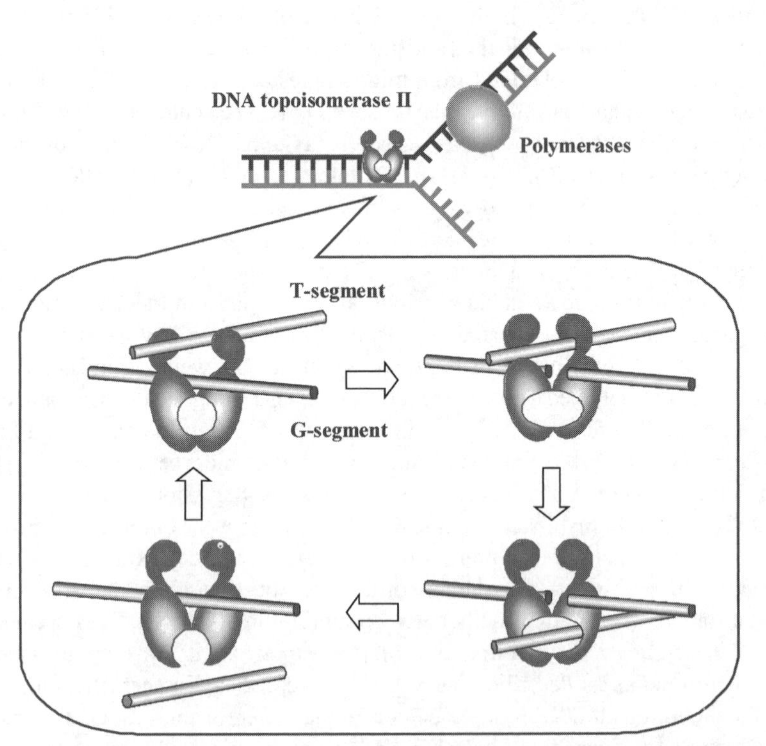

Figure 6.3 A molecular model for the catalytic reaction of DNA topoisomerase II. DNA topoisomerase II is a nuclear enzyme regulating DNA topology through strand breakage, strand passage, and ligation. Thus, it is extensively involved in DNA metabolism, including replication, transcription, recombination, and sister chromatid segregation. (Upper left) DNA topoisomerase II binds the G-segment DNA. (Upper right) Upon binding of ATP and the T-segment, the G-segment is split. (Lower right) The T-segment is transported through the break. (Lower left) Following transport, the G-segment is resealed and the T-segment is released.

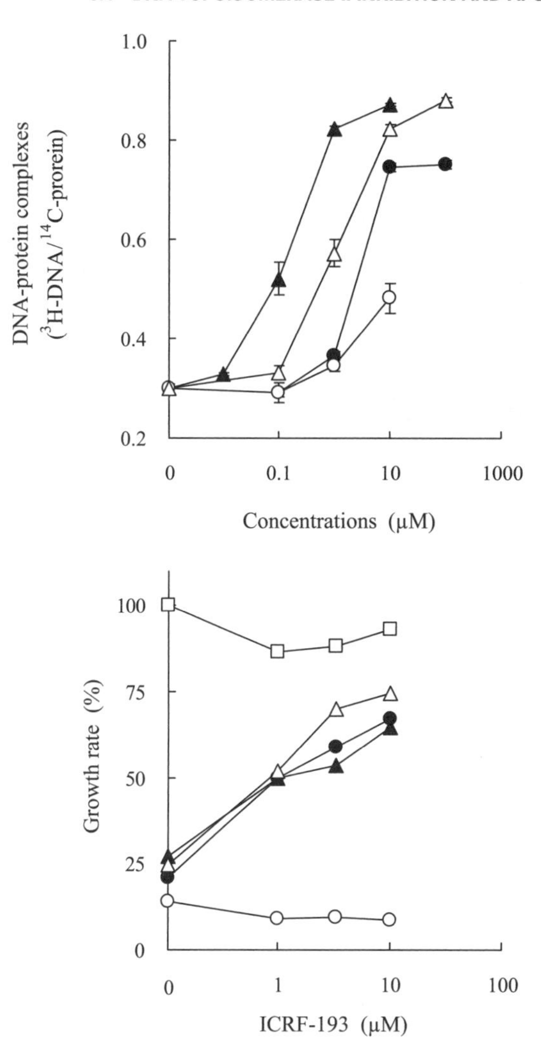

Figure 6.4 Cell growth inhibition mediated by stabilizing topoisomerase II-DNA complex. (Upper) DNA–protein complex formation in human leukemia CCRF-CEM cells. Cells were treated with agents for 1 h at 37 °C. The ability of agents to stabilized DNA–protein complexes was measured by the K-SDS precipitation assay. Amrubicin (closed circle), amrubicinol (closed triangle), DXR (open circle), etoposide (open triangle). Results are given as the average ± SD ($n = 3$). (Lower) Antagonistic effect of ICRF-193 on cell growth inhibition. CCRF-CEM cells were pretreated with ICRF-193 for 30 min and then incubated with both ICRF-193 and each agent. After 1 h, cells were reincubated for 3 days in the absence of agents. ICRF-193 alone (open square), + 5 μM amrubicin (closed circle), + 0.1 μM amrubicinol (closed triangle), + 1 μM DXR (open circle), + 5 μM etoposide (open triangle).

with the breakage–reunion reaction of topo II by trapping a covalent enzyme–DNA complex, termed the "cleavable complex," where DNA strands are broken and their 5′ termini are covalently linked to the enzyme.

Amrubicin, and its major metabolite amrubicinol, inhibited the decatenation of kinetoplast DNA by topo II and stimulated topo II-mediated DNA cleavage [30]. In cultured human leukemia CCRF-CEM cells, amrubicin, and amrubicinol, as well as etoposide, induced both DNA–protein complex formation and double-strand DNA breaks in a dose-dependent manner (Figure 6.4). The IC_{50} values of amrubicin, amrubicinol, DXR, and etoposide for CCRF-CEM cells were 3.3, 0.060, 0.40, and 2.3 μM, respectively. Accordingly, under conditions where cell growth was inhibited by amrubicin, amrubicinol, and etoposide, considerable amounts of DNA–protein complex were formed. In contrast, DXR was less effective in inhibiting cellular topo II under the same conditions although it has been shown to be a topo II inhibitor [30]. ICRF-193, a topo II catalytic inhibitor which lacks the ability to stabilize the cleavable complex [31], antagonized cell growth inhibition, DNA–protein complex formation, and double-strand DNA breaks induced by amrubicin, amrubicinol, or etoposide, but not by DXR (Figure 6.4). We also observed that both

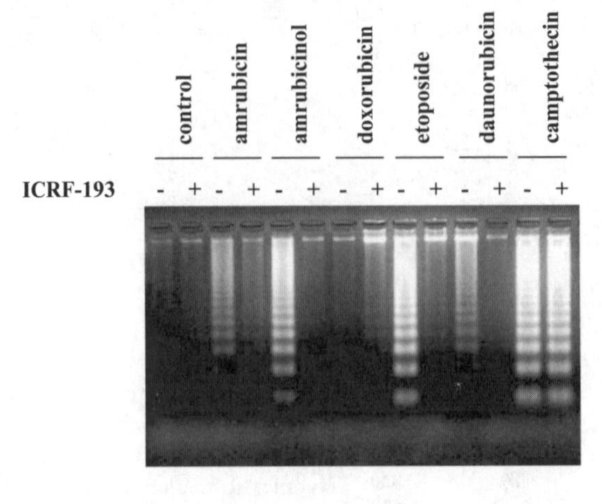

Figure 6.5 Amrubicin-induced apoptosis mediated by DNA topoisomerase II. Human leukemia U937 cells were preincubated with 1 μM ICRF-193 for 30 min and then incubated with both ICRF-193 and 20 μM amrubicin, 0.2 μM amrubicinol, 1 μM DXR, 10 μM etoposide, 1 μM DNR, or 1 μM camptothecin. After 1 h, cells were reincubated for 5 h in the absence of agents, and the DNA fragmentation was analyzed on a 2% agarose gel.

amrubicin and amrubicinol interacted with DNA by intercalation with lower potencies than DXR, and could not inhibit topo I [30]. Accordingly, amrubicin induced cell growth inhibition mainly by stabilizing the topo II–DNA complex.

Apoptosis is a specific mode of cell death with a characteristic pattern of morphological, biochemical,and molecular changes and is well recognized as a distinct pathologic mechanism in tumors responding not only to topo II inhibitors, but also to most antitumor agents. After treatment of human leukemia U937 cells with amrubicin, amrubicinol, DNR, or etoposide, nuclear condensation and fragmentation occurred, and agarose gel electrophoresis revealed internucleosomal DNA fragmentation [32], showing that cells underwent typical apoptosis. DNA fragmentation induced by amrubicin or amrubicinol was antagonized by ICRF-193, indicating that they induced apoptosis mediated by the inhibition of topo II (Figure 6.5). Measuring the populations of sub-G_1 cells by flow cytometric analysis after propidium iodide staining, there was a time-dependent and dose-dependent induction of apoptosis with amrubicin, or amrubicinol, accompanied with cell cycle arrest at G_2/M (Figure 6.6). A variety of key events in apoptosis converge at mitochondria, including the release of cytochrome *c*, loss of mitochondrial membrane potential ($\Delta\Psi_m$), and the participation of pro- and antiapoptotic Bcl-2 family proteins. The central component of the apoptotic machinery is a proteolytic system involving a family of caspases. There are two major pathways for inducing apoptosis: one that starts with the ligation of death receptors leading to caspase-8 activation and another that involves the mitochondrial release of cytochrome *c* enhancing caspase-9 activity (Figure 6.7). Both caspase-8 and -9 activate the same downstream caspases, such as caspase-3, -6, and -7. The activation of caspase-3/7, but not caspase-1, occurred upstream of the rapid reduction in $\Delta\Psi_m$ during apoptosis induced by amrubicin and amrubicinol. Both reduction in $\Delta\Psi_m$ and activation of caspase-3/7, as well as topo II inhibition, were common steps in apoptosis induced by amrubicin, amrubicinol, DNR, and etoposide; however, experiments with oligomycin, a mitochondrial F_0F_1-ATPase inhibitor, suggested that apoptosis induced by these four agents involved substantially different pathways. Indeed, oligomycin blocked the etoposide-induced increase in sub-G_1 without preventing caspase activation, and had no inhibitory effects on sub-G_1 in DNR-treated cells, whereas apoptosis-related changes caused by amrubicin or amrubicinol were suppressed in the presence of oligomycin.

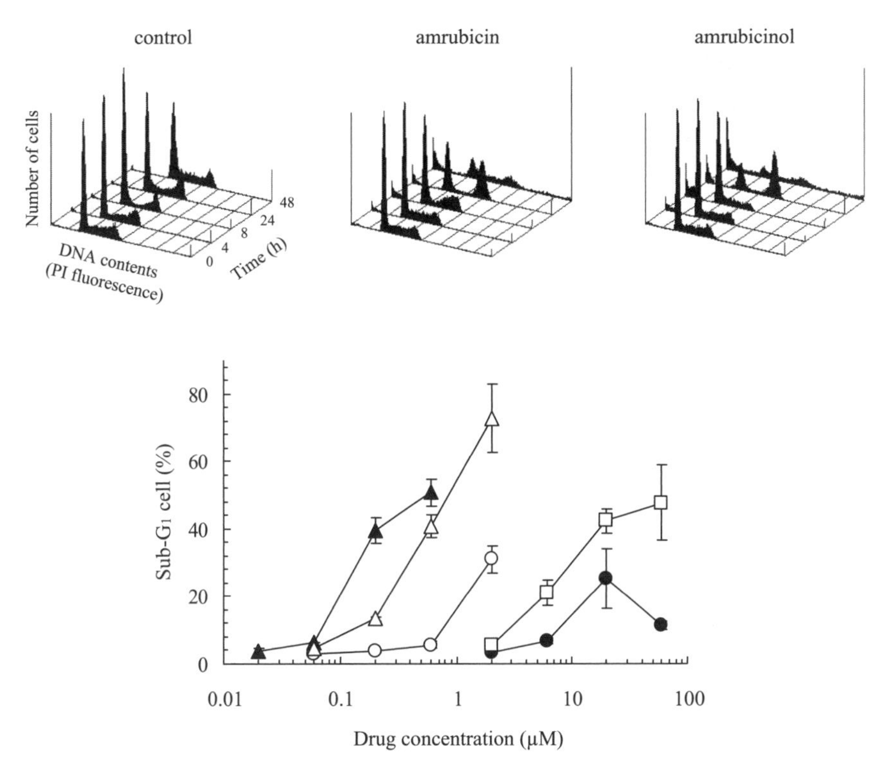

Figure 6.6 Time-dependent and dose-dependent development of apoptosis in cells. (Upper) Flow cytometric analysis of cells treated by amrubicin and amrubicinol. U937 cells were cultured for 1 h with 20 μM amrubicin or 0.2 μM amrubicinol. After removal of agents, cells were incubated in drug-free medium. At the indicated time points, fixed cells were stained with propidium iodide and analyzed by flow cytometry. (Lower) Dose-dependent induction of apoptosis. U937 cells were treated for 1 h with the indicated concentrations of amrubicin (closed circle), amrubicinol (closed triangle), DXR (open circle), DNR (open triangle), and etoposide (open square). After removal of agents, cells were incubated in drug-free medium for 24 h. The populations of sub-G_1 cells were determined by flow cytometry. Results are given as the average ± SD ($n = 2$).

6.5 AMRUBICIN METABOLISM: THE DISCOVERY OF AMRUBICINOL

6.5.1 Amrubicinol Functions as an Active Metabolite of Amrubicin

A major pathway of anthracycline's metabolism is the reduction of the C-13 carbonyl group to a hydroxyl group by reductases. Like the other anthracycline derivatives, amrubicin could be metabolized to a C-13 hydroxyl metabolite, amrubicinol [19]. It is generally regarded as an inactivation pathway, and the C-13 hydroxyl metabolites of DXR, DNR, and epirubicin are known to be much less cytotoxic than the corresponding parent drugs [33]. In contrast, amrubicinol was five to hundred times more active than amrubicin in inhibiting the growth of 17 human cancer cell lines, including both hematological malignancies and solid tumors [34]. No other metabolites were shown to be more active than amrubicinol *in vitro* (Table 6.2). Cellular incorporation and the potency of the incorporated amrubicin/amrubicinol were evaluated using four human cancer cell lines; the intracellular concentrations of amrubicinol were equal to those of amrubicin when the medium concentrations of amrubicinol were five

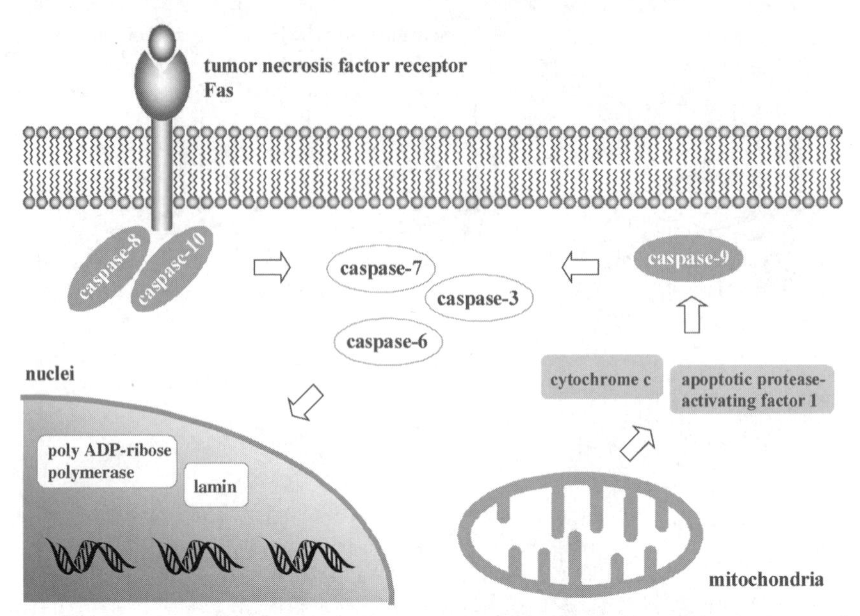

Figure 6.7 Two major pathways for inducing apoptosis. The ligation of death receptors leads to the caspase-8/10 activation, and the damaged mitochondrial releases cytochrome *c*, enhancing caspase-9 activity. Although the upstream events that activates caspase-8/9/10 are different but not mutually exclusive, the same downstream caspases, caspase-3/6/7, are commonly activated during apoptosis.

to ten times lower than those of amrubicin. The most probable explanation for the higher activity of amrubicinol is the cellular pharmacokinetic difference between them, with amrubicinol accumulating in cells at a higher level than amrubicin. Furthermore, the intracellular concentration of amrubicinol necessary to produce 50% cell growth inhibition was three to eight times lower than that of amrubicin in four human cancer cell lines tested, indicating that amrubicinol had higher activity than amrubicin at the same intracellular concentration. These findings suggested that amrubicinol exerted higher activity on intracellular target(s) than amrubicin. Amrubicinol was also 10 times more effective than the parental agent at causing the formation of a cleavable complex and inducing apoptosis in cells [30,32]; therefore, amrubicin was unique among the anthracycline derivatives in that C-13 hydroxyl metabolite inhibited the growth of cancer cells more effectively than the parent agent. As described below, amrubicinol appears to play an important role in the *in vivo*

TABLE 6.2 ***In vitro* Activity of Amrubicin Metabolites**[a]

	IC_{50} (μM)			
Drugs	CCRF-CEM	U937	PC-8	A549
Amrubicin	0.58 ± 0.03	0.48 ± 0.06	0.26 ± 0.16	0.062 ± 0.008
Amrubicinol	0.017 ± 0.008	0.0071 ± 0.0011	0.021 ± 0.015	0.0079 ± 0.0022
7-Deoxyamrubicin aglycone	1.1 ± 0.1	13 ± 0	1.3 ± 0.4	0.80 ± 0.21
Amrubicinol aglycone	0.79 ± 0.04	0.76 ± 0.08	0.76 ± 0.27	0.45 ± 0.25
7-Deoxyamrubicinol aglycone	0.73 ± 0.02	0.93 ± 0.00	0.92 ± 0.25	0.77 ± 0.16
9-Deaminoamrubicin	1.2 ± 0.3	2.3 ± 0.2	9.2 ± 5.4	0.70 ± 0.08

[a]CCRF-CEM and U937 are human leukemia cell lines, PC-8 and A549 are human lung cancer cell lines. Cells were cultured for 3 days with each agent. Results are given as the average ± SD ($n = 2$).

antitumor effect of amrubicin as an active metabolite although amrubicinol in itself did not show any favorable antitumor activity due to its non-selective distribution.

6.5.2 Tumor-Selective Metabolism of Amrubicin to Amrubicinol

Amrubicin administered intravenously at 25 mg kg^{-1} substantially prevented the growth of several human cancer xenografts, including SCLC cell lines (LX-1, Lu-24, and Lu-134), NSCLC cell lines (QG-56, Lu-99, LC-6, and L-27), gastric cancer cell lines (SC-6, SC-7, SC-9, St-4, St-15, and 4-1ST), and a breast cancer cell line (MX-1) [12,35]. To characterize the biological properties of amrubicinol, the concentrations of amrubicinol in several tissues of tumor-bearing mice given amrubicin 25 mg kg^{-1} were measured and the relationship between amrubicinol in tumors and the *in vivo* efficacy of amrubicin was evaluated [36]. Concentrations of amrubicinol in the tumors of these mice were higher than those of DXR in mice treated with DXR 12.5 mg kg^{-1} (Figure 6.8). In contrast, concentrations of amrubicinol in several normal tissues, including the heart, were lower than those of DXR. Amrubicinol was found to be a major metabolite in several human cancer xenografts treated with amrubicin, and the AUC of amrubicinol, but not amrubicin, in tumors closely correlated with the *in vivo* efficacy of amrubicin, as shown in

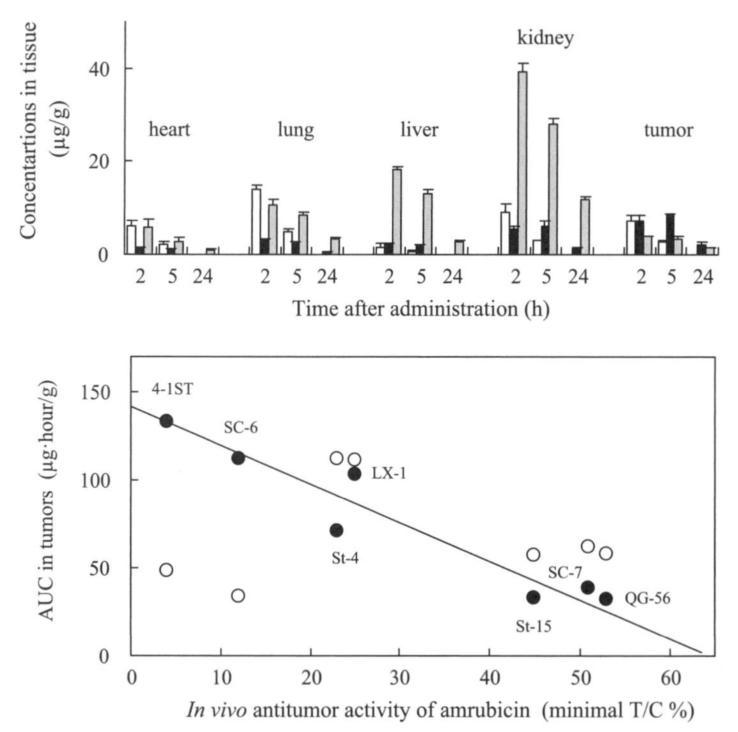

Figure 6.8 Amrubicinol functions as an active metabolite of amrubicin. (Upper) Concentrations of amrubicin, amrubicinol and DXR in tissues. Mice bearing 4-1ST tumors that received amrubicin (25 mg kg^{-1}) or DXR (12.5 mg kg^{-1}) were sacrificed at 2, 5, and 24 h after administration ($n = 2$ or 3). Amrubicin (white bar), amrubicinol (block bar), or DXR (gray bar) was extracted with methanol/chloroform (2:1) from tissues and analyzed by HPLC. Results are given as the average ± SD. (Lower) Correlation between the *in vivo* antitumor activities of amrubicin and the AUC of amrubicinol. AUC values of amrubicin (open circle) and amrubicinol (closed circle) were calculated by summing trapezoids. *In vivo* antitumor activity was represented as the value of minimal T/C%.

Figure 6.8 [36]. To estimate how the metabolism of amrubicin in tumors contributed to its antitumor activity, homogenates derived from various cancer cell lines were incubated with amrubicin *in vitro*, and the concentration of amrubicinol in mixtures was measured. The more sensitive these tumors were to amrubicin, the higher the metabolizing activity they showed [36]. These data indicated that concentrations of amrubicinol in tumors after treatment with amrubicin *in vivo* closely correlated with the metabolizing activities of amrubicin to amrubicinol in tumor homogenates *in vitro*. To assess the significance of the conversion of amrubicin to amrubicinol in tumors, the tumor-selective toxicity of *in vivo* administration of amrubicinol was compared to that of amrubicin. In contrast to amrubicin, amrubicinol by itself showed less selective antitumor activity in xenograft models, because amrubicinol was more distributed in normal tissues, such as the kidney and heart, than tumors leading to toxic death at a higher dose than MTD (12.5 mg kg^{-1}). Accordingly, the preferential metabolism of amrubicin to amrubicinol in tumors appeared to result in tumor-selective distribution of amrubicinol, leading to good *in vivo* efficacy of amrubicin in experimental therapeutic models. These results suggested that amrubicinol as an active metabolite played the most important role in the antitumor activity caused by amrubicin.

CBR is able to catalyze the NADPH-dependent reduction of a variety of xenobiotic ketones and quinones [37]. The xenobiotic substrates shown to be metabolized by CBR1 include anthracycline derivatives, such as DXR and DNR [37,38]. The role of CBR1 in xenobiotic metabolism remains to be elucidated; however, DNA sequence analysis in the promoter region of CBR1 revealed two xenobiotic response elements with potential regulatory functions [39]. According to this, the exposure of a human breast cancer cell line, MCF-7, to low concentrations of DXR caused a significant elevation of its reduction rate, accompanied with an increase of CBR1 protein levels [40]. Taken together, it might be suggested that tumors recognized anthacyclines as xenobiotics and induced CBR1 in response to them, leading to detoxification. It has been reported by de Cerain *et al.* that CBR activity was elevated in tumors with respect to normal tissues in 15 of 17 patients with lung cancer although no relationship was found between CBR activity and the tumor histology, grade, and stage [41]. Based on these findings, it could be speculated that amrubicin was activated and effective in some cancers which were resistant or refractory to conventional anthracyclines due to high CBR1 activity.

6.6 IMPROVED USAGE OF AMRUBICIN

Amrubicin administered intravenously more markedly prevented the growth of several human cancer xenografts than DXR [12,35]. To identify the most effective dosing schedule of amrubicin, antitumor activity was evaluated when amrubicin was administered repeatedly or in combination with other antitumor agents. The MTD of amrubicin could be administered three times at 10 day intervals [12]. Repeated administration of amrubicin exerted greater antitumor effects, including complete tumor loss, on 4-1ST tumors than a single administration (Figure 6.9). The MTD by 5 day administration in mice was estimated to be 7.5 mg kg^{-1} day^{-1} (total 37.5 mg kg^{-1}) for amrubicin, with no death due to toxicity or severe body weight loss [42]. Antitumor activities on some human cancer xenografts with 5 day administration were found to be higher than with a single administration (Figure 6.9), probably due to the high concentration of amrubicinol in tumors. Bone marrow suppression by amrubicin at MTD on a 5 day schedule was more severe than with a single administration although the time needed to recover from myelosuppression was similar between the two schedules. From these results, it was

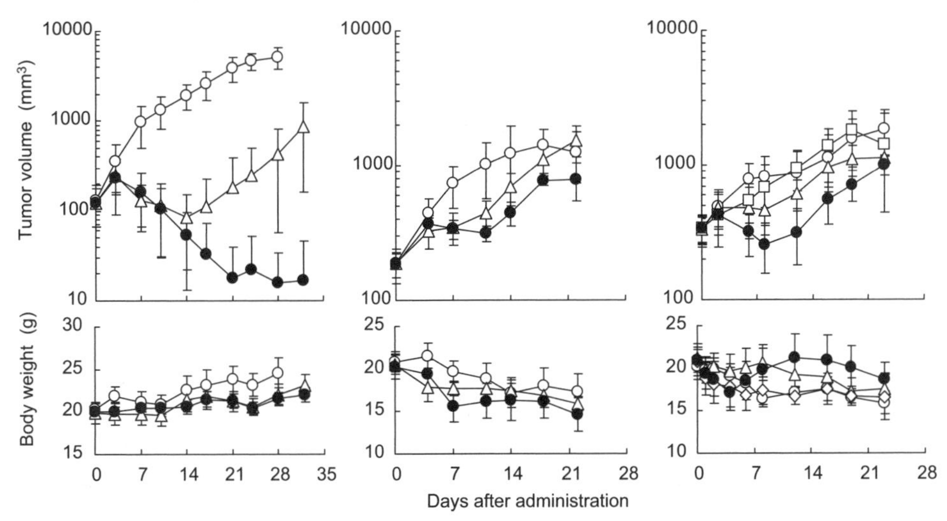

Figure 6.9 Improved antitumor effects of amrubicin administered consecutively or in combination with CDDP. (Left) Growth of human gastric cancer xenograft 4-1ST. Groups of six mice were untreated (open circle), given amrubicin intravenously at the MTD (25 mg kg^{-1}) with a single administration (open triangle), or three times every 10 days (days 0, 10, and 20, closed circle). (Middle) Growth of human SCLC xenograft LX-1. Groups of six mice were untreated (open circle), given amrubicin intravenously at the MTD (25 mg kg^{-1}) with a single administration (open triangle), or five consecutive days (7.5 mg kg^{-1} day^{-1}, days 0 to 5, closed circle). (Right) Growth of human SCLC xenograft LX-1. Groups of six mice were untreated (open circle), given amrubicin intravenously at the MTD (25 mg kg^{-1}, open triangle), CDDP intravenously at the MTD (10 mg kg^{-1}, open square), or amrubicin approximately 1 h before CDDP (closed circle). All data are shown as the average $\pm$ SD

demonstrated that amrubicin administered consecutively was more effective than a single administration.

The current standard for the first-line treatment of patients with NSCLC and ED-SCLC is platinum-based combination chemotherapy. As clinical trials of combination chemotherapy are often conducted in the presence of supporting experimental data, a comprehensive examination of amrubicin in combination with clinically available agents was conducted focusing on agents effective against lung cancers. First, multiple drug effects were quantitatively analyzed by calculating combination indexes (CIs), as described by Chou and Talalay [43], where CI values less than and greater than 1 indicated synergism and antagonism, respectively, whereas a value of 1 indicated addition. Synergy is defined as a combination of two agents which achieves an anti-proliferative effect greater than that expected by the simple addition of their effects. Such synergistic interactions between two agents may improve clinical therapeutic effect.

CDDP is commonly used in lung cancer chemotherapy, and is considered to be a key agent in the treatment of ED-SCLC as well as advanced NSCLC. In combination experiments, LX-1 cells were exposed simultaneously to amrubicinol and CDDP for 3 days [35]. Mean CI values at fraction affected of 0.5 and more, for the combination of CDDP with amrubicinol, were less than 1, indicating clear synergistic interaction. Simultaneous exposure of human SCLC cell line SBC-3 cells to amrubicinol and CDDP showed synergistic effects, as previously described by Takigawa *et al.* [44]. A SN-38 (an active metabolite of irinotecan)-resistant subline, SBC-3/SN-38, retained sensitivity to amrubicinol, and additive effects were also observed when the cells were simultaneously treated with amrubicinol and CDDP. Yamauchi *et al.* demonstrated that CDDP enhanced topo II inhibition by amrubicinol in a kinetoplast DNA decatenation assay, and amrubicinol increased the number of platinum–DNA adducts formed by CDDP in SBC-3 cells [45]. Next, to further evaluate the potential therapeutic effect of CDDP in combination with amrubicin, *in vivo* experiments were carried out using a human SCLC model. As shown in Figure 6.9, the use of CDDP in combination with amrubicin resulted in a significant inhibition of growth compared to CDDP alone or amrubicin alone in the treatment of LX-1 tumors [35]. While treatment with CDDP or amrubicin yielded a minimum T/C of 69% or 57%, respectively, the combination was 31% ($p<0.05$). The maximum decrease in body weight was within 10% in all groups, indicating that MTDs of CDDP as well as amrubicin were well tolerated by mice with this combination. Besides CDDP, the combinations of irinotecan, vinorelbine, trastuzumab (anti-HER2 monoclonal antibody), tegafur/uracil (Figure 6.1), and to a lesser extent, gemcitabine with amrubicin caused significant growth inhibition of human tumor xenografts without markedly enhancing body weight loss, compared with treatment using amrubicin alone at the MTD [35]. These results suggested that amrubicin appeared to be a possible candidate for combined use with CDDP, and this combination would be effective against SCLC.

6.7 CLINICAL TRIALS

6.7.1 Clinical Trials of Amrubicin as First-line Therapy in Patients with ED-SCLC

In April 2002, amrubicin hydrochloride was approved for the treatment of SCLC and NSCLC in Japan. As amrubicin is a highly active and promising agent with acceptable toxicity for previously untreated and relapsed patients with ED-SCLC, the clinical development of amrubicin for ED-SCLC will be focused on. Clinical studies of amrubicin are summarized in Tables 6.3 and 6.4.

The MTD of amrubicin was determined to be 130 mg m^{-2} in a single-dose schedule, 25 mg m^{-2} day^{-1} for 5 days, and 50 mg m^{-2} day^{-1} for 3 days [4,46–48]. In regards to the antitumor effect, no clear response was observed in studies using single or 5 day administration; however, three partial responses (PRs) were achieved in 13 patients with advanced NSCLC in the phase I study where amrubicin was administered by daily intravenous injection for three consecutive days every 3 weeks [48]. The dose-limiting toxicity (DLT) was defined as toxicity consisting of grade 4 neutropenia and leucopenia lasting 4 days or more, and grade 3 or 4 toxicity other than neutropenia, leucopenia, anorexia, nausea/vomiting, and alopecia. At dose level 1 (40 mg m^{-2} day^{-1}), one of four patients experienced grade 4 neutropenia and leucopenia, which did not last for 4 days or longer. At dose level 2 (45 mg m^{-2} day^{-1}), three of four patients also experienced grade 4 neutropenia, lasted for 4 days or longer in only one. No grade 4 leucopenia was observed at this dose. Dose-limiting leucopenia and neutropenia lasting for more than 4 days were observed in two and in all five patients at dose level 3 (50 mg m^{-2} day^{-1}), respectively. Although no grade 3 or 4 nonhematological toxicity was observed at dose level 1 or 2 in this study, grade 3 or 4 toxicities were noted in three of five patients at dose level 3; grade 3 nausea/vomiting and melaena and grade 4 hematemesis in one patient each. There was no toxicity to renal or cardiac function, but a mild effect on hepatic function was observed. Based on these findings and in consideration of convenience in practical therapy, a regimen of repeated doses for three consecutive days was also recommended for amrubicin. The recommended dose for phase II was determined to be 45 mg m^{-2} day^{-1} for 3 days every 3 weeks for previously untreated patients with lung cancer.

TABLE 6.3 Clinical Studies of Amrubicin in Patients with Previously Untreated ED-SCLC

Studies [references]	Regimens	Patients (*n*)	ORRs (%) [95% confidence interval]	MSTs (months) [95% confidence interval]
Yana et al. [49]	45 mg/m^2/day, day 1 to 3	Naïve (35)	75.8 [57.7–88.9]	11.7 [9.9–15.3]
Yamamoto et al. [50]	40 or 35 mg/m^2/day, day 1 to 3	Naïve (7)	71 [29–96]	9.4 [7.7–14.1]
		Relapsed (14)	14 [2–43]	6.0 [2.6–8.6]
Igawa et al. [51]	40 or 35 mg/m^2/day, day 1 to 3	Naïve, elderly or >PS2 (27)	70	6.6
Ohe et al. [52]	40 mg/m^2/day, day 1 to 3 Cisplatin at 60 mg/m^2, day 1	Naïve (41)	87.8 [73.8–95.9]	13.6 [11.1–16.6]
O'Brien et al. [53]	40 mg/m^2/day, day 1 to 3	Naïve (33)	61	11.1[7.9–14.5]
	40 mg/m^2/day, day 1 to 3 Cisplatin at 60 mg/m^2, day 1	Naïve (33)	77	11.1[7.3–16.3]
	Etoposide at 100 mg/m^2, day 1 to 3 Cisplatin at 75 mg/m^2, day 1	Naïve (33)	63	10.0[9.2–13.3]
Inoue et al. [55]	35 mg/m^2/day, day 1 to 3 Carboplatin at AUC 4.0, day 1	Naïve, elderly (36)	89 [79–99]	18.6 [16.1–19.4]

TABLE 6.4 Clinical Studies of Amrubicin in Patients with Relapsed ED-SCLC

Studies [references]	Regimens	Patients (*n*)	ORRs (%) [95% confidence interval]	MSTs (months) [95% confidence interval]
Kato et al. [60]	40 mg/m^2/day, day 1 to 3	Relapsed (35)	53	8.8
Hasegwa et al. [61]	40 mg/m^2/day, day 1 to 3	Sensitive (9)	55.6 [21.2–86.3]	11.0
		Refractory (17)	41.2 [18.4–67.1]	5.7
Onoda et al. [62]	40 mg/m^2/day, day 1 to 3	Sensitive (16)	52 [37–68]	11.6
		Refractory (44)	50 [25–75]	10.3
Ettinger et al. [63]	40 mg/m^2/day, day 1 to 3	Refractory (75)	21.3 [12.7–32.3]	6.0 [4.8–7.1]
Inoue et al. [64]	40 mg/m^2/day, day 1 to 3	Sensitive (17)	53	9.9
		Refractory (12)	17	5.3
	Topotecan 1.0 mg/m^2/ day, day 1 to 5	Sensitive (19)	21	11.7
		Refractory (11)	0	5.4
Jotte et al. [65]	40 mg/m^2/day, day 1 to 3	Sensitive (50)	44	9.2[5.7–12.0]
	Topotecan 1.5 mg/m^2/ day, day 1 to 5	Sensitive (26)	15	7.6[4.5–13.8]

In the first phase II study of amrubicin in previously untreated patients with ED-SCLC, three had a CR and 22 had a PR, for an ORR of 75.8% [49]. The median survival time (MST) was 11.7 months. Compared to the other agents, amrubicin demonstrated a much higher response rate, indicating that it is a promising agent with potential to overcome the therapeutic plateau of ED-SCLC. The 1 and 2 year survival rates were 48.5% and 20.2%, respectively. The major observed toxicity was hematologic. Grade 3 or 4 leucopenia and neutropenia occurred in 51.5% and 84.8%, respectively. Despite severe hematological toxicities, there was no febrile neutropenia or treatment-related death. Non-hematological toxicity of grade 3 and higher was not observed except for anorexia (9.1%) and alopecia (3.0%). No LEVF decrease was observed. Amrubicin monotherapy was assessed in patients with SCLC who were unable to tolerate platinum-based combination chemotherapy due to old age (>76 years), a poor performance status (PS, 3 or 4) [66], or complications [50]. Twenty-one patients were treated with amrubicin at 40 or 35 mg m^{-2} given on three consecutive days every 3 weeks. RR and MST in previously untreated patients were 71% and 9.4 months, respectively. Hematological toxicity was common and relatively severe, whereas non-hematological toxicity was relatively mild. Approximately half of all SCLC patients in Japan are >70 years, and as the populations of elderly SCLC patients are continuously increasing. Igawa *et al.* conducted a study to evaluate the efficacy of amrubicin as first-line chemotherapy for elderly and poor risk patients with ED-SCLC [51]. Twenty-seven patients who were >75 years had a PS of 2 or more were enrolled and evaluated in this study. The ORR, MST, and 1-year survival rate were 70%, 9.3 months, and 30%, respectively. Grade 3 or 4 hematologic toxicities were neutropenia (63%), leucopenia (56%), thrombocytopenia (15%), and anemia (19%). Febrile neutropenia was observed in four (15%) patients.

Amrubicin has been used in clinical studies in combination with conventional chemotherapeutic agents, such as CDDP, carboplatin, irinotecan, and topotecan [52–58]. In a phase I/II study of CDDP and amrubicin in previously untreated patients with ED-SCLC, four patients were enrolled at dose level 1 (amrubicin 40 mg m^{-2} day^{-1} on days 1 to 3 and CDDP 60 mg m^{-2} on day 1) and three patients at level 2 (amrubicin 45 mg m^{-2} day^{-1} and CDDP 60 mg m^{-2}) [52]. At level 2, grade 4 neutropenia persisting 4 days or more occurred in three patients and febrile neutropenia in one although no DLT was observed at level 1. Consequently, the MTD and the recommended dose were determined to be level 2 and level 1, respectively, so 41 patients were treated at the recommended doses. The ORR was 87.8% with four CRs and 32 PRs. The MST and 1-year survival rate were 13.6 months and 56.1%, respectively. Hematological toxicities, especially leucopenia and neutropenia, were common and relatively severe. Grade 3 or 4 leucopenia, neutropenia, thrombocytopenia, and anemia occurred in 65.9%, 95.1%, 24.4%, and 53.7%, respectively. Major non-hematological toxicities were gastrointestinal, including anorexia, nausea, and vomiting. The combination of CDDP and amrubicin has demonstrated an impressive overall response and MST in patients with previously untreated ED-SCLC. These results were comparable with those in the Japan Clinical Oncology Group (JCOG) 9511 trial where ORR and MST were 84.4% and 12.8 months in the CDDP plus irinotecan group, respectively [3].

A phase II study of amrubicin in combination with CDDP has also been conducted outside of Japan for previously untreated ED-SCLC, in which patients with ED-SCLC were randomized to three arms: (1) amrubicin alone (45 mg m^{-2} day^{-1} on days 1 to 3), (2) amrubicin (40 mg m^{-2} day^{-1} on days 1 to 3) combined with CDDP (60 mg m^{-2} on day 1), or (3) etoposide (100 mg m^{-2}/day on days 1 to 3) combined with CDDP (75 mg m^{-2} on day 1) [53]. Grade 3 and higher hematological toxicity in arms 1 to 3 was neutropenia (73%, 73%, 69%), thrombocytopenia (17%, 15%, 9.4%), anemia (10%, 15%, 3.1%), and febrile neutropenia (13%, 18%, 6%). The RR assessed by investigators was 61%, 77%, and

63% for arm 1, 2, and 3, respectively. The combination of CDDP and amrubicin was associated with the highest RR and further evaluation of this combination is warranted.

The JCOG is conducting a phase III study (JCOG 0509) comparing CDDP and amrubicin with CDDP and irinotecan for previously untreated ED-SCLC. Another phase III study of CDDP and amrubicin compared with CDDP and etoposide for previously untreated ED-SCLC is in progress mainly in China and Japan (ClinicalTrial.gov identifier, NCT00660504).

6.7.2 Clinical Trials of Amrubicin as Second-Line Therapy in Patients with ED-SCLC

Although a number of clinical trials have been carried out for relapsed SCLC using etoposide, irinotecan, paclitaxel, or picoplatin (Figure 6.1), every agent has shown only limited activity [59]. Unfortunately, recent targeted agents such as imatinib, bevacizumab (anti-VEGF monoclonal antibody), sorafenib, and gefitinib (Figure 6.1) have also failed to demonstrate the effectiveness of SCLC in the second-line setting. As amrubicin as a single agent was highly effective for previously untreated ED-SCLC, several studies have been conducted to evaluate its efficacy in the treatment of relapsed/refractory SCLC. Kato *et al.* reported that amrubicin at 45 mg m^{-2} on days 1 to 3 every 3 weeks showed not only promising activity but severe hematological toxicities in previously treated patients [60]. Four CRs and 14 PRs were observed among 34 patients treated, yielding an ORR of 53%. Grade 3 or 4 leucopenia, neutropenia, febrile neutropenia, and thrombocytopenia were observed in 76%, 97%, 35%, and 38%, respectively. On the other hand, 26 patients (9 sensitive and 17 refractory) were treated with amrubicin at 40 mg m^{-2} day^{-1} for three consecutive days in a phase II study conducted by Hasegawa *et al.* [61]. The RR was 46.2% (55.6% for sensitive, 41.2% for refractory). The MST was 9.4 months (11.0 months for sensitive, 5.7 months for refractory). Grade 4 leucopenia and neutropenia occurred in 42.3%, and 73.1%, respectively. Grade 3 febrile neutropenia occurred in 42.3%. Grade 3 or 4 thrombocytopenia occurred in 50.0%. Amrubicin monotherapy was considered an encouraging regimen for second-line treatment of SCLC. The Japanese Thoracic Oncology Research Group conducted a multicenter phase II study of amrubicin for the treatment of refractory or relapsed SCLC [62]. Among 60 patients (16 refractory and 44 sensitive), two achieved a CR and 29 had a PR, for an ORR of 52% (52% in sensitive and 50% in refractory). The MST and 1-year survival rate in the sensitive group and refractory group were 11.6 and 10.3 months, and 46% and 40%, respectively. Grade 3 or 4 hematologic toxicities were leucopenia (70%), neutropenia (83%), febrile neutropenia (5%), thrombocytopenia (20%), and anemia (33%). No cardiotoxicity, except for one transient atrial fibrillation, was observed.

A phase II study of amrubicin in the second-line setting has also been conducted outside of Japan by Ettinger *et al.*, who confirmed the safety and activity of amrubicin (40 mg m^{-2} day^{-1} for 3 days every 3 weeks) in the treatment of platinum-refractory SCLC [63]. The ORR and MST were 21.3% and 6.0 months, respectively. The most commonly grade 3 or 4 adverse events included neutropenia (67%), thrombocytopenia (41%), and anemia (30%). LEVF remained stable in patients treated with amrubicin, even at cumulative doses exceeding 750 mg m^{-2}.

As single-agent amrubicin showed promising efficacy with 20–50% ORRs and an acceptable safety profile when used as second-line therapy in patients with relapsed/refractory SCLC, two randomized phase II studies comparing amrubicin (40 mg m^{-2} day^{-1} for 3 days) with topotecan (1.0 or 1.5 mg m^{-2} day^{-1} for 5 days every 3 weeks) were conducted in this population [64,65]. One study with 60 Japanese patients achieved an ORR of 38% in the amrubicin arm (53% for sensitive and 17% for refractory) and that of 13% in the topotecan arm (21% for sensitive and 0% for refractory) [64]. The PFS on the amrubicin arm was 3.5 months (3.9 months, sensitive; 2.6 months, refractory), and on the topotecan arm was 2.2 months (3.0 months, sensitive; 1.5 months, refractory). Despite the lower response and shorter PFS of topotecan than amrubicin, the OS curve of the topotecan arm could be superimposed on that of the amrubicin arm. It was notable that most long survivors in the topotecan arm received amrubicin for third-line or later chemotherapy, and subsequent multivariate analysis revealed that amrubicin had the strongest effect to prolong OS of patients enrolled in this study. In the other study, 76 non-Japanese patients with ED-SCLC sensitive to first-line platinum-based chemotherapy were randomized to receive either amrubicin or topotecan [65]. Amrubicin significantly improved ORR versus topotecan (44% versus 15%, $p = 0.021$). The PFS and MST were 4.5 months and 9.2 months with amrubicin, and 3.3 momths and 7.6 months with topotecan. These results suggested that amrubicin might be superior to topotecan for relapsed ED-SCLC.

Pharmacokinetic parameters of amrubicin (45 mg m^{-2} day^{-1} for 3 days) in plasma were almost identical on days 1 and 3 [52]. The half-life at distribution phase, the half-life at elimination phase, the distribution volume, and the total body clearance were 0.09 h, 2.27 h, 51.9 L, and 14.2 L h^{-1} on day 3, respectively. The AUC of amrubicinol in red blood cells tended to increase on day 3. Combination with CDDP did not alter the pharmacokinetics of amrubicin and amrubicinol.

Amrubicin as a single agent and in combination with CDDP appears to be effective in treating Western as well as Japanese patients with naive ED-SCLC. In addition, its effectiveness in treating Japanese patients with relapsed ED-SCLC could be reproduced in Western patients with the disease.

6.8 CONCLUSIONS

Natural products have been a rich source of agents of value to medicine. Many antitumor agents have been discovered by screening natural products from plants, marine organisms, and microorganisms. Vincristine, paclitaxel, and etoposide are examples of plant-derived compounds employed in cancer treatment; DXR and DNR are antitumor agents derived from microbial sources. The introduction of these effective agents derived from nature into the cancer chemotherapy offer us a great opportunity to evaluate novel mechanism of action and to synthesize related compounds with novel chemical structures. Most clinically available anthracycline derivatives have been produced by fermentation or semisynthesis, while amrubicin has been discovered by screening totally synthetic 9-aminoanthracycline derivatives [11,12]. This unique approach made it possible to find a novel anthracycline derivative characterized by 9-amino group and simple sugar moiety at the 7-position.

To identify more potent and safer anthracycline derivative than DXR, we have conducted *in vivo* screening mainly [12]. We have evaluated the survival benefit for mice implanted with leukemia primarily, and the antitumor activity in human tumor xenograft models secondly. If our primary assay were *in vitro* or cell-free screening, amrubicinol but not amrubicin might be discovered as one of active candidate compounds. While amrubicinol by itself could not exert tumor-selective toxicity in xenograft models due to its higher systemic distribution and toxicity [36], it has been shown that the preferential metabolism of amrubicin to amrubicinol in tumors appeared to lead to good *in vivo* efficacy of amrubicin. Therefore, primary *in vivo* screening was useful to find antitumor agents which could be distributed and/or activated in tumors. To the best of my knowledge, amrubicin is the first anthracycline that is activated by the reduction of the C-13 carbonyl group to a hydroxyl group.

A large number of clinical trials of ED-SCLC have been conducted in the first-line setting and more; however, treatment advances are slow. Both new agents introduced around 1990 and recent molecular targeted agents have failed to improve the survival of patients with ED-SCLC. Therefore, there is a clear unmet need for novel and effective agents and/or combinations to treat naive and relapsed/refractory patients with ED-SCLC. In spite of the smaller number of patients with ED-SCLC, several clinical trials of amrubicin have been conducted in this population (Tables 6.3 and 6.4). Based on its clinical efficacy, amrubicin is recognized as one of the most promising agents at present as a monotherapy and in combination therapy with CDDP. Several phase III trials comparing amrubicin with the standard regimen for ED-SCLC are in progress.

The preferential conversion of amrubicin to its C-13 hydroxyl active metabolite, amrubicinol, in tumors appeared to result in more effective antitumor activity and less cardiotoxicity by amrubicin than conventional anthracycline derivatives such as DXR. As the major long-term side effect of anthracyclines is cardiotoxicity, we investigated the degree of cardiotoxicity of amrubicin compared with that of DXR in rabbits and dogs [14,15]. Amrubicin has exhibited less cardiotoxicity than DXR in these preclinical studies, and its cardiac safety profile of amrubicin in patients with ED-SCLC has been confirmed in clinical studies and the postmarketing experience [16]. Besides amrubicin was more effective in several human lung cancer xenograft models compared with DXR, its lower cardiotoxicity proved in preclinical studies also could promote the clinical development of amrubicin. The DLT of amrubicin was myelosuppression, especially neutropenia. Its reduction would make amrubicin more useful for patients with ED-SCLC who are elderly, have a poor PS, or are relapsed/refractory to standard platinum-based chemotherapy.

Amrubicin is anticipated to be a boon to patients suffering from ED-SCLC in the near future.

REFERENCES

1. Perkin, D. M., Bray, F. I., and Devesa, S. S. Cancer burden in the year 2000. The global picture. *Eur. J. Cancer* **2001**, *37*, S4–S66.
2. Tiseo, M. and Ardizzoni, A. Current status of second-line treatment and novel therapies for small cell lung cancer. *J. Thorac. Oncol.* **2007**, *2*, 764–772.
3. Noda, K., Nishiwaki, Y., Kawahara, M., Negoro, S., Sugiura, T., Yokoyama, A., Fukuoka, M., Mori, K., Watanabe, K., Tamura, T., Yamamoto, S., and Saijo, N. Irinotecan plus cisplatin compared with etoposide plus cisplatin for extensive small-cell lung cancer. *N Engl. J. Med.* **2002**, *346*, 85–91.
4. Ettinger, D. S. Amrubicin for the treatment of small cell lung cancer: does effectiveness cross the pacific? *J. Thorac. Oncol.* **2007**, *2*, 160–165.
5. von Pawel, J., Schiller, J. H., Shepherd, F. A., Fields, S. Z., Kleisbauer, J. P., Chrysson, N. G., Stewart, D. J., Clark, P. I., Palmer, M. C., Depierre, A., Carmichael, J., Krebs, J. B., Ross, G., Lane, S. R., and Gralla, R. Topotecan versus cyclophosphamide, doxorubicin, and vincristine for the treatment of recurrent small-cell lung cancer. *J. Clin. Oncol.* **1999**, *17*, 658–667.
6. O'Brien, M. E. R., Ciuleanu, T-E., Tsekov, H., Shparyk, Y., Čučeviá, b., Juhasz, G., Thatcher, N., Ross, G. A., Dane, G. C., and Crofts, T. Phase III trial comparing supportive care alone with supportive care with oral topotecan in patients with relapsed small-cell lung cancer. *J. Clin. Oncol.* **2006**, *24*, 5441–5447.
7. Löwenberg, M., Downing, J. R., and Burnett, A. Acute myeloid leukemia. *N Engl. J. Med.* **1999**, *341*, 1051–1062.
8. Cardoso, F., Bedard, P. L., Winer, E. P., Pagani, O., Senkus-Konefka, E., Fallowfield, L. J., Kyriakides, S., Costa, A., Cufer, T., and Albain, K. S. International guidelines for management of metastatic breast cancer: combination vs sequential single-agent chemotherapy. *J. Natl Cancer Inst.* **2009**, *101*, 1174–1181.
9. Michallet, A-S. and Coiffier, B. Recent developments in the treatment of aggressive non-Hodgkin lymphoma. *Blood Rev.* **2009**, *23*, 11–23.
10. Minotti, G., Menna, P., Salvatorelli, E., Cairo, G., and Gianni, L. Anthracyclines: molecular advances and pharmacologic developments in antitumor activity and cardiotoxicity. *Pharmacol. Rev.* **2004**, *56*, 185–229.

11. Ishizumi, K., Ohashi, N., and Tanno, N. Stereospecific total synthesis of 9-aminoanthracyclines: (+)-9-amino-9-deoxydaunomycin and related compounds. *J. Org. Chem.* **1987**, *52*, 4477–4485.
12. Morisada, S., Yanagi, Y., Noguchi, T., Kashiwazaki, Y., and Fukui, M. Antitumor activities of a novel 9-aminoanthracycline (SM-5887) against mouse experimental tumors and human tumor xenografts. *Japan. J. Cancer Res.* **1989**, *80*, 69–76.
13. Shioiri, T., Izawa, K., and Konoike, T. *Pharmaceutical Process Chemistry*, Wiley-VCH, Weinheim, **2010**, chapter 10.
14. Suzuki, T., Minamide, S., Iwasaki, T., Yamamoto, H., and Kanda, H. Cardiotoxicity of a new anthracycline derivative (SM-5887) following intravenous administration to rabbits: comparative study with doxorubicin. *Invest. New Drugs* **1997**, *15*, 219–225.
15. Noda, T., Watanabe, T., Kohda, A., Hosokawa, S., and Suzuki, T. Chronic effects of a novel synthetic anthracycline derivative (SM-5887) on normal heart and doxorubicin-induced cardiomyopathy in beagle dogs. *Invest. New Drugs* **1998**, *16*, 121–128.
16. Spigel, D. Amrubicin (AMR) does not reduce LEVF with cumulative dose >1000 mg/m^{-2} in 2nd-line treatment of small cell lung cancer (SCLC): a pooled analysis of two phase II trials. **2009**, 13th World Conference on Lung Cancer, D6.7.
17. Forrest, G. L., Gonzalez, B., Tseng, W., Li, X., and Mann, J. Human carbonyl reductase overexpression in the heart advances the development of doxorubicin-induced cardiotoxicity in transgenic mice. *Cancer Res.* **2000**, *60*, 5158–5164.
18. Olson L. E., Bedja, D., Alvey, S. J., Cardounel, A. J., Gabrielson, K. L., and Reeves, R. H. Protection form doxorubicin-induced cardiac toxicity in mice with a null allele of carbonyl reductase 1. *Cancer Res.* **2003**, *63*, 6602–6606.
19. Tani, N., Yabuki, M., Komuro, S., and Kanamaru, H. Characterization of the enzyme involved in the in vitro metabolism of amrubicin hydrochloride. *Xenobiotica* **2005**, *35*, 1121–1133.
20. Morisada, S., Yanagi, Y., Kashiwazaki, Y., and Fukui, M. Toxicological aspects of a novel 9-aminoanthracycline, SM-5887. *Japan. J. Cancer Res.* **1989**, *80*, 77–82.
21. Noguchi, T, Ichii, S, Morisada, S, Yamaoka, T, and Yanagi, Y. Tumor-selective distribution of an active metabolite of the 9-aminoanthracycline amrubicin. *Japan. J. Cancer Res.* **1998**, *89*, 1061–1066.
22. Obara, N., Imagawa, S., Nakano, Y., Yamamoto, M., Noguchi, T., and Nagasawa, T. Hematological aspects of a novel 9-aminoanthracycline, amrubicin. *Cancer Sci.* **2003**, *94*, 1104–1106.
23. Kassner, N., Huse, K., Martin, H-J., Gödtel-Armbrust, U., Metzger, A., Meineke, I., Brockmöller, J., Klein, K., Zanger, U., Maser, M.E., and Wojnowski, L. Carbonyl reductase 1 is a predominant doxorubicin reductase in the human liver. *Drug Metab. Dispos.* **2008**, *36*, 2113–2120.
24. Gonzalez-Covarrubias, V., Zhang, J., Kalabus, J.L., Relling, M.V., and Blanco, J. G. Pharmocogenetics of human carbonyl reductase 1 (CBR1) in livers from black and white donors. *Drug Metab. Dispos.* **2009**, *37*, 400–407.
25. Matsunaga, Y., Hamada, A., Okamoto, I., Sasaki, J., Moriyama, E., Kishi, H., Matsumoto, M., Hira, A., Watanabe, H., and Saito, H. Pharmacokinetics of amrubicin and its active metabolite amrubicinol in lung cancer patients. *Ther. Drug Monitoring* **2006**, *28*, 76–82.
26. Tanaka, M., Bateman, R., Rauh, D., Vaisberg, E., Ramachandani, S., Zhang, C., Hansen, K.C., Burlingame, A.L., Trautman, J.K., Shorkat, K.M., and Adams, C. L. An unbiased cell morphology-based screen for new, biologically active small molecules. *PLoS Biol.* **2005**, *3*, e128.
27. Judson, I., Radford, J.A., Harris, M., Blay, J-Y., van Hoesel, Q., le Cesne, A., van Ooterom, A.T., Clemons, M.J., Kamby, C., Hermans, C., Whittaker, J., Donato di Paola, E., Verweij, J., and Nielsen, S. Randomised phase II trial of pegylated liposomal doxorubicin (DOXIL®/CAELYX®) versus doxorubicin in the treatment of advanced or metastatic soft tissue sarcoma: a study by the EORTC Soft Tissue and Bone Sarcoma Group. *Eur. J. Cancer* **2001**, *37*, 870–877.
28. O'Brien, M. E. R., Wigler, N., Inbar, M., Rosso, R., Grischke, E., Santoro, A., Catane, R., Kieback, D. G., Tomczak, P., Ackland, S. P., Orlandi, F., Mellars, L., Alland, L., and Tendler, C. Reduced cardiotoxicity and comparable efficacy in a phase III trial of pegylated liposomal doxorubicin HCl (CAELYXTM/Doxil®) versus conventional doxorubicin for first-line treatment of metastatic breast cancer. *Ann. Oncol.* **2004**, *15*, 440–449.
29. D'Arpa, P. and Liu, L. F. Topoisomerase-targeting antitumor drugs. *Biochimica et Biophysica Acta* **1989**, *989*, 163–177.
30. Hanada M., Mizuno S., Fukushima A., Saito Y., Noguchi T., Yamaoka T. A new antitumor agent amrubicin induces cell growth inhibition by stabilizing topoisomerase II-DNA complex. *Japan. J. Cancer Res.* **1998**, *89*, 1229–1238.
31. Tanabe, K., Ikegami, Y., Ishida, R., and Andoh, T. Inhibition of topoisomerase II by antitumor agents bis (2, 6-dioxopiperazine) derivatives. *Cancer Res.* **1991**, *51*, 4903–4908.
32. Hanada M., Noguchi T., and Yamaoka T. Amrubicin induces apoptosis in human tumor cells mediated by the activation of caspase-3/7 preceding a loss of mitochondrial membrane potential. *Cancer Sci.* **2006**, *97*, 1396–1403.
33. Limonta M., Biondi, A., Giudici, G., Specchia, G., Catapano, C., Masera, G., Barbui, T., and D'Incalci, M. Cytotoxicity and DNA damage caused by 4-demethoxydaunorubicin and its metabolite 4-demethoxy-13-hydoroxydaunorubicin in human acute myeloid leukemia cells. *Cancer Chemother. Pharmacol.* **1990**, *26*, 340–342.
34. Yamaoka T., Hanada M., Ichii S., Morisada S., Noguchi T., and Yanagi Y. Cytotoxicity of amrubicin, a novel

9-aminoanthracycline, and its active metabolite amrubicinol on human tumor cells. *Japan. J. Cancer Res.* **1998**, *89*, 1067–1073.

35. Hanada, M., Noguchi, T., and Yamaoka, T. Amrubicin, a novel 9-aminoanthracycline, enhances the antitumor activity of chemotherapeutic agents against human cancer cells in vitro and in vivo. *Cancer Sci.* **2007**, *98*, 447–454.
36. Noguchi, T., Ichii, S., Morisada, S., Yamaoka, T., and Yanagi, Y. In vivo efficacy and tumor-selective metabolism of amrubicin to its active metabolite. *Japan. J. Cancer Res.* **1998**, *89*, 1055–1060.
37. Oppermann, U. Carbonyl reductases: the complex relationships of mammalian carbonyl- and quinine-reducing enzymes' and their role in physiology. *Ann. Rev. Pharmacol. Toxicol.* **2007**, *47*, 293–322.
38. Ohara, H., Miyabe, Y., Deyashiki, Y., Matsuura, K., and Hara, A. Reduction of drug ketones by dihydrodiol dehydrogenases, carbonyl reductase and aldehyde reductase of human liver. *Biochem. Pharmacol.* **1995**, *50*, 221–227.
39. Lakhman, S. S., Chen, X., Gonzalez-Covarrubias, V., Schuetz, E. G., and Blanco, J. G. Functional characterization of the promoter of human carbonyl reductase 1 (CBR1). Role of XRE elements in mediating the induction of CBR1 by ligands of the aryl hydrocarbon receptor. *Mol. Pharmacol.* **2007**, *72*, 734–743.
40. Gavelová, m., Hladíková, j., Vildová, L., Novotná, R., Vondráček, j., Krčmář, p., Machala, M., and Skálová, l. Reduction of doxorubicin and oracin and induction of carbonyl reductase in human breast carcinoma MCF-7 cells. *Chemico-Biological Interactions*, **2008**, *176*, 9–18.
41. de Cerain, A. L., Marín, a., Idoate, M. A., Tuñón, M. T., and Bello, J. Carbonyl reductase and NADPH cytochrome P450 reductase activities in human tumoral versus normal tissues. *Eur. J. Cancer* **1999**, *35*, 320–324.
42. Noguchi, T., Ichii, S., Morisada, S., Yamaoka, T., and Yanagi, Y. Evaluation of amrubicin with a 5 day administration schedule in a mouse model. *Japan J. Cancer Chemother.*, **1999**, *26*, 1305–1312.
43. Chou, T-C. and Talalay, P. Quantitative analysis of dose-effect relationships: the combined effects of multiple drugs or enzyme inhibitors. *Adv. Enzyme Regul.* **1984**, *22*, 27–55.
44. Takigawa, N., Takeyama, M., Shibayama, T., Tada, A., Kawata, N., Okada, C., Aoe, K., Kozuki, T., Hotta, K., Tabata, M., Kiura, K., Ueoka, H., Tanimoto, M., and Takahashi, K. The combination effect of amrubicin with cisplatin or irinotecan for small-cell lung cancer cells. *Oncol. Rep.* **2006**, *15*, 837–842.
45. Yamauchi, S., Kudoh, S., Kimura. T., Hirata, K., and Yoshikawa, J. Additive effects of amrubicin with cisplatin on human lung cancer cell lines. *Osaka City Med. J.* **2002**, *48*, 69–76.
46. Inoue, K., Ogawa, M., Horikoshi, N, Mukaiyama, T., Itoh, Y., Imajoh, K., Ozeki, H., Nagamine, D., and Shinagawa, K. Phase I and pharmacokinetic study of SM-5887, a new anthracycline derivative. *Invest. New Drugs* **1989**, *7*, 213–218.
47. Kurata T., Okamoto, I., Tamura, K., and Fukuoka, M. Amrubicin for non-small-cell lung cancer and small-cell lung cancer. *Invest. New Drugs* **2007**, *25*, 499–504.
48. Sugiura, T., Ariyoshi, Y., Negoro, S., Nakamura, S., Ikegami, H., Takada, M., Yana, T., and Fukuoka, M. Phase I/II study of amrubicin, a novel 9-aminoanthracycline, in patients with advanced non-small-cell lung cancer. *Invest. New Drugs* **2005**, *23*, 331–337.
49. Yana, T., Negoro, S., Takada, M., Yokota, S., Takada, Y., Sugiura, T., Yamamoto, H., Sawa, T., Kawahara, M., Katakami, N., Ariyoshi, Y., and Fukuoka, M. Phase II study of amrubicin in previously untreated patients with extensive-disease small cell lung cancer: West Japan Thoracic Oncology Group (WJTOG) study. *Invest. New Drugs* **2007**, *25*, 253–258.
50. Yamamoto. M., Yanase, N., Yanaihara, T., Onoda, S., Ishii, K., Hagiri, S., Ryuge, S., Wada, M., Kato, E., and Masuda, N. Amrubicin (Calsed®) monotherapy for patients with small-cell lung cancer: study in cases unfit for combination chemotherapy. *Japan J. Lung Cancer* **2005**, *45*, 329–333.
51. Igawa, S., Ryuge, S., Fukui, T., Otani, S., Kimura, Y., Kanato, K., Takakura, A., Kubota, M., Mistufuji, H., Katagiri, M., Yanase, N., and Masuda, N. Amrubicin for treating elderly and poor-risk patients with small-cell lung cancer. *Int. J. Clin. Oncol.* **2010**, *15*, 147–452.
52. Ohe, Y., Negoro, S., Matsui, K., Nakagawa, K., Sugiura, T., Takada, Y., Nishiwaki, Y., Yokota, S., Kawahara, M., Saijo, N., Fukuoka, M., and Ariyoshi, Y. Phase I-II study of amrubicin and cisplatin in previously untreated patients with extensive-stage small-cell lung cancer. *Ann. Oncol.* **2005**, *16*, 430–436.
53. O'Brien, M., Konopa, K., Lorigan, P., Bosquee, L., Marshall, E., Bustin, F., Margerit, S., Fink, C., Stigt, J. A., Dingemans, A. M. C., Hasan, B., Van Meerbeeck, J., and Baas, P. Randomised phase II study of amrubicin as single agent or in combination with cisplatin versus cisplatin etoposide as first-line treatment in patients with extensive-stage small cell lung cancer - EORTG 08062. *Eur. J. Cancer*, **2011**, *47*, 2322–2330.
54. Fukuda, M., Nakamura, Y., Kasai, T., Nagashima, S., Nakatomi, K., Doi, S., Nakano, H., Takatomi, H., Fukuda, M., Kinoshita, A., Soda, H., Tsukamoto, K., Oka, M., Kohno, S., Nagasaki Thoracic Oncology Group. A phase I study of amrubicin and carboplatin for previously untreated patients with extensive-disease small cell lung cancer. *J. Thorac. Oncol.* **2009**, *4*, 741–745.
55. Inoue, A., Yamazaki, K., Maemondo, M., Suzuki, T., Kimura, Y., Kanbe, M., Isobe, H., Nishimura, M., Saijo, Y., and Nukiwa, T. A phase I study of amrubicin combined with carboplatin for elderly patients with small-cell lung cancer. *J. Thorac. Oncol.* **2006**, *1*, 551–555.

56. Inoue, A., Ishimoto, O., Fukumoto, S., Usui, K., Suzuki, T., Yokouchi, H., Meamondo, M., Kanbe, M., Ogura, S., Harada, T., Oizumi, S., Harada, M., Sugawara, S., Fukuhara, T., and Nukiwa, T. A phase II study of amrubicin combined with carboplatin for elderly patients with small-cell lung cancer: North Japan Lung Cancer Study Group trial 0405. *Ann. Oncol.*, **2010**, *21*, 800–803.
57. Oshita, F., Saito, H., and Yamada, K. Dose escalation study of amrubicin in combination with fixed-dose irinotecan in patients with extensive small-cell lung cancer. *Oncology*, **2007**, *74*, 7–11.
58. Shibayama, T., Hotta, K., Takigawa, N., Tada, A., Ueoka, H., Harita, S., Kiura, K., Tabata, M., Segawa, Y., Nogami, N., Kuyama, S., Shinkai, T., and Tanimoto, M. A phase I and pharmacological study of amrubicin and topotecan in patients of small-cell lung cancer with relapsed or extensive-disease small-cell lung cancer. *Lung Cancer* **2006**, *53*, 189–195.
59. Kim, Y. H. and Mishima, M. Second-line chemotherapy for small-cell lung cancer (SCLC). *Cancer Treatment Rev.*, **2010**, DOI: 10.1016/j.ctrv.2010.05.004
60. Kato, K., Nikihara, H., Ohe, Y., Yamamoto, N., Sekine, I., Kunitoh, H., Kubota, K., Nishikawa, Y., Saijo, N., and Tamura, T. Phase II trial of amrubicin in patients with previously treated small cell lung cancer (SCLC). *J. Clin. Oncol.* **2006**, *24*, 7061.
61. Hasegawa, Y., Takeda, K., Kashii, T., Kawano, Y., Katayama, H., Sumitani, M., Takifuji, N., and Negoro, S. Clinical experience of amrubicin hydrochloride (Calsed®) monotherapy in previously treated patients with small-cell lung cancer. *Japan. J. Lung Cancer* **2005**, *45*, 811–815.
62. Onoda, S., Masuda, N., Seto, T., Eguchi, K., Takiguchi, Y., Isobe, H., Okamoto, H., Ogura, T., Yokoyama, A., Seki, N., Asaka-Amano, Y., Harada, M., Tagawa, A., Kunitake, H., Yokoba, M., Uematsu, K., Kuriyama, T., Kuroiwa, Y., and Watanebe, K. Phase II trial of amrubicin for treatment of refractory or relapsed small-cell lung cancer: Thoracic Oncology Research Group study 0301. *J. Clin. Oncol.* **2006**, *24*, 5448–5453.
63. Ettinger, D. S., Jotte, R., Lorigan, P., Gupta, V., Garbo, L., Alemany C., Conklings, P., Spigel, D. R., Dudek, A. Z., Shah, C., Salgia, R., McNally, R., Renschler, M. F., and Oliver, J. W. Phase II study of amrubicin as second-line therapy in patients with platinum-refractory small-cell lung cancer. *J. Clin. Oncol.* **2010**, *28*, 2598–2603.
64. Inoue, A., Sugawara, S., Yamazaki, K., Maemondo, M., Suzuki, T., Gomi, K., Takanashi, S., Inoue, C., Inage, M., Yokouchi, H., Watanabe, H., Tsukamoto, T., Saijo, Y., Ishimoto, O., Hommura, F., and Nukita, T. Randomized phase II trial comparing amrubicin with topotecan in patients with previously treated small-cell lung cancer: North Japan Lung Cancer Study Group trial 0402. *J. Clin. Oncol.* **2008**, *26*, 5401–5406.
65. Jotte, R., Conkling, P., Reynolds, C., Galsky, M. D., Klein, L., Fitzgibbons, J. F., McNally, R., Renschler M. F., and Oliver, J. W. Randomized phase II trial of single-agent amrubicin or topotecan as second-line treatment in patients with small-cell lung cancer sensitive to first-line platinum-based chemotherapy. *J. Clin. Oncol.* **2010**, *29*, 287-293.

CHAPTER 7

THE DISCOVERY OF DUAL IGF-1R AND IR INHIBITOR FQIT FOR THE TREATMENT OF CANCER

Meizhong Jin, Elizabeth Buck, and Mark J. Mulvihill

7.1 BIOLOGICAL RATIONAL FOR TARGETING THE IGF-1R/IR PATHWAY FOR ANTI-CANCER THERAPY

The type I insulin-like growth factor receptor (IGF-1R) is a receptor tyrosine kinase that has been implicated in the development and progression of various human cancers. Receptor activation can promote tumor cell proliferation and survival pathways. IGF-1R can couple strongly to the PI3K-AKT cellular survival pathway through the adaptor proteins insulin receptor substrates 1/2 (IRS-1/2), and IGF-1R signaling plays a significant role in the growth and survival of multiple human cancers including hepatocellular carcinoma (HCC), Ewing's sarcoma (EwS), multiple myeloma (MM), and nonsmall cell lung carcinoma (NSCLC) [1–3]. IGF-1R activity is required for the cellular transforming capabilities of a number of oncogenes including Ras [4]. Expression of IGF-1R and overexpression of its ligands IGF-I and IGF-II have been observed in human cancers and are associated with disease incidence, progression, and prognosis [5,6]. Ablation of IGF-1R signaling through either genetic or pharmacological methods has been shown to reduce tumor cell proliferation and survival for select tumor models [7]. Furthermore, it has been shown that IGF-1R signaling is associated with acquired resistance of tumor cells to chemo or radiation therapies, and molecular targeted therapies including epidermal growth factor receptor (EGFR) inhibitors and human epidermal growth factor receptor 2 (HER2) inhibitors [8–17].

More recent data has demonstrated that signaling through the structurally and functionally related insulin receptor (IR) also plays a role in tumor growth. IR can promote tumor cell survival and proliferation and induce cellular transformation *in vitro* [18]. IR expression can also promote tumor growth *in vivo* [19]. Ablation of pancreatic islet cells in the Alloxan-induced diabetes model is accompanied by reduced growth of xenografted tumors [20,21], and the administration of insulin can promote the growth of rat mammary tumors [22]. Overexpression of IR is observed in a number of tumor types including breast, ovarian, and thyroid, where autocrine or paracrine expression of IGF-II, through activation of IR homodimers, has been shown to drive tumor cell proliferation [23,24]. IGF-II has been shown to signal through both the IR-A IR isoform and IR/IGF-1R heterodimers, in addition to its stimulation of IGF-1R. Epidemiologic studies also support a role for IR in cancer, as elevated levels of insulin or C-peptide is a poor prognostic indicator for prostate and breast cancer patients [7,25,26]. Inhaled insulin has also been associated with increased lung cancer risk [27].

Case Studies in Modern Drug Discovery and Development, Edited by Xianhai Huang and Robert G. Aslanian.

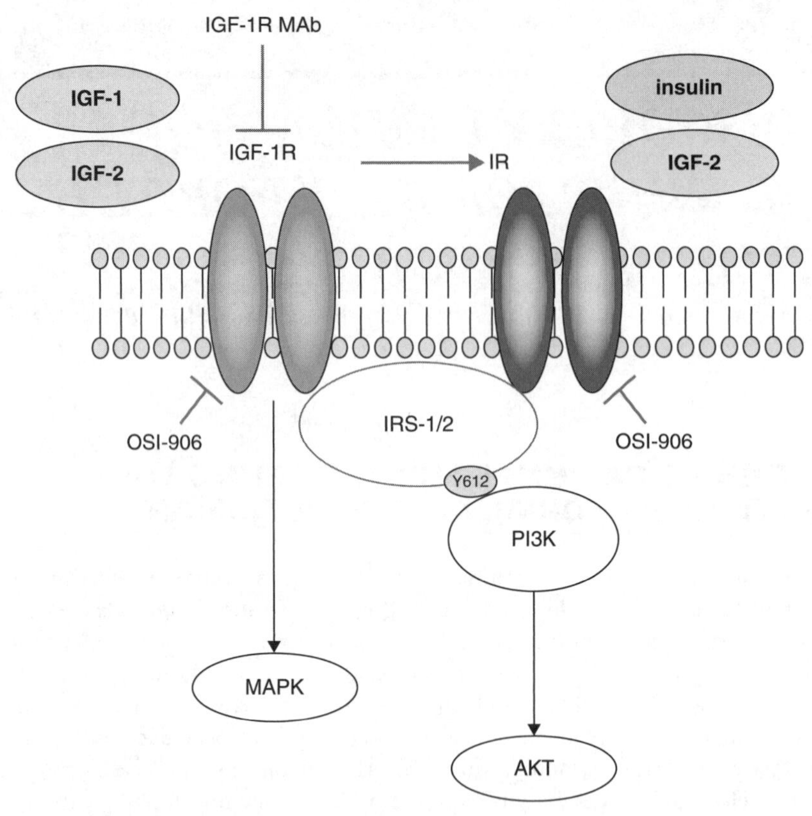

Figure 7.1 IGF-1R and IR cellular signaling cascades, highlighting the varying approaches that can be used to target this axis. Treatment with an IGF-1R specific antibody may be associated with a compensatory increase in IR activity. In contrast, a small molecule tyrosine kinase inhibitor such as OSI-906 can effectively co-inhibit both IGF-1R and IR.

There is evidence for functional reciprocity between IGF-1R and IR. For both osteoblasts and adipocytes, compensatory signaling through the insulin-IR-IRS1-AKT pathway can maintain growth and differentiation upon ablation of IGF-1R [28,29]. It has been recently reported by OSI that human tumor cells frequently co-express both IGF-1R and IR, and IR activity is upregulated upon IGF-1R inhibition by specific anti-IGF-1R antibodies [19]. The inability of IGF-1R neutralizing antibodies to inhibit IR is associated with incomplete AKT pathway inhibition in many cancer types including NSCLC, ovarian carcinoma (OvCa), EwS, colorectal carcinoma (CRC), and adrenocortical carcinoma (ACC). Collectively, these data indicate that co-targeting both IGF-1R and IR may yield superior and broader antitumor efficacy as compared to specific targeting of IGF-1R alone for some tumor types. Moreover, these data provide a rationale for potential differentiation of dual inhibitors of IGF-1R and IR kinase activity, compared to the IGF-1R-selective monoclonal antibodies currently in clinical development (Figure 7.1).

7.2 DISCOVERY OF OSI-906

7.2.1 Summary of OSI-906 Discovery

Due to the significance of IGF-1R and IR in oncogenesis, OSI Pharmaceuticals, Inc. invested in a small molecule drug discovery platform that targeted IGF-1R and IR kinase activities. The initial efforts centered around an imidazo[1,5-*a*]pyrazine scaffold [30–32]. Compound **1** represents an early hit for the series with a benzyloxyphenyl moiety at the C1 position.

TABLE 7.1 Evolution of Imidazo[1,5-*a*]Pyrazine-Derived IGF-1R/IR Inhibitors

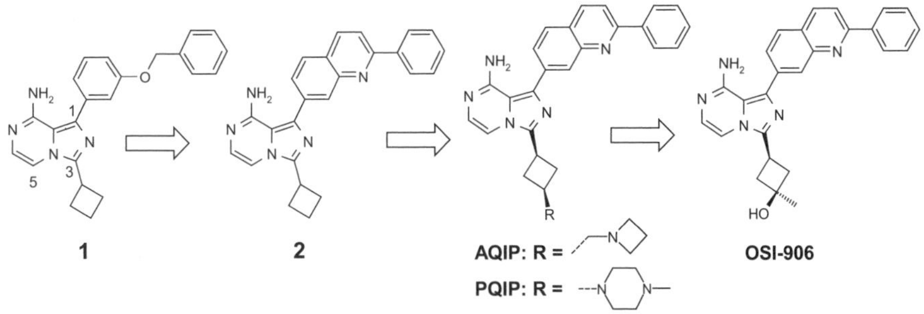

1 ⇨ 2 ⇨ AQIP: R = / PQIP: R = ⇨ OSI-906

Compound	IGF-1R cellular mechanistic IC_{50} (nM)[a]	Microsomal stability (ER)	
		Mouse	Human
1	1160	0.96	0.93
2	86	0.88	0.85
AQIP	20	0.52	0.28
PQIP	19	0.53	0.59
OSI-906	24	0.54	0.55

[a]IGF-1R potency in NIH 3T3/huIGF-1R cells.

Medicinal chemistry exploration driven by structure-based drug design (SBDD) led to the identification of a 2-phenylquinolin-7-yl moiety as an optimal group at the C1 position as shown in compound **2**. This moiety binds to a hydrophobic back pocket of IGF-1R, forming a critical H-bond to Lys1003 via the quinoline nitrogen and places the terminal phenyl ring in contact with several hydrophobic residues including F980, F1124, F1017, G1125, and A1021. These key interactions led to a significant increase in IGF-1R potency for the quinolinyl series over that of the benzyloxyphenyl series, as exemplified by compounds **1** and **2** (Table 7.1) and suggest that a more optimal bioactive conformation was achieved.

The C3 position highlighted an additional key SAR feature, where substitution at this position impacted both potency and drug metabolism and pharmacokinetic (DMPK) properties of the molecule [30–32]. A bridging cyclobutyl moiety was found to be an optimal C3 substituent. It is a compact cycloalkyl moiety (minimizes molecular weight and log *P* versus other larger cycloaklyl options such as cyclohexyl), occupies the ribose binding pocket where it makes critical hydrophobic interactions with V983 and L975, acts as a linker to distal groups that access a solvent exposed region of the protein and when substituted at the C3 position with the examples described within, maintains a plane of symmetry. Extensive analoging in this region of the molecule yielded advanced lead compounds such as AQIP [30], PQIP [31], and eventually OSI-906 [32], which features a cyclobutyl moiety substituted with a *cis*-tertiary alcohol. OSI-906 is the first and only small molecule dual IGF-1R/IR inhibitor currently in phase III clinical trials. Some key IGF-1R binding interactions of OSI-906 with the IGF-1R kinase domain are highlighted in Figures 7.2a and 7.2b.

7.2.2 OSI-906 Clinical Aspects

OSI-906 is currently in advanced clinical development. Phase I studies for OSI-906 as a single agent have identified a maximum tolerated dose (MTD) for both continuous and intermittent dosing schedules. Inhibition of IGF-1R and IR targets in tissues and peripheral blood was evidenced by monitoring for phosphorylation of IGF-1R and IR on peripheral

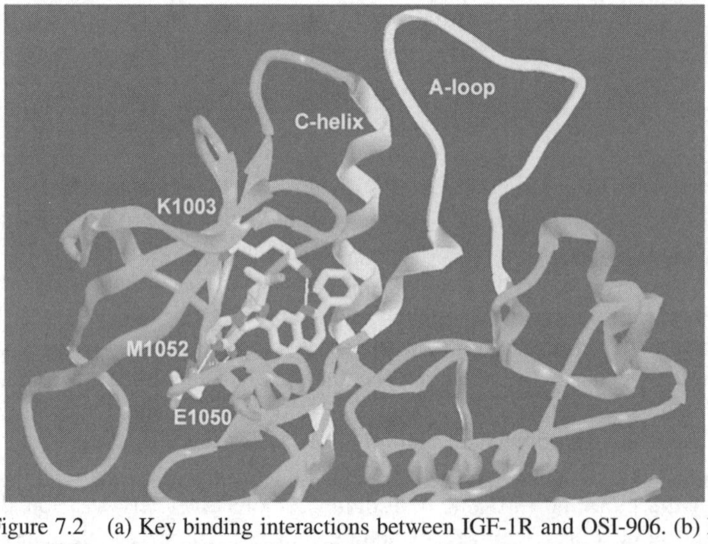

Figure 7.2 (a) Key binding interactions between IGF-1R and OSI-906. (b) Modeled structure of OSI-906 in complex with IGF-1R with (a) key hydrogen bonding interactions highlighted; (b) C-helix highlighted in yellow and (c) activation loop (A-loop) highlighted in white. (See color version of the figure in Color Plate section)

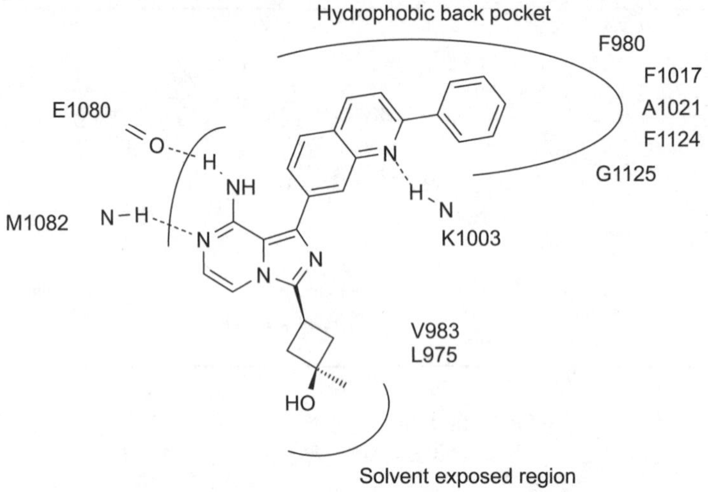

blood mononuclear cells (PBMCs) and for changes in circulating IGF-1 and IGFBP3 levels. Preliminary evidence for antitumor activity was observed, including both long-term stable disease and antitumor response for a patient with ACC. Interestingly, ACC is associated with elevated expression of IGF-II ligand. As preclinical data has provided a rationale for combining an EGFR inhibitor with an IGF-1R/IR inhibitor due to compensatory signaling, current efforts are ongoing in a phase I study to determine the MTD for OSI-906 in combination with the EGFR inhibitor erlotinib. Advanced phase II and phase III studies are also currently ongoing for OSI-906 as a single agent in ACC and HCC, where preclinical data have highlighted the importance for dual IGF-1R and IR targeting, and also in combination with paclitaxel for the treatment of ovarian cancer.

7.3 OSI-906 BACK UP EFFORTS

As OSI-906 advanced though late stage preclinical and early clinical studies, we initiated back-up efforts both to expand and further diversify our IGF-1R/IR small-molecule inhibitor library and to identify a series of advanced agents that were poised to progress into the development stage behind OSI-906 if warranted. A major challenge associated with a backup program is that one is limited to addressing preclinical liabilities associated with the most advanced agent, which may in some cases be species specific and therefore may not emerge as a liability in the human clinical setting. Therefore, the goal of our backup efforts centered around identifying a series of late stage drug-like dual IGF-1R/IR inhibitors with a different chemical scaffold to that of OSI-906 (in case of the emergence of a core-related issues) and which demonstrated a comparable if not superior drug-like profile to OSI-906 and therefore met the following target candidate profile.

- High degree of kinase selectivity especially against targets such as vascular endothelial growth factor receptor (VEGFR) and cell cycle associated kinases (i.e., Aurora kinases) to avoid potential dose-limiting off-target toxicities.
- Inhibition of ligand-induced phosphorylation of IGF-1R and IR in cell-based assays with an IC_{50} value of <50 nM.
- Metabolic stability assessment in both human and mouse liver microsomes with an *in vitro* extraction ratio (ER) of <0.7 in order to filter compounds that are predicted to be extensively metabolized and cleared by the liver via first-pass drug metabolism.
- High permeability (PAMPA $\geq 100 \times 10^{-6}$ cm s^{-1}, pH $= 5$–7.4) to achieve good drug absorption.
- Oral bioavailability %F ≥ 30 in rodent and nonrodent species both to enable *in vivo* efficacy and toxicology studies via oral administration and to provide preclinical precedence for oral dosing in humans.
- Sustained inhibition ($\geq$12 h) of IGF-1R and IR phosphorylation in tumor xeno-graft models without inducing sustained hyperglycemia (blood glucose level <300 mg dL^{-1}).
- *In vivo* efficacy in tumor xenograft models without inducing sustained hyperglycemia.
- Clear correlation between drug exposures, PD effects and efficacy.
- Therapeutic index >1 in multiple species in order to demonstrate tolerability in rodent and nonrodent species at doses exceeding the predicted efficacious dose.
- No inhibition of major cytochrome P450 (CYP) isoforms ($IC_{50} > 10\,\mu$M) to avoid any potential CYP enzyme-mediated drug–drug interactions.
- No *in vitro* mutagenicity (negative in the Ames test $\pm$ S9 fraction) to avoid genotoxicity.

The efforts on our initial OSI-906 backup program led to the discovery of dual IGF-1R/IR inhibitor FQIT as one of the several lead agents that met the desired target candidate profile. Our drug discovery and medicinal chemistry efforts leading to FQIT are described within.

7.4 THE DISCOVERY OF FQIT

7.4.1 Lead Generation Strategy

Our investment in the imidazo[1,5-*a*]pyrazine chemotype as a tunable kinase template, utilized to create selective IGF-1R/IR [30–32] and mTOR [33] inhibitors, led to further exploration of the chemical reactivity of this novel and underexploited scaffold. As

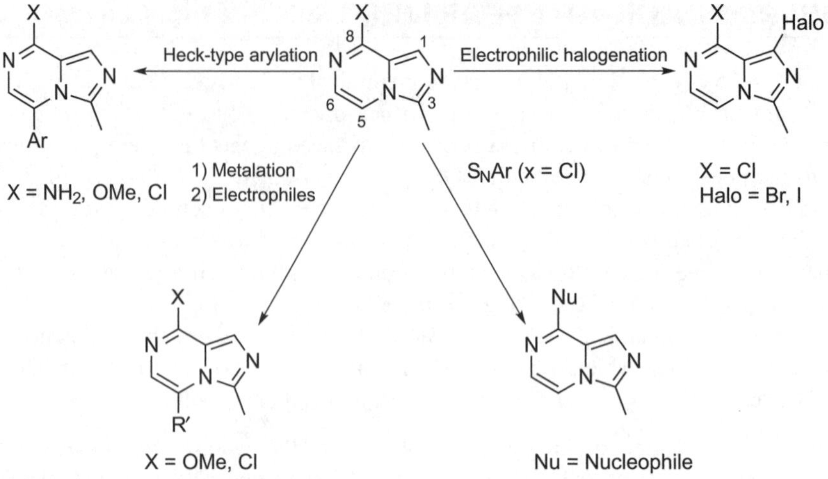

Heck-type arylation

Electrophilic halogenation

X = NH_2, OMe, Cl

1) Metalation
2) Electrophiles

S_NAr (x = Cl)

X = Cl
Halo = Br, I

X = OMe, Cl

Nu = Nucleophile

Figure 7.3 Chemical reactivity of the imidazo[1,5-*a*]pyrazine scaffold.

summarized in Figure 7.3, in addition to the C1 carbon as the major site for electrophilic substitutions and the C8 position as the site for S_NAr reactions (when X is a leaving group such as chloro), the exploration led to the discovery that the C5 carbon is also reactive under certain conditions. For example, under palladium catalyzed conditions a Heck-type direct arylation occurs at the C5 position, presumably due to partial double bond-like characteristics of C5=C6 within the aromatic system [34]. It was also demonstrated that the C5-H proton is the most acidic proton when the C3 position is occupied by groups such as simple alkyls. Selective deprotonation was achieved and subsequent quench with a range of electrophiles afforded various C5-substituted compounds in good yields [35]. These newly discovered chemistries, while providing excellent methodologies for the installation of various functionalities at the C5 position, highlighted the reactivity of the C5-H and/or the C5=C6 structural unit under selected conditions. These results shed light on an observed biotransformation noted upon incubation in hepatic microsomes and the formation of a minor M-24 metabolite among selected imidazo[1,5-*a*]pyrazine derivatives as a result of oxidation of the C5=C6 bond followed by a subsequent hydrolytic cleavage.

During our drug discovery efforts, various cores that were bioisosteric to the imidazo [1,5-*a*]pyrazines were explored. The imidazo[5,1-*f*][1,2,4]triazine scaffold was of particular interest since it closely mimics the imidazo[1,5-*a*]pyrazine scaffold and therefore allows for the transfer of key pharmacophoric elements and replaces the C5 carbon of the imidazo[1,5-*a*]pyrazine with a nitrogen atom (Figure 7.4) and therefore blocking the C5 site of metabolism. The medicinal chemistry effort towards a series of imidazo[5,1-*f*][1,2,4] triazine-based inhibitors of IGF-1R and IR is reported here, and particularly, the discovery of FQIT as a potent, selective, orally bioavailable dual IGF-1R and IR inhibitor [36]. Through extensive preclinical studies including *in vivo* efficacy in mouse xenograft models and pharmacokinetics (PK) and toxicology in multiple species, this agent has demonstrated overall comparable drug-like qualities to that of the clinical agent, OSI-906.

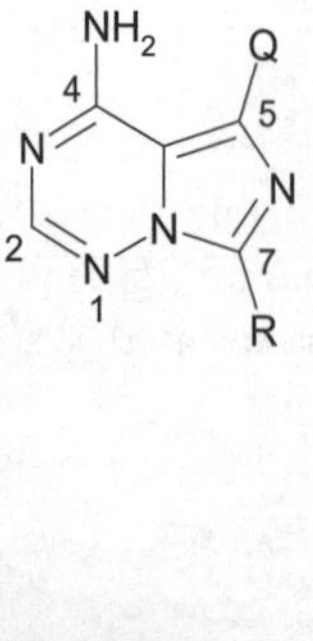

Figure 7.4 5, 7-disubstituted imidazo[5,1-*f*][1,2,4]triazine.

7.4.2 Small Molecule Dual IGF-1R/IR Inhibitor Drug Discovery Cascade

A general *in vitro* and *in vivo* IGF-1R/IR small molecule inhibitor centric drug discovery cascade is described in Figure 7.5. Compounds were profiled in an enzyme-linked immunosorbent assay (ELISA)-based cell assay utilizing NIH-3T3 cells over-expressing human IGF-1R (LISN) to determine IGF-1R cellular mechanistic potencies. Furthermore, compounds were profiled in various *in vitro* assays to determine such ADME properties as microsomal stability (ER), CYP inhibition, and permeability (PAMPA). Key compounds were also profiled for selectivity in a Caliper and/or Invitrogen kinase panel. Compounds with favorable potency, absorption, distribution, metabolism, excretion (ADME), and selectivity properties were then progressed into various phenotypic assays that measured the ability of the compounds to inhibit proliferation and/or induce apoptosis in IGF-1R/IR-, IGF-1R-, and IR-driven cell lines, including for example, the colorectal tumor cell line GEO as well as IGF-1R and IR direct complementation (DC) cell lines, respectively. Compounds with promising *in vitro* profiles from these assays were further advanced into *in vivo* studies, which included PK studies in rodents with both i.v. and p.o. dosing regimens. Compounds with adequate PK properties progressed to evaluation in various pharmacodynamic (PD) and tumor growth inhibition (TGI) studies. Robust *in vivo* efficacy combined with good tolerability with a clear PK to PD correlation then triggered additional advanced profiling that included a variety of toxicological and IND-track enabling studies.

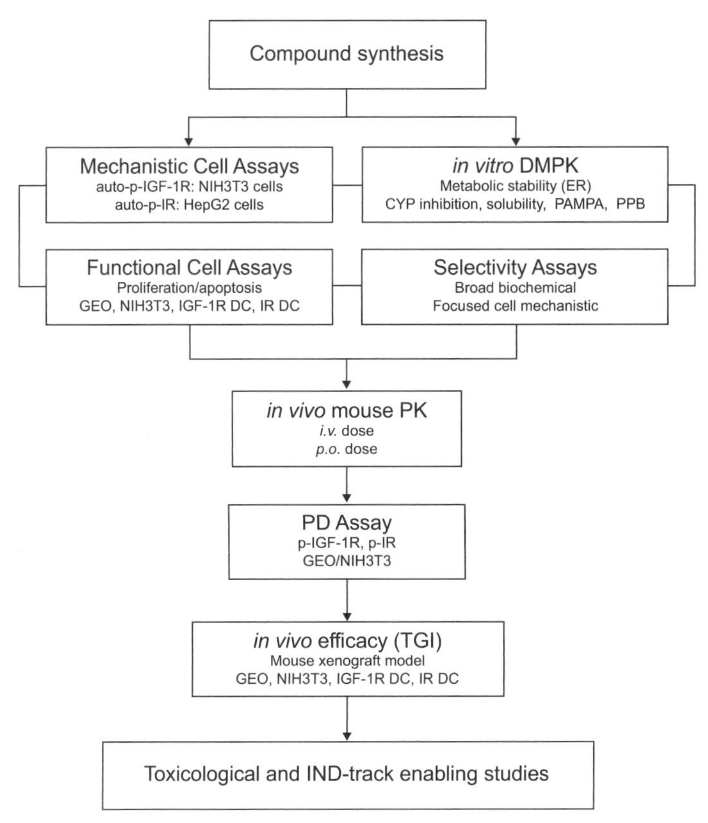

Figure 7.5 General *in vitro* and *in vivo* IGF-1R/IR drug discovery cascade.

7.4.3 Initial Proof-of-Concept Compounds

Initially, in order to determine the viability of the 5,7-disubstituted imidazo[5,1-*f*][1,2,4] triazines as a bioisosteric template to the established imidazo[1,5-*a*]pyrazines, two imidazotriazine proof-of-concept (PoC) compounds, **3** and **22**, were synthesized and compared head to head with imidazo[1,5-*a*]pyrazine early hit **1** and lead compound **2**. As shown in Table 7.2, compounds **3** and **22** showed activity against IGF-1R both biochemically and cellularly. However, a approximately three- to fourfold of loss in potency was observed when compared to imidazo[1,5-*a*]pyrazine counterparts **1** and **2**, respectively. This decrease in potency is speculated to be due to a weaker hinge hydrogen bonding interaction due to a reduction in the electron density of the donor and acceptor in the imidazo[5,1-*f*][1,2,4] triazine chemotype versus that of the imidazo[1,5-*a*]pyrazine chemotype. A desolvation penalty due to the introduction of the extra nitrogen atom in the imidazo[5,1-*f*][1,2,4] triazine scaffold may also play a contributing role. Interestingly, compound **22** was still approximately seven- to ninefold more potent than compound **3**, which correlated with the earlier SAR trend established in the imidazo[1,5-*a*]pyrazine series. This suggested that the SAR in this region of the molecule was likely transferable from imidazo[1,5-*a*]pyrazine series to imidazo[5,1-*f*][1,2,4]triazine series. Since the quinolinyl moiety was a key potency driving pharmacophore in the imidazo[1,5-*a*]pyrazine series, efforts focused on further optimizing the quinoline/Lys1003 interaction as a means of improving potency for the new series. Additionally, both compounds **3** and **22** displayed poor microsomal stability (ER >0.85). This instability was suspected to be due to extensive metabolism of the cyclobutyl moiety as noted with earlier unoptimized analogues and could be alleviated through the incorporation of key substituents in the solvent exposed region of the molecule.

TABLE 7.2 ***In vitro*** **IGF-1R Potency and Microsomal Stability of Compounds 3 and 22 and their Imidazo[1,5-*a*]Pyrazine Counterparts 1, 2**

1: X = CH
3: X = N

2: X = CH
22: X = N

Compound	IGF-1R biochemical[a] IC_{50} (μM)	IGF-1R cellular[b] IC_{50} (μM)	Microsomal stability (ER) Mouse	Microsomal stability (ER) Human
1	0.61	1.2	0.96	0.93
3	1.9	3.0	0.96	0.95
2	0.079	0.086	0.88	0.85
22	0.27	0.33	0.89	0.91

[a] 100 μM ATP.

[b] Cellular mechanistic potency in NIH 3T3/huIGF-1R cell line.

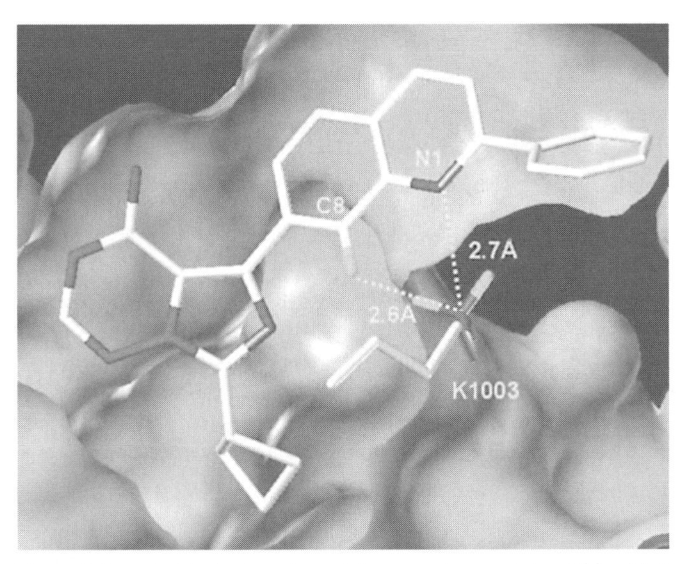

Figure 7.6 Modeled interaction of the quinoline moiety of **22** with the catalytic lysine (K1003) of IGF-1R. Altering the inhibitor structure from PQIP (PDB ID: 3D94) by deleting the attachment off the cyclobutyl moiety and modifying the C5 position of the imidazopyrazine core from CH to N yields the depicted model.

In order to further increase the potency of the imidazotriazine series through optimization of the binding interaction of the quinolinyl moiety with the Lys1003 residue, the team turned to further assessment of imidazopyrazine/IGF-1R and IR co-crystal structures [37]. Detailed evaluation of the interaction of the quinoline with Lys1003 revealed that a proton from the Lys1003 amine points directly at the C8-H position in a lowest energy rotamer of the amine (depicted in Figure 7.6). This observation led to the hypothesis that a hydrogen bond acceptor at the C8 position of the quinolinyl moiety could strengthen the binding interaction to Lys1003 through the formation of an additional hydrogen bond and lead to enhanced IGF-1R potency. Moreover, further evaluation suggested that the space adjacent to the quinoline C8 position is sterically congested, limiting replacements of the C8-H to either N8 or C8-F. It was eventually decided to pursue a fluorine substitution at this position based on the following factors: (1) fluorine is metabolically inert while serving as a hydrogen bond acceptor; (2) fluorine has small Van der Waals volume; (3) a fluorine at the C8 position approaches the basic amine on Lys1003 in a optimal distance for hydrogen bonding versus a ring nitrogen atom at that position.

7.4.4 Synthesis of 5,7-Disubstituted Imidazo[5,1-*f*][1,2,4] Triazines

Two synthetic approaches were implemented for the synthesis of the 5,7-disubstituted imidazo[5,1-*f*][1,2,4]triazines as IGF-1R/IR inhibitors [38]. As shown in Figure 7.7, synthetic approach 1 featured the installation of substituents at the C5 position (Q) earlier in the synthesis and thus provided a key common intermediate that allowed for analoging at the C7 position by incorporating different "R" groups. Synthetic approach 2 featured a key C5 halogenated intermediate that enabled rapid analoging at the C5 position primarily via palladium catalyzed cross-coupling reactions. Subsequently, several modified routes to approach 2 were implemented that took advantage of various commercially available starting materials.

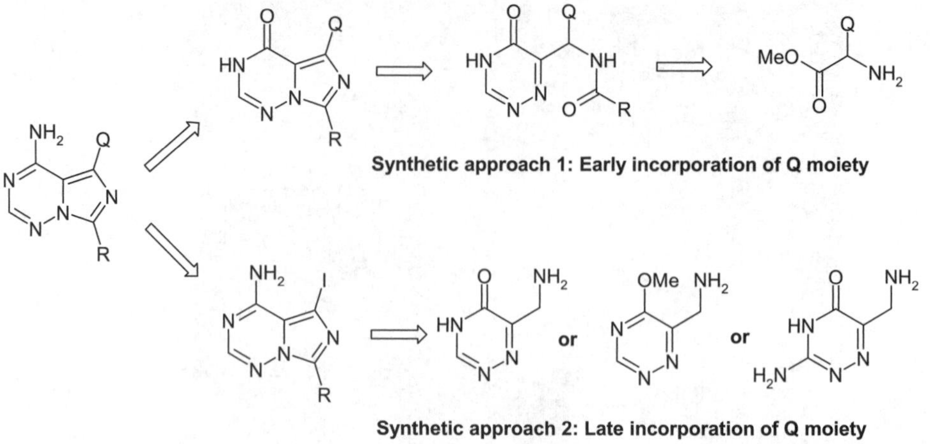

Synthetic approach 1: Early incorporation of Q moiety

Synthetic approach 2: Late incorporation of Q moiety

Figure 7.7 Synthetic approaches to 5,7-disubstituted imidazo[5,1-*f*][1,2,4]triazines.

The detailed synthetic routes are illustrated in Schemes 7.1–7.3, which highlight the synthesis of compound **3**, an early stage PoC compound for this series. Compound **3** was synthesized via synthetic approach 1 from methyl amino[3-(benzyloxy)phenyl]acetate **4**. As shown in Scheme 7.1, key steps included a hydrazonoformic hydrazide [$CH(=NHNH_2)NHNH_2$]-mediated cyclization [39] reaction that converted amide **6** to triazinone **7** in moderate yield. Deamination via the diazonium salt using sodium nitrite followed by $POCl_3$-mediated cyclization afforded the desired bicyclic imidazotriazinone **8**. Finally, treatment of **8** with $POCl_3$ and 1,2,4-triazole in pyridine and subsequent ammonolysis in a one-pot fashion provided target compound **3**.

While this initial synthetic approach led to the early installation of C-5 substituents and allowed for analoging at the C7 position by utilizing different acids or acid derivatives in the amide coupling step, this approach was not suitable for rapid analoging at the C5 position. In order to enable late stage analoging at the C5 position, intermediate **9**, which incorporated a halogen at the C5 position as a handle for further analoging, was targeted. The initial synthesis of compound **9** commenced from the cyclization of ester **10** and

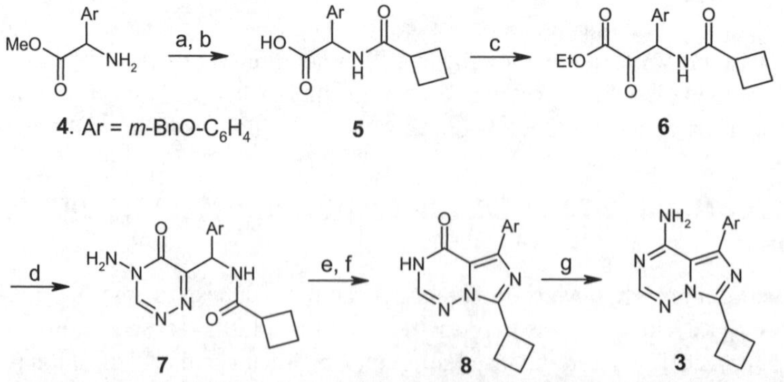

4. Ar = *m*-BnO-C_6H_4

Scheme 7.1 Synthesis of compound **3** via synthetic approach 1. *Reagents and conditions:* (a) cyclobutanecarbonyl chloride, $NaHCO_3$, THF, 0 °C ~ rt, 83%; (b) 1M NaOH, THF/H_2O (1:1), 84%; (c) (i) EtO_2CCOCl, pyridine, DMAP, THF, reflux; (ii) NaOEt, EtOH, reflux, 16%; (d) 1M N_2H_4 in THF, $HC(=NH)NH_2$.HCl, EtOH, 0°C ~ −20 °C ~ rt, 45%; (e) $NaNO_2$, conc. HCl, EtOH/H_2O, 0 °C ~ rt, 83%; (f) $POCl_3$, 55 °C, 100%; (g) 1,2,4-triazole, $POCl_3$, pyridine, rt, then 1M NH_3 in *i*-PrOH, 0 °C ~ rt, 39%.

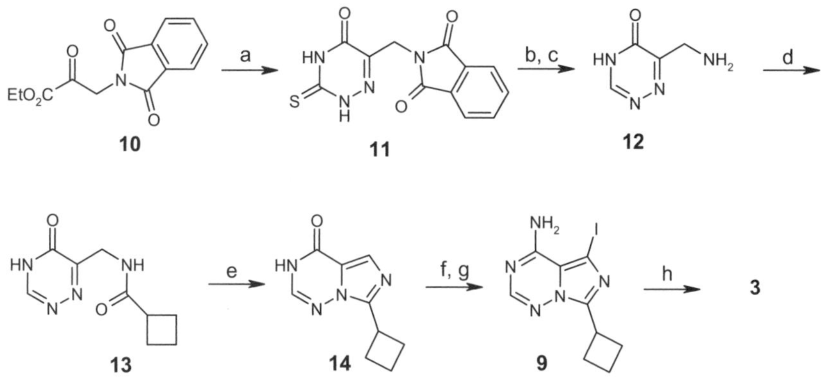

Scheme 7.2 Synthesis of compound **3** via synthetic approach 2 – route 1. *Reagents and conditions*: (a) thiosemicarbazide, EtOH, 80 °C, 3 h, then DIEA, 40 °C, 16 h, 81%; (b) Raney Ni (10 eq.), EtOH, reflux, 70%; (c) anhydrous hydrazine, DCM/EtOH (1:1), rt; (d) cyclobutanecarbonyl chloride, DIEA, DMF, 0 °C ~ rt, 57% (2 steps); (e) $POCl_3$, 55 °C, 41%; (f) 5 eq. NIS (5 eq.), DMF, rt ~ 55 °C, 53%; (g) 1,2,4-triazole, $POCl_3$, pyridine, rt, then 1M NH_3 in *i*-PrOH, 0 °C ~ rt, 82%; (h) [3-(benzyloxy) phenyl]boronic acid, $PdCl_2$(dppf), K_2CO_3, Dioxane/H_2O (4:1), 100 °C (microwave), 30 min, 72%.

thiosemicarbazide (Scheme 7.2). Key steps included desulfurization of compound **11** using Raney nickel followed by cleavage of the phthalimide protecting group to give amino-methyl-triazinone **12**. This compound proved to be a versatile intermediate since various C-7 substituents could be readily installed at this stage via a carboxylic acid or equivalent thereof. After amide formation and $POCl_3$-mediated cyclization, iodination and ammonolysis provided key intermediate **9**, from which various groups could be introduced at the C-5 position by palladium catalyzed cross coupling reactions. For example, compound **3** was readily synthesized in good yield via Suzuki coupling of [3-(benzyloxy)phenyl]boronic acid with iodo-imidazotriazine intermediate **9**.

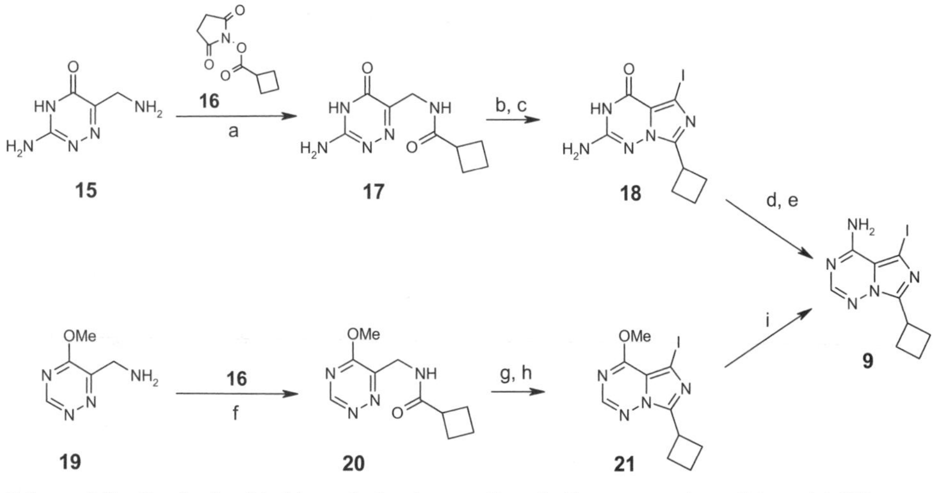

Scheme 7.3 Synthesis of imidazotriazine intermediate **9**. *Reagents and conditions*: (a) 1M $NaHCO_3$, THF/MeCN (1:1), rt, 83%; (b) $POCl_3$, 1,2-dichloroethane, reflux, 90%; (c) NIS, DMF, rt, 75%; (d) *t*-butylnitrite, 5% DMF in MeCN, rt, 91%; (e) 1,2,4-triazole, $POCl_3$, pyridine, rt, then 1M NH_3 in *i*-PrOH, 0 °C ~ rt, 82%. (f) 10% aq. $NaHCO_3$, THF, rt, 72%; (g) $POCl_3$, DMF/MeCN, rt, 55%; (h) NIS, DMF, 55 °C, 68%; (i) 7N NH_3 in MeOH, rt, 89%.

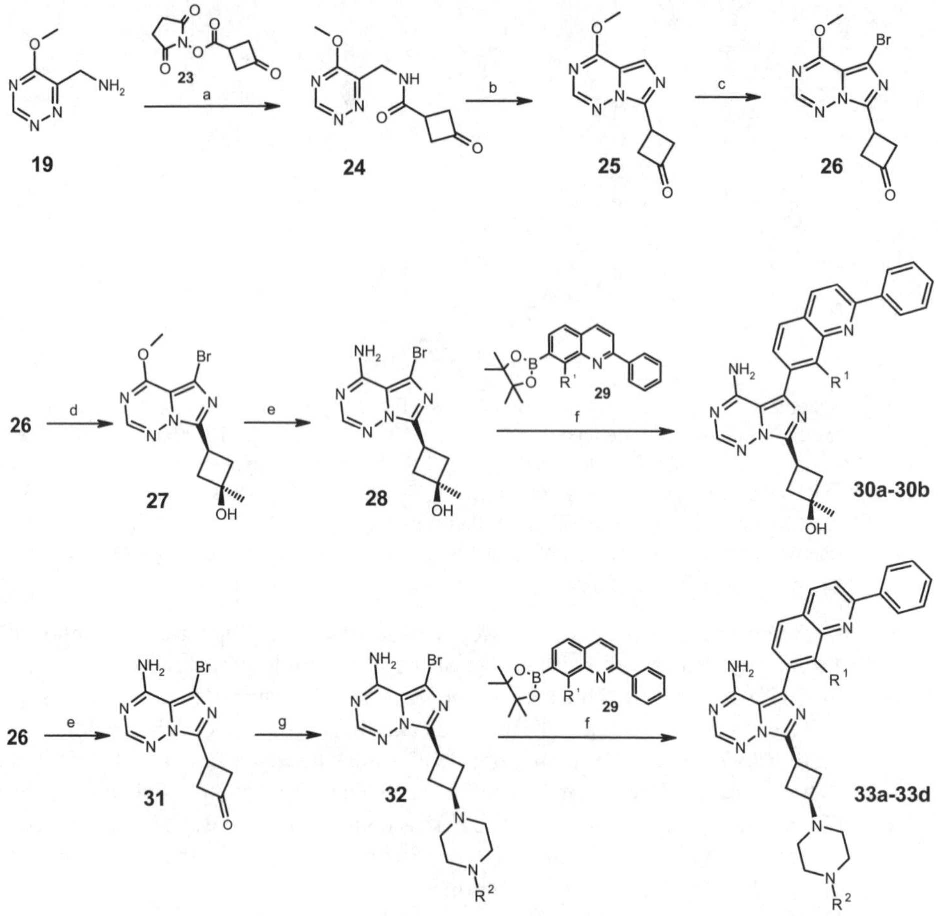

Scheme 7.4 General synthesis of compounds **30**, **33.** *Reagents and conditions*: (a) 10% aq. $NaHCO_3$, THF, rt, 65%; (b) $POCl_3$, DMF/MeCN, rt; (c) NBS, DMF, 55%, 2 steps; (d) MeMgCl, THF, −78 °C; (e) 2N NH_3 in *i*PrOH, 50 °C, 65-75%, 2 steps from **26**; (f) $PdCl_2$(dppf), K_2CO_3, dioxane-water (4:1, v:v), 95 °C, 60-70%; (g) 1-methylpiperazine or 1-formylpiperazine, $NaBH(OAc)_3$, THF, rt, 72-88%, 2 steps from **26**.

With two established routes in place, alternative synthetic routes to key intermediate **9** were developed and focused on eliminating the use of Raney-nickel. As shown in Scheme 7.3, starting from triazinone **15**, key intermediate **9** was prepared in a five step synthesis in good overall yield. In a similar fashion, **9** could be prepared in four steps starting from aminomethylmethoxytriazine **19**. In both cases, an activated ester **16** was used in the amide coupling step that facilitated the purification since no coupling reagent was required.

Efforts around the imidazo[5,1-*f*][1,2,4]triazine series were based on the structural insights and SAR developed around the earlier imidazo[1,5-*a*]pyrazine series, since the observation from PoC compounds suggested that the SAR between the two series was essentially transferable. The C5 substituent was maintained as the 2-phenylquinolin-7-yl moiety, incorporating C8-F variations. The C7 substituents were limited to several preferred analogs that showed favorable ADME/DMPK properties and maintained both IGF-1R and IR target potency within the previously established imidazopyrazine series. The synthesis of key analogs based on this strategy is illustrated in Scheme 7.4. Coupling of starting material aminomethyl-methoxy-triazine **19** with the activated cyclobutanone ester **23** provided

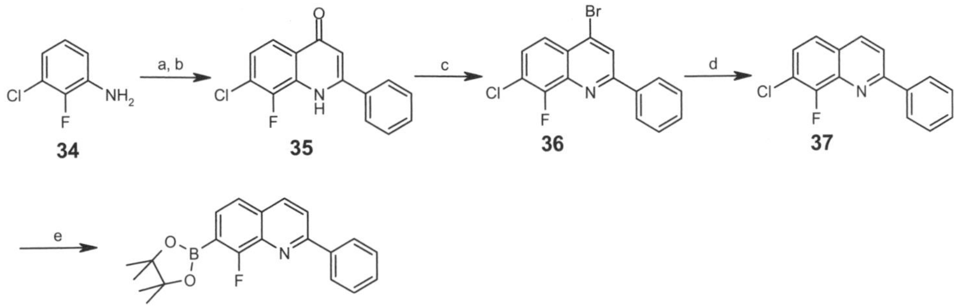

Scheme 7.5 Synthesis of boronate **29b**. *Reagents and conditions*: (a) Ethyl benzoylacetate, PTSA, toluene, reflux; (b) Polyphosphoric acid, 175 °C, 69%, 2 steps; (c) Phosphorus oxybromide, MeCN, 100 °C, 92%; (d) *n*-BuLi, THF, −100 °C; then acetic acid, 55%; (e) $Pd(OAc)_2$, KOAc, 1,3-bis(2,6-diisopropylphenyl)imidazol-2-ylidene hydrochloride, bis(pinacolato)diboron, dioxane, 80 °C, 82%.

amide **24**. Subsequent $POCl_3$-mediated cyclization followed by bromination using *N*-bromosuccinimide (NBS) afforded the versatile intermediate **26**. The cyclobutanone moiety of **26** was converted to a tertiary-alcohol via a Grignard reaction with MeMgCl yielding the *cis*-isomer **27** in a highly stereoselective fashion. Subsequent ammonolysis of **27** gave compound **28** with C4-NH_2 functionality. Finally, compounds **30a–30b** were obtained after a Suzuki coupling of **28** with quinolinyl boronates **29** (**29a**: $R^1 = H$; **29b**: $R^1 = F$). Alternatively, common intermediate **26** was subjected to ammonolysis followed by reductive amination to provide compound **32**, which was progressed to a Suzuki coupling with quinolinyl boronates **29** to give final compounds **33a–33d**. The quinolinyl boronate **29b** was synthesized via various methods [40], one of which is shown in Scheme 7.5. Aniline **34** was subjected to ethyl benzoylacetate in the presence of *p*-toluenesulfonic acid (PTSA) followed by treatment with polyphosphoric acid to afford quinolinone **35**. Treatment of **35** with phosphorus oxybromide afforded brominated intermediate **36**. A subsequent *n*-butyl lithium-mediated Li/Br exchange followed by quenching with acetic acid afforded the desired quinoline **37**. Conversion of **37** to boronate **29b** proceeded smoothly under a palladium catalyzed condition.

7.4.5 Lead Imidazo[5,1-*f*][1,2,4] Triazine IGF-1R/IR Inhibitors and Emergence of FQIT

Compounds **30a–30b** and **33a–33d** were tested against both IGF-1R and IR in cell based mechanistic assays and the results are shown in Table 7.3. The addition of a fluorine atom at the C8 position of the quinoline ring consistently provided an increase in potency among matched pairs, in line with the enhanced Lys1003 binding affinity hypothesis. It is also of significance to note that these compounds inhibited IR and IGF-1R with similar potencies and showed improved *in vitro* microsomal stability ($ER < 0.7$) when compared to initial PoC compound **22**. From our earlier medicinal chemistry efforts around the imidazo[1,5-*a*] pyrazine series, we determined that the C3 position of the cyclobutyl moiety of compound **2** was a metabolic hotspot, undergoing metabolic transformation to the M+16 hydroxy derivative [32]. Therefore, substitution at this position affording analogues such as **30a–30b** and **33a–33d**, blocked that site of metabolism, which was reflected by improved *in vitro* metabolic stability upon incubation in microsomes and therefore lower ERs.

Based on acceptable *in vitro* potencies and ADME profiles, imidazotriazine compounds **30b, 33b,** and **33d** were prioritized for mouse PK evaluation at $5\,mg\,kg^{-1}$ for i.v.

TABLE 7.3 ***In vitro*** **Profiling of Compounds 30a–30b, 33a–33d**

Cpd	R^1	R^2	IGF-1R cell mechanistic[a] IC_{50} (μM)	IR cell mechanistic[b] IC_{50} (μM)	Microsomal stability (ER) Mouse	Microsomal stability (ER) Human	CYP3A4 inh. IC_{50} (μM)
30a	H		0.15	0.70	0.62	0.71	>20
30b	F		0.017	0.076	0.43	0.55	>20
33a	H	CHO	0.026	0.26	0.24	0.66	>20
33b	F	CHO	0.008	0.048	0.44	0.65	>20
33c	H	CH_3	0.025	0.32	0.52	0.64	>20
33d	F	CH_3	0.014	0.068	0.44	0.50	>20

[a]NIH 3T3/huIGF-1R cell line.

[b]HepG2 cell line.

TABLE 7.4 Permeability (PAMPA) and Mouse PK[a] of 30b (FQIT), 33b and 33d

	PAMPA (10^{-6} m s^{-1})		5 mg kg^{-1} i.v. dose		25 mg kg^{-1} p.o. dose		
Cpd	pH 5.0	pH 7.4	Cl (mL min^{-1} kg^{-1})	V_{ss} (L kg^{-1})	C_{max} (μM)	$AUC_{0-\infty}$ (ngh mL^{-1})	F (%)
30b	1090	1100	4	1.0	20.5	160985	162
33b	204	1050	7	1.2	3.1	10426	18
33d	145	672	21	4.9	1.9	5331	27

[a]Compounds were dosed as the freebase in female CD-1 mice.

dosing and 25 mg kg^{-1} for oral dosing. The key PK parameters for these compounds are summarized in Table 7.4. All three compounds displayed a suitable i.v. profile, with low to moderate clearances and volumes of distribution. However, compounds **33b** and **33d** displayed lower oral exposures (C_{max} and AUC) and bioavailabilities as compared to **30b**. The apparent oral bioavailability in excess of 100% for **30b** may indicate saturation of a clearance mechanism. Based on its overall *in vitro* and DMPK profile, **30b (FQIT)** was selected for further profiling.

7.5 *IN VITRO* PROFILE OF FQIT

7.5.1 Cellular and Antiproliferative Effects as a Result of IGF-1R and IR Inhibition

The ability of FQIT to inhibit IGF-1R and IR tyrosine kinase activity in intact GEO cells was investigated. This colon cancer cell line harbors an active IGF-II autocrine loop as indicated by significant phosphorylation of IGF-1R and IR without stimulation with an exogenous IGF-I or IGF-II ligand [31]. This cell line therefore represents an IGF-1R/IR-driven mechanism in which signaling pathways and functional effects of both IGF-1R and IR inhibition can be assessed both *in vitro* and *in vivo*. FQIT effectively inhibits basal IGF-1R and IR activity in a dose-dependent fashion (Figure 7.8a). Cells were cultured with 10% serum-containing medium with the indicated concentrations of FQIT for 2 h at 37°C. The cell lysates were then analyzed for phosphorylated IGF-1R, IR, protein kinase B

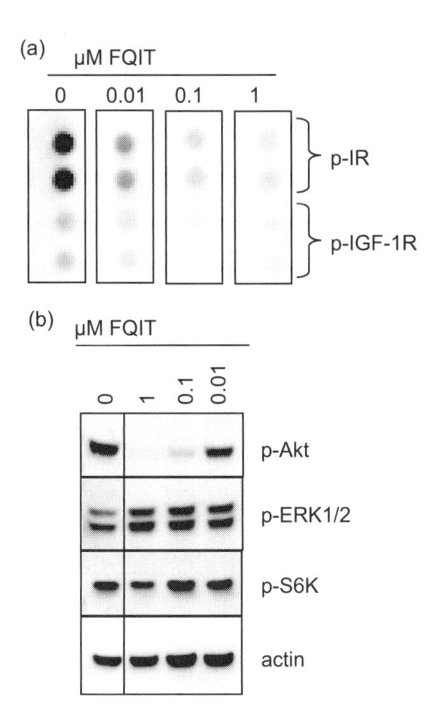

Figure 7.8 Inhibition of cellular signaling pathways by FQIT in GEO cells. (a) Cell lysates were analyzed for phosphorylated IGF-1R and IR protein content by RTK arrays. (b) Inhibition of AKT, ERK1/2, and S6K phosphorylation was determined through Western blot analysis.

(PKB/AKT), extracellular signal-regulated kinase (ERK1/2), and S6K proteins. FQIT effectively inhibits downstream AKT activation but shows little to no effect on ERK or p70S6K activation (Figure 7.8b). As previously demonstrated, IGF-1R is not well coupled to ERK signaling in this cell line [41]. In summary, FQIT potently inhibits IGF-1R, IR, and downstream AKT activation in GEO colorectal carcinoma cells with nanomolar potency. FQIT also displays potent antiproliferative effects in GEO cells correlating with IR and IGF-1R inhibition (EC_{50} = 130 nM).

In order to determine the importance of dual inhibition of IGF-1R and IR for FQIT activity, the ability for FQIT to inhibit the proliferation of IGF-1R- and IR-driven DC tumor cell lines was assessed. IGF-1R and IR DC tumor cell lines were generated from a mouse mammary tumor driven by HER2 under doxycyclin-directed expression, where loss of HER2 upon doxycyclin withdrawal was accompanied by the introduction of either IGF-1R or IR, along with the ligand IGF-II [18]. Because these cell lines are specifically driven by their respective targets, where both IGF-1R and IR were found to maintain tumor growth, the IGF-1R and IR DC tumor models, as well as tumor cell lines derived from them, provide a platform for *in vitro* and *in vivo* target validation and assessment of the activity of pharmacological inhibitors of these receptors. The antiproliferative activity of FQIT against IGF-1R and IR DC tumor cell lines was assessed for 72 h following dosing serial dilutions of FQIT. FQIT potently inhibited the proliferation of cell lines derived from IGF-1R or IR DC tumors (Figure 7.9). Collectively, these data demonstrate the ability for FQIT to be active against either IGF-1R- or IR-driven tumors.

7.5.2 Cellular Potency in the Presence of Plasma Proteins

To predict efficacious plasma levels *in vivo*, whole plasma from mouse, rat, rhesus monkey, and human was included in the human IGF-1R cellular autophosphorylation assay to functionally assess the influence of plasma protein binding on the biological activity of FQIT across these species. FQIT was assayed by quantification of the level of tyrosine

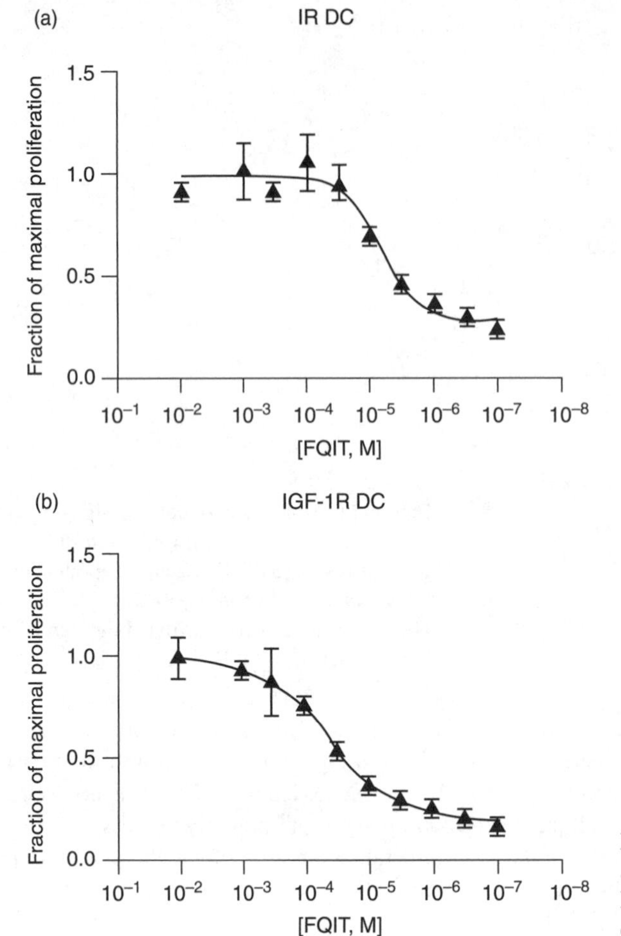

Figure 7.9 Inhibition of proliferation by varying concentrations of FQIT for IGF-1R and IR DC tumor cell lines.

phosphorylation in the presence and absence of compound, using antibody capture ELISA in NIH 3T3/huIGF-1R (LISN) cells. Cells were serum-starved and incubated with compound for 2 h. Whole plasma from mouse, rat, rhesus monkey, and human was included at the time of compound addition.

As shown in Table 7.5, significantly different plasma protein-binding effects were observed between species with FQIT in the cellular IGF-1R shift assay. The protein binding potency shift in the presence of mouse plasma was approximately 75-fold, whereas the protein-binding shift observed with rhesus monkey and human plasma was approximately 10- and 12-fold. These differential plasma protein shifts of FQIT potency suggest that the apparent potency of the compound to inhibit IGF-1R and IR *in vivo* will be greater in humans than in mice by up to sixfold. The differential potency shifts in the presence of plasma may

TABLE 7.5 Cell-based Potency of FQIT in IGF-1R Mechanistic Assays and Influence of Plasma Protein-Binding Across Species

FQIT	No plasma	+90% Mouse plasma	+90% Rat plasma	+50% Rhesus monkey plasma	+90% Human plasma
Human IGF-1R cell IC_{50} (nM)	17	1275	917	165	213

TABLE 7.6 Plasma Protein Binding of FQIT at 10 μM in Different Species[a]

Species	% Free	% Bound
Mouse	1.50	98.50
Rat	3.41	96.59
Rhesus monkey	2.75	97.25
Human	2.73	97.27

[a]Data are mean of ($n = 6$) replicates, from ultracentrifugation assay using pooled mixed gender plasma.

be used to estimate equivalent exposures in other species compared to those required for efficacy in mouse models when assessing the therapeutic window.

As a follow up to the aforementioned shift assay, direct measurement binding of FQIT to plasma proteins from various species was also conducted as measured by % bound drug by ultracentrifugation (Table 7.6). Results from the plasma protein-binding study were consistent with the observed differential plasma protein-binding shifts for mouse, rhesus monkey, and human, with rat being the exception. As an aside, it has been our experience that determining protein binding via either the shift assay, ultracentrifugation, or equilibrium dialysis methods can routinely produce conflicting results. This emphasizes the challenges associated with transferring *in vitro* results to the *in vivo* setting and in this case highlights the complexity of accurately estimating *in vivo* free drug levels through *in vitro* protein-binding experiments. Ideally, correlating *in vitro* protein binding and therefore free drug estimates with actual drug concentrations *in vivo* required to inhibit the target of interest through careful PD analysis provides the most accurate results and reflects our practice.

7.5.3 *In Vitro* Metabolism and CYP450 Profile

FQIT displays good metabolic stability across species as evidenced by favorable microsomal ERs of < 0.70 as shown in Table 7.7. In short, the metabolic stability assay incubates compound at 10 μM for 120 min in liver microsomes from various species supplemented with cofactors for glucuronidation. Liver microsomes are subcellular fractions that contain membrane-bound drug metabolizing enzymes. This assay can be used to calculate various PK related parameters, including half-life ($T_{1/2}$), intrinsic clearance (Cl_{int}), and scaled hepatic clearance (Cl_h). An "Extraction Ratio" (ER) is calculated with the formula of $ER = Cl_h/\text{hepatic blood flow}$. Treatment of FQIT in the metabolic stability assay resulted in the formation of only minor metabolites (<5% compare to parent compound level) from the different species. The lack of any major metabolites and therefore the presence of the intact

TABLE 7.7 *In Vitro* Microsomal Stability (ER) of FQIT in Multiple Species

Species	Gender	Microsomal stability (ER)
Mouse	Female	0.43
Rat	Male	<0.2
Rat	Female	<0.2
Dog	Male	0.42
Rhesus monkey	Male	0.67
Human	Mixed	0.55

TABLE 7.8 CYP450 Inhibition Data for FQIT[a]

CYP isoform	IC_{50} (μM)
2C9	14.9
1A2	>25
2D6	>25
3A4	>25

[a]Data are based on assays employing isoform-specific substrates, each at K_m, and LC-MS/MS quantitation except for 1A2 which is a fluorescence assay.

parent molecule FQIT when incubated in microsomes is consistent with the low rate of clearance (4 mL min^{-1} kg^{-1}) observed upon dosing in mice and suggests that excess first pass clearance via the liver should not be expected. The profiles also suggests that the dog and rhesus monkey closely mirror the human *in vitro* metabolite profile and are therefore suitable as potential nonrodent toxicology species.

The CYP450 profile of FQIT was evaluated in human microsomes. FQIT does not significantly inhibit any major CYP450 isoforms including CYP3A4, 1A2, 2D6, and 2C9 (Table 7.8). An assay to determine the time-dependant inhibition of CYP3A4 was also carried out by preincubating FQIT in human liver microsomes at a range of concentrations (0.1 and 25 μM) for 30 min, with and without NADPH (the reduced form of nicotinamide adenine dinucleotide phosphate (NADP)), followed by adjusting concentration of microsomes following standard protocols. The data indicate that FQIT does not show any significant time-dependent inhibition of CYP3A4, with an IC_{50} value of greater than 25 μM. The potential for FQIT to show clinical drug–drug interactions cannot be directly predicted from the available *in vitro* data although the data suggest that the probability of interactions arising from inhibition of these enzymes is low.

7.6 PHARMACOKINETIC PROPERTIES OF FQIT

7.6.1 Formulation and Salt Study

Initially, for the mouse PK studies, the free base of FQIT was dosed as a solution in PEG-400/25 mM tartaric acid. Unfortunately, the free base has limited solubility under these conditions (e.g., ~10 mg mL^{-1}). A preliminary salt screen was conducted in an attempt to increase solubility and yielded the hydrochloride salt, which has an improved solubility of 60 mg mL^{-1} in 40% w/v hydroxypropyl-β-cyclodextrin (Trappsol®). This solubility was sufficient for *in vivo* efficacy and toxicology studies. Further analysis by NMR verified that FQIT (HCl salt) forms a 1:1 complex with Trappsol® (data not shown).

7.6.2 Pharmacokinetics Following Intravenous Administration

The PK profiles of FQIT have been evaluated following i.v. administration in the female CD-1 mouse, female Sprague Dawley rat and the male rhesus monkey. The PK parameters obtained from noncompartmental modeling following i.v. dosing are summarized in Table 7.9. There is a notably lower elimination half-life in the rhesus monkey compared

TABLE 7.9 Median Pharmacokinetic Parameters for FQIT Following Intravenous Administration in Different Species

Species	Dose (mg kg^{-1})	CL (mL min^{-1} kg^{-1})	V_{ss} (L kg^{-1})	$AUC_{0\text{-}\infty}$ (ngh mL^{-1})	Elimination $t_{½}$ (h)
Mouse (F)[a]	5	4	1.00	19897	2.85
Rat (F)[a]	5	4	0.97	19534	3.21
Rhesus monkey (M)[b]	5	15	0.55	5634	0.47

[a]FQIT dosed as the free base.

[b]FQIT dosed as the HCl salt.

to the two rodent species, as a result of both increased clearance and a lower volume of distribution at steady-state, V_{ss}.

7.6.3 Pharmacokinetics Following Oral Administration

The pharmacokinetic properties of FQIT following oral administration have been evaluated in the female CD-1 mouse, female Sprague Dawley rat, and the male rhesus monkey. The pharmacokinetic parameters at a range of doses administered are summarized in Table 7.10. In a direct comparison in the female CD-1 mouse, the HCl salt gave an increase in exposure and bioavailability compared to the free base, when both were dosed in 40% w/v Trappsol®. This combination of salt form and formulation was subsequently used in mouse efficacy studies, rhesus monkey PK, and toxicology studies. In each species, the calculated oral bioavailability increases with dose and in several cases is significantly higher than 100%, which indicates that the AUC is nonlinear with greater than dose-proportional increases over the range of doses examined. This is likely to be due to saturation of clearance mechanism(s) at higher doses.

The pharmacokinetic profiles have also been determined in tissues of nontumor-bearing mice at a dose of 10 mg kg^{-1} (efficacious dose in mice, see *in vivo* efficacy section), as shown in Figure 7.10. In general, there is a strong correlation between plasma and tissue concentrations. Compared to plasma, the concentrations in adipose and liver tissue are higher, those in lung are similar, and in muscle are lower. All tissue concentrations are below the limit of quantitation at 24 h, indicating that no tissue accumulation may be expected at this dose in the mouse. The pharmacokinetic parameters after repeat oral administration at a range of doses were carried out in mouse, rat, and rhesus monkey (data not shown). There was no evidence of increase or decrease in plasma or tissue concentrations compared to data from single doses.

TABLE 7.10 Median Pharmacokinetic Parameters for FQIT Following Single Oral Administration in Different Species

Species	Dose (mg kg^{-1})	C_{max} (μM)	$AUC_{0\text{-}\infty}$ (ngh mL^{-1})	F (%)	Elimination $t_{½}$ (h)
Mouse (F)[a]	25	35.19	240013	241	12.68
Rat (F)[b]	5	1.00	4560	23	2.42
	25	11.35	62415	64	3.83
Rhesus monkey (M)[a]	30	10.81	31383	97	2.45
	100	32.20	259221	163	2.68

[a]FQIT dosed as the HCl salt.

[b]FQIT dosed as the free base.

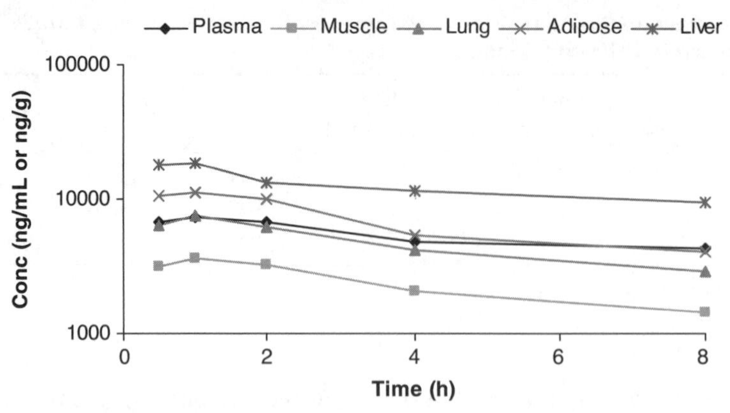

Figure 7.10 Comparison of plasma and tissue PK profiles for FQIT following a single oral administration at $10\,\mathrm{mg\,kg^{-1}}$ in the female CD-1 mouse. Data are median ($n = 3$) at each timepoint and error bars are omitted for clarity. (See color version of the figure in Color Plate section)

7.7 *IN VIVO* PROFILE OF FQIT

7.7.1 *In Vivo* Pharmacodynamic and PK/PD Correlation

Pharmacodynamic studies were performed in the GEO colon carcinoma xenograft model, where effects on phosphorylation of tumor IGF-1R and IR in relation to plasma drug levels were evaluated. As shown in Figure 7.11, following a $10\,\mathrm{mg\,kg^{-1}}$ single oral dose of FQIT, sustained inhibition of tumor IGF-1R phosphorylation (>70%) was observed up to 8 h, corresponding to drug plasma levels of >4 μM. This value correlates with the plasma concentration being above the IGF-1R mechanistic IC_{50} in the presence of plasma protein (shift assay) for the entire 8 h time period. Drug levels dropped to 0.38 μM by 16 h and 0.19 μM by 24 h, with partial recovery of pIGF-1R content (~50% inhibition at 24 h). Similar inhibitory effects of FQIT on tumor IR phosphorylation were observed.

7.7.2 *In Vivo* Efficacy

To evaluate the *in vivo* efficacy of FQIT, a TGI study was undertaken in the GEO mouse xenograft model. FQIT was evaluated on a *qd* (once-daily) and bid (twice-daily) oral dosing

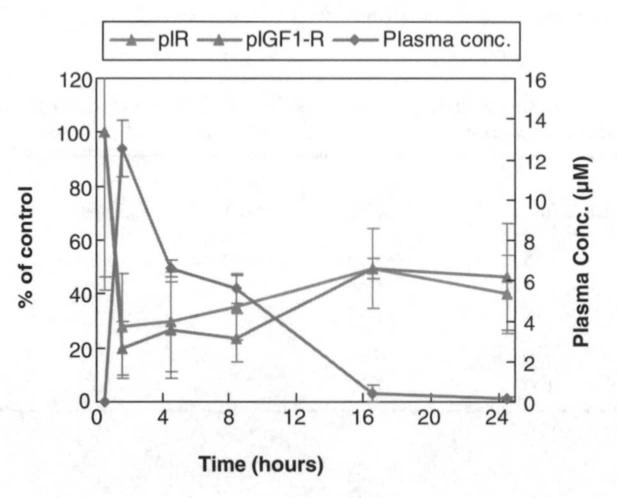

Figure 7.11 Correlation of inhibition of IGF-1R and IR phosphorylation and plasma drug exposure in GEO tumor xenografts following oral dosing with $10\,\mathrm{mg\,kg^{-1}}$ FQIT. The blue line corresponds to mean ± SE plasma concentrations of FQIT at indicated time following $10\,\mathrm{mg\,kg^{-1}}$ *qd* dose. Red and green line represents mean ± SE pIGF-1R and pIR content in GEO tumors and expressed as a percentage of control pIGF-1R or pIR content from vehicle-treated animals, respectively. (See color version of the figure in Color Plate section)

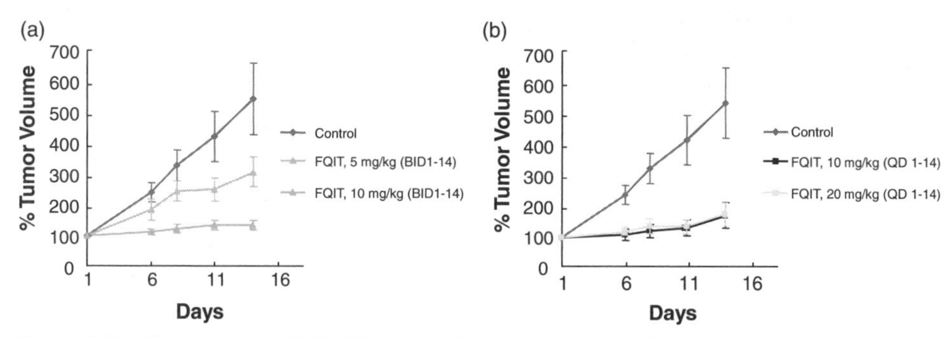

Figure 7.12 Dose–response TGI efficacy of FQIT in GEO xenograft models. Plotted data are mean tumor volumes expressed as a percentage of initial volume ± SE. FQIT was dosed on twice-daily schedule (a) or once-daily schedule (b) for 14 days. (See color version of the figure in Color Plate section)

schedule (Figure 7.12). A dose of 10 mg kg^{-1}*qd* and 20 mg kg^{-1}*qd* provided comparable TGI (85%) [42] with minimal effects on body weight (3% body weight loss). The maximum tolerated dose (MTD) for FQIT on the *qd* dose schedule appears to be ≥20 mg kg^{-1}. FQIT also demonstrated robust efficacy on the *bid* dosing schedule (FQIT 10 mg kg^{-1}*bid* gave significant TGI of 91%) and was well tolerated.

In the TGI study described above, tumors from control and FQIT-treated animals were removed after the last dose to investigate target inhibition in tumor tissue (Figure 7.13). FQIT at 20 mg kg^{-1}*qd* resulted in >70–90% sustained inhibition of tumor IGF-1R phosphorylation for a full 24 h post last dose. On a *bid* dosing schedule, 5 mg kg^{-1}*bid* provided less tumor pIGF-1R inhibition (40–50%, data not shown) that correlated with only 31% TGI. Increasing the dose to 10 mg kg^{-1}*bid* resulted in significant inhibition of tumor pIGF-1R (70–90%) for 24 h correlating with greater TGI (91%), mimicking the 20 mg kg^{-1}*qd* dose. Taken together, these results indicate a clear dose response and a strong PD to TGI correlation. Anti-tumor activity of FQIT was extended into additional tumor models. For example, in a human IGF-1R overexpressing NIH 3T3 xenograft model (LISN), FQIT demonstrated 100% TGI when dosed at a well-tolerated dose of 10 mg kg^{-1}*bid* for 14 days (data not shown). Overall, FQIT displays good efficacy in IGF-1R- and IGF-1R/IR-driven tumor models and is well tolerated. Such models allowed for us to link FQIT *in vitro* mechanistic and functional IGF-1R and IR inhibitory activities to *in vivo* PD effects including tumor growth inhibition.

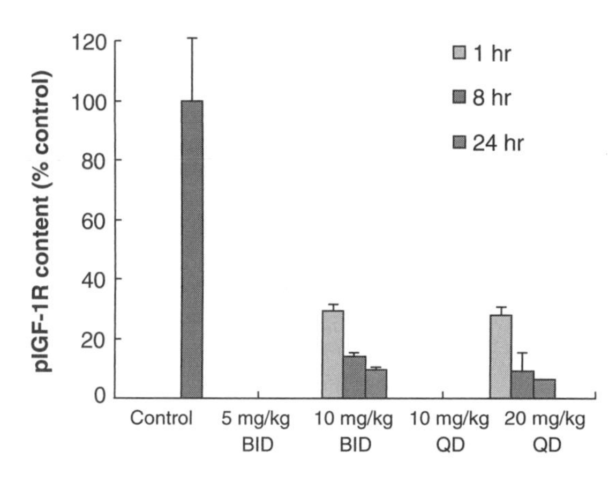

Figure 7.13 Inhibition of IGF-1R phosphorylation in GEO tumor xenografts following oral dosing with FQIT. Phospho-IGF-1R in GEO tumors expressed as a percentage of control pIGF-1R content from vehicle treated animals at 1, 8, and 24 h after 14 days of treatment with FQIT at various doses. Data are mean ± SE. (See color version of the figure in Color Plate section)

7.8 SAFETY ASSESSMENT AND SELECTIVITY PROFILE OF FQIT

7.8.1 Effects on Blood Glucose and Insulin Levels

Clinical experience with IGF-1R inhibitors, including both neutralizing antibodies and small-molecule tyrosine kinase inhibitors, has shown hyperglycemia upon treatment, consistent with the mechanism of action for these agents. For OSI-906, elevated levels of insulin and glucose are reported at the MTD, but such effects are transient and reversible upon cessation of treatment. To assess the effects of FQIT treatment on glucose homeostasis *in vivo*, blood glucose and insulin levels were monitored in a single-dose study and after a multiple-dose TGI study in preclinical mouse models. In the single-dose study, the efficacious dose of 10 mg kg^{-1} FQIT showed only a transient elevation of blood glucose (> 300 mg dL^{-1}) at the earliest time point measured, with rapid return to baseline by 1 h. Plasma insulin levels were transiently increased up to 8 h and returned to normal levels by 16 h post dose.

To assess effects on blood glucose and insulin after repeat dosing, blood glucose and insulin were measured after the last dose post 14 days of dosing (end of TGI study). After dosing FQIT at 10 mg kg^{-1} *qd* for 14 days, the blood glucose levels were indistinguishable from untreated control mice, while plasma insulin was transiently increased for 8 h after dosing and returned to normal levels by 24 h. Thus, the FQIT 10 mg kg^{-1} repeat dose glucose and insulin profiles are similar to those observed after a single dose. This suggests that repeated dosing of FQIT does not exacerbate hyperglycemia or hyperinsulinemia in mice.

7.8.2 Oral Glucose Tolerance Test

To evaluate the acute metabolic effects of FQIT *in vivo*, an oral glucose tolerance test (OGTT) was performed in mice treated with vehicle alone or with FQIT. As shown in Figure 7.14, after a 4 h fasting period, mice were dosed orally with vehicle or FQIT at an efficacious dose of 10 mg kg^{-1} for 1 h before an oral glucose challenge. Blood glucose before challenge was elevated following treatment with FQIT at 10 mg kg^{-1} to 239 mg dL^{-1} compared to mean blood glucose of 155 mg dL^{-1} in vehicle control mice. Upon administration of the glucose load, blood glucose was elevated for 2 h before return to control levels. At 2 h post the glucose challenge, plasma insulin levels were comparable to control levels. In summary, in an OGTT, the efficacious dose of 10 mg kg^{-1} of FQIT induced a transient increase in blood glucose and did not significantly increase insulin levels.

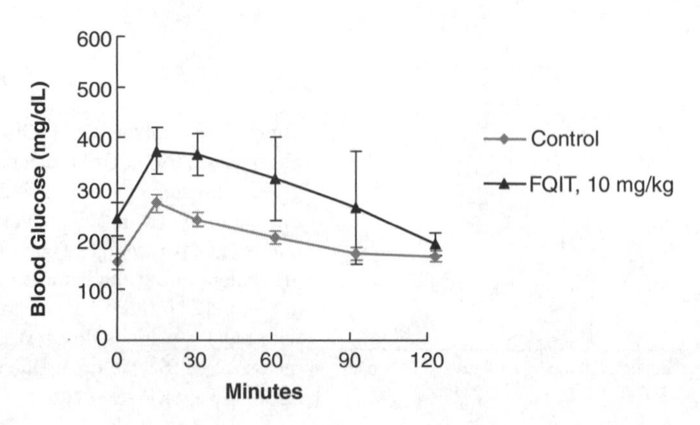

Figure 7.14 Oral glucose tolerance test with FQIT in mice. Plotted data are average blood glucose values obtained following a single oral dose of 10 mg kg^{-1} in the *nu/nu* CD-1 mouse after the glucose challenge (2 g kg^{-1}) of FQIT.

7.8.3 Ames, Rodent, and Nonrodent Toxicology Studies

In order to further evaluate the safety profile of FQIT beyond repeat dosing in mice, FQIT was profiled both for genotoxicity in an *in vitro* mutagenicity assay and for toxicity upon repeat dosing in the rat and rhesus monkey. FQIT was determined to be nonmutagenic in a mini-salmonella typhimurium reverse mutation (AMES ± S9 fraction) assay. In a 14 day rat toxicology study and a 5 day rhesus monkey toxicology study, FQIT was well tolerated and showed no detectable off-target toxicological effects, even at doses and exposures above those predicted to be required for efficacy in these species.

7.8.4 Selectivity Profile of FQIT

FQIT was evaluated against a broad range of 68 receptors including enzymes, receptors, and ion channels at a concentration of 10 μM in a general receptor-binding screen and did not reveal any significant off-target activities. Furthermore, FQIT has been assayed *in vitro* for inhibitory activity against 167 purified protein kinases representing the tyrosine and serine/threonine kinase families using an in-house Caliper EZ Reader mobility shift assay followed by counterscreening at Invitrogen for more rigorous dose response analysis. A representative list of kinases included in the Caliper selectivity profiling assay is summarized in Table 7.11. In short, FQIT is a potent and highly selective dual inhibitor of IGF-1R and IR.

The exquisite selectivity of FQIT might be rationalized from a modeling perspective based on the isosteric PQIP structure (PDB ID: 3D94) (Figure 7.15) [37]. It was hypothesized that like PQIP and OSI-906, FQIT targets an intermediate conformation of the protein that features an inactive orientation of the C-helix (0P form) but an orientation of the activation loop more associated with the phospho-protein (3P form)

TABLE 7.11 FQIT Kinase Selectivity Profile[a]

Kinase	Inhibition (%)	Kinase	Inhibition (%)	Kinase	Inhibition (%)
IGF-1R	97.5	ERK1	−3.9	PAK2	5.7
IR	82.0	FGFR1	6.4	PDGFRα	10.8
ABL	24.5	FGFR2	4.3	PKA	11.5
ALK	−0.2	FLT3	14.2	PKBα	−4.0
AMPKa1	3.7	FYN	12.8	PKG	6.0
AURORA-A	21.4	GSK3β	17.4	PRKD2	−4.0
AURORA-B	17.8	JAK2	−4.3	PYK2	8.9
AURORA-C	2.9	KDR	18.0	RET	−4.7
AXL	7.6	LTK	3.8	ROCK1	−6.3
BLK	−3.8	MAPK1	6.6	RON	−3.7
BTK	5.0	MAPKAPK2	1.4	ROS	8.6
c-KIT	−14.9	MARK4	1.1	RSK1	2.0
CAMKIV	3.3	MELK	14.5	S6K	6.1
CDK1	4.3	MER	11.5	SGK	8.0
c-RAF	13.8	MET	−19.6	SRC	15.5
EGF-R	3.2	MSK1	4.7	STK3	13.1
EPHA1	−8.0	NEK2	8.7	SYK	−6.5
EPHB1	3.7	P38α	−0.8	YES	6.6

[a]A representative list of kinases included in the caliper EZ reader mobility shift assay. Assays were conducted with the concentration of ATP at Km and concentration of FQIT at 1 μM.

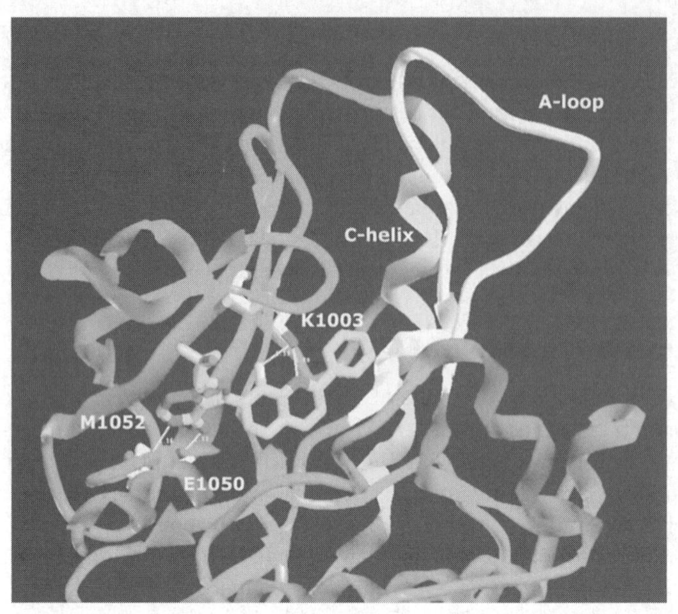

Figure 7.15 Modeled structure of FQIT in complex with IGF-1R with (a) key hydrogen bonding interactions highlighted; (b) C-helix highlighted in yellow, and (c) activation loop (A-loop) highlighted in white.

through its interactions with the C-helix. Similar to PQIP and OSI-906, the terminal phenyl ring of FQIT interacts with several hydrophobic residues in IGF-1R including F980 (P-loop), F1124 and G1125 (DFG motif), and F1017 and A1021 (C-helix). FQIT displays a high degree of selectivity since induction of this intermediate conformation appears quite rare in kinases and residues are generally less conserved in the C-helix region across different kinases. FQIT inhibits IR kinase activity with similar potency to that of the IGF-1R since these two proteins are >80% homologous in the kinase domain and are 100% homologous in the ATP-binding site. The high degree of selectivity and potent dual inhibitory activity against IGF-1R and IR distinguish both FQIT and OSI-906 from selective IGF-1R targeting monoclonal antibodies as well as nonselective multikinase small molecule IGF-1R and IR inhibitors.

7.9 SUMMARY

In summary, a series of 5,7-disubstituted imidazo[5,1-*f*][1,2,4]triazine compounds were developed as dual IGF-1R/IR inhibitors. From this series, FQIT emerged as a highly potent and selective IGF-1R/IR dual inhibitor with favorable drug-like properties. Key strategies applied to the discovery of FQIT included the bioisosteric core replacement where the imidazo[5,1-*f*][1,2,4]triazine chemotype was envisioned to serve as an isosteric alternative to imidazo[1,5-*a*]pyrazines, eliminating the potentially metabolically reactive C5 and C5=C6 structural unit while maintaining critical pharmacophores and thus taking advantages of existing, transferable SAR to facilitate the drug discovery process. Moreover, SBDD insights were incorporated to optimize binding interactions. For example, a specific structural feature to the imidazo[5,1-*f*][1,2,4]triazine series was the incorporation of the C8-F in the quinoline moiety, designed to assimilate an extra hydrogen bond interaction with Lys1003 at the lowest energy conformation where a consistent and significant potency gain was observed. A streamlined testing cascade of IGF-1R and IR *in vitro* and *in vivo* models allowed for the rapid assessment of PK, PD, efficacy, and safety for lead agent profiling including FQIT. Overall, FQIT possesses a profile comparable to that of OSI-906, including excellent PK and tolerability in multiple species and robust *in vivo* antitumor activity in mouse xenograft tumor models.

ACKNOWLEDGMENTS

We would like to thank Dr. Jing Wang for kindly providing the modeling pictures in Figures 7.2b and 7.15.

REFERENCES

1. Kaiser, U., Schardt, C., Brandscheidt, D., Wollmer, E., and Havemann, K. Expression of insulin-like growth factor receptors I and II in normal human lung and in lung cancer. *J. Cancer Res. Clin. Oncol.* **1993**, *119*, 665–668.
2. Kondo, M., Suzuki, H., Ueda, R., Osada, H., Takagi, K., Takahashi, T., and Takahashi, T. Frequent loss of imprinting of the H19 gene is often associated with its overexpression in human lung cancers. *Oncogene* **1995**, *10*, 1193–1198.
3. Rubin, R. and Baserga, R. Insulin-like growth factor-I receptor. Its role in cell proliferation, apoptosis, and tumorigenicity. *Lab. Invest.* **1995**, *73*, 311–331.
4. Sell, C., Rubini, M., Rubin, R., Liu, J. P., Efstratiadis, A., and Baserga, R. Simian virus 40 large tumor antigen is unable to transform mouse embryonic fibroblasts lacking type 1 insulin-like growth factor receptor. *Proc. Natl Acad. Sci.* **1993**, *90*(23),11217–11221.
5. LeRoith, D. and Roberts, C. T. Jr., The insulin-like growth factor system and cancer. *Cancer Lett.* **2003**, *195*, 127–137.
6. Ma, J., Giovannucci, E., Pollak, M., Leavitt, A., Tao, Y., Gaziano, J. M., and Stampfer, M. J. A prospective study of plasma C-peptide and colorectal cancer risk in men. *J. Natl. Cancer Inst.* **2004**, *96*, 546–553.
7. Pollak, M. Insulin and insulin-like growth factor signalling in neoplasia. *Nat. Rev. Cancer* **2008**, *8*, 915–928.
8. Jerome, L., Alami, N., Belanger, S., Page, V., Yu, Q., Paterson, J., Shiry, L., Pegram, M., and Leyland-Jones, B. Recombinant human insulin-like growth factor binding protein 3 inhibits growth of human epidermal growth factor receptor-2-overexpressing breast tumors and potentiates herceptin activity in vivo. *Cancer Res.* **2006**, *66*, 7245–7252.
9. Lu, Y., Zi, X., and Pollak, M. Molecular mechanisms underlying IGF-I-induced attenuation of the growth-inhibitory activity of trastuzumab (Herceptin) on SKBR3 breast cancer cells. *Int. J. Cancer* **2004**, *108*, 334–341.
10. Lu, Y., Zi, X., Zhao, Y., Mascarenhas, D., and Pollak, M. Insulin-like growth factor-I receptor signaling and resistance to trastuzumab (Herceptin). *J. Natl. Cancer Inst.* **2001**, *93*, 1852–1857.
11. Chakravarti, A., Loeffler, J. S., and Dyson, N. J. Insulin-like growth factor receptor I mediates resistance to anti-epidermal growth factor receptor therapy in primary human glioblastoma cells through continued activation of phosphoinositide 3-kinase signaling. *Cancer Res.* **2002**, *62*, 200–207.
12. Gooch, J. L., Van Den Berg C. L., and Yee, D. Insulin-like growth factor (IGF)-I rescues breast cancer cells from chemotherapy-induced cell death--proliferative and anti-apoptotic effects. *Breast Cancer Res. Treatment* **1999**, *56*, 1–10.
13. Jones, H. E., Goddard, L., Gee, J. M., Hiscox, S., Rubini, M., Barrow, D., Knowlden, J. M., Williams, S., Wakeling, A. E., and Nicholson, R. I. Insulin-like growth factor-I receptor signalling and acquired resistance to gefitinib (ZD1839, Iressa) in human breast and prostate cancer cells. *Endocrine-Related Cancer* **2004**, *11*, 793–814.
14. Knowlden, J. M., Hutcheson, I. R., Barrow, D., Gee, J. M., and Nicholson, R. I. Insulin-like growth factor-I receptor signaling in tamoxifen-resistant breast cancer: a supporting role to the epidermal growth factor receptor. *Endocrinology* **2005**, *146*, 4609–4618.
15. Lu, Y., Zi, X., Zhao, Y., Mascarenhas, D., and Pollak, M. Insulin-like growth factor-I receptor signaling and resistance to trastuzumab (Herceptin). *J. Natl. Cancer Inst.* **2001**, *93*, 1852–1857.
16. Nahta, R., Yuan, L. X., Zhang, B., Kobayashi, R., and Esteva, F. J. Insulin-like growth factor-I receptor/human epidermal growth factor receptor 2 heterodimerization contributes to trastuzumab resistance of breast cancer cells. *Cancer Res.* **2005**, *65*, 11118–11128.
17. Turner, B. C., Haffty, B. G., Narayanan, L., Yuan, J., Havre, P. A., Gumbs, A. A., Kaplan, L., Burgaud, J. L., Carter, D., Baserga, R., and Glazer, P. M. Insulin-like growth factor-I receptor overexpression mediates cellular radioresistance and local breast cancer recurrence after lumpectomy and radiation. *Cancer Res.* **1997**, *57*, 3079–3083.

18. Giorgino, F., Belfiore, A., Milazzo, G., Costantino, A., Maddux, B., Whittaker, J., Goldfine, I. D., and Vigneri, R. Overexpression of insulin receptors in fibroblast and ovary cells induces a ligand-mediated transformed phenotype. *Mol. Endocrinol.* **1991**, *5*, 452–459.
19. Buck, E., Gokhale, P. C., Koujak, S., Brown, E., Eyzaguirre, A., Tao, N., Rosenfeld-Franklin, M., Lerner, L., Chiu, M., Wild, R., Epstein, D., Pachter, J. A., and Miglarese, M. R. Compensatory insulin receptor (IR) activation on inhibition of insulin-like growth factor-1 receptor (IGF-1R): rationale for cotargeting IGF-1R and IR in cancer. *Mol. Cancer Ther.* **2010** *9*, 2652–2664.
20. Heuson, J. C. and Legros, N. Effect of insulin and of alloxan diabetes on growth of the rat mammary carcinoma in vivo. *Eur. J. Cancer* **1970**, *6*, 349–351.
21. Heuson, J. C. and Legros, N. Influence of insulin deprivation on growth of the 7,12-dimethylbenz(a) anthracene-induced mammary carcinoma in rats subjected to alloxan diabetes and food restriction. *Cancer Res.* **1972**, *32*, 226–232.
22. Heuson, J. C., Legros, N., and Heimann, R. Influence of insulin administration on growth of the 7,12-dimethylbenz(a)anthracene-induced mammary carcinoma in intact, oophorectomized, and hypophysectomized rats. *Cancer Res.* **1972**, *32*, 233–238.
23. Sciacca, L., Costantino, A., Pandini, G., Mineo, R., Frasca, F., Scalia, P., Sbraccia, P., Goldfine, I. D., Vigneri, R., and Belfiore A. Insulin receptor activation by IGF-II in breast cancers: evidence for a new autocrine/paracrine mechanism. *Oncogene* **1999**, *18*, 2471–2479.
24. Vella, V., Pandini, G., Sciacca, L., Mineo, R., Vigneri, R., Pezzino, V., and Belfiore, A. A novel autocrine loop involving IGF-II and the insulin receptor isoform-A stimulates growth of thyroid cancer. *J. Clin. Endocrinol. Metab.* **2002**, *87*, 245–254.
25. Cox, M. E., Gleave, M. E., Zakikhani, M., Bell, R. H., Piura, E., Vickers, E., Cunningham, M., Larsson, O., Fazli, L., and Pollak, M. Insulin receptor expression by human prostate cancers. *Prostate* **2009**, *69*, 33–40.
26. Pollak, M. Targeting insulin and insulin-like growth factor signalling in oncology. *Curr. Opin. Pharmacol.* **2008**, *8*, 384–392.
27. Kling, J. Inhaled insulin's last gasp? *Nat. Biotechnol.* **2008**, *26*, 479–480.
28. Entingh-Pearsall, A. and Kahn, C. R. Differential roles of the insulin and insulin-like growth factor-I (IGF-I) receptors in response to insulin and IGF-I. *J. Biol. Chem.* **2004**, *279*, 38016–38024.
29. Fulzele, K., DiGirolamo, D. J., Liu, Z., Xu, J., Messina, J. L., and Clemens, T. L. Disruption of the insulin-like growth factor type 1 receptor in osteoblasts enhances insulin signaling and action. *J. Biol. Chem.* **2007**, *282*, 25649–25658.
30. Mulvihill, M., Ji, Q., Coate, H., Cooke, A., Dong, H., Feng, L., Foreman, K., Rosenfeld-Franklin, M., Honda, A., Mak, G., Mulvihill, K., Nigro, A., O'Connor, M., Pirrit, C., Steinig, A., Siu, K., Stolz, K., Sun, Y., Tavares, P., Yao Y., and Gibson, N. Novel 2-phenylquinolin-7-yl-derived imidazo[1,5-a]pyrazines as potent insulin-like growth factor-I receptor (IGF-IR) inhibitors. *Bioorg. Med. Chem.* **2008**, *16*, 1359–1375. AQIP: *cis*-3-(3-azetidin-1-ylmethylcyclobutyl)-1-(2-phenylquinolin-7-yl)imidazo[1,5-a]pyrazin-8-ylamine
31. Ji, Q., Mulvihill, M., Rosenfeld-Franklin, M., Cooke, A., Feng, L., Mak, G., O'Connor, M., Yao, Y., Pirritt, C., Buck, E., Eyzaguirre, A., Arnold, L., Gibson, N., and Pachter, J. A novel, potent, and selective insulin-like growth factor-I receptor kinase inhibitor blocks insulin-like growth factor-I receptor signaling in vitro and inhibits insulin-like growth factor-I receptor dependent tumor growth in vivo. *Mol. Cancer Ther.* **2007**, *6*, 2158–2167. PQIP: *cis*-3-[3-(4-methyl-piperazin-l-yl)-cyclobutyl]-1-(2-phenyl-quinolin-7-yl)-imidazo[1,5-a] pyrazin-8-ylamine
32. Mulvihill, M., Cooke, A., Rosenfeld-Franklin, M., Buck, E., Foreman, K., Landfair, D., O'Connor, M., Pirrit, C., Sun, Y., Yao, Y., Arnold, L., Gibson, N., and Ji, Q. Discovery of OSI-906: a selective and orally efficacious dual inhibitor of the IGF-1 receptor and insulin receptor. *Future Med. Chem.* **2009**, *1*, 1153–1171.
33. Crew, A.P., Bhagwat, S.V., Dong, H., Bittner, M.A., Chan, A., Chen, X., Coate, H., Cooke, A., Gokhale, P., Honda, A., Jin, M., Kahler, J., Mantis, C., Mulvihill, M.J., Tavares-Greco, P.A., Volk, B., Wang, J., Werner, D.S., Arnold, L.D., Pachter, J.A., Wild, R., and Gibson, N.W. Imidazo[1,5-a]pyrazines: orally efficacious inhibitors of mTORC1 and mTORC2, *Bioorg. Med. Chem. Lett.* **2011**, *21*, 2092–2097.
34. Wang, J., McCubbin, J., Jin, M., Laufer, R., Mao, Y., Crew, A., Mulvihill, M., and Snieckus, V. Palladium-catalyzed direct heck aArylation of dual p-deficient/p-excessive heteroaromatics, synthesis of C-5 arylated imidazo[1,5-a]pyrazines. *Org. Lett.* **2008**, *10*, 2923–2926.
35. Board, J., Wang, J., Crew, A., Jin, M., Foreman, K., Mulvihill, M., and Snieckus, V. Synthesis of substituted imidazo[1,5-a]pyrazines via mono-, di-, and directed remote metalation strategies. *Org. Lett.* **2009**, *11*, 5118–5121.
36. Jin, M., Gokhale, P., Cooke, A., Foreman, K., Buck, E., May, E., Feng, L., Bittner, M., Kadalbajoo, M., Landfair, D., Siu, K., Stolz, K., Werner, D., Laufer, R., Li, A., Dong, H., Steinig, A., Kleinberg, A., Yao, Y., Pachter, J., Wild, R., and Mulvihill, M. J. Discovery of an orally efficacious imidazo[5,1-*f*][1,2,4]triazine dual inhibitor of IGF-1R and IR. *ACS Med. Chem. Lett.* **2010**, *1*, 510–515. Compound **9b** in this manuscript is referred to FQIT (*cis*-3-[4-amino-5-(8-fluoro-2-phenyl-quinolin-7-yl)-imidazo[5,1-*f*][1,2,4]triazin-7-yl]-1-methyl-cyclobutanol) herein.
37. Wu, J., Li, W., Craddock, B. P., Foreman, K. W., Mulvihill, M. J., Ji, Q. S., Miller, W. T., and Hubbard, S. R. Small-molecule inhibition and

activation-loop *trans*-phosphorylation of the IGF1 receptor. *Embo J.* **2008**, *27*(14),1985–1994.

38. Werner, D. S., Dong, H., Kadalbajoo, M., Laufer, R.S., Tavares-Greco, P.A., Volk, B.R., Mulvihill, M. J., and Crew, A. P. Synthetic approaches to 5,7-disubstituted imidazo[5,1-*f*][1,2,4]triazin-4-amines. *Tetrahedron Lett.* **2010**, *51*, 3899–3901.
39. Draber, W., Timmler, H., Dickore, K., and Donner, W. *Liebigs Ann. Chem*, **1976**, 2206.
40. Arnold, L. D., Cesario, C., Coate, H., Crew, A. P., Dong, H., Foreman, K., Honda, A., Laufer, R., Li, A., Mulvihill, K. M., Mulvihill, M. J., Nigro, A., Panicker, B., Steinig, A. G., Sun, Y., Weng, Q., Werner, D. S., Wyle, M. J., and Zhang, T. Preparation of 6,6-bicyclic ring substituted heterobicyclic protein kinase inhibitors. *PCT Int. Appl.* **2005**, WO 2005097800.
41. Buck, E., Eyzaguirre, A., Rosenfeld-Franklin, M., Brown, E., O'Connor. M., Yao, Y., Pachter, J., Miglarese, M., Epstein, D., Iwata, K., Haley, J. D., Gibson, N. W., and Ji, Q. Feedback mechanisms promote cooperativity for small molecule inhibitors of epidermal and insulin-like growth factor receptors. *Cancer Res.* **2008**, *68*, 8322–8332.
42. Female *nu/nu* CD-1 mice were used for xenograft studies. To assess antitumor efficacy, cells were implanted s.c. in the right flank. Tumors were allowed to establish to $200 \pm 50\,mm^3$ before randomization into treatment groups. Tumor volumes were determined twice weekly from caliper measurements by $V = (\text{length} \times \text{width}^2)/2$. TGI was determined by $\%TGI = \{1 - [(T_t/T_0)/(C_t/C_0)]/1 - [C_0/C_t]\} \times 100$, where T_t = tumor volume of treated animal × at time t, T_0 = tumor volume of treated animal × at time 0, C_t = median tumor volume of the control group at time t, and C_0 = median tumor volume of the control group at time 0. Mean %TGI was calculated for the entire dosing period for each group. Significant antitumor activity is defined as mean %TGI >50%.

CHAPTER 8

DISCOVERY AND DEVELOPMENT OF MONTELUKAST (SINGULAIR®)

Robert N. Young

This chapter will chronicle the nearly 20-year effort that eventually resulted in the discovery and bringing to market in 1998 of montelukast sodium (Singulair®) as a safe and effective therapy for asthma and allergic rhinitis. It does not purport to be a totally inclusive record of all studies associated with the discovery and development but rather to highlight the strategies and thinking that went into the project and to show the many issues that were faced along the way and how the teams sought to face and ultimately solve them. Many hundreds of researchers and dedicated scientists and clinicians were implicated in the effort and it is not possible to acknowledge or describe the efforts of them all. We do salute their efforts, nonetheless, as do the millions of patients whose lives have been improved with the access to this treatment.

8.1 INTRODUCTION

To fully appreciate the contexts of the project, it is necessary to start at the beginning when the leukotrienes (LTs) were first discovered. For a more complete review of the field see the book *Leukotrienes and Lipoxygenases* published by Elsevier in 1989 [1].

In 1938, two physiologists, Feldberg and Kellaway, published a paper characterizing an unstable substance they observed in dog and monkey lungs treated with cobra venom that was later termed "slow reacting substance" [2]. Subsequently, Brockelhurst in the 1960s showed a similar if not the same substance that could be crudely isolated from perfusions of the lungs of immunologically challenged sensitized guinea pigs which he named "slow reacting substance of anaphylaxis (SRS-A)" [3]. As the names implied, the substance caused the slow contraction of smooth muscles in the lung and other tissues such as ileum or vas deferens and the contractions were strong and sustained in contrast to the rapid and short-lived contractions induced by contractile agents such as histamine. They and others came to hypothesize that this substance might play a role in the pathophysiology of asthma and other allergy-related diseases. SRS-A was exquisitely potent but was produced in only minute quantities by sensitized tissues and thus proved to be an elusive and unstable substance which resisted purification and further characterization. It was almost 40 more years before the chemical composition of SRS-A was elucidated. The introduction of modern techniques such as high performance liquid chromatography (HPLC) allowed purification and revealed a distinctive UV chromophore reminiscent of a conjugated triene structure [4]. Parallel studies had shown that neutrophils could convert

Case Studies in Modern Drug Discovery and Development, Edited by Xianhai Huang and Robert G. Aslanian.

arachidonic acid to several metabolites including a dihydroxyl compound that also had the characteristic triene chromophore [5]. This led researchers such as Bengt Samuelsson at the Karolinska Institute in Stockholm, Sweden, to suspect that SRS-A and this new "triene" might be derived from a common unstable epoxide intermediate [6] (see Figure 8.1). The study of the incorporation of radio-labeled putative biosynthetic precursors and partial synthesis allowed Samuelsson and co-workers in 1979 to propose a structure for SRS-A, as a novel hybrid structure where a cysteine-containing element was conjugated with a 20 carbon fatty acid triene derived from arachidonic acid (**1**) [6]. Samuelsson coined the name "leukotriene" (LT) for the substance based on the biosynthetic source from leukocytes and the triene structure. The initially proposed structure(s) of SRS were indefinite with respect to the exact nature of the cysteine-containing element and the stereochemistry about the chiral centers (5-hydroxyl and 6-S-cysteinyl) and of the

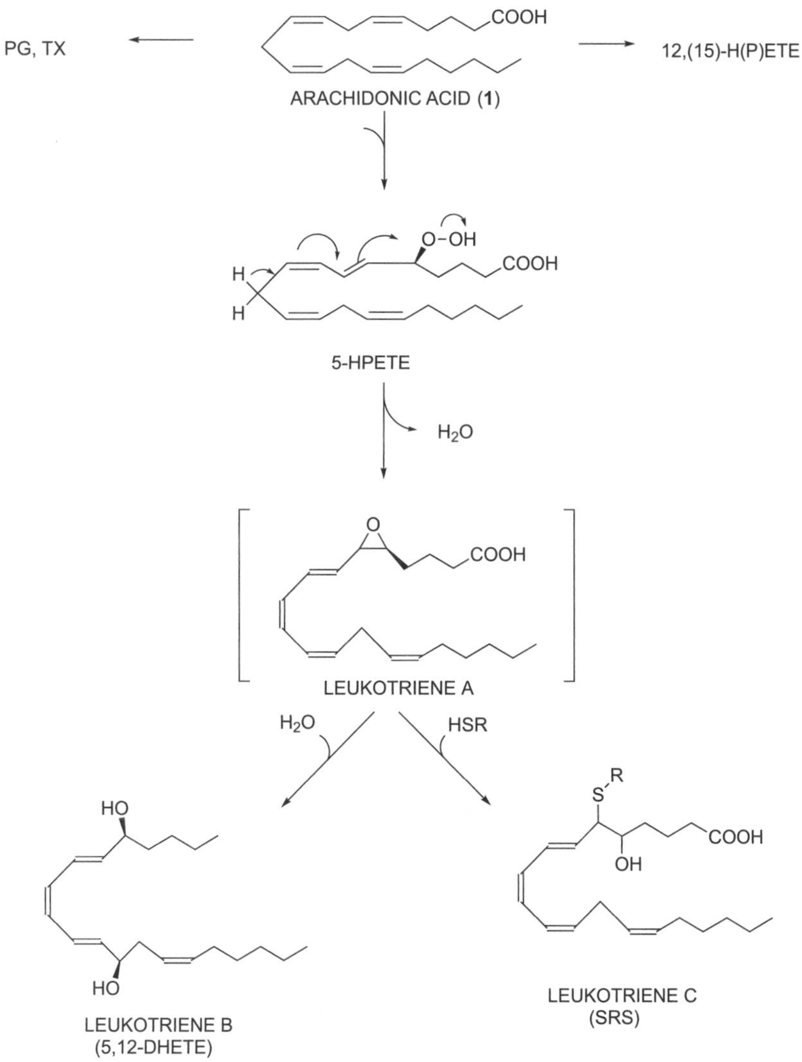

Figure 8.1 Proposed biosynthesis and structures of leukotriene B and SRS.

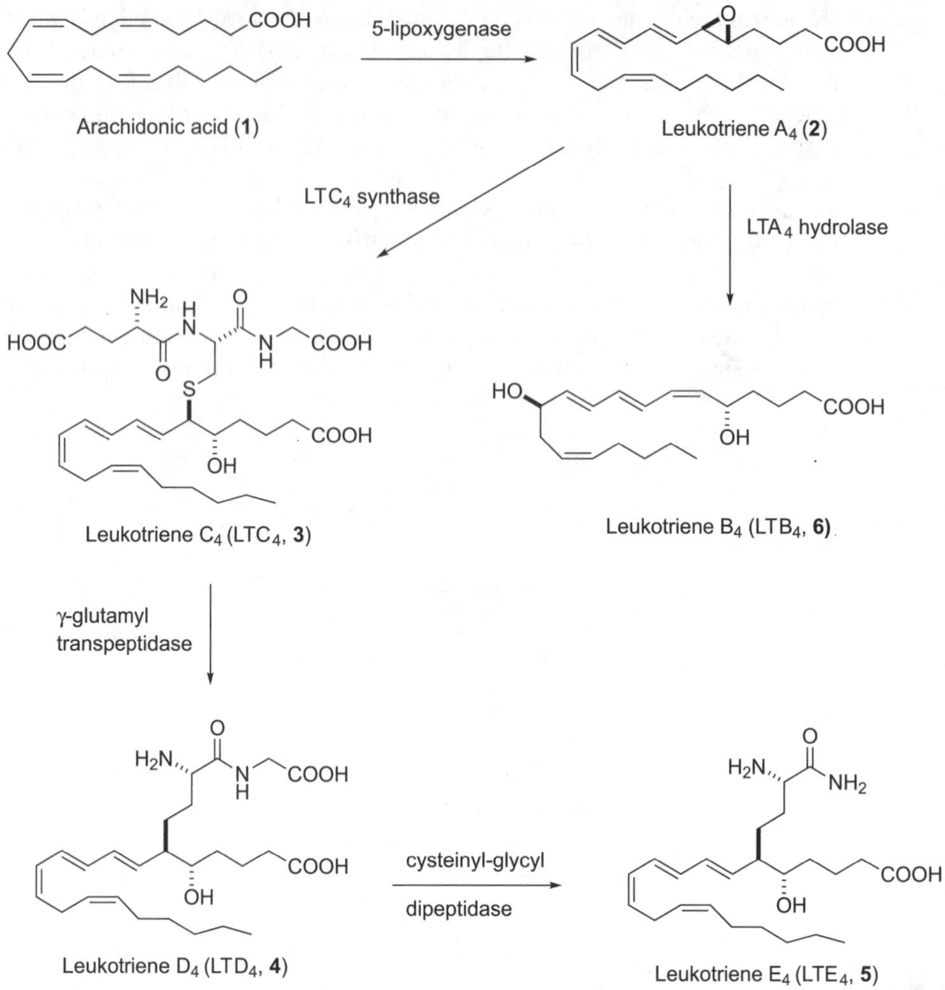

Figure 8.2 Biosynthesis of the leukotrienes.

double bonds (Figure 8.1). The structures were rapidly confirmed and clarified by total synthesis in the laboratories of Corey at Harvard University [7] and at Merck Frosst in Montreal [8], and SRS-A was found to consist of a variable mixture of three compounds bearing either *S*-glutathione (named LTC4 (**3**), where the 4 represented the number of double bonds in the molecule), *S*-cysteinyl-glycine (LTD_4) (**4**) or *S*-cysteine (LTE_4) (**5**) at C-6 (Figure 8.2) [9]. The dihydroxy-leukotriene was called LTB_4 (**6**) and it was found to exert a potent chemotactic effect on eosinophils and neutrophils and other inflammatory cells and was subsequently recognized to be the likely structure of another previously described substance which was known as the eosinophil chemotactic factor of anaphylaxis (ECF-A) [10]. The first syntheses of a leukotriene were published less than 6 months after the structure proposal [7,8] and subsequent improved syntheses (particularly by researchers at Merck Frosst [11] who made the compounds available for free to bona fide researchers around the world) rapidly made SRS-A leukotrienes widely available for study and served to stimulate a resurgence in interest in the role of SRS-A in human asthma. Subsequently, total synthesis also allowed characterization of the *in vivo* human and animal metabolites of LTs [13], the synthesis of radio-labeled LTs, and the development of analytical techniques such as mass spectrometry [14], radio-immunoassays (RIA) [1,15], and enzyme-linked immunoassays (ELISA) [1,16] for the study of the production of leukotrienes in pathological situations. Work with the synthetic LTs in many laboratories around the world served to confirm that these substances were indeed extremely potent contractile agents for smooth muscle (subnanomolar potency) [17] and that they could induce a variety of effects, such as increased permeability of lung vasculature leading to edema [18]; increased mucus secretion from airway epithelial mucus glands [19] and deceased mucociliary activity leading to decreased mucus transport [20]; induction of smooth muscle hypertrophy [21]; stimulation of influx of inflammatory cells into the lung (e.g., mast cells and eosinophils) [22]; concurrent with production of cationic peptides such as "major basic protein" from eosinophils and epithelial cell damage [23]; and release of tachykinins from C-fibers in the lung (properties associated with the development of hyper-reactivity of the airways) [24]. Studies on the production of LTs *in vivo* indicated that these substances were produced in a variety of inflammatory environments [25] and that excreted LT metabolites increased during asthma attacks [26]. LTs were felt to be largely pathological and no "normal" physiological role for leukotrienes could be found other than the hypothesis that LTs might be part of a vestigial protection mechanism evolved as a crude defense against parasitic infections in the lung and perhaps other tissues "open" to the outside world such as the gastrointestinal tract [27]. All these studies served to support an important role for leukotrienes in the pathophysiology of asthma in humans and led to a growing consensus that a blocker of leukotriene action, either a biosynthesis inhibitor or an antagonist at the putative receptor(s) might provide a much needed new therapy for treatment of asthma. The largely pathological role suggested that such a drug could be very safe and without mechanism-based side effects.

At the time of the discovery of the leukotriene structures, preferred treatments for asthma were limited to the acute use of nonspecific bronchodilators such as theophylline and β-receptor agonists such as salbutamol that were used to blunt or abort the episodic lung contractions of "asthma attacks." For more chronic use, corticosteroids, such as dexamethasone, were used to treat what was considered to be the underlying inflammation in the lung thought to be ultimately responsible for the disease. Merck was an early pioneer in the development of corticosteroids for treatment of inflammation and later developed aerosolized steroids for the treatment of asthma. Indeed Merck was first to market cortisone in 1948 and later hydrocortisone in 1952 [28]. In the 1960s, Merck introduced inhaled dexamethasone sodium as a treatment for asthma [28]. Although effective, all these treatments were associated with worrisome side effects such as tachycardia with theophylline and the β-agonists and a multitude of liver, bone, and skin effects with steroids (especially systemically administered steroids). The side effects for β-agonists and steroids could be mitigated through administration as aerosols but many doctors were still reluctant to prescribe chronic treatment of children with steroids for fear of adrenal suppression and growth retardation. Another treatment used at the time, especially in children due to its safety profile, was inhaled sodium cromoglycate that was said to "stabilize mast cells" and thus inhibit mediator release [29]. However, efficacy was marginal at best and the relatively large recommended doses were difficult to administer especially to young children. Indeed administration of aerosols was a major issue for treatment in general and for children and for the elderly in particular in that there was often poor compliance and outcomes of aerosol therapy due to difficulties to coordinate inhalation with activation of the devices. The time was right for development of a safe and effective orally absorbed drug to treat asthma.

Studies confirmed Samuelsson's hypothesis that both LTB4 and the trio of cysteinyl LTs were biosynthesized from arachidonic acid through the common intermediacy of the unstable epoxide, LTA4 (**2**). A single enzyme, 5-lipoxygenase was found to effect the two-step conversion of AA to LTA4 via an intermediate 5-hydroperoxyeicosatetraenoic acid (5-HPETE) [30]. Other enzymes then converted LTA_4 to LTB_4 (LTA_4 hydrolase) [31] or to LTC_4 (LTC_4 synthase) [32] and thence to LTD4 (γ-glutamyl transpeptidase) and to LTC_4 (cysteinyl-glycyl dipeptidase) (Figure 8.2). A variety of evidence, including the specific binding of radio-labeled LTs to lung and inflammatory cell membranes, indicated that the LTs exerted their effects through interaction with specific membrane-associated receptors [33].

8.2 DRUG DEVELOPMENT STRATEGIES

Thus, a variety of potential drug targets were possible. At Merck Frosst (and at many other companies), it was proposed that blockade of 5-LO would abort the entire pathway and thus should be an excellent target with maximum therapeutic potential. On the other hand, it was demonstrated that LTD_4 was the most potent of the cysteinyl-LTs [34] and thus the LTD_4 receptor could also be an excellent target to block many of the activities of LTs. It was decided to embark in both directions at once with the major effort to be directed towards the 5-LO inhibitor. What followed on the inhibitor side was a multi-decade long effort starting at Merck Frosst in 1980 that lead to the discovery of many excellent inhibitors that almost inevitably were found to show unacceptable safety profiles. At Merck, six-candidate 5-LO inhibitors were identified and brought into development but not to clinic [35]. An alternative target (a 5-LO-associated protein necessary for cellular LT biosynthesis named 5-lipoxygenase activating protein or FLAP) was identified in the mid-1980s [36] and led to two clinical candidates, MK-866 (**7**) [37] and MK-0591 (**8**) [38], but eventually the antagonist approach was found to be most

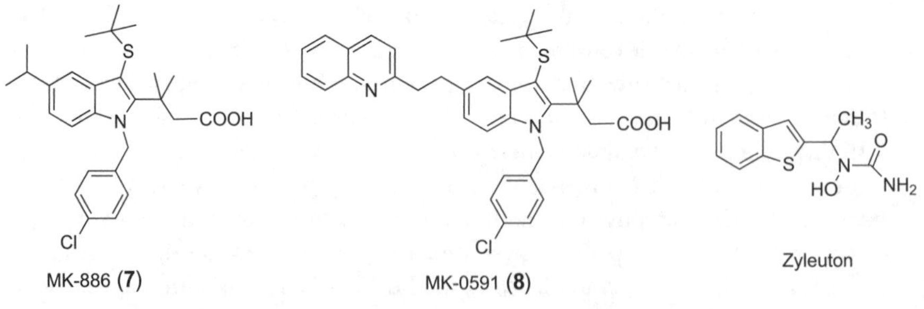

Structures of MK-886, MK-0591 and Zyleuton

productive. Abbott laboratories identified a 5-LO inhibitor, zileuton, which made it to the marketplace under the name Zyflo but high dose (600 mg four times a day); drug interactions and an incidence of liver side effects [39] have limited its wide use. As this chapter follows, the development of the LTD_4 receptor antagonist, montelukast, we will focus on rather than describe the inhibitor project. It should be noted however that until the availability of suitable clinical candidates it was not known which approach would be best or even if LT blockade would have any useful clinical benefit at all.

8.3 LTD_4 ANTAGONIST PROGRAM

8.3.1 Lead Generation and Optimization

In 1980, when this project initiated, there was widespread skepticism among asthma researchers that blocking any one mediator was likely to derive a truly beneficial clinical effect as asthma was a "multimediator" disease. Inflammatory cells were known to produce other mediators besides LTs including prostaglandins and histamine and it was generally known that antihistamines and prostaglandin blockers were not beneficial, and indeed inhibition of PG biosynthesis with aspirin often exacerbated asthma symptoms [40]. Corticosteroids however, which are demonstrably effective, are known to cause a general suppression of inflammatory cell activation and thus to suppress all mediator release (among other effects). Only a clinical study in asthmatic patients with a potent and specific antileukotriene molecule could prove or disprove the potential utility of this class of drug. The search for an SRS-A receptor antagonist had in fact predated the leukotriene structure elucidation by a number of years. To test compounds researchers had laboriously isolated crude SRS-A from lung perfusates from sensitized guinea pigs to allow them to screen selected compounds for their ability to block SRS-A-induced contraction of guinea pig ileum tissue in organ baths. In this manner, FPL-55712 (**9**, Figure 8.3), a compound related to the asthma drug sodium cromoglycate, had been shown to be an SRS-A antagonist [41]. Similar studies had been ongoing at Merck Frosst and some laborious screening had already been carried out. The availability of synthetic LTD_4 allowed the definitive proof that FPL-55712 was indeed an LTD_4 antagonist and also allowed development of *in vitro* assays and more effective and "higher throughput" screening to go ahead.

8.3.2 *In Vitro* and *In Vivo* Assays

As synthetic leukotrienes and radio-labeled LTD_4 became available, it became possible to set up higher throughput *in vitro* screening assays and to evaluate the *in vivo* effects of LTD_4 and the blockade by antagonists. [^{3}H]-LTD_4 binding to lung membranes from guinea pigs or humans was developed [42]. Biological activity could be further evaluated by measuring the ability of compounds to antagonize contractions induced by LTD_4 (or other agonists) of isolated guinea pig ileum, guinea pig trachea, or human tracheal tissue [43]. Compounds could also be evaluated for their ability to inhibit contractions induced in tracheal tissues from sensitized guinea pigs by an antigen or in human tracheal tissues by a goat-anti-human IGE antibody. A number of *in vivo* assays were developed or adapted for assay of compounds to inhibit LTD4 or antigen-induced effects in animals. Compounds were evaluated for their ability to block LTD_4 or antigen-induced bronchoconstriction in either normal or sensitized anesthetized guinea pigs after either i.v. or intraduodenal (i.d.) administration. Compounds were also evaluated for their ability to block dyspnea induced by an aerosolized antigen in conscious hyper-reactive rats after oral dosing [44]. This assay was abandoned in later years due to difficulties in maintaining the colony and observations that dyspnea was largely due to mucous secretion in the lungs rather than bronchoconstriction. Another useful and unique model was developed at Merck Frosst using specially trained squirrel monkeys where LTD_4-induced or antigen-induced bronchoconstrictions could be evaluated in conscious animals [45]. These animals were trained to sit in specially designed chairs and to wear a mask that allowed introduction of aerosols or LTD_4 or antigen. Some were naturally allergic and reacted to antigen presentation very much like a human would do. Compounds could be dosed i.v. or p.o. or by aerosol directly to the lung and responses could be observed over several hours. Finally, compounds could be evaluated for

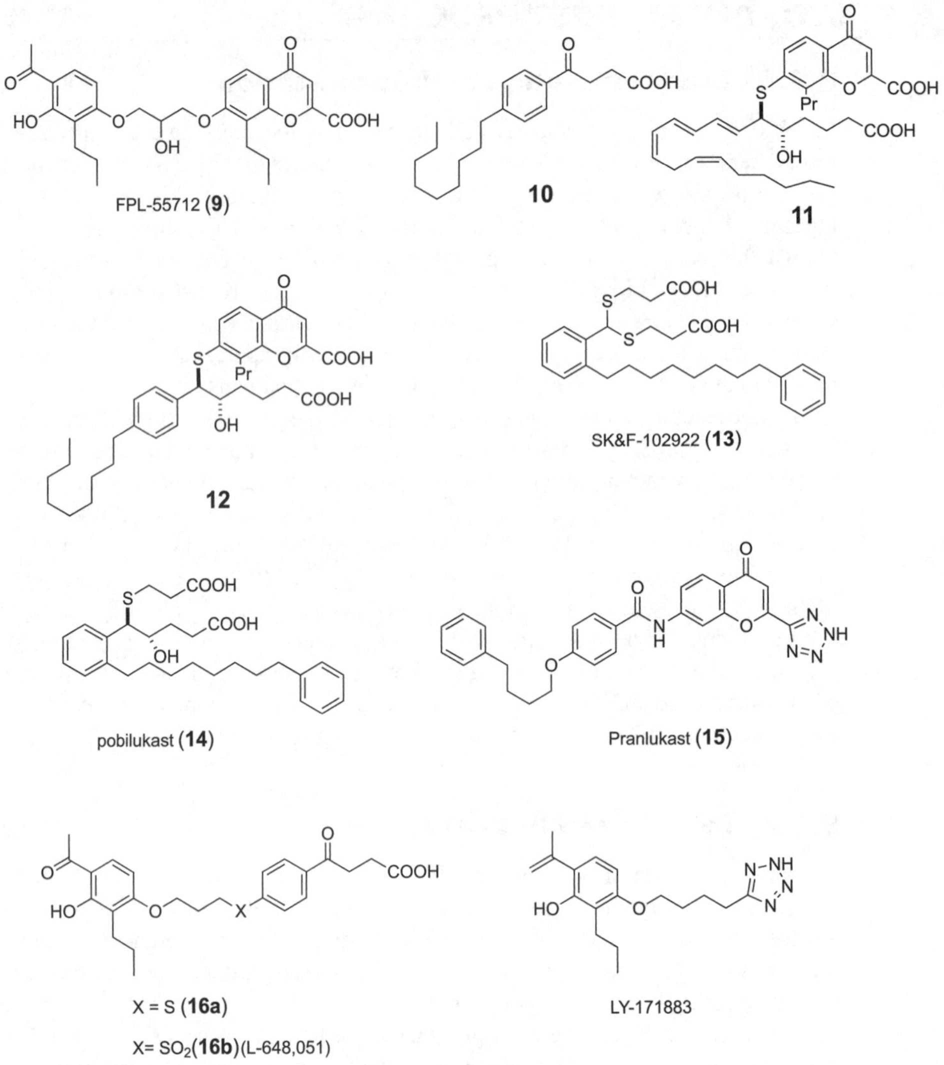

FPL-55712 (**9**) **10** **11**

12 SK&F-102922 (**13**)

pobilukast (**14**) Pranlukast (**15**)

X = S (**16a**)
X= SO_2(**16b**)(L-648,051)
LY-171883

Figure 8.3 Some first generation LTD4 antagonists.

their abilities to block either LTD_4, other mediator (e.g., histamine or methacholine) or antigen-induced bronchoconstrictions in a special colony of allergic sheep in the laboratories of Dr. William Abraham at the University of Miami [46]. In these animals it was possible to observe effects over many hours and to determine efficacy against the so-called early (or immediate phase) or late phase responses as well as to determine effects on induced airway hyper-reactivity. Due to the complex digestive tracts of the sheep, compounds were usually dosed either i.v. or by aerosol.

8.4 THE DISCOVERY OF MONTELUKAST (SINGULAIR®)

8.4.1 First-Generation Antagonists (Figure 8.3)

At the beginning of the program in 1980, all screening was for functional blockade of LTD_4-induced contractions on guinea pig smooth muscle tissues in organ baths. Thus, as the program began, we had FPL-55712 and the LTD_4 structure to use as leads. Screening at Merck Frosst also revealed a "lead structure" 4-[4-nonylphenyl]-4-oxo-butanoic acid (**10**) as a moderately potent LTD_4 antagonist inhibiting LTD_4-induced contractions of guinea pig ileum. In addition, a number of analogs of LTD_4 were synthesized and a structure activity relationship (SAR) for agonist activity was built up using both functional and $[^3H]$-LTD_4-binding assays. Conclusions from these studies were that at least one acidic functionality was required as well as a second polar group that could be acidic or nonacidic (the C- amide derived from LTD_4 was equi-active with LTD_4 while the cysteinyl-glycyl amide was 10-fold less active). There was need of an extended lipophilic group of a length similar to that of LTD_4 with at least a C-7 double bond, and a hydroxyl group at C-5 with appropriate absolute and relative stereochemistry at C-5 and C-6 was critical for agonist activity [47]. Flexibility and the multitude of rotatable bonds in the overall LTD_4 structure obviated any attempts to define a clear active conformation, but SAR suggested a crude model for the putative receptor-binding site (Figure 8.4) that we tried to use to advance and optimize the lead antagonist structures that were then at hand. The acid group in **10** and the chromone carboxylic acid part of FPL-55712 were considered to occupy the acidic-binding site in the receptor and the nonyl group in **10** and propylphenyl groups in **9** were considered to lie in the lipophilic pocket. FPL-55712 while quite potent (pA2 of about 7) did not show good *in vivo* activity in animal asthma models nor acceptable oral absorption. We thus tried to meld the two structure types together. Cognizant of the LTD_4 structure and of the role of a second polar element in LTD_4, a number of structures were synthesized based on **9** where a variety of bipolar chains were attached to leukotriene backbones or nonyl–phenyl groups including some where the chromone element was used (e.g., **11** and **12**) [48]. Many of these showed comparable or improved potency compared to FPL-55712, but none exhibited good *in vivo* properties and the approach was suspended. It is notable however that workers at Smith Kline and French also followed this approach and eventually identified compounds **13** and **14** which were not only potent LTD_4 antagonists but also showed good oral absorption and

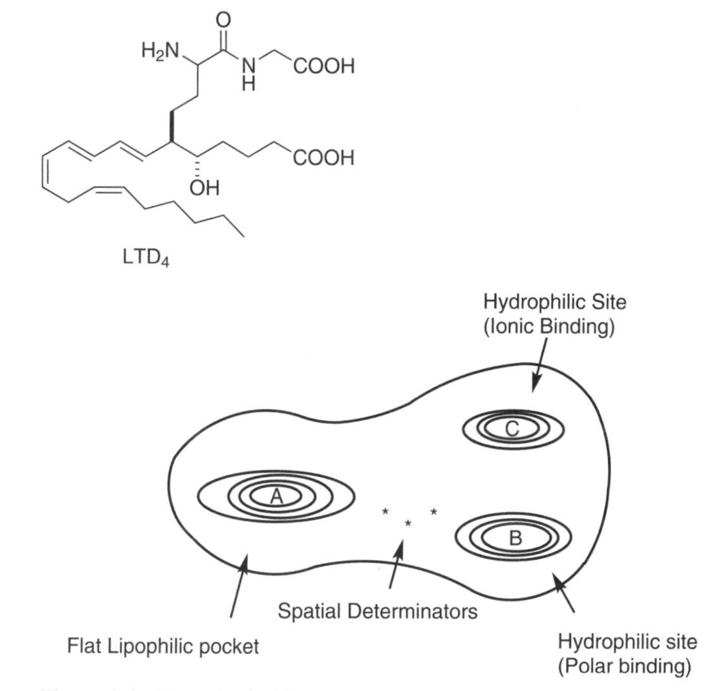

Figure 8.4 Hypothetical LTD4 receptor model.

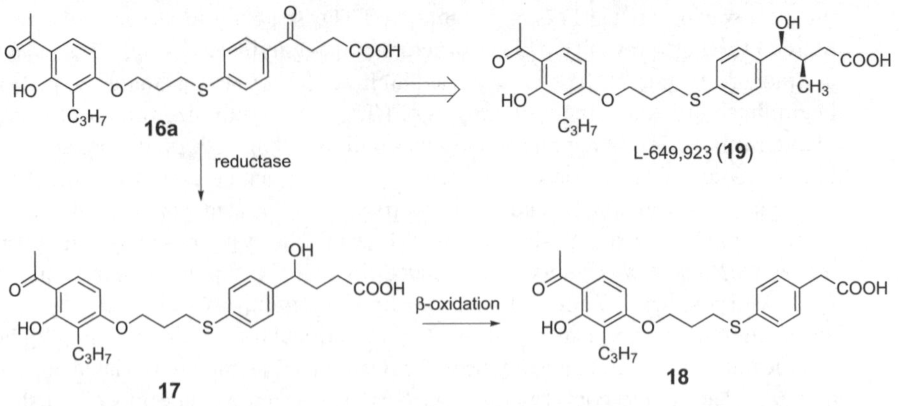

Figure 8.5 Metabolism of **16a** and evolution to L-649,923 (**19**).

in vivo activity [49]. **14** (later named pobilukast) was found to be 100-fold more potent than FPL-55712 and later shown to be clinically active [50]. Ono in Japan followed a somewhat similar approach and identified the compound **15** (ONO-1078; pranlukast) [51] that was eventually licensed to SmithKline Beechams for the US market but was never approved. It was however approved in Japan where it reached the market in 1995 (the first LTD_4 antagonist to do so).

However, the next phase of research at Merck Frosst was directed towards attempting to prepare analogs of FPL-55712 with improved metabolic stability, and in particular where the chromone ring system was replaced (as this system was assumed to be the major site of instability). Noting similarities of FPL-55712 (**9**) and compound **10**, a number of analogs were prepared where the chromone ring system was replaced with a phenylpropionic acid such as in **16**. Numerous analogs were prepared and evaluated *in vitro* for LTD4 antagonism and *in vivo* in a guinea pig bronchoconstriction model. Notably, both compounds **16a** and **16b** showed good *in vitro* activity and *in vivo* blockade of LTD_4-induced bronchoconstriction when dosed intravenously (i.v.) but only **16a** showed activity when dosed intraduodonally (i.d.). Exploratory metabolism studies showed that **16a** was rapidly metabolized via reduction (to **17** and β-oxidation to the phenylacetic acid **18** (Figure 8.5). Analogs were prepared and evaluated for *in vivo* metabolic stability and oral absorption, eventually leading to the discovery of compound **19** (L-649,923) [52] which was chosen for further developments. The sulphone analog **16b** (L-648,051), while not orally active (later attributed to rapid first pass metabolism and elimination in the liver), was shown to exert superior topical properties especially for blockade of LTD_4- or antigen-induced contraction of human tracheal preparations [53]. It was particularly notable that **16b** effectively blocked anti-IGE-induced contractions of human tissue in the micromolar range of concentrations, while it could only partially block antigen-induced contractions in guinea pig tracheal preparations. Later, it was revealed that human tracheal tissues express the LTD_4 receptor (Cys-LT1) almost exclusively, while guinea pigs express both the Cys-LT1 and Cys-LT2 (or LTC_4) receptors [54]. These species-specific differences may have at least in part been responsible for the different efficacies observed and the experience serves to emphasize the importance of using human tissue wherever possible to confirm the validity (or lack of validity) of animal models of disease. These compounds were also evaluated for efficacy in blocking LTD4-induced or ascaris antigen-induced bronchoconstriction in conscious squirrel monkeys where orally administered L-649,923 (**19**) (1.5–5 $mg\,kg^{-1}$ p.o.) and nebulized L-648,051 (**16b**) (0.1% solution over 5 min) were effective [52,55].

Both L-648,051 and L-649,923 were approved for development, the former as a powder aerosol and the latter as an orally administered compound. They both passed preliminary safety evaluations and were entered into clinical trials. Notably L-649,923 was found to cause hepatomegaly (liver weight increases) and hepatic enzyme induction in rats at high doses [56], considered to be an adaptive rather than toxic effect but an effect that would complicate the development of leukotriene antagonists in years to come. L-649,923 was first tested in man in 1985 and was studied both for its ability to antagonize aerosolized LTD_4-induced bronchoconstriction in human subjects and for its ability to block antigen-induced bronchoconstriction in asthmatic patients (studies modeled on the squirrel monkey results) [57,58]. The compound was well absorbed with a relatively short half-life. It was found to shift a dose response to LTD_4 by 3.8-fold to higher doses when administered at the maximum allowable dose of 1000 mg orally. It had no effect on a dose response to histamine indicating that it was indeed selective for LTD_4 [57]. At a similar dose, the compound inhibited antigen-induced bronchoconstriction but produced only a small reduction in the early response to an antigen but not for specific airway conductance. It also had no effect on the late response leading to the conclusion that either the compound was not a sufficiently potent antagonist to diminish the effect of endogenous LTD_4 *in vivo* or that LTD_4 does not play a major role in the airway response to the antigen challenge [58]. Thus, clinical efficacy was deemed inadequate and the development was stopped and the whole concept of LTD_4 in asthma was called into question. In 1986, L-648,051 passed safety evaluation and entered clinical trials dosed both i.v. and as a dry powder aerosol. It was hoped that direct application to the lung tissue might provide a greater measure of activity. As expected, the compound showed a very short half-life when dosed i.v. as had been observed in animals. The aerosol however was well tolerated and L-648,051 at 12 mg powder aerosol dose was shown to partially block the LTD_4 response and not histamine [59]. Unfortunately, it also only weakly blocked antigen-induced bronchoconstriction [60] and further development was stopped. About this time, Eli Lilly discovered the antagonist, LY-171,883 (Figure 8.3) [61], with a profile comparable to that of L-649,923. LY-171,883 that also gave disappointing results in clinical trials [62,63] and many researchers in the field began to question the importance of leukotrienes in the etiology of asthma. Indeed companies such as Lilly suspended their programs based on these results. The view at Merck, however, was that the relative impotency of the compounds so far tested (as evidenced by about fourfold shifts in the LTD_4 dose response curves achieved at maximum tolerated or deliverable doses) had not adequately tested the hypothesis and it was decided one would need to achieve at least a 10-fold shift to properly evaluate the role of leukotriene D_4 in asthma.

8.4.2 Discovery of MK-571

8.4.2.1 Medicinal Chemistry Effort Leading to the Discovery of MK-571 While the optimization of L-648,051 and L-649,923 was being done, there was a parallel effort to screen the extensive Merck compound sample collection going on. The effort would appear laughably slow in today's world but it, nonetheless, proved to be effective. Compounds were manually selected from scanning computer printouts of structures with selections made with the "intuitive eye" of the scanning chemist (usually RNY). Considering the extended π-system of LTD_4 and the various polar functions of the natural and unnatural known ligands, compounds were selected for testing knowing our testing capacity was rather small (20–100 compounds per week). The selections were sent from Montreal to the sample collection in Rahway, New Jersey, where the staff dutifully located and weighed out samples which were shipped back to Montreal. The screening was done largely by testing compounds for their ability to block the contractions induced by LTD_4 on strips of guinea pig ileum tissue in organ baths equipped with tensiometers. The optimized rig had 10 organ baths set up in an arc and the LTD_4 was added by a robotized syringe. Increasing amounts of LTD_4 were added to a bath containing a set concentration (usually 10 μM) of the test compound and the shift in the dose–response curve was recorded. If a good shift was observed, lower concentrations were evaluated and a pA2 value determined. Potent compounds could also be evaluated on guinea pig tracheal ring preparations or on human trachealis. Using these techniques, >10,000 compounds were evaluated over several years. Later, a $[^3H]$-LTD_4-binding assay was set up to measure displacement of radioligand from lung membrane preparations, but not before the key "hit" structure had been identified. A number of moderate "hits" were identified and confirmed and some preliminary SAR was evaluated and eventually one compound, 2-(2-(3-pyridyl)-ethenyl)quinoline (**20**), was selected for optimization based on its simplicity and potency. Notably, the compound was found to have an IC_{50} in the $[^3H]$-LTD_4-binding assay of 6 μM (only sixfold less potent than L-649,923) and it showed activity when dosed orally in the "asthmatic rat" model with an ED_{50} of 3 mg kg^{-1} (only twofold less potent than L-649,923). A hypothesis was developed that the structure might fit in the LTD_4 receptor in the putative, flat lipophilic pocket that recognized the extended conjugation (triene) of LTD_4 and thus it was suggested that appropriately placed chains bearing carboxylic acids or H-bond acceptors (such as amides) might be expected to boost the potency considerably (Figure 8.4) [47]. An initial foray into preparing substituted pyridyl analogs led to synthetic difficulties and quickly convinced us to evaluate substituted phenyl analogs instead. Happily the pyridine could be replaced with a phenyl ring without loss of potency and such compounds could be easily prepared by reaction of 2-methyl-quinoline with readily available substituted benzaldehydes [64]. A series of phenol analogs were prepared and initial indications were that the meta-analog (**21b**) was quite potent (IC_{50} 0.56 μM) and much more potent than the para- (**21c**) or the ortho-analogs (**21a**) (Table 8.1). Thus, meta-substituted compounds were further evaluated. In spite of the increased activity of the phenol **20** on the receptor, it was less potent when evaluated in the rat assay (ED_{50} 10 mg kg^{-1}) and an evaluation of blood samples from orally dosed rats showed little free drug in the blood and rather the *O*-glucuronide was found (a common fate of phenolic drugs). The phenol provided a convenient handle for attachment of chains bearing polar functions however and a series of *O*-alkanoic acids and esters were prepared leading to the observation that the *O*-acetic and *O*-propionic esters (**22** and **23**) were both

TABLE 8.1 Initial Structure Activity Studies Based on Lead Structure 20

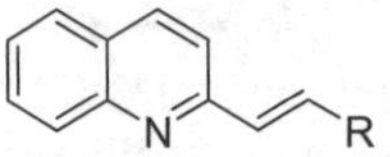

Compound	R	$[^3H]$-LTD_4 binding (GP lung) IC50, μM
20	3-pyridyl	6 ± 4
	phenyl	6 ± 2
21a	2-hydroxylphenyl	>50
21b	3-hydroxylphenyl	0.56 ± .2
21c	4-hydroxylphenyl	>50

TABLE 8.2 Structure Activity Studies in the Styryl Quinoline Series [47]

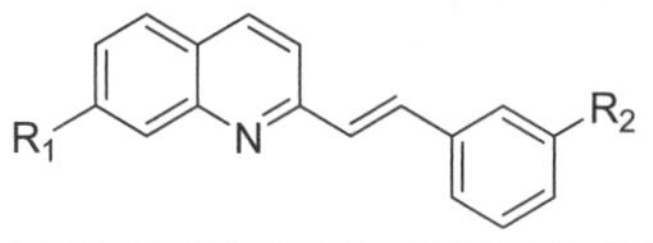

Compound	R_1	R_2	$[^3H]$-LTD_4 binding GP lung IC_{50} nM	Hyperreactive rat[44] ED_{50} (mg/kg)
20	H	OH	560 ± 200	10
22	H	OCH_2COOCH_3	1000 ± 890	2.0
23	H	$OCH_2CH_2CH_2COOC_2H_5$	580 ± 380	1.5
24	5-Cl	$OCH_2CH_2CH_2COOH$	1430 ± 1400	-
25	6-Cl	$OCH_2CH_2CH_2COOH$	270 ± 190	40% @ 1.5 mg/kg
26	7-Cl	$OCH_2CH_2CH_2COOH$	39 ± 41	41% @ 0.5 mg/kg
27	7-Cl	SCH_2CH_2COOH / SCH_2CH_2COOH	3 ± 1.4	43% @ 0.15 mg/kg
28	7-Cl	$SCH_2CH2COOH$ / $SCH_2CH_2COON(CH_3)_2$	0.8 ± 0.6	0.07

potent on the receptor and in the rat model (Table 8.2). Again, when blood samples from dosed rats were evaluated, the dosed drugs were not found but rather the corresponding acids were observed. These acids were however also active on the receptor. Several of these acid derivatives showed excellent bioavailability and duration in the blood of rats and dogs and were considered as possible development candidates. At this time, however, we became somewhat concerned that the unsubstituted quinoline functionality common to all these compounds might be a source of toxicity through metabolic oxidation. Additionally, overlay of computer-generated models of LTD_4 and compound **23** suggested that there could be further room for lipophilic binding through substitution of the quinoline in the 5, 6, or 7 position. Such substitution might serve to suppress potential oxidative metabolism on the quinoline. A number of substituted quinoline and 1,4 quinazoline analogs were prepared and in particular, a series of 3′-phenoxypropionic acids with varying quinoline substitutions were evaluated (Table 8.2, compounds **24–26**). We were pleased to find that alkyl or halogen substitution was not only tolerated but 7-halogen substitution (e.g., compound **25**) led to compounds with about 10-fold greater potency at the LTD_4 receptor (Table 8.2). Knowing that LTD_4 contains two polar chains and **25** only one, the question was asked: "What if a second acidic chain were incorporated into the structure?" This was readily achieved by reacting the precursor 7-chloro-2[3′-formylphenylethenyl}-quinoline with 3-thiopropionic acid to form the thioacetal **27** in a manner that at the time had been employed in SKF-102922 (**13**) [65]. Compound **27** was significantly more potent in the receptor-binding assay (IC_{50} = 3 nM). However, the oral activity in the squirrel monkey model of LTD_4-induced bronchoconstriction was not as good as expected despite having good pharmacokinetics in rats and monkeys. Lipophilic acids were well known to bind to serum albumin and while such binding can be useful to provide sustained blood levels and duration of action in the body, we considered that the suboptimal *in vivo* activity of **27** might be due to inability to its effectively penetrate tissues due to excessive binding to plasma proteins. Measurement of plasma-protein binding (PPB) using the equilibrium dialysis method confirmed the extremely high degree of binding (>99.9%) and we therefore attempted to design analogs with reduced binding while maintaining the potency. Knowing that for LDT_4 itself, the C1 carboxyl group could be converted to an amide without loss of binding potency [47], we explored a series of mono-amide analogs of **27**. We felt that by varying the amide substitution, we might modulate the physical properties of the molecules while hopefully retaining the LTD_4 receptor-binding potency. A number of mono-amides were prepared and as hoped these compounds generally showed diminished levels of PPB (95–99%) while retaining LTD_4 receptor-binding potency. Eventually, the mono-dimethylamide **28** (L-660,711; MK-571) was identified as a compound with the optimal combination of subnanomolar potency on the LTD_4 receptor (IC_{50} 0.8 nM for inhibition of LTD_4 binding on the guinea-pig lung membrane), good oral absorption and bioavailability in several species, good half-lives, moderated PPB, and excellent oral activity in rat and monkey asthma models [66]. In the squirrel monkey, MK-571 effectively blocked LTD_4-induced bronchoconstriction 4 h after an oral dose of 0.1 mg kg^{-1}. In addition, it blocked the bronchoconstriction induced by aerosolized antigen exposure in allergic monkeys 4 h after a dose of 0.5 mg kg^{-1} [67]. Furthermore, when MK-571 was formulated as a solution that could be administered by intravenous infusion or by aerosol to antigen-challenged allergic sheep, it was found to block both early- and late-phase bronchoconstriction as well as induced hyperreactivity [68,69].

8.4.2.2 Synthesis and Preclinical Development of MK-571 MK-571 had been relatively readily prepared in only four steps from 7-chloroquinaldine (see Scheme 8.1) [64] and indeed Dr. Robert Zamboni single handedly prepared several hundred grams in keeping with of the depth of his leadership in this project. However, the synthesis had one major flaw from a process chemistry point of view and that was the nonselective introduction of the propionate and dimethylamino-propionate side chains, both introduced in the same reaction by reacting equal amounts of methyl 3-mercaptopropionate and 3-mercaptopropionic acid *N,N*-dimethylamide with a boron trifluoride catalyst. This gave a 1:2:1 mixture of the three possible adducts which were readily separated by column chromatography and then the ester amide was hydrolyzed to provide MK-571. The prospect of performing this chromatography on a kilogram (or potentially ton) scale was not greeted with enthusiasm by the process development chemists and so they devised a more tractable stepwise synthesis wherein the intermediate aldehyde was first reacted with trimethylsilylchloride and 3-mercaptopropionic acid *N,N*-dimethylamide to form the TMS hemithioacetal which was then reacted in a following step to provide the unsymmetrical dithioacetal which could be purified by crystallization and then finally hydrolyzed to give the required drug (Scheme 8.2) and thus no chromatography was needed [70]. Scale-up in the pilot pant provided the drug in kilogram quantities for development. MK-571 could be formulated as a crystalline sodium salt as a tablet for oral dosing and also as a solution in buffered saline for intravenous administration.

8.4.2.3 Clinical Development of MK-571 [71] MK-571 was taken into safety assessment in rats and dogs where it was shown to have a safety profile appropriate for introduction into man. MK-571 entered clinical trials in 1989 and was shown to be well absorbed in human volunteers and to have a half-life of elimination and pharmacokinetic properties suggesting the possibility of bid or tid dosing [72,73]. The compound was

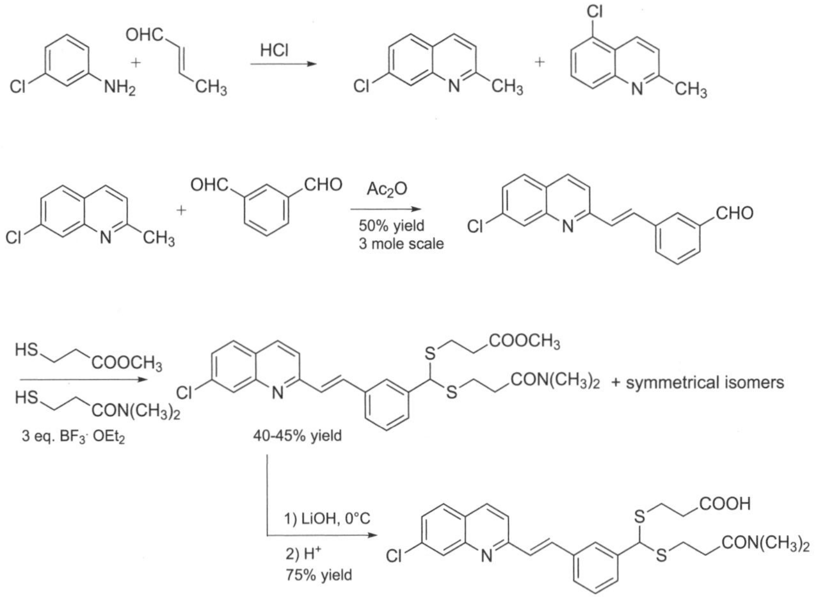

Scheme 8.1 Initial medicinal chemistry synthesis of **MK-571** [70].

generally well tolerated with no significant side effects different from those observed for placebo. The initial clinical evaluation was shepherded by Dr. Dorothy Margolski in the Merck Clinical Pharmacology Department [71]. The clinical pharmacology group sought to understand the properties of a new drug as completely as possible in the early phase development. Thus, Dr. Margolski resolved to test the efficacy of MK-571 for blocking the LTD_4 challenge, and ultimately antigen challenge by administering the drug as a constant i.v. infusion as had been done in the sheep model. In this way, they felt one could accurately

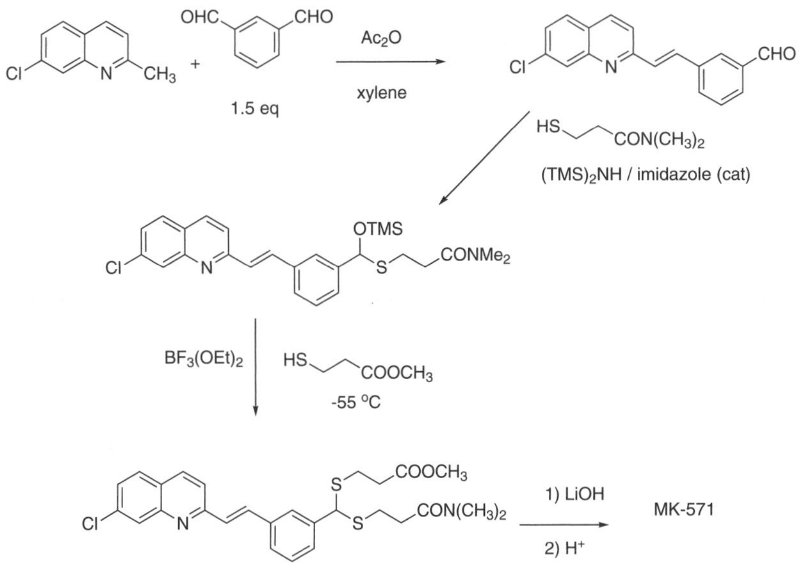

Scheme 8.2 Process synthesis of **MK-571** [70].

evaluate the blood levels needed to provide (hopefully) a profound block of LTD_4- (and antigen-) induced bronchoconstriction. Thus, the activity could be associated with a specific drug blood level which could then be subsequently targeted for oral dosing as a desired trough level and appropriate doses chosen for subsequent oral asthma studies in phase 2. Infusion studies in phase 1 in otherwise healthy asthmatic patients showed that doses of 28 or 227 mg of MK-571 infused so as to produce plasma concentrations of 2 and 20 $\mu g\ ml^{-1}$, profoundly shifted or blocked the bronchoconstriction induced by increasing doses of inhaled LTD4 such that at the higher dose no response to LTD_4 was noted even when the agonist was exposed at 10^{-4} molar concentration. A similar infusion study in asthmatic patients was done at total infused doses of 37.5, 165, and 450 mg (yielding estimated MK-571 plasma levels of 1, 3.3, and 13 $\mu g\ ml^{-1}$) and was shown to inhibit from 43% to 88% of the immediate bronchoconstriction (early phase reaction) induced by an inhaled antigen. The late phase bronchoconstriction reaction was inhibited from 25% to 63%. Other i.v. infusion studies showed for the first time that LTD_4 antagonists had efficacy against exercise-induced bronchoconstriction in asthmatics and that MK-571 caused bronchodilation in moderately severe asthmatic patients. These impressive outcomes showed that LTD_4 was a critical mediator of asthma pathophysiology and set the stage for true asthma studies in phase 2. MK-571 performed well in phase 2A [74,75] and then Phase 2B studies in asthmatic patients [76]. The research team felt reason to celebrate the possibility that MK-571 could be a truly useful drug for the treatment of asthma. The celebratory mood was unfortunately quashed by news emanating from the safety assessment department which was continuing its studies of the compound by treating rats and mice for more extended periods and at higher doses. They observed that rats treated for extended periods of time with high oral doses of MK-571 showed signs of liver changes including increased liver weights and increases in peroxysomal enzyme activities [77]. These effects were even more enhanced in mice while little effect was seen in monkeys. While these changes were considered to be an adaptive response rather than overt toxicity, there were other compounds in the historical record (including LY-171883 [78]) which had shown similar responses and had been associated with an increased incidence of liver carcinogenesis [79]. The prospect of waiting 2 years while such studies were carried out on MK-571 was not considered worth the risk and management decided to terminate the development on MK-571. This was a great disappointment to the discovery team, but, nonetheless, the compound had proven the potential of an LTD_4 antagonist for treatment of asthma if only a "clean" compound could be found.

8.4.3 Discovery of MK-0679 (29)

8.4.3.1 Medicinal Chemistry Effort Leading to the Discovery of MK-0679 One troubling prospect that needed to be confronted was the possibility that blocking LTD_4 receptors was somehow mechanistically responsible for the observed liver changes. Indeed similar changes had been observed for other LTD4 antagonists L-649,928 and LY-171883 and others had postulated a role for leukotrienes in liver injury in mice [80]. However, MK-571 only showed these effects at high doses and high systemic exposure despite being many times more potent and thus the effects did not seem to correlate with potency on the LTD_4 receptor. The search was therefore on for an LTD_4 antagonist which would be free of these effects. This search did not need to go far because MK-571 was itself a mixture of enantiomers and the question that immediately came to mind was whether only one or both enantiomers were responsible for the observed liver changes. In fact the two enantiomers of MK-571 had been prepared and evaluated earlier, but the biological activity of the two compounds was very similar and at the time there was no clear reason to select one enantiomer over the other [81,82]. With the liver issue at hand, the two enantiomers were revisited, this time to assess their ability to induce liver weight increases and liver enzyme elevations in mice. Dosed at up to 400 mg kg^{-1} p.o. in mice, the *S*-enantiomer (L-668,018) caused liver weight increases and peroxysomal enzyme activity elevation similar to what had been observed for MK-571, while the *R*-enantiomer (MK-0679) (**29**) was found to be essentially devoid of such effects [77]. The *S*-enantiomer was slightly more potent *in vitro* with IC_{50} 0.77 nM versus 3.2 nM for MK-0679 ([^{3}H]-LTD_4-binding assay) but was not significantly more active *in vivo* in a rat asthma model possibly because of the superior pharmacokinetics of the *R*-enantiomer. The expectation was that this pharmacokinetic advantage would also extend to human. Previous clinical studies had shown that when racemic MK-0571 was dosed in humans (i.v.) and both enantiomers were monitored by a quantitative enantioselective assay, the *R*-enantiomer was eliminated significantly slower than was the *S*-enantiomer [72] (similar to what was observed in rats). Thus, the decision was taken to initiate development of L-668,019, the *S*-enantiomer of MK-571.

8.4.3.2 Synthesis and Preclinical Development of MK-0679 (L-668,019, Verlukast; Venzair™)

The original preparation of the enantiomer MK-0697 was complex, multistep, and involved careful chromatography to derive pure material. It was not practical for large-scale production [74]. To prepare quantities of MK-0679, the Merck process research group devised a remarkably simple, efficient, and cost-effective synthesis in a very short time after the compound was declared a formal candidate for development. The synthesis [83] (see Scheme 8.3) involved only three steps (from 7-chloro-2-methylquinoline) via the achiral but diasterotopic diester **30**. They reasoned that if one of the ester groups could be selectively hydrolyzed (enzymatically), one could derive a

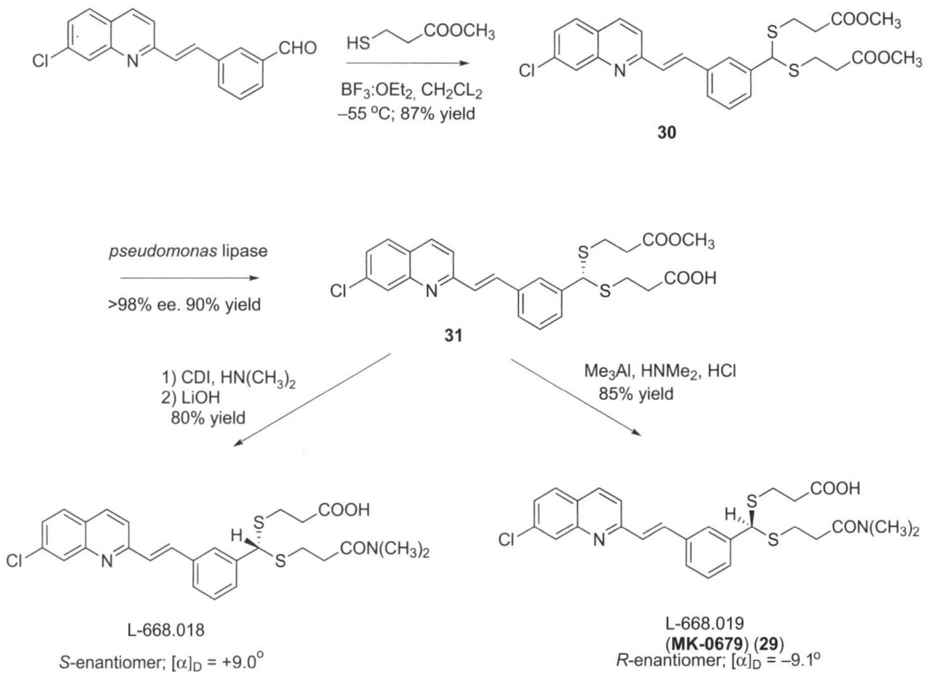

Scheme 8.3 Process synthesis of MK-0679 [83].

chiral mono-ester carboxylic acid Y. Depending on the absolute stereochemistry obtained then either the acid or ester group could be converted to the dimethyl amide thus deriving MK-0679. A survey of a variety of available esterases and lipases identified a *pseudomonas* lipase enzyme from *Pseudomonas cepacia* LPL-80 which very efficiently and effectively hydrolyzed only one enantiotopic ester to give the chiral mono-ester which could be purified by crystallization to give **31** in 80% yield and > 99% enantiomeric purity. Indeed the entire hydrolysis reaction was run as a heterogeneous reaction where the starting ester was stirred vigorously as slurry with the enzyme and a surfactant, Triton-X-100. Over time the slurry went partially into a solution before precipitating again as the mono-ester product that could be filtered off in excellent purity and yield. The filtrate could be recycled for the next batch. To produce the desired *R*-enantiomer, the ester moiety of **31** was reacted with dimethylamine hydrochloride and trimethylaluminum to give MK-0679 (**29**) directly in 85% yield. If the *S*-enantiomer were desired, the same mono-ester could be converted to the amide ester by reaction with carbonyl-diimidazole and dimethyl amine, followed by hydrolysis of the ester. This remarkable three step synthesis was much more efficient than the previous racemic synthesis and led Dr. Paul Reider of Process Research at Merck, Rahway, New Jersey, to comment that if he were ever called on to prepare the racemic MK-571 again, he would prefer to make the two enantiomers by the chiral route and mix them together as the final step!

The synthesis was scaled up to provide the kilogram quantities needed to repeat safety assessment and provide material for formulation development. All this proceeded smoothly and MK-0679 was ready to enter clinical evaluation in less than a year after the suspension of development of MK-571!

8.4.3.3 Clinical Development of MK-0679 (Verlukast)

MK-0679 entered into clinical trials in 1990 and in phase 1 studies was found to be generally well tolerated. It was almost completely absorbed and had a half-life consistent with at least three times daily dosing [84]. In keeping with the preclinical pharmacology and excellent pharmacokinetics, MK-0679 was found to have clinical efficacy almost identical to that which had been obtained with MK-571 [85]. In addition, a landmark study examined MK-0679 in aspirin-intolerant asthmatics [86], patients whose asthma could be dramatically exacerbated when exposed to aspirin and other nonsteroidal anti-inflammatory drugs. The underlying etiology of this syndrome was poorly understood but there were suggestions that in these patients blockade of cyclo-oxygenase enzymes might somehow stimulate leukotriene LT synthesis and/or release. Studies ongoing at the time and subsequently published showed that these patients did indeed excrete high levels of leukotriene metabolites in their urine [87]. When aspirin-intolerant patients were treated with MK-0679, their baseline respiratory function (FEV1) increased a remarkable 18% and there was a highly significant shift in their bronchoconstrictor dose–response curve to inhaled lysine-aspirin [86,88]. These results served to dramatically demonstrate the role of leukotrienes in asthma in this subset of patients and further bolstered the potential place for a safe leukotriene antagonist in the treatment of asthma. Based on the excellent activity in clinical trials, MK-0679 was given the generic name verlukast. Although the original goal of the program had been a once a day oral drug, the potency and human pharmacokinetics suggested that it would require twice or possibly three times a day dosing. Nonetheless, verlukast was considered to be a viable drug candidate and was continued in more extensive safety and clinical trials. In 6 week, phase 2 chronic asthma trials, verlukast showed efficacy as measured by a number of parameters such as increases in FEV1 measurements, decreased symptom scores and beta-agonist usage when dosed orally 250 mg twice a day [89]. However, a small percentage (approximately 3%) of treated patients also showed elevation in serum transaminases. In light of Merck's goal to develop a drug for chronic treatment of asthma in both adults and children, the decision was taken in 1991 to abandon the development of MK-0679. The observed enzyme elevations were particularly disconcerting to the discovery and development team, because no evidence of significant serum transaminase elevations had been observed in safety studies which at that time had extended for up to 1 year in rats and primates and at doses many times higher than had been used in these clinical trials. Extensive studies were undertaken to try to understand the mechanism of this apparent toxicity. In spite of these efforts, no substantiated explanation could be uncovered. However, the studies on MK-571 and MK-0679 had proven the potential value of an LTD_4 receptor antagonist for treatment of asthma and thus efforts to find an optimal drug were continued.

8.4.4 Discovery of Montelukast (L-706,631, MK-0476, Singulair®)

While verlukast was in preclinical and clinical development, efforts had continued to be made to find possible back-up candidates with emphasis on structural diversity, increased potency, and improved pharmacokinetics. Initially, efforts had been directed towards replacing the dithioacetal moiety as this had been shown to be a site of metabolism for MK-571 and MK-679 [90]. As well, efforts were directed to replacement of the vinyl group bridging the quinoline and phenyl moieties in MK-571 and MK-0679. This had been partly motivated by observed photoisomerization and the potential for thiol addition to the vinyl group in MK-571 [91]. With the demise of MK-0679, these efforts were redoubled in earnest. Extensive SAR was developed through modifications around these sites in the molecules as well as investigation of chain lengths and substitutions.

Replacement of the vinyl group by a variety of saturated spacers such as $-CH_2-X-$, ($X = CH_2$, O or S) generally led to an approximately 10-fold loss in binding potency (Table 8.3, compounds **32, 33, 34**). Replacement of one sulfur atom in the dithioacetal moiety with a methylene group and addition of alkyl substitution into the carbon chain was

TABLE 8.3 Some Nonvinyl Analogs of MK-571

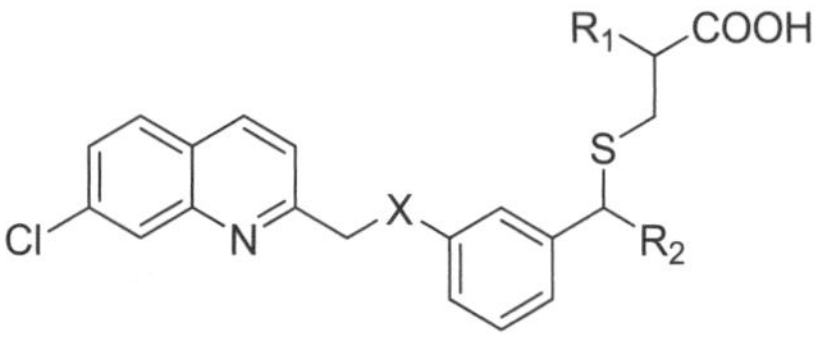

Compound	X	R_1	R_2	[³H]-LTD4 binding GP lung IC_{50} nM
MK-571			$S(CH_2)_2CON(CH_3)_2$	1
32	CH_2	H	$S(CH_2)_2CON(CH_3)_2$	31
33	S	H	$S(CH_2)_2CON(CH_3)_2$	75
34	O	H	$S(CH_2)_2CON(CH_3)_2$	15
35	O	H	$-(CH_2)_2(CH(CH_3))CON(CH_3)_2$	10
36	O	H	$-(CH_2)_2$-o-Phenyl-$CON(CH_3)_2$	1.5
37	O	CH_3	$-(CH_2)_2$-o-Phenyl-$CON(CH_3)_2$	0.5

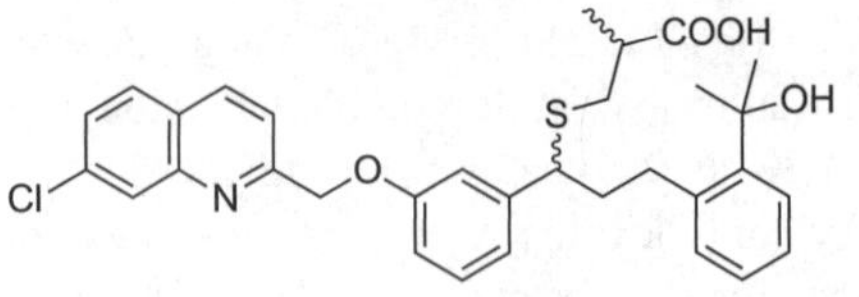

39

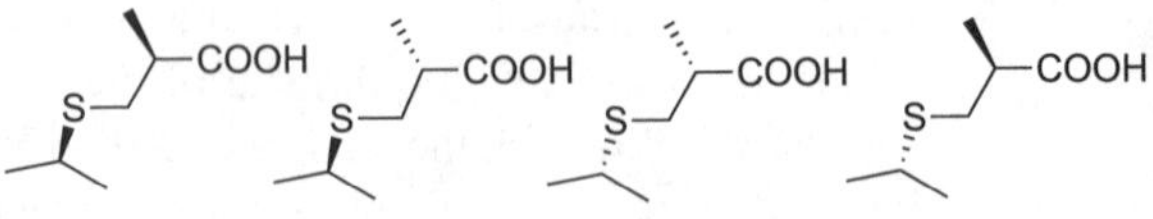

LTD4 binding (nM) (G.P. lung)	6	18	3	0.25
pA2 G.P. trachea	8.8	8.3	9.1	9.4
FACO* activity increase @ 800 mg/kg p.o. in mice	-7%	10%	128%	155%

* Fatty Acyl Co-A Oxidase activity in liver compared to vehicle treated mice at 400 mg/kg for 4 days

Figure 8.6 Correlation of potency at the LTD4 receptor and liver enzyme effects with substitution and stereochemsirty.

found to lead to retention or even an increase in potency (compound **35**) and alkyl substitution on the thioether chain also led to increases in potency. Most importantly, when a phenyl group was inserted into the carbon chain, a dramatic boost in activity was noted (Table 8.3, **36, 37**) [92]. Optimal compounds were several fold more potent than verlukast, but when pharmacokinetics were evaluated in rats they were found to have significantly shorter half-lives than verlukast. This was attributed to metabolism and hydrolysis of the amide moiety, and therefore, a more stable replacement was sought. A study was done evaluating intrinsic potency and clearance rates in rat, and somewhat surprisingly, it was found that the amide moiety could be replaced with a wide variety of substituents. Many relatively polar and nonpolar groups were tolerated and a compound incorporating a dimethylcarbonyl group on the phenyl ring and an α-methyl group on the thioether side chain was found to have optimal properties in the ether linked series. The optimum compound **39** consisted of a mixture of four diastereomers and these were individually prepared and evaluated more extensively. As had been seen before with MK-571, the pair with the *R*-configuration at the benzylic center was peroxysomal-enzyme inducers in mice, while the other pairs were free of this activity but somewhat less potent (Figure 8.6). Unfortunately, neither of this pair of compounds had an overall profile of activity and pharmacokinetic properties superior to verlukast. Considering the likelihood that the methylene-ether linking group in these compounds was a site for metabolism and considering that a 10-fold loss in potency had been incurred when the vinyl linker in verlukast was replaced by the ether linker, it was decided to re-visit the vinyl series and to apply what had been learned from these SAR studies. A series of analogous thioethers were synthesized and evaluated both *in vitro* and *in vivo* and an isomer pair *S*-thioether **40** (L-695,499) and *R*-thioether **41** were particularly interesting. While **40** was free of enzyme-inducing properties, **41** was exquisitely potent while also being a very potent enzyme inducer (Figure 8.7). The vinyl series in general exhibited excellent pharmacokinetics with good half-lives in the rat [92].

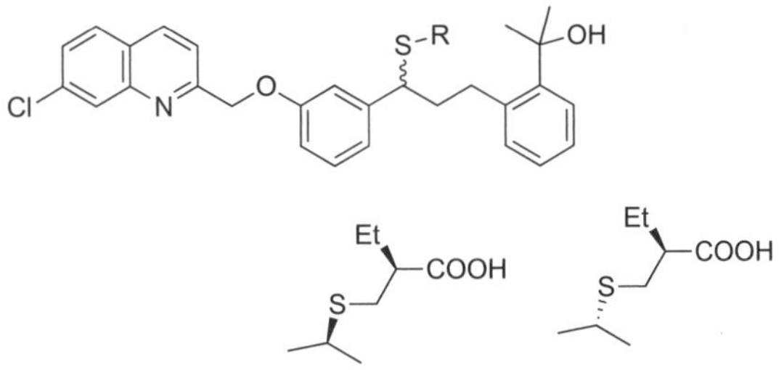

	L-695,499 (**40**)	L-697,008 (**41**)	MK-0679
LTD4 binding (nM) (G.P. lung)	0.5	0.13	4.6
(U-937 cell; human)	2.0	0.1	8
pA2 G.P. trachea	8.7	10.0	8.8
FACO* activity increase @ 800 mg/kg p.o. in mice	38%	607%	29%

* Fatty Acyl Co-A Oxidase activity in liver compared to vehicle treated mice at 400 mg/kg for 4 days

Figure 8.7 Correlation of potency at the LTD4 receptor and liver enzyme effects with substitution and stereochemistry.

It was decided to determine if the peroxysomal-enzyme induction activity could be dissociated from the *R*-thioether stereochemistry so as to take advantage of this superior potency at the LTD_4 receptor. The enzyme activity we observed to be increased in the livers of treated rats was determined to be fatty acyl Co-A oxidase (FACO) [93] and it was known that peroxysomes in the liver recognize and β-oxidize fatty acids as an adaptive process [94]. Over the concurrent years while these efforts were underway, studies had shown that a class of nuclear receptors known as the peroxysome proliferator-activated receptor (PPAR) mediate the activation and proliferation of peroxysomes in the liver [95–97]. Thus, it seemed coincidental that the PPAR receptor activity should correlate by stereospecifically recognizing the *R*-thioalkanoic acid chain in our compounds. Since the binding factors controlling PPAR interaction and the interaction with the LTD_4 receptor with these compounds were undoubtedly different, it seemed likely that structural elements could be introduced into the potent *R*-series of compounds which would disrupt PPAR binding but preserve LTD_4 receptor binding. Thus, an extensive parallel SAR effort was undertaken where structural modifications were introduced into the molecule, the LTD_4 antagonist potency was confirmed, and if acceptable, the mouse pharmacokinetics were determined (to ensure that adequate exposure could be achieved so that observed *in vivo* liver effects would be valid). If acceptable, sufficient quantities were resynthesized (about 2 g each) to allow dosing mice for 4 days at 200 or 400 mg kg^{-1}. Livers were examined for weight increases and peroxysomal enzyme activity (FACO) was determined and compared to controls. This effort was carried out over most of a year as a close collaboration between the Merck Research Laboratories Safety Assessment Group in West Point Pennsylvania under the direction of Dr. Darryl Patrick and the discovery group at Merck Frosst in Montreal, Canada [98]. Between three and five compounds were identified, validated, and synthesized in scale and tested in mice each month. Considering the large effort required to prepare the compounds and the need to ensure the drugs were delivered on time, each month one of the Montreal researchers was chosen to "win a free trip to Pennsylvania" so the compounds could be guaranteed to be delivered to the Safety

Assessment Department on time. Changes to both of the polar side chains were examined but changes to the alkanoic acid side chain proved to be most instructive. Working on the assumption that the PPAR recognizes fatty acids and that steric bulk in the vicinity of the carboxyl group might impair binding to the PPAR, changes were made on the alkanoic acid chain incorporating small alkyl substitutions in defined positions and with defined absolute and/or relative stereochemistry. A selection of the most pertinent compounds from this study is presented in Table 8.4. As can be seen from the results, effects on liver weights and on FACO enzyme activity were generally well correlated and alpha alkyl substitution (and particularly if the branched center had the *S* configuration) was associated with significant increases in both effects. Effects of β-substitution were less pronounced and most importantly, compounds with only β,β-di-substitution were essentially without effect on either liver weights or enzyme activity induction. Generally, most of these compounds retained potent subnanomolar activity on the LTD_4 receptor. This led to a more extensive evaluation of β,β-di-substituted analogs and of the longer chain butyric acid series. This series was particularly attractive as there was no theoretical possibility of β-thiol elimination for these compounds. The compounds that were both intrinsically potent and essentially free of liver effects at 400 mg kg^{-1} in mice were further evaluated for pharmacokinetics in several species, including mice, rats, and squirrel monkeys, and also for the effect of addition of plasma proteins or plasma on potency in an $[^3H]$-LTD_4 receptor-binding assay. This "protein shift" was deemed to be representative of the relative degree of attenuation of activity one might expect *in vivo* in a proteinaceous environment and therefore of the expected translation of *in vitro* to *in vivo* potency. In this assay, unlike MK-571 that showed up to 20-fold shift with human plasma, compound **42** was essentially unshifted on addition of either 0.05% human serum albumin, 1% human plasma or 1% squirrel monkey plasma [100]. Compound **42** (L-706,631, MK-0476) was extensively evaluated and was determined to exhibit the best overall *in vitro* and *in vivo* profile. Most notably, the compound *significantly inhibited LTD_4-induced bronchoconstriction in conscious squirrel monkeys 4 h after an oral dose of 0.01 mg kg^{-1}*. This represented an at least 10-fold potency enhancement compared to what had been observed with MK-571 and MK-0679. MK-0476 also showed excellent *in vitro* activity versus LTD_4 and/or antigen stimulation of human, sheep, guinea pig, and monkey tissues and cells and *in vivo* in guinea pigs, sheep, and monkeys [100]. With these data in hand, MK-0476 was selected for development in 1991. In that, the generic nomenclature required the suffix–lukast and the discovery of MK-0476 in the Montreal labs of Merck, it was given the generic name **montelukast**.

8.5 SYNTHESIS OF MONTELUKAST

8.5.1 Medicinal Chemistry Synthesis

The medicinal chemistry synthesis of montelukast (**42**) (Scheme 8.4) followed the convergent strategy that had been developed to prepare the variety of analogs that led up to the discovery of MK-0476 [92,93,99]. This strategy made use of synthetic methodologies that had been discovered and developed in the 1980s and some of which have been more recently been recognized through the award of several Nobel Prizes in chemistry (Corey in 1990 and Heck in 2010), such as enantioselective reductions of ketones, palladium catalyzed couplings of aryl halides with allylic alcohols, and enantioselective aldol condensations. The efficiency and selectivity of these relatively new reactions were critical to the rapid preparation of the compounds in Table 8.4 and were

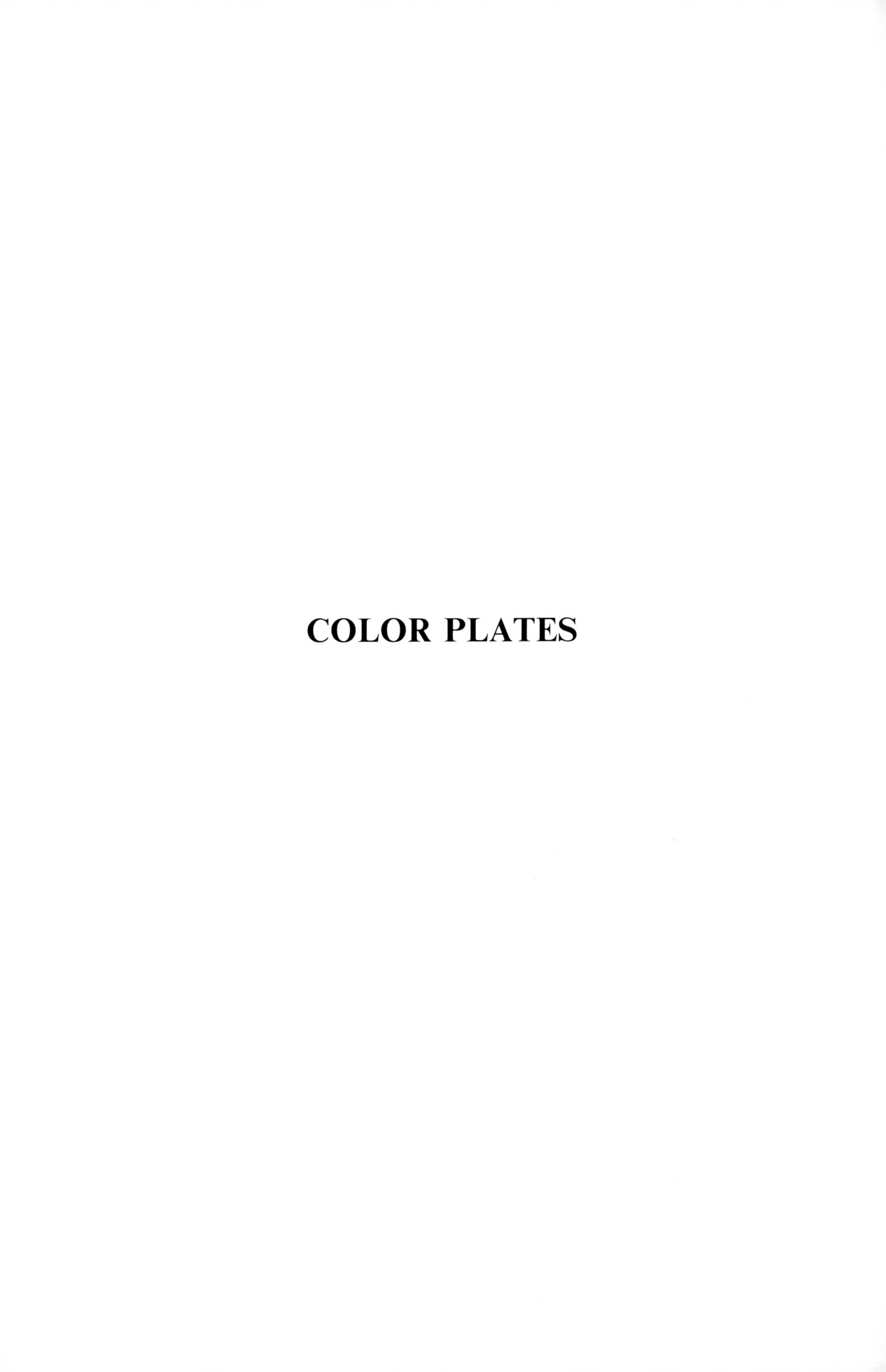

COLOR PLATES

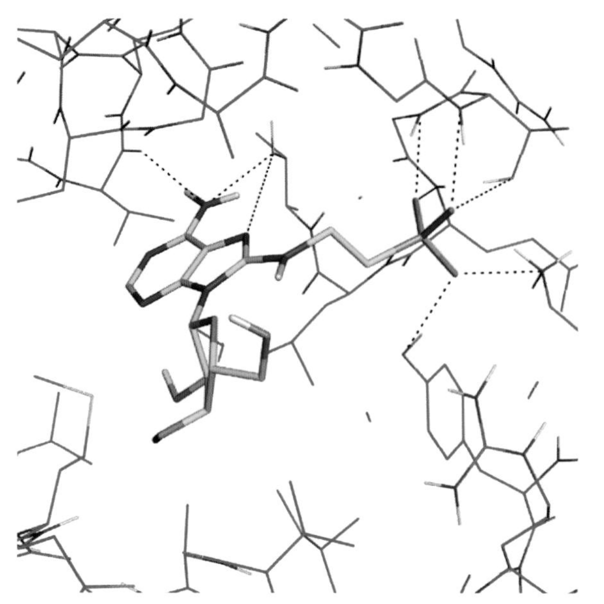

Figure 4.4 X-ray structural analysis of **1.6** bound to FBPase.

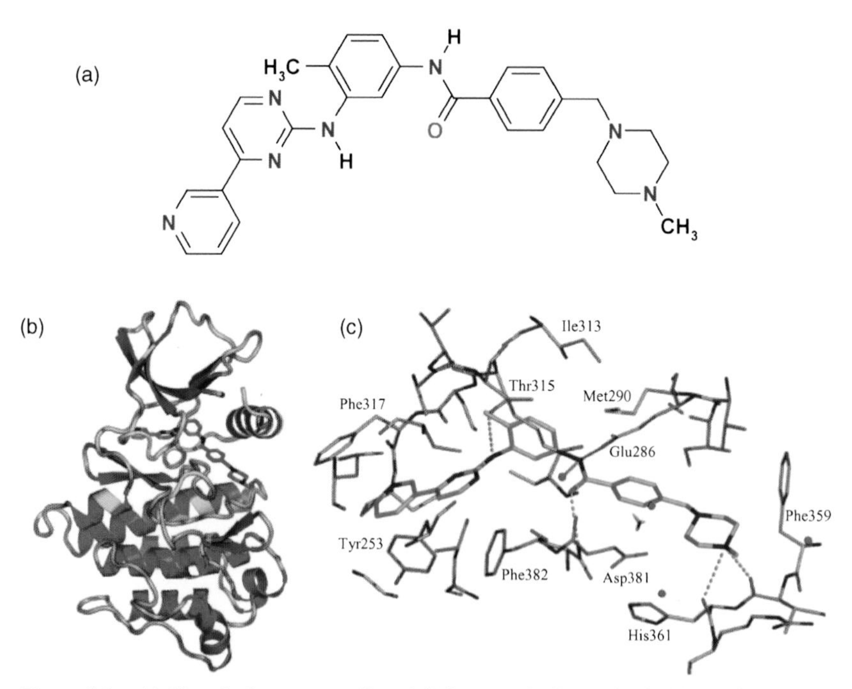

Figure 5.3 (a) Chemical structure of imatinib in pose similar to that in 3b and 3c. (b) Ribbon diagram showing the binding of imatinib (green C atoms, blue N atoms and red O atom) within the ATP-binding cleft between the two lobes of the ABL kinase SH1 domain (helices in red, strands in blue, loops and turns in gray), with the locations of mutants isolated from imatinib-resistant patients shown in yellow. (c) Details of the binding of imatinib (color-coded as in 3b) to ABL kinase (gray C atoms, blue N atoms and red O atoms; conserved water molecules shown as red spheres) showing potential hydrogen bonds as orange dotted lines and, clearly showing the hydrogen bond between the imatinib-NH and the oxygen atom of the threonine315 CH(Me)OH sidechain, that is not possible for the $CH(Me)CH_2CH_3$ isoleucine sidechain of the T315I mutant enzyme. (Adapted from [49] with permission from Elsevier.)

(b)

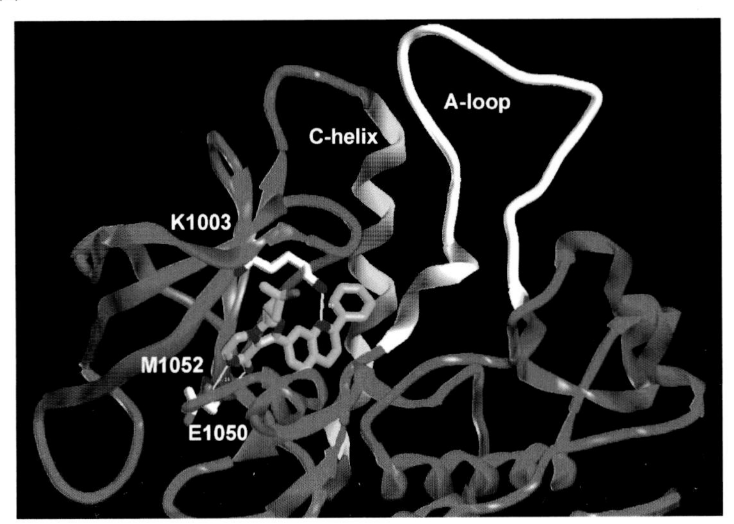

Figure 7.2b Modeled structure of OSI-906 in complex with IGF-1R with (a) key hydrogen bonding interactions highlighted; (b) C-helix highlighted in yellow and (c) activation loop (A-loop) highlighted in white.

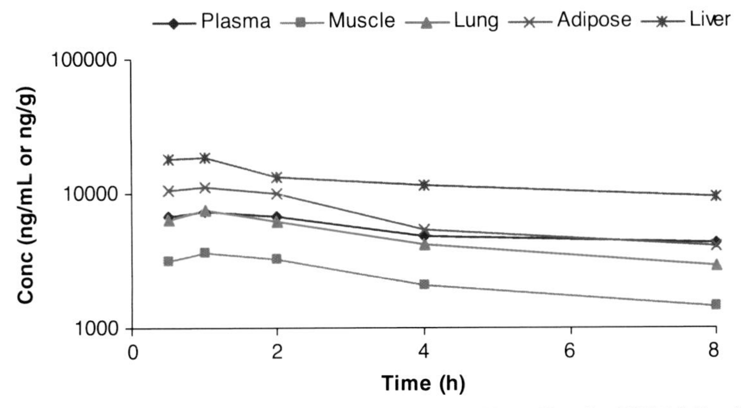

Figure 7.10 Comparison of plasma and tissue PK profiles for FQIT following a single oral administration at 10 mg kg^{-1} in the female CD-1 mouse. Data are median ($n = 3$) at each timepoint and error bars are omitted for clarity.

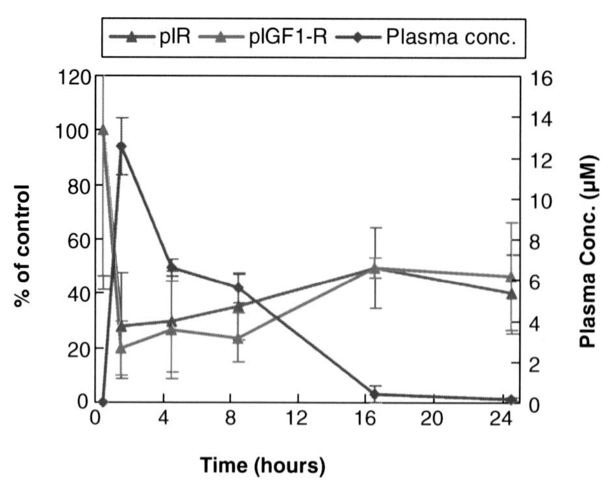

Figure 7.11 Correlation of inhibition of IGF-1R and IR phosphorylation and plasma drug exposure in GEO tumor xenografts following oral dosing with $10\,\mathrm{mg\,kg^{-1}}$ FQIT. The blue line corresponds to mean ± SE plasma concentrations of FQIT at indicated time following $10\,\mathrm{mg\,kg^{-1}}$ *qd* dose. Red and green line represents mean ± SE pIGF-1R and pIR content in GEO tumors and expressed as a percentage of control pIGF-1R or pIR content from vehicle-treated animals, respectively.

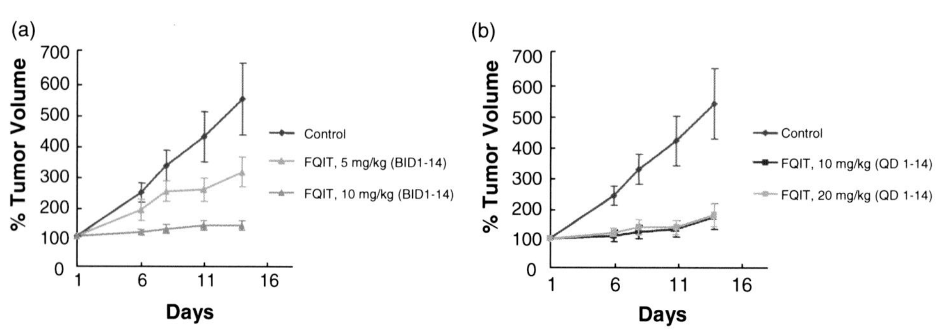

Figure 7.12 Dose–response TGI efficacy of FQIT in GEO xenograft models. Plotted data are mean tumor volumes expressed as a percentage of initial volume ± SE. FQIT was dosed on twice-daily schedule (A) or once-daily schedule (B) for 14 days.

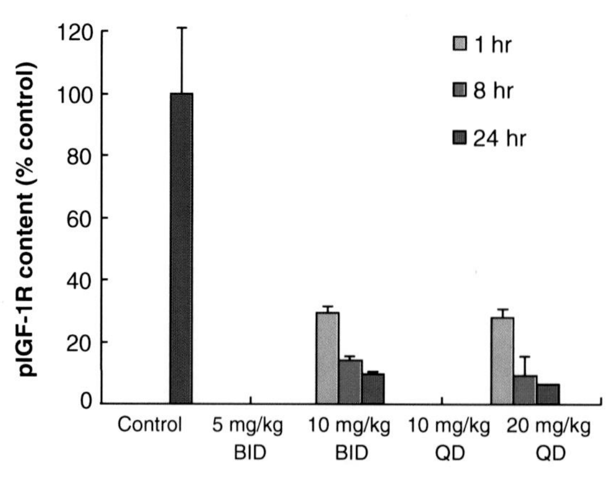

Figure 7.13 Inhibition of IGF-1R phosphorylation in GEO tumor xenografts following oral dosing with FQIT. Phospho-IGF-1R in GEO tumors expressed as a percentage of control pIGF-1R content from vehicle treated animals at 1, 8, and 24 h after 14 days of treatment with FQIT at various doses. Data are mean ± SE.

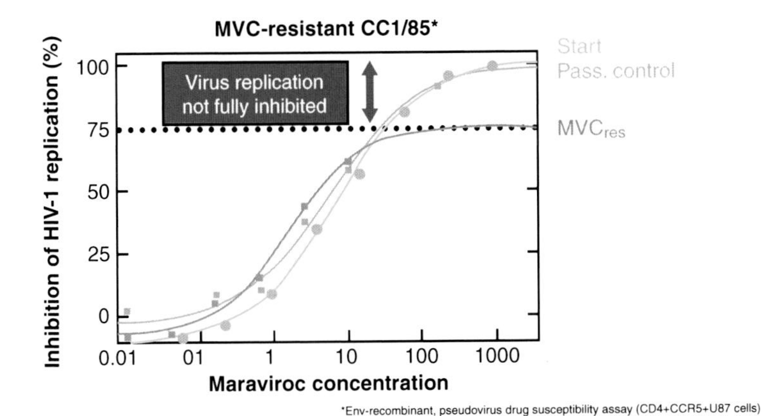

Figure 9.3 Susceptibility of pseudoviruses derived from CC1/85 to maraviroc. CCR5 tropic virus strain CC1/85 was serially passaged in peripheral blood mononuclear cells in the presence or absence of maraviroc. Susceptibility to MVC of resultant viruses was determined using the Phenosense™ HIV Entry Assay. Start = input virus; MVC_{res} = virus passaged in the presence of maraviroc; Pass. control = virus passaged in the absence of maraviroc. Adapted from Ref. [50].

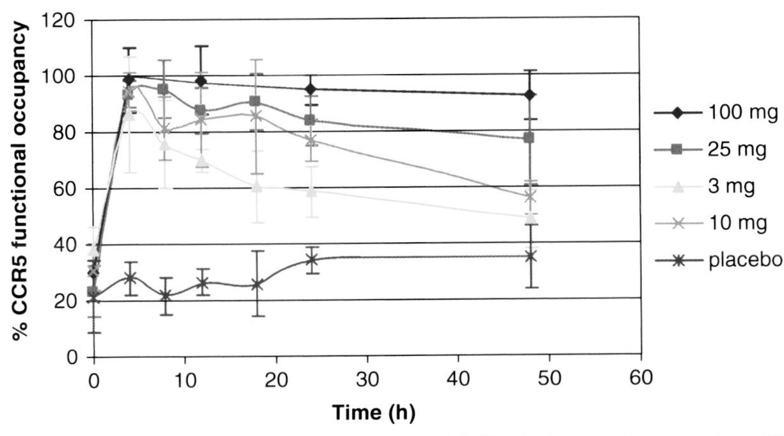

Figure 9.6 Dynamic functional occupancy of CCR5 in humans by maraviroc. CCR5 receptor occupancy was evaluated using an *ex vivo* MIP-1β internalization assay. Peripheral blood mononuclear cells were isolated from blood samples taken at time indicated following single doses to healthy volunteers. Reproduced from Ref. [29].

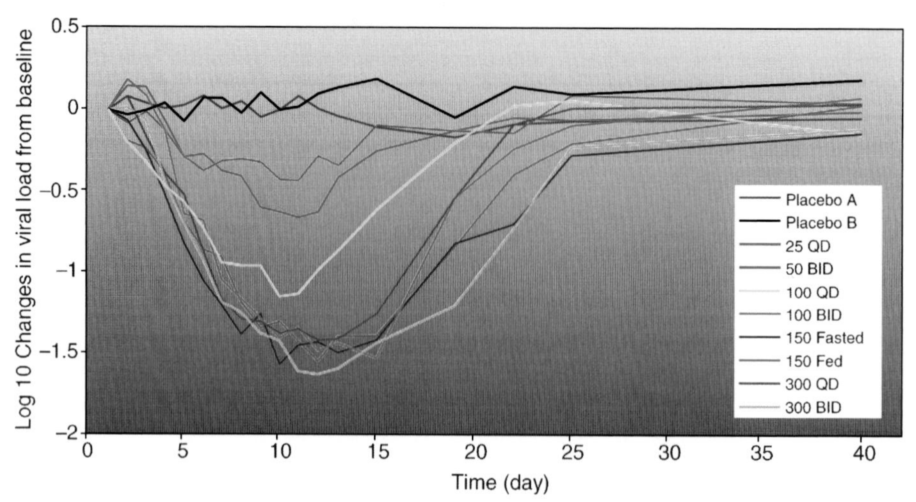

Figure 9.7 Phase 2a dose-ranging studies: dose-dependent reduction in viral load following 10 days of monotherapy. Subjects who were antiretroviral therapy naïve, or have been off therapy for at least 8 weeks, received maraviroc or placebo for 10 days at the doses indicated. HIV-RNA was monitored during dosing and for a 30 day follow-up period after the last dose. QD = once daily; BID = twice daily. Reproduced from Ref. [28].

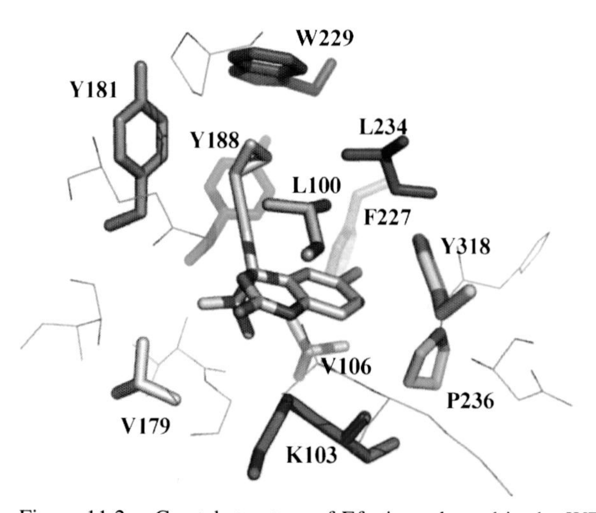

Figure 11.2. Crystal structure of Efavirenz bound in the WT-RT binding site.

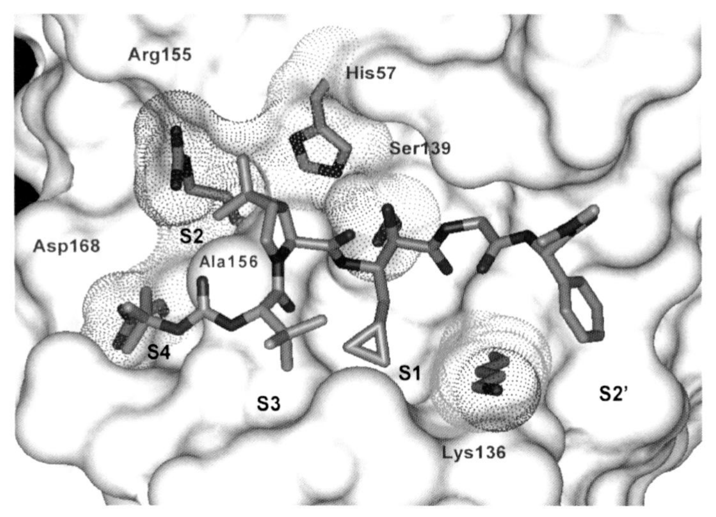

Figure 12.4 X-ray crystal structure of compound **24** (SCH-6) bound to HCV NS3 protease.

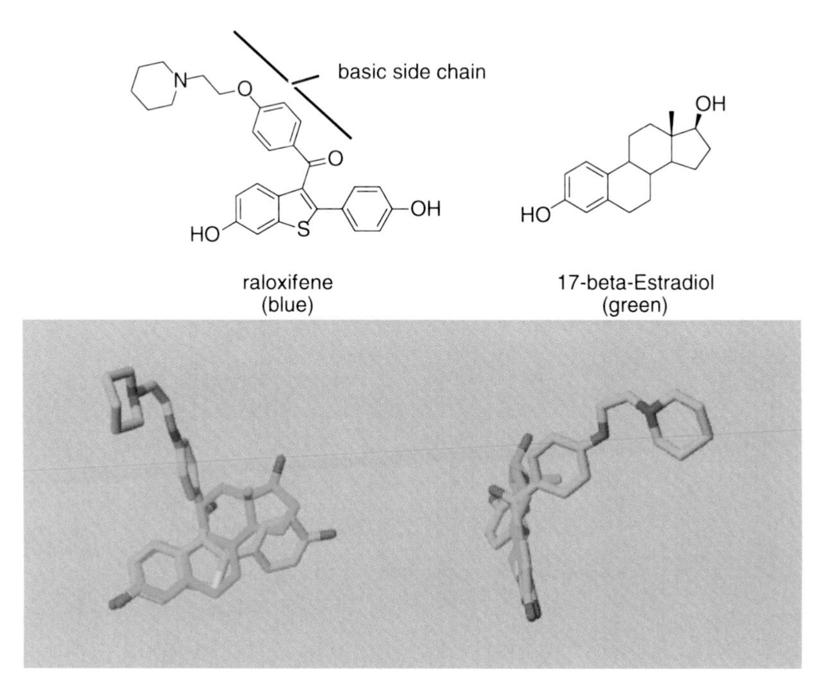

Figure 15.2 Key structural features and three-dimensional overlay of 17-beta-estradiol and raloxifene.

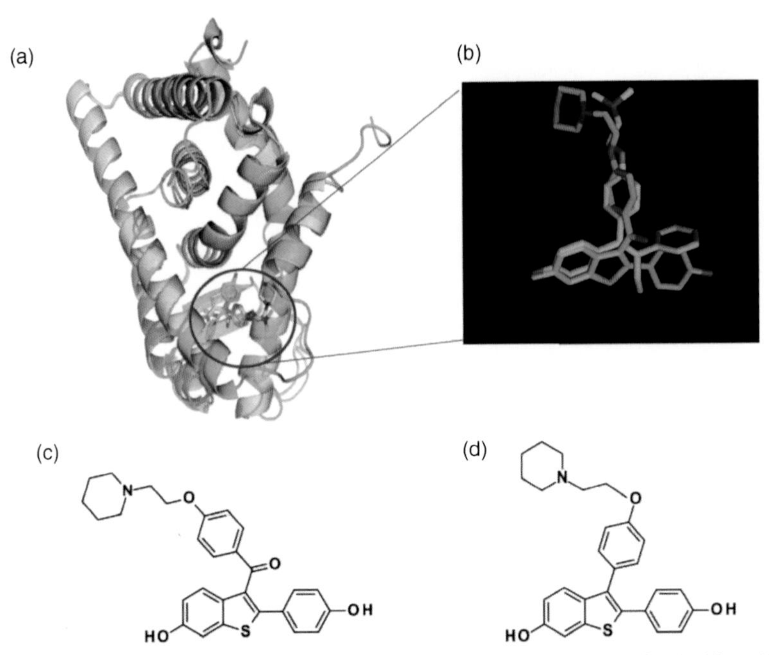

Figure 15.3 (A) Superimposed protein-ligand crystal structures of raloxifene (yellow) and 4-hydroxytamoxifen (teal) in the LBD of ERalpha. (B) Overlay of raloxifene and 4-hydroxytamoxifen in their protein bound state. (C) Structure of raloxifene. (D) Structure of raloxifene analog with the hinge region removed.

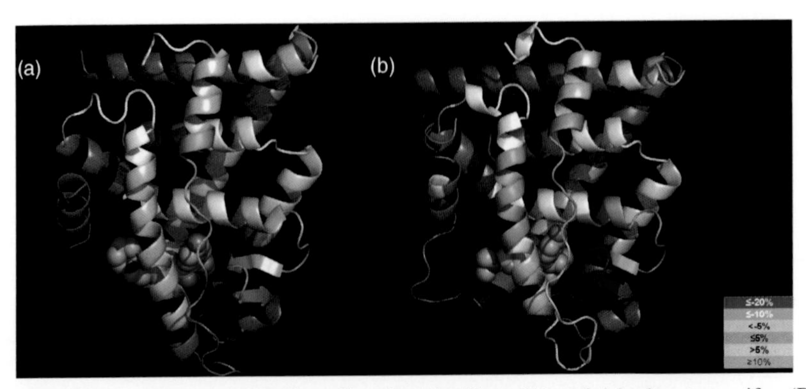

Figure 15.4 ER-ligand HDX profiles for raloxifene (A) and 4-hydoxytamoxifen (B) [13].

TABLE 8.4 Effects of Thioalkanoic Acid Chain Substitution on Receptor Potency and Liver Effects

Thioalkanoic acid chain	LTD4 binding GP IC_{50} (nM)	LWI[a]	PEI[b]
	0.1	+63%	+608%
	0.6	+9%	+188%
	0.3	+11%	+24%
	0.4	+12%	+109%
	0.4	+27%	+673%
	0.3	+10%	+91%
	2.3	+32%	+393%
	0.7	+3%	−10%
	0.3	+2%	+25%
42	0.5	0%	+16%
MK-571 (**28**)	1.5	+38%	+318%
verlukast (**29**)	3.1	0%	+65%

[a]Liver weight increase in mice dosed po 4 days at 400 mg kg^{-1} (except L-668,018 which was dosed at 200 mg kg^{-1}.

[b]Peroxysomal enzyme induction at same doses.

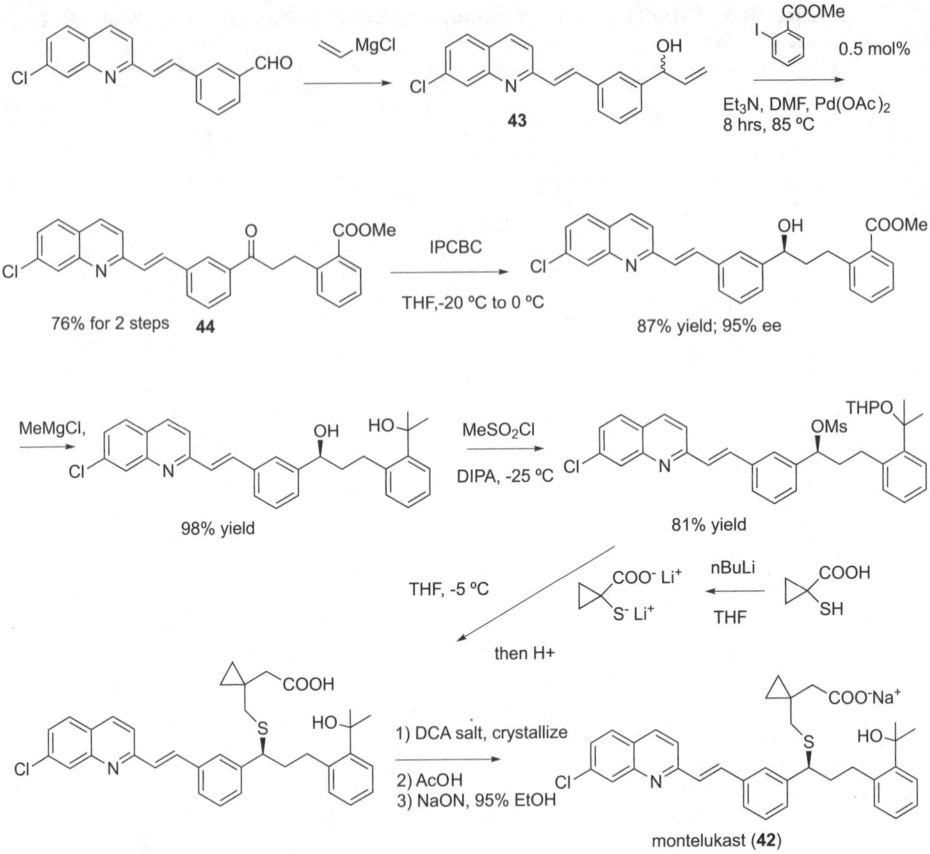

Scheme 8.4 Medicinal chemistry synthesis of montelukast (**42**).

further applied (with modifications) for the synthesis of MK-0476. The formation of the backbone of the molecule was prepared using Heck coupling [101] which was very effective and efficient. Thus, 2[2-[3-formylphenyl-ethylene]-7-chloroquinoline was reacted with vinyl Grignard reagent and the resulting allylic alcohol was reacted in a palladium-catalyzed coupling with an 2-iodo-methyl benzoate to give the ketone which was then reduced enantioselectively using the Corey chiral oxazaborilidine catalyst [102,103]. The required thiol was prepared in 9 steps from 1,1-dicarbomethoxy-cyclopropane and then reacted with the mesylate to install the chain with the required stereochemistry. Hydrolysis then yielded the MK-0476.

8.5.2 Process Chemistry Synthesis [104,105] (Schemes 8.5 and 8.6)

The process chemistry group at MRL in Rahway, New Jersey, under the direction of Dr. Paul Reider at that time, was built on the medicinal chemistry synthesis to devise an elegant and scalable synthesis of montelukast. Considering the complexity of the structure, the synthesis was a true *tour de force* and allowed preparation of large quantities and eventually manufacturing on ton scales. The development synthesis was highly convergent and similar to the medicinal chemistry but with no chromatography required and all purifications done by crystallization. A very efficient four-step synthesis of the required 3,3-cyclopropyl-4-thiolbutanoic acid side chain was developed. Using the same 1,1-cyclopropanedimethanol as the starting material, the problem of selectively and efficiently introducing the required thiol and carboxyl groups was elegantly solved by conversion first to the cyclic sulfite in 90% yield by reaction with thionyl chloride. The product was then directly reacted with sodium cyanide in DMF-toluene at 70°C to give the (hydroxymethyl)cyclopropaneacetonitrile in 87.5% yield. This alcohol was then directly converted to the mesylate by reaction with methanesulfonyl chloride and triethylamine in toluene-DMF. *In situ* displacement of the mesylate was effected by addition of thiolacetic acid and triethylamine to directly give the crude thioacetate in 93% yield. This material was then azeotropically dried with toluene and then hydrolyzed with sodium hydroxide (5 N). After acidification and toluene extraction, the 4-mercapto-3,3-cyclopropyl-butanoic acid was obtained in 82% yield. The product could be further purified by recrystallization from toluene-hexane. Thus, the required thiol was obtained in four steps in an overall yield of about 60%! (Scheme 8.5).

Like the earlier small scale synthesis, the process chemistry synthesis started with reaction of 2(2-[3-formylphenyl]ethenyl]-7-chloroquinoline (used in the synthesis of MK-571 and MK-0679) with vinyl magnesium bromide in THF-toluene at 0°C to give the racemic allylic alcohol **43** in 92% yield which was reacted directly and without isolation with 2-iodomethylbenzoate with 0.5% palladium acetate as a catalyst in acetonitrile with triethylamine over 8 h to give the ketone **44** in 76% yield for the two steps. The product was purified by crystallization. The ketone was then reduced stereospecifically to the *R*-alcohol **45** using bis-(+)-α-pinenylboranylchloride prepared *in situ* from ca 70% ee α-pinene and chloroborane. In spite of the low optical purity α-pinene (which is very cheap to buy), the yield was 87% with 95% ee which could be enhanced to 99.5% ee by recrystallization! This apparently incongruous result is explicable as the pinene–borane complex which does the reduction involves *two pinene molecules* and therefore one expects that 70% optical purity α-pinene would form a mixture of complexes in a theoretical ratio of (+ , +):(+ ,−):(−,−) of 74:24:2. The (+ ,−) complex reacts very sluggishly and thus the product ratio is determined by the (+ , +): (−,−) ratio which is 97:3. This predicts a 94% ee and 95% was observed. The chiral

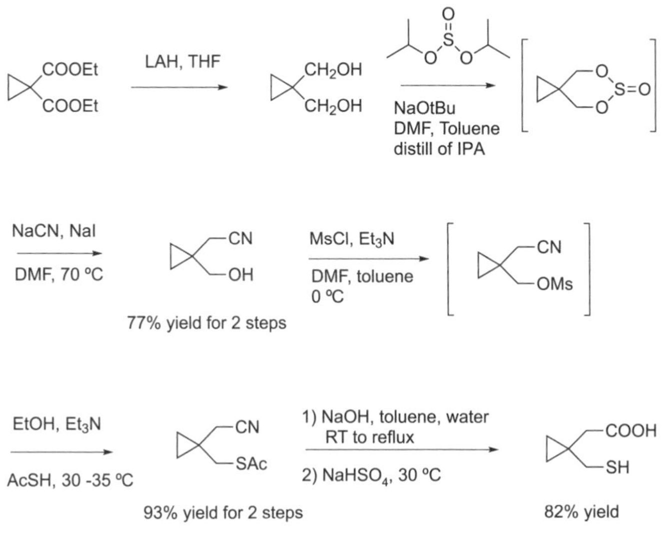

COOEt
COOEt
LAH, THF
CH_2OH
CH_2OH
NaOtBu
DMF, Toluene
distill of IPA
S=O

NaCN, NaI
DMF, 70 °C
CN
OH
77% yield for 2 steps
MsCl, Et_3N
DMF, toluene
0 °C
CN
OMs

EtOH, Et_3N
AcSH, 30 -35 °C
CN
SAc
93% yield for 2 steps
1) NaOH, toluene, water
RT to reflux
2) $NaHSO_4$, 30 °C
COOH
SH
82% yield

Scheme 8.5 Process synthesis of the carboxymethylcyclopropylmethyl thiol.

alcohol was reacted with methyl magnesium bromide and cerium trichloride at 0°C to give the tertiary alcohol **46** in excellent yield (89%). The process group found a method to selectively convert the secondary alcohol to the mesylate **47** by careful reaction with methanesulfonyl chloride and diisoproplylethylamine in acetonitrile at −25°C to give the desired mesylate, after direct crystallization, in 81% yield (Scheme 8.6). Thus, the multistep alcohol protection and deprotection used in the initial medicinal chemistry synthesis was avoided (and of course no chromatographic purification was needed).

The two parts were then merged by first conversion of the thiol acid to the dilithium salt by reaction in THF with two equivalents of *n*-butyllithium. The mesylate in THF was then added at −5°C. The product salt was acidified with tartaric acid and the crude product free acid isolated by extraction into ethyl acetate. Purification was effected by conversion to the dicyclohexylamine (DCA) salt which crystallized readily and gave pure product salt in 79% yield and > 99.8% ee optical purity. The pure DCA salt was then broken with acetic acid and converted in toluene to its sodium salt with sodium hydroxide 1% aqueous ethanol. After filtering and concentration, the pure crystalline montelukast sodium salt was obtained in 98% yield by adding acetonitrile and filtration. This amazing synthesis provided many kilograms of compound for safety assessment studies, formulation development, and clinical studies. Scale up to the pilot plant and eventually to the manufacturing plant followed essentially the same synthetic process.

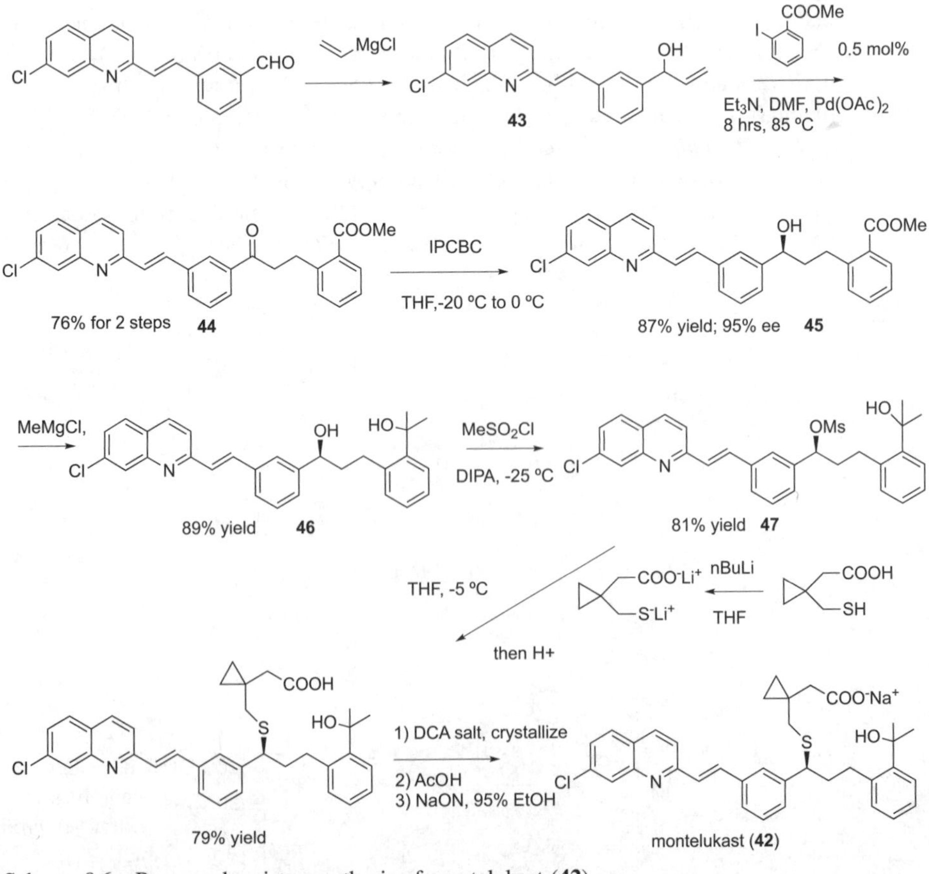

Scheme 8.6 Process chemistry synthesis of montelukast (**42**).

8.6 ADME STUDIES WITH MK-0476 (MONTELUKAST)

MK-0476 exhibited superior pharmacokinetics and excellent bioavailability and half-lives in all species tested [99,100]. *In vitro* metabolism studies were done using mice, rats, monkeys, and human (adult and pediatric) liver microsomes. A number of oxidized metabolites were observed in microsomal incubations with montelukast. The metabolites were identified as putative diastereomeric sulfoxides (**48**), benyzylic alcohols (C-21 hydroxyl) (**49**), and diols formed by oxidation of one of the geminal methyl groups (C-35-hydroxyl) (**50**) [106]. In addition, an acyl-glucoronide (**51**) was observed when glucoronyl transferase was added. A hydroxylated phenyl metabolite (**52**) was also characterized by mass spectroscopy and NMR (Figure 8.8). To confirm structures, authentic samples were synthesized [107]. Animal studies (mice, rats) generally showed the same spectrum of metabolites but also showed the dicarboxylic acid metabolite (53) derived from further oxidation of the diol. These studies indicated that montelukast was extensively metabolized (about > 95%) and that the major route of elimination was via the bile. Subsequently, human clinical ADME studies were devised using [^{14}C]-montelukast and with sampling of bile effluent through aspiration with a gastropic probe [108]. Thus, most of the same metabolites were observed in human subjects and confirmed by comparison with the authentic samples. In the human ADME trials after dosing radioactive montelukast, most of the radioactivity in the plasma was unchanged montelukast and only small amounts

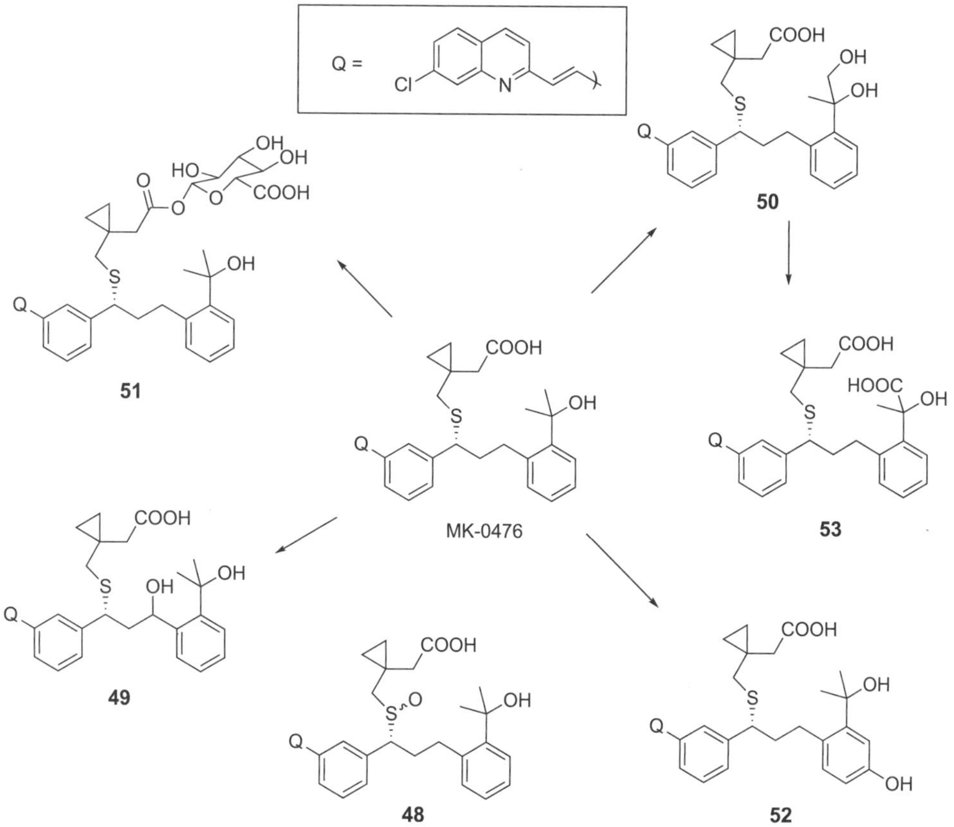

Figure 8.8 Identified metabolites of montelukast (**MK-0476**).

of two pairs of diastereomeric metabolites, the benzylic (or C-21) hydroxyl compounds (**49**), and the hydroxymethyl (or C-36) compounds (**50**) were identified as circulating in human plasma. The major biliary metabolite was shown to be the dicarboxylic acid. *In vitro* studies with human microsomes showed very similar activity in human and pediatric microsomes and identified P450 isozymes 3A4, 2C9, and 2A6 as important in the formation of the major metabolites [109].

8.7 SAFETY ASSESSMENT OF MONTELUKAST

Montelukast was evaluated extensively in safety studies in animals to support and allow subsequent clinical studies to proceed. Longer term safety studies in animals and ultimately in humans supported NDA filing and FDA approval. These studies were supported by extensive toxicokinetics studies to ensure high exposure of drug and metabolites in the safety species. Many of these studies are only available through FDA reports [110] and on the label [111]. Montelukast was initially evaluated in rats and mice for acute toxicity and was found to be tolerated at doses up to 5 g kg^{-1}, and the LD50 in mice was estimated to be between 2 and 5 mg kg^{-1} and > 5 mg kg^{-1} in rats! In more chronic testing, it was evaluated in rats, mice, and monkeys where exposures after oral (p.o.) dosing were high and dose proportional in rat (with AUC up to 4795 μg min ml^{-1} and C_{max} of 15.7 μg ml^{-1} at 200 mg kg^{-1}), in mice (AUC 9004 μg min ml^{-1} and C_{max} 34.2 μg ml^{-1}), and monkey (AUC 35456 μg min ml^{-1} and C_{max} 60.4 μg ml^{-1}). Intravenous doses were also examined up to 10 mg kg^{-1} in these three species. In medium and long-term chronic toxicity testing in rats and mice (up to 1 year), the no observable adverse effect level (NOAEL) was 50 mg kg^{-1}. In adult monkeys, the NOAEL for 1 year studies was 150 mg kg^{-1}. Safety testing of montelukast was also geared to allow rapid approval for use by pediatric patients (viewed as an important medical need by the development team) and therefore safety testing was also done in infant monkeys (4 weeks of age). They showed a toxicity profile (after 3 months dosing) similar to that observed for adult monkeys although they were somewhat more sensitive and the NOAEL level in that study was 50 mg kg^{-1}. Thus, the FDA conclusions were that "...NOAELs observed in all repeat dose toxicity studies demonstrated wide margins of safety relative to proposed therapeutic doses for all observed toxicity." Teratogenicity studies in rats (up to 400 mg kg^{-1} day^{-1}) and rabbits (up to 300 mg kg^{-1} day^{-1}) showed "no evidence of embryo-fetal toxicity or teratogenicity." Montelukast was tested in lifetime studies in mice (at 100 mg kg^{-1} day^{-1}) and rats (at 200 mg kg^{-1} day^{-1}) for tumorigenic potential and "was regarded as negative for tumorigenic activity in both the mouse and the rat." Montelukast has a core structure with extended π-orbital conjugation and thus a strong UV absorption. It was therefore tested for phototoxic potential in mice dosed at 500 mg kg^{-1} and found to be negative.

8.8 CLINICAL DEVELOPMENT OF MONTELUKAST

8.8.1 Human Pharmacokinetics, Safety, and Tolerability

Montelukast entered phase 1 clinical trials in 1992 where it was gratifyingly found to be well absorbed and well tolerated. Initially dosed to male volunteers in single and rising doses as capsules from 20 to 800 mg and as a solution at 200 mg, montelukast was shown to be well tolerated with only side mild and transient effects and no laboratory abnormalities noted [111]. The solution and capsule (200 mg each) achieved similar plasma concentrations and T_{max} (2–4 h). Absorption was quite dose proportional and food was found to mildly enhance and delay absorption. The apparent half-life of 4–5 h and excellent exposures achieved supported further development and the possibility of once a day dosing. Subsequently, absolute bioavailability was determined in adult males and females comparing drug levels after intravenous administration with those from oral administration of a 10 mg tablet. Very similar pharmacokinetics were found for each gender with elimination half-lives of 5.1 and 4.9 h and bioavailability of 66% and 58%, respectively [112]. Again side effects were generally mild and no laboratory adverse experiences were noted. Evaluation of pharmacokinetics in young and elderly adults showed no apparent age-related differences which could justify modifying dosages with age and little accumulation (<15%) of montelukast over a 7 day dosing period at 10 mg day^{-1} [113]. In keeping with the desire to expedite development for the pediatric asthmatic population, pharmacokinetics and tolerability studies were also done in children, initially from ages 6 to 14. Children were also found to absorb and tolerate montelukast very well. Doses of 5 mg day^{-1} in children 6–14 were found to yield comparable pharmacokinetic profiles as did 10 mg day^{-1} in adults [114]. Considering the experiences with MK-0679 and the observed liver enzyme elevations observed with MK-0679 only after longer term dosing, the team anxiously awaited results from longer term multiple dosing studies with montelukast. Happily, longer term exposures even at high doses of 900 mg day^{-1} for 7 days [114] and up to 200 mg day^{-1} for 22 weeks dosing produced no significant adverse effects. Analysis of data from long-term exposures in both pediatric (6–14) and adult patients did not reveal any dose-related adverse clinical or laboratory effects [115]. It is notable that several cases of over-dosage were reported including a case where a 3-year-old child took 80 mg and a 5 year old child took 135 mg unintentionally. The first was managed at home with observation alone and the latter was managed in an emergency department. In neither case were there any symptoms! [116].

8.8.2 Human Pharmacology

Based on receptor potency and pharmacokinetics, it was anticipated that montelukast could be a low dose once a day drug and a number of early clinical studies were undertaken first to show efficacy against a LTD_4 challenge in mildly asthmatic individuals [117]. In this study, aerosolized LTD_4-induced bronchoconstriction responses were recorded 4 h after single oral doses of 5 to 250 mg montelkast (trial A) and also 20 h after 40 or 200 mg montelukast (trial B). The drug treatments were compared to placebo and the intention was to determine the shift in the amount of LTD_4 needed to produce a >50% drop in specific airway conductance (sGAW). In the first trial *none of the drug-treated patients showed a 50% drop in sGAW* (even those treated with 5 mg) and the estimated minimum shift in the LTD_4 dose–response curves for 5 mg dose was between >85 and >240-fold! At this dose, the blood levels of drug were averaged as 0.12 μg ml^{-1}. In trial B, at the 40 mg dose only two patients out of six showed a >50% drop in sGAW and in these patients 18- and 45-fold shifts in LTD_4 dose response were observed. For these two, the blood levels of drug after challenge were <0.029 and 0.30 μg ml^{-1}. For the other four patients, shifts were >45- to > 131-fold and trough blood levels were higher. Clearly montelukast was effective as an LTD_4 antagonist in humans and once a day dosing was feasible. In another later study, montelukast was tested for potency and efficacy against an antigen-induced bronchoconstriction in asthmatic patients. In this study, montelukast was given at 10 mg, 36 and 12 h before challenge and was shown to block 75% of the early asthmatic response to an antigen challenge and 54% of the late asthmatic response [118]. In other studies, montelukast was shown to block exercise-induced bronchoconstriction after single oral doses of 100 mg (50% block of drop in FEV1) [119].

Thus, the pharmacological efficacy was determined and it remained to define a minimum maximally clinically effective dose in native asthma in phase 2b studies to develop a regime for the critical phase 3 studies to follow.

8.8.3 Phase 2 Studies in Asthma

A number of phase 2 studies were carried out and are too numerous to detail here. Results are detailed in the montelukast label [120] and in the FDA-drug approval package [110]. Initially, however, it was decided to define the minimum effective dose in adult asthmatic patients dosed once a day over a 6 week period. After much debate, oral doses of 10, 100, or 200 mg once daily and 10 and 50 mg doses twice daily were selected. These carefully controlled double-blinded trials involved a 3 week placebo run-in period to deal with any placebo effect before blinded dosing started. At the end of 6 weeks of treatment, there was a 1 week washout period [121]. Remarkably (and to some considerable consternation), the treatment effects at all doses were the same and no dose or dosing interval effects were seen! All doses caused a significant improvement in chronic asthma symptoms with maximum efficacy seen within 1 h after the first administered dose and with an average 10.3% increase in FEV1 sustained over the 6 week period. Other parameters such as daytime symptom score, β-agonist usage, and morning peak expiratory flow rates (PEFR) were all significantly improved. Notably, it was also found that the montelukast-induced bronchodilation was additive to that induced by aerosolized β-agonist. After the washout period, the effects reverted to that of the placebo treatment. All doses were generally well tolerated without important clinical or laboratory adverse experiences. However, before setting doses for phase 3 studies, it was necessary to define the minimum maximally effective dose, and as all were essentially identical, it was necessary to initiate further phase 2b dose ranging studies to show an inactive or lesser active dose before initiating phase 3 studies. Two simultaneous studies were done to study the efficacy of once-daily bedtime dosing of montelukast with a lower dose range, one in chronic asthma [122] and the other in exercise-induced asthma (EIA) [123]. In the chronic asthma study, doses of 2, 10, and 50 mg per day were studied. All doses showed benefit but the 2 mg dose while trending to significance was not significantly different from placebo, whereas the 10 and 50 mg dose were similar and significant ($p = < 0.050$). In the second EIA [123] study, patients were administered doses of 0.4, 2, 10, and 50 mg montelukast or placebo for 2 days and exercise challenge was commenced after a further 20 to 24 h and then again after a further 32 to 36 h after the last dose. The 10 and 50 mg doses significantly blocked the AUC of the fall in FEV1, while the lower doses showed nonsignificant block. Little effect was evident after 32–36 h for any of the doses. Thus, the 10 mg per day dose at bedtime was selected for phase 3 studies. Dose selection for larger pediatric trials was based on extensive evaluation of adult and pediatric pharmacokinetic measurements that had shown a good correlation of AUC and body weight. Specific age ranging studies were carried out to confirm the performance of the selected dosage forms in children where a 5 mg chewable tablet was selected and bioequivalence with the adult 10 mg dose was demonstrated. These studies are well reviewed and the reader is referred to Knorr et al. [124].

8.8.4 Phase 3 Studies in Asthma

Many phase 3 studies were carried out to support the registration of montelukast with the FDA and with worldwide regulatory authorities. It is not appropriate to try to summarize all these studies here, but they are well documented and reviewed in the montelukast FDA-approved label [120], in the registration package [110] and elsewhere [125]. A few key

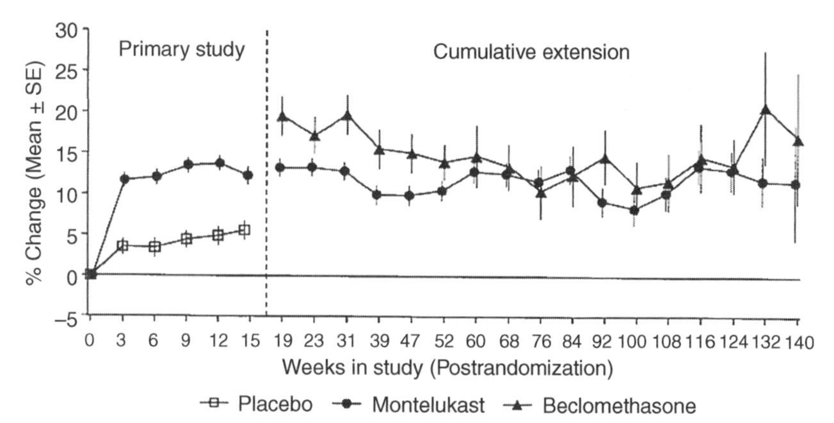

Figure 8.9 Mean percent change from pre-randomized baseline in FEV1 over time (Reprinted from Ref. [129] with permission).

studies will be discussed. Two pivotal trial in adults (>/= 15 years) compared montelukast to placebo over 12 weeks of treatment [126,127] and showed significant improvements in all monitored parameters including FEV1 and morning and evening PEFR. Significant improvements in daytime asthma symptoms, reductions in β-agonist usage, nocturnal awakenings, and asthma exacerbations were noted as well. The treatment effects were seen after the first dose and no tolerance developed over the trials. As with the phase 2 trials, when treatment was ceased, symptoms returned to the placebo level. In other studies, montelukast was compared with aerosolized corticosteroids and was found to have a more rapid onset of action but not to achieve the same levels of efficacy [e.g., 127]. Similar to findings in adults, in pediatric patients aged 6–14 years, once a day 5 mg doses were found to be significantly effective relative to placebo over an 8 week trial [128]. It is notable, however, that when patients from these controlled trials were followed in open-label extensions for up to up to 140 weeks, the apparent advantage of beclomethasone decreased and overall there was a high degree of concordance for the ability of both montelukast and beclomethasone to provide asthma control over the long term (Figure 8.9) [129]. This may reflect a better level of compliance for patients taking a once a day oral drug compared to an aerosol. Eventually, the NDA for montelukast was filed with the FDA and with the European regulatory authorities in 1997. The drug was approved for treatment of asthma first in Mexico in the summer of 1997 and then in Finland (which served as the rapporteur state for the European Union) in August 1997. The first launch of the new drug was in Finland and the very first prescription written in Espoo, Finland October 1, 1997. A copy of that first prescription is presented in Figure 8.10. Approval in the rest of the EU countries followed in December 1997 and US approval was given February 23, 1998. Montelukast, now known by the trade name Singulair®, was one of the few drugs to be approved both for adults and for children (aged 6–14) from the outset. It is now approved in over 70 countries around the world. Development did not cease with approval however and trials continued to better define the utility of montelukast and to demonstrate safety and efficacy in younger children. A 12 week placebo controlled trial in children from ages 2 to 5 years subsequently demonstrated significantly improved multiple asthma efficacy endpoints, and improved parameters of asthma control [130]. Montelukast use is now supported for treatment of children as young as 6-month old. One important study in 6- to 8-year-old children followed growth rates for those treated with montelukast (5 mg once daily), placebo, and inhaled beclomethasone (200 μg twice daily). The patients were tracked over 56 weeks and while linear growth rates

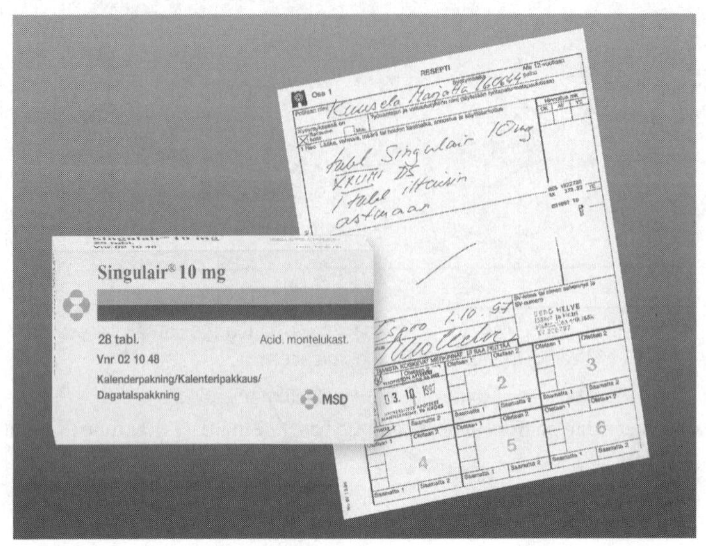

Figure 8.10 The world's first prescription and package of Singulair® issued and purchased in Espoo, Finland, October 1, 1997.

were similar for montelukast and placebo, they were significantly lower for those taking beclomethasone [131] (Figure 8.11).

Other studies have looked at the co-administration of montelukast and aerosolized steroids and shown that montelukast can offer added benefit in combination with steroids and can also allow the dose of steroids to be tapered down [132–134]. However, abrupt replacement of steroid with montelukast is not recommended and in the first period after introduction to the market and experience in several million patients was evaluated, a number of montelukast-treated patients developed a rare inflammatory condition known as Chugg-Strauss Syndrome [135,136]. On evaluation, it was proposed that the abrupt cessation of steroid treatment was likely responsible and that this syndrome was underlying in these patients and controlled until the steroid treatment was withdrawn [137].

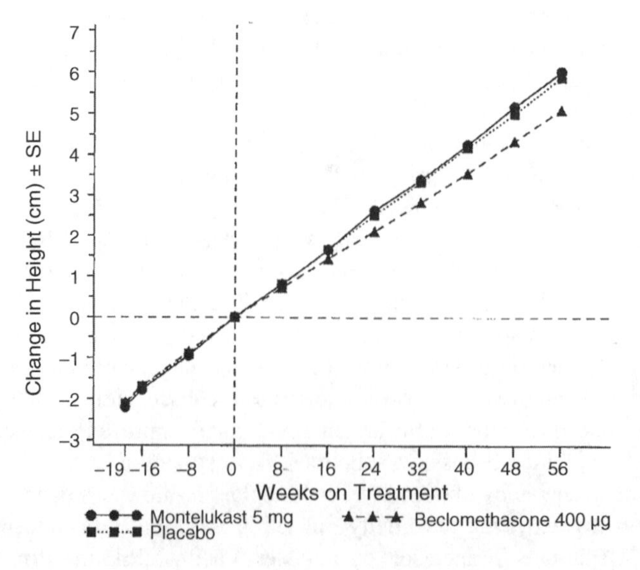

Figure 8.11 Mean +/− change in height from the randomization visit (week 0 to week 56. Error bars are contained in the symbols (Reprinted from Ref. [131] with permission).

8.8.5 Effects of Montelukast on Inflammation

Studies have shown that montelukast treatment in adults and children leads to a steady decline in the prominent asthma-related inflammatory eosinophils in peripheral blood [126,127] and in airways [138]. Montelukast also caused a decrease in exhaled nitric oxide in asthmatic children [139]. These studies and other animal studies support an anti-inflammatory effect for montelukast.

8.8.6 Montelukast and Allergic Rhinitis

Allergic rhinitis (AR) (or hay fever) is a condition of the airways, more localized to the nasal area and mucous membranes, which has many similarities with asthma and often co-occurs with asthma. It affects 20–40 million people in the USA including many children and can be very debilitating. AR may be seasonal (often related to the prevalence of specific plant pollens in the air) or perennial where it is likely related to the presence of molds or animal or insect allergens which persist in the environment. Like asthma, it can manifest an early or immediate response and a late phase or delayed response. Many of the same inflammatory cells found in the asthmatic lung (basophils, eosinophils, mast cells, neutrophils) are found in the nasal passages of AR patients and a similar battery of cytokines and mediators, including histamine, prostaglandins, and cysteinyl leukotrienes, are released and contribute to the symptoms. Nasal steroids are used to treat AR and also, unlike asthma, antihistamines can provide relief. The presence of leukotrienes suggested a possible role for montelukast in the treatment of AR, and subsequent to the approval of montelukast for asthma, a whole series of trials were undertaken to study montelukast alone and in combination with antihistamines and inhaled corticosteroids for treatment of AR. Several recent articles review these many trials [140,141]. Montelukast showed an excellent safety profile in these studies and the side effect profiles were generally indistinguishable from placebo (where such comparisons were available). In summary, montelukast alone was found to control symptoms similarly and sometimes superior (night time symptoms) when compared to antihistamines such as loratidine but was generally less effectively than nasal steroids such as fluticasone. When montelukast was dosed in combination with antihistamines, effects were additive and in some trials comparable to nasal steroids. These studies allowed Merck to obtain approval from the FDA for the use of Singulair® for treatment of allergic rhinitis and it is now approved for treatment of patients 2 years of age and older for treatment of seasonal AR for patients 6 months and older for treatment of perennial AR. In addition, a special 4 mg sprinkles formulation was developed for treatment of very young children (for asthma or AR) that can be added to baby formula or soft food.

8.9 SUMMARY

8.9.1 Impact on Society

Singulair® has proved to be a very successful addition to the available therapies for treatment of asthma and allergic rhinitis and has touched and improved the lives of millions of people since it became available in the world market. Its use and sales have grown steadily over the last 12 years and it is one of the best selling drugs on the market. The acceptance and utility has been enhanced by its excellent safety and tolerability profile and its availability to treat children as young as 6 months of age. Merck was awarded the Prix Galien Canada Innovative Product 2000 and also the Prix Galien Research. Singulair® was also recognized with the Prix Galien MEDEC in France for the best drug of 2000 and the Prix Galien

Portugal for the best drug launched in 1999. In addition, the impact that this discovery has had on the lives and health of children was recognized in 2003 by the Heroes of Chemistry Award of the American Chemical Society given to three of the chemists involved in the discovery; Marc Labelle, Robert Young and Robert Zamboni.

8.9.2 Lessons Learned

The program which resulted in the bringing of Singulair® to market spanned 20 years and many of the participants literally grew up with the project and in doing so learned many valuable lessons along the way. We all came to realize the enormous complexity and intensity of effort that must be applied to reach what is a most elusive goal. All my colleagues in Discovery were driven to succeed not just with a drug candidate to be handed off to others but a candidate with the properties that would see it through and make it into the Pharmacopia where it would alleviate suffering and hopefully change lives. A great level of persistence was needed to identify flaws in compounds along the way, define the issues, and regroup to find a better compound to address the problem. Most importantly, we were fortunate to have an enlightened and science evidence-driven research management led by Dr. Ed Scolnick that recognized the potential of such a drug and impressed upon those of us in Discovery just how good and safe it had to be to succeed. When the early compounds in the project (L-648,051 and L-949,923) failed to provide clinically relevant efficacy, we realized that the compounds were not sufficiently potent in humans to adequately test the mechanism and management agreed to continue the effort. It is important to realize that in that era, the initial enthusiasm for leukotriene blockers in asthma waned dramatically when the rather disappointing clinical results for these early compounds and for the Eli Lilly antagonist, LY-171883 became known. Many began to feel that asthma was too complex and a multi-mediator disease such that blockade of any one mediator would not offer real benefit. In the same time period, antagonists of platelet-activating factor (PAF) were also being developed and they too showed no efficacy in asthma [for a timely review see 142].

Another difficulty that the whole field faced was the observation of liver-based side effects that so frequently were found with LTD4 antagonists in animals or people. Many researchers felt there must be some mechanism-based reason for these toxicities and effects. The Singulair® story taught us that when faced with such imponderables, one must first characterize and determine if the effects are indeed mechanism-based (e.g., by determining if the toxicity tracks with potency) and if not then try to understand the biochemical or physiological bases for the effects and set up toxicity assays to develop an independent parallel SAR. In this way, one can effectively determine the structural parameters associated with the undesired properties and those parameters that mitigate or eliminate the effects. One can then feed this information into the compound optimization.

Another lesson of the project was the value of animal and human clinical pharmacology studies where drug is given by i.v. infusion so as to provide a steady state level of drug in the blood stream which can then be associated with a quantifiable physiological response. In the case of montlukast and its progenitors, we were blessed with excellent solubility and tolerability to allow such experiments to be carried out. These studies determined effective blood levels to help determine clinical target levels at trough (24 h after dosing) to support once-a-day dosing.

Perhaps the most important lesson to draw from the story of Singulair® is the importance of safety, tolerability, and ease of dosing in the success of a drug for treatment of a chronic disease. This is doubly important for treatment of children. Montelukast was not the first leukotriene antagonist to reach the market. Pranlukast (Onon, Azlaire™, Smith Kline Beecham and Ono) was first approved in Japan in 1995 and zifirlukast (Accolate™,

AstraZeneca) was approved in the USA in October 1996. Despite being second or third to the market Singulair® rapidly grew in sales and use to dominate the sector.

8.10 PERSONAL IMPACT

Millions of people have taken Singulair® to treat their asthma and allergic rhinitis since it became available. From the many stories of how it changed lives, the following is perhaps the most dramatic.

Denis Brown is a physician living in Summerland, British Columbia, Canada, who has had personal experience with the benefits of Singulair®. Denis suffers from cold air-induced asthma that for him has been particularly problematic as he is an avid mountain climber and hiker. Thanks in part to Singulair® he was able to realize a life-long dream, to reach the south summit of Mount Everest! He was originally from South Africa and a life-long hiker and climber. In South Africa, his asthma was not a big problem but after immigrating to Canada and attempting more and more demanding climbs, he found his success was impaired by his asthma and attendant bronchoconstriction brought on by exposure to cold air. He still tried to climb whenever he could, helped by liberal amounts of bronchodilators such as Ventolin®. He made his first attempt to climb Everest in 1991 and his second in 1994 (the north side). During these first two attempts, he acted as physician to Canadian climbing groups. In both cases, he was concerned about the dangers to his health and he decided he would have to climb without oxygen to avoid the possibility that if he were to have an asthma attack during the climb, and if he were to run short on oxygen, he could be in real trouble. In the event, his asthma hindered his abilities and he was forced to halt both climbs before reaching the summit.

In 1998, Singulair® became available on the market and Denis thought he might try to see if it could control his asthma sufficiently to allow him to finally summit the mountain. He presented his idea to Merck and they were very interested and agreed to help sponsor his climb. The next winter he skied and snow shoed as much as possible to get as much cold air training and found his asthma was indeed well controlled with Singulair®. In March 1999, he joined a British climbing group, again as their physician. In fact, it turned out he was acting as physician to the whole base camp of more than 300 climbers from countries all over the world. It was exhausting work and he was always fearful he might catch some bug from a sick climber and his expedition would be over again. They planned the attempt for April and May of 1999 and luckily Denis was able to stay fit. Once again, he decided it would be most prudent to climb without oxygen (the others in the group decided to use oxygen). They decided to take the south route and on the first attempt, starting May 2 at camp 4, in sight of the summit, the team leader developed hemiparesis and cardiovascular problems. Although the team was only hours away from the summit, Denis convinced them they needed to get the sick climber down immediately and so they turned back and carried him down to base camp. He was flown off to hospital in Katmandu by helicopter and happily survived without further problems. In May 13, 1999, they began their second attempt from camp 4 setting off in the very early morning (again Denis was without oxygen) and at 1 pm he reached the south summit (see the photo below, Figure 8.12). Soon after, the weather closed in and they were caught in a snowstorm. It took 7 h to return to the camp. During the decent, one climber simply vanished and was never seen again. Needless to say this was a life changing experience and one Denis will always remember.

Denis still uses Singulair® frequently, especially in winter and he continues to ski, snow shoe and hike although he is now over 50 years of age. He stated in interview, "I have noted that asthmatic patients tend to back off from exercise and I council them to try to do as

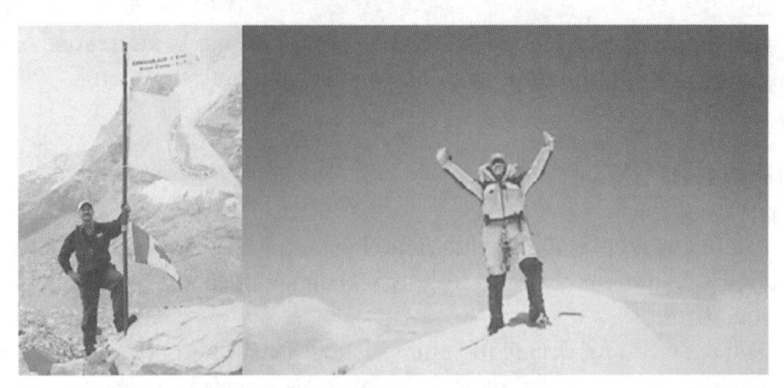

Figure 8.12 Denis Brown at Base Camp and at south summit of Everest in 1999.

much as they can and to push themselves so as to improve their lung function. Asthmatics do not need to be sedentary and if necessary, with drugs like Singulair®, can achieve much more than they think they can" (From a telephone interview with Dr. Denis Brown, Summerland, BC, March 15, 2011).

REFERENCES

1. ROKACH, J. *Leukotrienes and Lipoxygensases, Chemical, Biological and Clinical Aspects* (ed J. Rokach), Elsevier, Amsterdam, 1989.
2. (a) FELDBERG, W., and KELLAWAY, C. H. Liberation of histamine and formation of lyscithin-like substances by cobra venom. *J. Physiol.* **1938**, *94*, 187–226. (b) FELDBERG, W., HOLDEN, H. F., and KELLAWAY, C. H. The formation of lyscithin and of a muscle-stimulating substance by snake venoms. *J. Physiol.* **1938**, *94*, 232–248.
3. BROCKLEHURST, W. E., The release of histamine and formation of a slow reacting substance (SRS-A) during anaphylactic shock. *J. Physiol.* **1960**, *151*, 416–435.
4. MORRIS, H. R., TAYLOR, G. W., PIPER, P. J., SIROIS, P., and TIPPINS, J. R. Slow-reacting substance of anaphylaxis: purification and characterization. *FEBS Lett.* **1978**, *87*, 203–206.
5. BORGEAT, P. and SAMUELSSON, B. Metabolism of arachidonic acid in polymorphonuclear leukocytes. Structural analysis of novel hydroxylated compounds. *J. Biol. Chem.* **1979**, *254*, 7865–7869.
6. MURPHY, R. C., HAMMARSTRÖM, S., and SAMUELSSON, B. LEUKOTRIENE C: a slow-reacting substance from murine mastocytoma cells. *Proc. Natl. Acad. Sci. USA* **1979**, *76*, 4275.
7. COREY, E. J., CLARK, D. A., GOTO, G., MARFAT, A., MIOSKOWSKI, C., SAMUELSSON, B., and HAMMARSTRÖM, S. Stereospecific total synthesis of a "slow reacting substance" of anaphylaxis, leukotriene C-1. *J. Am. Chem. Soc.* **1980**, *102*, 1436–1439.
8. ROKACH J. GIRARD Y, GUINDON Y, ATKINSON J. G. LAUE, M., YOUNG, R. N., MASSON, P., and HOLME, G. The synthesis of a leukotriene with SRS-like activity. *Tetrahedron Lett.* **1980**, *21*, 1485–1488.
9. SAMUELSSON, B., and HAMMARSTRÖM, S. Nomenclature for leukotrienes. *Prostaglandins* **1980**, *19*, 645–646.
10. CZARNETZKI, B. M., and ROSENBACH, T. From eosinophil chemotactic factor of anaphylaxis to leukotriene B4—chemistry, biology and functional significance of eosinophil chemotactic leukotrienes in dermatology. *Dermatologica* **1989**, *179*Suppl 1, 54–59.
11. (a) ROKACH, J., ZAMBONI, R., LAU, C. K., and GUINDON, Y. The stereospecific synthesis of leukotriene A4 (LTA4), 5-epi-LTA4, 6-epi-LTA4 and 5-epi,6-epi-LTA4. *Tetrahedron Lett.* **1981**, *22*, 2759–2762; (b) ROKACH, J., ZAMBONI, R., and GUINDON, Y. Synthesis of the four optical isomers of LTA4 *Tetrahedron Lett.* **1981**, *22*, 2763–2766; (c) ROKACH, J., YOUNG, R. N., KAKUSHIMA, M., LAU, C. K., SEGUIN, R., FRENETTE, R., and GUINDON, Y. Synthesis of leukotrienes new synthesis of natural leukotriene A4, *Tetrahedron Lett.* **1981**, *22*, 979–982.
12. FOSTER, A., FITZSIMMONS, B., and LETTS, L. G. The synthesis of *N*-acetyl-leukotriene E4 and its effects on cardiovascular and respiratory function of the anesthetized pig. *Prostaglandins* **1986**, *31*, 1077–1086.
13. DELORME, D., GIRARD, Y., and ROKACH, J. Total synthesis of leukotriene E4 metabolites and precursors to radiolabeled forms of those metabolites. *J. Org. Chem.* **1989**, *54*, 3635–3640.
14. MAMER, O., JUST, G., LI, C.-S., PRÉVILLE, P., WATSON, S., YOUNG, R., and YERGEY, J. A. Enhancement of mass spectrometric detection of LTC4, LTD and LTE by derivatization. *J. Am. Soc. Mass Spectrom.* **1994**, *5*, 292–298.
15. (a) YOUNG, R. N., KAKUSHIMA M., and ROKACH, J. Studies on the preparation of conjugates of leukotriene C4 with proteins for the development of an immunoassay for SRSA (1). *Prostaglandins* **1982**, *23*, 603–613; (b) HAYES, E. C., GIRARD, Y., LOMBARDO, D. L., MAYCOCK, A. L., ROKACH, J., ROSENTHAL, A. S., YOUNG, R. N., EGAN R. W., and ZWEERINK, H. J.

Measuring leukotrienes of slow reacting substance of anaphylaxis: development of a specific radioimmunoassay. *J. Immunol.* **1983**, *131*, 429–433; (c) YOUNG, R. N., ZAMBONI, R., and ROKACH, J. Studies on the conjugation of leukotriene B4 with proteins for development of a radioimmunoassay for leukotriene B4. *Prostaglandins*, **1983**, *26*, 605–613; (d) J. ROKACH, HAYES, E. C., GIRARD, Y., LOMBARDO, D. L., MAYCOCK, A. L., ROSENTHAL, A. S., YOUNG, R. N., ZAMBONI, R., and ZWEERINK, H. J. The development of sensitive and specific radioimmunoassays for leukotrienes H. *J. Prostaglandins Leukotrienes Med.* **1984**, *13*, 21–25.

16. MILLER, D. K., SADOWSKI, S., DESOUSA, D., MAYCOCK, A. L., LOMBARDO, D., YOUNG, R. N., and HAYES, E. Development of enzyme-linked immunosorbant assays for measurement of leukotrienes and prostaglandins. *J. Immunol. Methods* **1985**, *81*, 169–185.
17. (a) LEWIS, R. A., AUSTEN, K. F., DRAZEN, J. M., CLARK, D. A., MARFAT, A., and COREY, E. J. Slow reacting substances of anaphylaxis: identification of leukotrienes C-1 and D from human and rat sources. *Proc. Natl Acad. Sci. USA*, **1980**, *77*, 3710–3714; (b) MORRIS, H. R., TAYLOR, G. W., PIPER, P. J., and TIPPINS, J. R. Structure of slow-reacting substance of anaphylaxis from guinea-pig lung. *Nature (London)* **1980**, *285*, 104–106.
18. (a) DRAZEN, J. M., AUSTEN, K. F., LEWIS, R. A., CLARK, D. A., GOTO, G., MARFAT, A., and COREY, E. J. Comparative airway and vascular activity of leukotriene C-1 and D in vivo and *in vitro*. *Proc. Natl Acad. Sci. USA*, **1980**, *77*, 4345–4358; (b) PIPER, P. J. Leukotrienes: potent mediators of airway constriction. *Int. Arch. Allergy Immunol.* **1985**, *76*(Suppl.I) 43–48; (c) SNYDER, D. W. and FLEISCH, J. H. Leukotriene receptor antagonists as potential therapeutic agents. *Ann. Rev. Pharmacol. Toxicol.* **1989**, *29*, 123–143.
19. HOFFSTEIN, S. T., MALO, P. E., BUGELSKI, P., and WHEELDON, E. B. Leukotriene D_4 (LTD_4) induces mucus secretion from goblet cells in the guinea pig respiratory epithelium. *Exp. Lung Res.* **1990**, *16*, 711–725.
20. BISGAARD, H., and PEDERSEN, M. SRS-A leukotrienes decrease the activity of human respiratory cilia. *Feder. Proc. Am. Soc. Exp. Biol.* **1983**, *42*, 1381. Abstract 6381;LUNDGREN, J. D., SHELHAMER, J. H. and KALINER, M. A.The role of eicosanoids in respiratory mucus hypersecretion. Ann. Allergy **1985**, 55, 5–8, 11.
21. LEIKAUF, G. D., CLAESSON, H. E., DOUPNIK, C. A., HYBBINETTE, S. and GRAFTSTROM, R. C. Cysteinyl leukotrienes enhance growth of human airway epithelial cells. *Am. J. Physiol.* **1990**, *259*, L255–L261.
22. (a) MUNOZ, N. M., DOUGLAS, I., MAYER, D., HERRNREITER A., ZHU, X., and LEFF. A. R. Eosinophil chemotaxis inhibited by 5-lipoxygenase blockade and leukotriene receptor antagonism. *Am. J. Respir. Crit. Care Med.* **1997**, *155*, 1398–1403; (b) BUSSE, W. W. Leukotrienes and Inflammation. *Am. J. Respirol. Crit. Care Med.* **1998**, *157*, S210–S213.
23. CHUNG, K. F. Role of inflammation in the hyperreactivity of the airways in asthma. *Thorax* **1986**, *41*, 657–662.
24. (a) BLOOMQUIST, E. I., and KREAM, R. M. Release of substance P from guinea-pig trachea leukotriene D_4. *Exp. Lung Res.* **1990**, *16*, 645–659; (b) ELLIS, J. L., and UNDEM, B. J. Role of peptidoleukotrienes in capasaicin-sensitive sensory fibre-mediated responses in guinea-pig airways. *J. Physiol. (London)* **1991**, *436*, 469–484; (c) BISGAARD, H., GROTH, S., and MADSEN, F., Bronchial hyperreactivity to leucotriene D_4 and histamine in exogenous asthma. *Br. Med. J.* **1985**, *290*, 1468–1471.
25. HENDERSON, W. R. JR. The role of leukotrienes in inflammation. *Ann. Internal Med.* **1994**, *121*, 684–698.
26. (a) OOSAKI, R., MIZUSHIMA, Y., KAWASAKI, A., KASHII, T., MITA, H., SHIDA, T., AKIYAMA, K., and KOBAYASHI, M. Urinary excretion of leukotriene E4 and 11-dehydrothromboxane B2 in patients with spontaneous asthma attacks. *Int. Arch. Allergy Immunol.* **1997**, *114*, 373–378;(b) KUMLIN, M., DAHLÉN, B., BJÖRCK, T., ZETTERSTRÖM, O., GRANSTRÖM, E., and DAHLÉN, S. E. Urinary excretion of leukotriene E4 and 11-dehydro-thromboxane B2 in response to bronchial provocations with allergen, aspirin, leukotriene D4, and histamine in asthmatics. *Am. Rev. Respir. Dis.* **1992**, *146*, 96–103.
27. MACHADO, E. R., UETA, M. T., LOURENÇO, E. V., ANIBAL, F. F., SORGI, C. A., SOARES, E. G., ROQUE-BARREIRA, M. C., MEDEIROS, A. I., and FACCIOLI, L. H. Leukotrienes play a role in the control of parasite burden in murine strongyloidiasis. *J. Immunol.* **2005**, *175*, 3892–3899.
28. LEMKE, T. L., and WILLIAMS, D. A. in *Foyles Principles of Medicinal Chemistry*; 5th edition, (ed. William O. Foye) Chapter 33, Lippincott, Williams and Wilkins, Philadelphia, 2008, p. 889.
29. NORRIS, A. A. Pharmacology of sodium cromoglycate. *Clin. Exp. Allergy* **1996**, *26*, s5–s7.
30. FORD-HUTCHINSON, A. W., GRESSER, M., and YOUNG, R. N. 5-Lipoxygenase. *Ann. Rev. Biochem.* **1994**, *63*, 383–417.
31. ORNING, L., and HAMMARSTRÖM, S. Inhibition of leukotriene C and leukotriene D biosynthesis. *J Biol. Chem.* **1980**, *255*, 8023–8026.
32. BERNSTRÖM, K., and HAMMARSTRÖM, S. Metabolism of leukotriene D by porcine kidney, *J. Biol. Chem.* **1981**, *256*, 9573–9578.
33. (a) BUCKNER, C. K., KRELL, R. D., LARAVUSO, R. B., COURSIN, D. B., BERNSTEIN, P. R., and WILL, J. A. Pharmacological evidence that human intralobar airways do not contain different receptors that mediate contractions to leukotriene C_4 and leukotriene D_4. *J. Pharmacol Exp Thera.*, **1986**, *237*, 558–562; (b) COLEMAN, R. A., R. M. EGLEN, R. L. JONES J, NARUMIYA S., SHIMIZU T., SMITH W. L., DAHLÉN S.-E., DRAZEN J. M., GARDINER P. J., JACKSON W. T., JONES T. R., KRELL R. D., and NICOSIA S. Prostanoid and leukotriene receptors: a progress report from the IUPHAR working parties on classification and nomenclature. *Adv. Prostaglandin Thromboxane Leukotriene Res.* **1995**, *23*, 283–285.

34. Lynch, K. R., O'Neill, G. P., Liu, Q., Im, D. S., Sawyer, N., Metters, K. M., Coulombe, N., Abramovitz, M., Figueroa, D. J., Zeng, Z., Connolly, B. M., Bai, C., Austin, C. P., Chateauneuf, A., Stocco, R., Greig, G. M., Kargman, S., Hooks, S. B., Hosfield, E., Williams, D. L. Jr., Ford-Hutchinson, A. W., Caskey, C. T. and Evans, J. F. Characterization of the human cysteinyl leukotriene CysLT1receptor. *Nature* **1999**, *399*, 789–793.
35. Young R. N. Inhibitors of 5-lipoxygenase: a therapeutic potential yet to be realized? *Eur. J. Med. Chem.* **1999**, *34*, 671–685.
36. (a) Miller, D. K., Gillard, J. W., Vickers, P. J., Sadowski, S., Léveillé, C., Mancini, J. A., Charleson, P., Dixon, R. A. F., Ford-Hutchinson, A. W., Fortin, R., Gauthier, J. Y., Rodkey, J., Rosen, R., Rouzer, C., Sigal, I. S., Strader, C. D., and Evans, J. F. Identification and isolation of a membrane protein necessary for leukotriene production. *Nature* **1990**, *343*, 278–281; (b) Dixon, R. A. F., Diehl, R. E., Opas, E., Rands, E., Vickers, P. J., Evans, J. F., Gillard, J. W., and Miller, D. K. Requirement of a 5-lipoxygenase-activating protein for leukotriene synthesis. *Nature* **1990**, *343*, 282–284.
37. Gillard, J., Ford-Hutchinson, A. W., Chan, C. C., Charleson, S., Denis, D., Foster, A, Fortin, R, Leger, S, McFarlane, C. S., Morton, H., Piechuta, H., Riendeau, D., Rouzer, C. A., Rokach, J., Young, R., MacIntyre, D. E., Peterson, L., Bach, T., Eiermann, G., Hopple, S., Humes, J., Hupe, L., Luell, S., Metzger, J., Meurer, R., Miller, D. K., Opas, E., and Pacholok, S. L-663,536 (MK-886) (3-[1-(4-chlorobenzyl)-3-t-butyl-thio-5-isopropylindol-2-yl]-2,2-dimethylpropanoic acid), a novel, orally active leukotriene biosynthesis inhibitor. *Canadian J. Physiol. Pharmacol.* **1989**, *67*, 456–464.
38. Prasit, P., Belley, M., Blouin, M., Brideau, C., Chan, C., Charleson, S., Evans, J. F., Frenette, R., Gauthier, J. Y., Guay, J., Gillard, J. W., Grimm, E., Ford-Hutchinson, A. W., Hutchinson, J. H., Fortin, R., Jones, T. R., Mancini, J., Leger, S., McFarlane, C. S., Piechuta, H., Riendeau, D., Roy, P., Tagari, P., Vickers, P. J., Young, R. N., and Zamboni, R. A. New class of leukotriene biosynthesis inhibitors: the discovery of MK-0591, *J. Lipid Mediators.* **1993**, *6*, 239–244.
39. Wenzel, S. E., and Kamada, A. K. Zileuton: the first 5-lipoxygenase inhibitor for the treatment of asthma. *Ann. Pharmacother.* **1996**, *30*, 858–864.
40. Varghese, M., and Lockey, R. F. Aspirin-exacerbated asthma. *Allergy Asthma Clin. Immunol.* **2006**, *4*, 75–83.
41. (a) Adams, G. K., and Lichenstein, L. M. Antagonism of antigen-induced contraction of guinea pig and human airways. *Nature* **1970**, *270*, 255–257; (b) Sheard, P., Lee, T. B., and Tattersall, M. L. Further studies on the SRS-A antagonist FPL 55712. *Monogr. Allergy.* **1977**, *12*, 245.
42. (a) Pong, S-S., and DeHaven, R. N. Characterization of a leukotriene D4 receptor in guinea pig lung. *Proc. Natl. Acad. Sci. USA.* **1983**, *80*, 7415–7419; (b) Lewis, M. A., Mong, S., Vessella, R. A., and Crooke, S. T. Identification and characterization of leukotriene D4 receptors in adult and fetal human lung, *Biochem. Pharmacol.* **1985**, *34*, 4311–4317.
43. Piper, P. J., Samhoun, M. N., Tippins, J. R., Williams, T. J., Palmer, A., and Peck, M. J. Pharmacological studies on pure SRS-A, SRS and synthetic leukotriene C4 and D4. in *SRS-A and Leukotrienes.* (ed P. J. Piper) Wiley, Chichester, **1981**, pp. 81–99.
44. Brunet, G., Piechuta, H., Hamel, R., Holme, G., and Ford-Hutchinson, A. W. Respiratory responses to leukotrienes and biogenic amines in normal and hyperreactive rats, *J. Immunol.* **1983**, *131*, 434–438.
45. McFarlane, C. S., Piechuta, H., Hall, R. A., and Ford-Hutchinson, A. W. Effects of a contractile prostaglandin antagonist (L-640,035) upon allergen-induced bronchoconstriction in hyperreactive rats and conscious squirrel monkeys. *Prostaglandins* **1982**, *131*, 434–438.
46. Abraham, N. M., Delehunt, J. C., Yerger, L., and Marchett, E. B. Characterization of late-phase response after antigen challenge in allergic sheep. *Am. Rev. Respir. Dis.* **1983**, *128*, 839–844.
47. Young, R. N. Structural analysis of sulfido-peptide leukotrienes: application to the design of potent and specific antagonists of leukotriene D4. *Adv. Prostaglandin Thromboxane Leukotriene Res.* **1987**, *19*, 643–646.
48. (a) Girard, Y., and Rokach, J.Leukotriene antagonists 1988, US Patent #4.761,425; (b) Coombs, W., Frenette, R., Guindon, Y., and Young, R. N. Unpublished results.
49. Gleason, J. G., Hall, R. F., Perchonock, C. D., Erhard, K. F., Frazee, J. S., Ku, T. W., Kondrad, K., McCarthy, M. E., Mong, S., Crooke, S. T., Chi-Rosso, G., Wasserman, M. A., Torphy, T. J., Muccitelli, R. M., Hay, D. W., Tucker, S. S. and Vickery-Clark, L. High-affinity leukotriene receptor antagonists. Synthesis and pharmacological characterization of 2-hydroxy-3-[(2-carboxyethyl)thio]-3-[2-(8-phenyloctyl)phenyl] propanoic acid. *J. Med. Chem.* **1987**, *30*, 959–961.
50. Christie, P. E., Smith, C. M., and Lee, T. H. The potent and selective sulfidopeptide leukotriene antagonist, SK&F 104353, inhibits aspirin-induced asthma. *Am. Rev. Respir. Dis.* **1991**, *144*, 957–958.
51. Nakagawa, N., Obata, T., Kobayashi, T., Okada, Y., Nambu, F., Terawaki, T., and Aishita, H. In vivo pharmacologic profile of ONO-1078: a potent, selective and orally active peptide leukotriene (LT) antagonist Japan. *J. Pharmacol.* **1992**, *60*, 217–225.
52. Jones, T. R., Young, R. N., Champion, E., Charette, L., Denis, D., Ford-Hutchinson, A. W., Frenette, R., Gauthier, J. Y., Guindon, Y., Kakushima, M., Masson, P., McFarlane, C., Piechuta, H., Rokach, J. and Zamboni, R. L-649,923, Sodium (βS*, γR*)-4-(3-(4-acetyl-3-hydroxy-2-propylphenoxy)-propylthio)-γ-hydroxy-β-methylbenzenebutanoate, a selective, orally active leukotriene receptor antagonist. *Can. J. Physiol. Pharmacol.* **1986**, *64*, 1068–1075.

53. Jones, T. R., Guindon, Y., Young, R. N., Champion, E., Charette, L., Denis, D., Ethier, D., Hamel, P., Ford-Hutchinson, A. W., Fortin, R., Letts, G., Masson, P., McFarlane, C., Piechuta, H., Rokach, J., Yoakim, C., DeHaven, R. N., Maycock, A. and Pong, S-S. L-648,051, sodium 4-[3-(4-acetyl-3-hydroxy-2-propylphenoxy)-propylsulfonyl]-γ-oxo-benzenebutanoate: a leukotriene D4 receptor antagonist. *Can. J. Physiol. Pharmacol.* **1986**, *64*, 1535–1542.
54. Mong, S., Wu, H. L., Scott, M. O., Lewis, M. A., Clark, M. A., Weichman, B. M., Kinzig, C. M., Gleason, J. G., and Crooke, S. T. Molecular heterogeneity of leukotriene receptors: correlation of smooth muscle contraction and radioligand binding in guinea-pig lung. *J. Pharmacol. Exp. Ther.* **1985**, *234*, 316–325.
55. Young R. N. The development of new anti-leukotriene drugs: L-648,051 and L-649,923, specific leukotriene D_4 antagonists. *Drugs Future* **1988**, *13*, 745–759.
56. Sanders, J. E., Eigenberg, D. A., Bracht, L. J., Wang, W. R., and van Zwieten M. J. Thyroid and liver trophic changes in rats secondary to liver microsomal enzyme induction caused by an experimental leukotriene antagonist (L-649,923). *Toxicol. Appl. Pharmacol.* **1988**, *95*, 378–387.
57. Barnes, N., Piper, P. J., and Costello, J. The effect of an oral leukotriene antagonist L-649,923 on histamine and leukotriene D4-induced bronchoconstriction in normal man. *J. Allergy Clin. Immunol.* **1987**, *79*, 816–821.
58. Britton, R., Hanley, S. P., and Tattersfield A. E. The effect of an oral leukotriene D4 antagonist L-649,923 on the response to inhaled antigen in asthma. *J. Allergy Clin. Immunol.* **1987**, *79*, 811–816.
59. Evans, J. M., Barnes, N. C., Zakrzewski, J. T., Sciberras, D. G., Stahl, E. G., Piper, P. J., and Costello, J. F. L-648,051, a novel cysteinyl-leukotriene antagonist is active by the inhaled route in man. *Br. J. Clin. Pharmacol.* **1989**, *28*, 125–135.
60. Bel, E. H., Timmers, M. C., Dijkman, J. H., Stahl, E. G., and Sterk, P. J. The effect of an inhaled leukotriene antagonist, L-648,051, on early and late asthmatic reactions and subsequent increase in airway responsiveness in man. *J. Allergy Clin. Immunol.* **1990**, *85*, 1067–1075.
61. Marshall, W. S., Goodson, T., Cullinan, G. J., Swanson-Bean, D., Haisch, K. D., Rinkema, L. E., and Fleisch, J. H. Leukotriene receptor antagonists. 1. Synthesis and structure-activity relationships of alkoxyacetophenone derivatives. *J. Med. Chem.* **1987**, *30*, 682–689.
62. Fuller, R. F., Black, P. N., and Dollery, C. T. Effect of the oral leukotriene D4 antagonist LY171883 on inhaled and intradermal challenge with antigen and leukotriene D_4 in atopic subjects. *J. Allergy Clin. Immunol.* **1998**, *83*, 939–944.
63. Israel, E., Juniper, E. F., Callaghan, J. T., Mathur, P. N., Morris, M. M., Dowell, A. R., Enas, G. G., Hargreave, F. E., and Drazen, J. M. Effect of a leukotriene antagonist, LY171883, on cold air-induced broncho-constriction in asthmatics. *Am. Rev. Respir. Dis.* **1989**, *140*, 1348–1353.
64. Zamboni, R., Belley, M., Champion, E., Charette, L., DeHaven, R., Frenette, R., Gauthier, J. Y., Jones, T. R., Leger, S., Masson, P., McFarlane, C. S., Metters, K., Pong, S. S., Piechuta, H., Rokach, J., Therien, M., Williams, H. W. R., and Young, R. N. Development of a novel series of styrylquinoline compounds as high-affinity leukotriene D4 receptor antagonists: synthetic and structure–activity studies leading to the discovery of (+/−)-3-[[[3-[2-(7-chloro-2-quinolinyl)-(E)-ethenyl] phenyl][[3-(dimethylamino)-3-oxopropyl]thio]methyl] thio]propionic acid. *J. Med. Chem.* **1992**, *35*, 3832–3844.
65. Perchonock, C. D., McCarthy, M. E., Erhard, K. F., Gleason, J. G., Wasserman, M. A., Muccitelli, R. M., DeVan, J. F., Tucker, S. S., and Vickery, L. M. Synthesis and pharmacological characterization of 5-(2-dodecylphenyl)-4,6-dithianonanedioic acid and 5-[2-(8-phenyloctyl)phenyl]-4,6-dithianonanedioic acid: prototypes of a novel class of leukotriene antagonists. *J. Med. Chem.* **1985**, *28*, 1145–1147.
66. Young, R. N., Zamboni, R., Belley, M., Champion, E., Charette, L., Dehaven, R., Frenette, R., Ford-Hutchinson, A. W., Gauthier, J. Y., Jones, T. R., Leger, S., McFarlane, C. S., Masson, P., Piechuta, H., Pong, S. S., Rokach J., and Williams, H. L-660,711: a potent selective and orally active antagonist of leukotriene D4. in *New Trends in Lipid Mediators Research* (eds U. Zor, Z. Naor, A. Danon) Basel, Karger, 1989, Vol. *3*, pp. 62–66.
67. Jones, T. R., Zamboni, R., Belley, M., Champion, E., Charette, L., Ford-Hutchinson, A. W., Frenette, R., Gauthier, J. Y., Leger, S., Masson, P., McFarlane, C. S., Piechuta, H., Rokach, J., Williams, H., Young, R. N., Dehaven R. N., and Pong, S. S. Pharmacology of L-660,711 (MK-571): a novel potent and selective leukotriene D4 receptor angatonist. *Can. J. Physiol. Pharmacol.* **1989**, *67*, 17–28.
68. Solér, M., Sielczak, M., and Abraham, W. M. Separation of late bronchial responses from airway hyperresponsiveness in allergic sheep. *J. Appl. Physiol.* **1991**, *70*, 617–623.
69. Abraham, W. M., and Stevenson, J. S. Lung inflammatory cell changes after local antigen-challenge in allergic sheep with and without late airway responses. *FASEB J.*, **1988**, *2*, a1057.
70. McNamara, J. M., Leezer, J. L., Bhupathy, M., Amato, J. S., Reamer, R. A., Reider, P. J., and Grabowski, E. J. J. Synthesis of unsymmetrical dithioacetals: an efficient synthesis of a Novel LTD_4 antagonist, L-660,711. *J. Org. Chem.* **1989**, *54*, 3718–3721.
71. Margoski, D. J. Clinical experience with MK-571: a potent and specific LTD4 receptor antagonist. *Ann. New York Acad. Sci.* **1991**. *629*, 148–156.
72. Depré, M., Margolskee, D. J., Hecken, A., Hsieh, J. S. Y., Buntinx, A., De Schepper, P. J., and Rogers, J. D. Dose-dependent kinetics of the enantiomers of MK-

571, an LTD_4-receptor antagonist. *Eur. J. Clin. Pharmacol.* **1992**, *43*, 431–433.
73. Depré, M., Margolskee, D. J., Hsieh, J. Y., Van Hecken, A., Buntinx, A., De Lepeleire, I., Rogers, J. D. and De Schepper, P. J. Plasma drug profiles and tolerability of MK-571 (L-660,711): a leukotriene D4 receptor antagonist, in man. *Eur. J. Clin. Pharmacol.* **1992**, *43*, 427–430.
74. Gaddy, J. N., Margolskee, D. J., Bush, R. K., Williams, V. C., and Busse, W. W. Bronchodilation with a potent and selective leukotriene D4 (LTD4) receptor antagonist (MK-571) in patients with asthma. *Am. Rev. Respir. Dis.* **1992**, *146*, 358–363.
75. Gaddy, J., McCreedy, W., Margolskee, D., Williams, V., and Busse, W. A potent leukotriene D4 antagonists (MK-571) significantly reduces airway obstruction in mild to moderate asthma. *J. Allergy Clin. Immunol.* **1991**, *87*, 308.
76. Margolskee, D., Bodman, S., Dockhorn, R., Israel. E., Kemp, J., Mansmann, H., Minotti, D. A., Spector, S., Stricker, W., Tinkelman, D., Townley, R., Winder, J., and Williams, V. The therapeutic effects of MK-571 a potent and selective leukotriene (LT)D-4 receptor antagonist in patients with chronic asthma [abstract]. *J. Allergy Clin. Immunol.* **1991**, *87*, 309.
77. Grossman, S. J., DeLuca, J. G., Zamboni, R. J., Keenan, K. P., Patrick, D. H., Herold, E. G., van Zwieten, M. J., and Zacchei, A. G. Enantioselective induction of peroxisomal proliferation in CD-1 mice by leukotriene antagonists. *Toxicol. Appl. Pharmacol.* **1992**, *116*, 217–224.
78. Eacho, P. I., Foxworthy, P. S., Johnson, W. D., Hoover, D. M., and White, S. L. Hepatic peroxisomal changes induced by a tetrazole-substituted akoxyacetophenone in rats and comparison with other species. *Toxicol. Appl. Pharmacol.* **1986**, *83*, 430–437.
79. Moody, D. E., Reddy, J. K., Lake, B. G., Popp, J. A., and Reese, D. H. Peroxisome proliferation and non-genotoxic carcinogenesis: commentary on a symposium. *Fundamental Appl. Toxicol.* **1991**, *6*, 233–248.
80. Nagai, H., Shimazawa, T., Yakuo, I., Aoki, M., Koda, A., and Kasahara, M. Role of peptide-leukotrienes in liver injury in mice. *Inflammation* **1989**, *13*, 673–680.
81. Young, R. N., Gauthier, J. Y., Thérien M., and Zamboni, R. Asymmetric dithioacetals III: the preparation of the enantiomers of 3-(((3-(2-(7-chloroquinolin-2-yl)-(E) -ethenyl) phenyl)3-dimethylamino-3-oxopropylthio)methyl)thio) propionic acid (L-660,711). An antagonist of leukotriene D4. *Heterocycles* **1989**, *28*, 967.
82. Gauthier, J. Y., Jones, T., Champion, E., Charette, L., Dehaven, R., Ford-Hutchinson, A. W., Hoogsteen, K., Lord, A., Masson, P., Piechuta, H., Pong, S. S., Springer, J. P., Thérien, M., Zamboni, R., and Young, R. N 3-((((3-(2-(7-Chloroquinolin-2-yl-(E)-ethenyl) phenyl)-3-dimethylamino-3-oxopropylthio)methyl) thio)propionic acid: a potent and specific leukotriene D4 receptor antagonist, stereospecific synthesis, assignment of absolute configuration and biological activity of the entantiomers. *J. Med. Chem.* **1990**, *33*, 2841–2845.
83. Bhupathy, M., Hughes, D. L., Amato, J. S., Bergan, J. J., Leazer, J. L., Lovelace, T. C., McNamara, J. M., Reamer, R. A., Sidler, D. R., Grabowski, E. J. J., Reider, P. J. and Shinkai, I. Chemoenzymatic synthesis of a novel LTD_4 antagonist. *Pure Appl. Chem.* **1992**, *64*, 1939–1944.
84. Cheng, H., Schwartz, J. I., Lin, C., Amin, R. D., Seibold, R. J., Lasseter, K. C., Ebel, D. L., Tocco, D. J., and Rogers, D. J. The bioavailability and nonlinear pharmacokinetics of MK-679 in humans. *Biopharma. Drug Dispos.* **1994**, *15*, 409–418.
85. Impens, N., Reiss, T. F., Teahan, J. A., Desmet, M., Rossing, T. H., Shingo, S., Zhang, J., Schandevyl, W., Verbesselt, R., and Dupont. A. G. Acute bronchodilation with intravenously administered leukotriene D_4 receptor antagonist, MK-0679. *Am. Rev. Respir. Dis.* **1993**, *147*, 1442–1446.
86. Dahlen, B., D. J. Margolskee, O. Zetterstrom, and S.-E. Dahlen. Effect of the leukotriene receptor antagonist MK-0679 on baseline pulmonary function in aspirin sensitive asthmatic subjects. *Thorax* **1993**, *48*: 1205–1210.
87. Christie, P. E., Tagari, P., Ford-Hutchinson, A. W., Charlesson, S., Chee, P., Arm, J. P., and Lee, T. H. Urinary leukotriene E_4 concentrations increase after aspirin challenge in aspirin-sensitive asthmatic subjects. *Am. Rev. Respir. Dis.* **1991**, *143*, 1025–1029.
88. Dahlen, B., Kumlin, M., Margolskee, D. J., Larsson, C., Blomqvist, H., Williams, V. C., Zetterstrom, O., and Dahlen. S.-E. The leukotriene-receptor antagonist MK-0679 blocks airway obstruction induced by inhaled lysine-aspirin in aspirin sensitive asthmatics. *Eur. Respir. J.* **1993**, *6*, 1018–1026.
89. Margolskee, D., Friedman, B., Williams, V., Botto, A., Noonan, N., Altman, L., Bone, R., Dockhorn, R., Ellis, E., Eschenbacher, W., Findlay, S., Grant, J., Grossman, J., Hendles, L., Izrael, E., Kemp, J., Nelson, H., Pearlman, D., Stricker, W., Tinkelman, D., Townley R., Vandewalker, M., Wanderer, A., Weisberg, G., and Winder, J. The therapeutic effects of MK-0679: a selective leukotriene D4 receptor antagonist, in patients with chronic asthma. *8th International Conference on Prostaglandins and Related Compounds*, **1992**, July 26–31, Montreal, Abstract 639.
90. Nicoll-Griffith, D., Yergey, J., Trimble, L., Williams, H., Rasori, R. and Zamboni, R. In vitro and in vivo biotransformations of the potent leukotriene D4 antagonist verlukast in the rat. *Drug Metab. Dispos.* **1992**, *20*, 383–389.
91. Nicoll-Griffith, D. A., Gupta, N., Twa, S. P. Williams, H., Trimble L. A., and Yergey J. A. Verlukast (MK-0679) conjugation with glutathione by rat liver and kidney cytosols and excretion in the bile. *Drug Metab. Dispos.* **1995**, *23*, 1085–1093.

92. LABELLE, M., PRASIT, P., BELLEY, M., BLOUIN, M., CHAMPION, E., CHARETTE, L., DELUCA, J. G., DUFRESNE, C., FRENETTE, R., GAUTHIER, J. Y., GRIMM, E., GROSSMAN, S. J., GUAY, D., HEROLD, E. G., JONES, T. R., LAU, C. K., LEBLANC, Y., LEGER, S., LORD, A., MCAULIFFE, M., MCFARLANE, C., MASSON, P., METTERS, K. M., OUIMET, N., PATRICK, D. H., PERRIER, H., PICKETT, C. B., PIECHUTA, H., ROY, P., WILLIAMS, H., WANG, Z., XIANG, Y. B., ZAMBONI, R. J., FORD-HUTCHINSON, A. W. and YOUNG, R. N. The discovery of a new structural class of potent orally active leukotriene D4 antagonists. *Bioorg. Med. Chem. Lett.* **1992**, *2*, 1141–1146.
93. LABELLE, M., BELLEY, M., CHAMPION, E., GORDON, R., HOOGSTEEN, K., JONES, T. R., LEBLANC, Y., LORD, A., MCAULIFFE, M., MCFARLANE, C., MASSON, P., METTERS, K. M., NICOLL-GRIFFITH, D., OUIMET, N., PIECHUTA, H., ROCHETTE, C., SAWYER, N., XIANG, Y. B., YERGEY, J., FORD-HUTCHINSON, A. W., PICKETT, C. B., ZAMBONI, R. J. and YOUNG, R. N. The discovery of L-699,392, a novel potent and orally active leukotriene D4 receptor antagonist. *Bioorg. Med. Chem. Lett.* **1994**, *4*, 463–468.
94. GROSSMAN, S. J., DELUCA, J. G., ZAMBONI, R. J., KECNAN, K. P., PATRICK, D. H., HEROLD, E. G., VAN ZWIETEN, M. J., and ZACCHEI, A. G. Enantioselective induction of peroxisomal proliferation in CD-1 mice by leukotriene antagonists. *Toxicol. Appl. Pharmacol.* **1992**, *116*, 217.
95. LAZAROW, P. B., and DE DUVE, C. A fatty acyl-CoA oxidizing system in rat liver peroxisomes; enhancement by clofibrate, a hypolipidemic drug. *Proc. Natl Acad. Sci. USA* **1976**, *73*, 2043.
96. HASHIMOTO, T., in *Peroxisomes in Biology and Medicine*, (eds H. D. Fahimi and H. Sies) Springer Verlag, Berlin, **1987**, pp. 97–104.
97. GREEN, S. Receptor-mediated mechanisms of peroxisome proliferators. *Biochem. Pharmacol.* **1992**, *43*, 393–401.
98. ZHU, Y., ALVARES, K., HUANG, Q., RAO, M. S. and REDDY, J. K. Cloning of a new member of the peroxisome proliferator-activated receptor gene family from mouse liver. *J. Biol. Chem.* **1993**, *268*, 26817–26820.
99. LABELLE, M., BELLEY, M., GAREAU, Y., GAUTHIER, J. Y., GUAY, D., GORDON, R., GROSSMAN, S. G., JONES, T. R., LEBLANC, Y., MCAULIFFE, M., MCFARLANE, C., MASSON, P., METTERS, K. M., OUIMET, N., PATRICK, D. H., PIECHUTA, H., ROCHETTE, C., SAWYER, N., XIANG, Y. B., PICKETT, C. B., FORD-HUTCHINSON, A. W., ZAMBONI, R. J. and YOUNG, R. N. Discovery of MK-0476: a potent and orally active leukotriene D_4 receptor antagonist devoid of peroxisomal enzyme induction. *Bioorg. Med. Chem. Lett.* **1995**, *5*, 283–288.
100. JONES, T. R., LABELLE, M., BELLEY, M., CHAMPION, E., CHARETTE, L., EVANS, J., FORD-HUTCHINSON, A. W., GAUTHIER, J. Y., LORD, A., MASSON, P., MCAULIFFE, M., MCFARLANE, C. S., METTERS, K. M., PICKETT, C., PIECHUTA, H., ROCHETTE, C., RODGER, I. W., SAWYER, N., YOUNG, R. N., ZAMBONI, R. and ABRAHAM, W. M. Pharmacology of montelukast sodium (Singulair™), a potent and selective leukotriene D4 receptor antagonist. *Can. J. Physiol. Pharmacol.* **1995**, *73*, 191–201.
101. MELPOLER, J. B., and HECK, R. F. Palladium-catalyzed arylation of allylic alcohols with aryl halides. *J. Org. Chem.* **1976**, *41*, 265.
102. COREY, E. J., BAKSHI, R. K., RAMAN, K., and SHIBATA, S. Highly enantioselective borane reduction of ketones catalyzed by chiral oxazaborolidines. Mechanism and synthetic implications. *J. Am. Chem. Soc.* **1987**, *109*, 5551.
103. MATHRE, D. J., JONES, T. K., XAVIER, L. C., BLAELDOCK, T. J., REAMER, R. A., MOHAN, J. J., TURNER JONES, E. T., HOOGSTEEN, K., BAUM, M. W., and GRABOWSKI, E. J. J. A practical enantioselective synthesis of alpha,alpha-diaryl-2-pyrrolidinemethanol. Preparation and chemistry of the corresponding oxazaborolidines. *J. Org. Chem.* **1991**, *56*, 751.
104. KING, A. O., CORLEY, E. G., ANDERSON, R. K., LARSEN, R. D., VERHOEVEN, T. R., REIDER, P. J., XIANG, Y. B., BELLEY, M., LEBLANC, Y., LABELLE, M., PRASIT, P., and ZAMBONI, R. J., An efficient synthesis of LTD4 antagonist L-699,392. *J. Org. Chem.* **1993**, *58*, 3731–3735.
105. BHUPATHY, M., MCNAMARA, J. M., SIDLER, D. R., VOLANTE, R., and BERGAN, J. Process for the preparation of leukotriene anatgonists. US patent # 5614632, March 25, **1997**.
106. CHAURET, N., YERGEY, J., TRIMBLE, L., and NICOLL-GRIFFITH D. In vitro biotransformation of MK-0476, a new potent LTD4 antagonist. in *Proceedings of the 10th International Symposium on Microsomes and Drug Oxidations*, **1994**, 22, p. 612.
107. DUFRESNE C., GALLANT M., GAREAU Y., RUEL R., TRIMBLE L., and LABELLE M. Synthesis of montelukast (MK-0476) metabolic oxidation products. *J. Org. Chem.* **1996**, *61*, 8518–8525.
108. BALANI, S. K., XU, PRATHA, X. V., KOSS, M. A., AMIN, R. D., DUFRESNE, C., MILLER, R. R., ARISON, B. H., DOSS, G. A., CHIBA, M., FREEMAN, A., HOLLAND, S. D., SCHWARTZ, J. I., LASSETER, K. C., GERTZ, B. J., ISENBERG, J. I., ROGERS, J. D., LIN, J. H., and BAILLIE. T. A. Metabolic profiles of montelukast sodium (Singulair): a potent cysteinyl leukotriene1 receptor antagonist, in human plasma and bile. *Drug Metab. Dispos.* **1997**, *25*, 1282–1287.
109. CHIBA M., XU X., NISHIME J. A., BALANI S. K., and LIN J. H. Hepatic microsomal metabolism of montelukast, a potent leukotriene D4 receptor antagonist, in humans. *Drug Metab. Disposl* **1997**, *25*, 1022–1031.
110. Drug Approval Package: Singulair (Montelukast Sodium) NDA# 020829 [http://www.accessdata.fda.gov/drugsatfda_docs/nda/98/020829s000_Singulair TOC.cfm]
111. SCHOORS, D. F., DE SMET, M., REISS, T., MARGOLSKEE, D., CHENG, H., LARSON, P., AMIN, R., and SOMERS, G. Single dose pharmacokinetics, safety and tolerability of MK-0476, a new leukotriene D4-receptor antagonist, in healthy volunteers. *Br. J. Clin. Pharmacol.* **1995**, *40*, 277–280.
112. CHENG, H., LEFF, J. A., AMIN, R., GERTZ, B. J., DE SMET, M., NOONAN, N., ROGERS, J. D., MALBECQ, W., MEISNER,

D., and Somers, G. Pharmacokinetics, bioavailability, and safety of montelukast sodium (MK-0476) in healthy males and females. *Pharma. Res.* **1996**, *13*, 445–448.

113. Zhao, J. J., Rogers, J. D., Holland, S. D., Larson, P., Amin, J. D., Haesen, R., Freeman, A., Merz, S. M., and Cheng, H. Pharmacokinetics and bioavailability of montelukast sodium (MK-0476) in healthy young and elderly volunteers. *Biopharma. Drug Dispos.* **1997**, *18*, 743–824.
114. Knorr, B., Larson, P., Nguyen, H. H., Holland, S., Reiss, T. F., Chervinsky, P., Blake, K., van Nispen, C. H., Noonan, G., Freeman, , A., Haesen, R., Michiels, N., Rogers, J. D., Amin, R. D., Zhao, J., Xu, X., Seidenberg, B. C., Gertz, B. J., and Spielberg, S. Montelukast dose selection in 6- to 14-year-olds: comparison of single-dose pharmacokinetics in children and adults, *J. Clin. Pharmacol.* **1999**, *39*, 786–793.
115. Storms, W., Michele, T. M., Knorr, B., Noonan, G., Shapiro, G., Zhang, J., Shingo, S., and Reiss. T. F. Clinical safety and tolerability of montelukast, a leukotriene receptor antagonist, in controlled clinical trials in patients aged $\geq$ 6 years. *Clin. Exp. Allergy* **2001**, *31*, 77–87.
116. Cobb, D. B. Abbot, C. L., Watson, W. A., and Fernandez, M. C. High-dose montelukast exposures in a 3-year-old and a 5-year-old child. *Veter. Human Toxicol.* **2002**, *44*, 91–92.
117. De Lepeleire, I., Reiss, T. F., Rochette, F., Botto, A., JZhang, J., Kundu, K., and Decramer, M. Montelukast causes prolonged, potent leukotriene D_4-receptor antagonism in the airways of patients with asthma. *Clin. Pharmacol. Thera.* **1997**, *61*, 83–92.
118. Diamant, Z., Grootendorst, D. C., Veselic-Charvat, M., Timmers, C., De Smet, M., Leff, J. A., Seidenberg, B. C., Zwinderman, A. H., Peszek, I., and Sterk, P. J. The effect of montelukast (Mk-0476): a cysteinyl leukotriene receptor antagonist, on allergen-induced airway Responses and sputum cell counts in asthma. *Clin. Exp. Allergy* **1999**, *29*, 42–51.
119. Reiss, T. F., Hill, J. B., Harman, E., Zhang, J., Tanaka, W. K., Bronsky, E., Guerreiro, D., and Hendeles. L. Increased urinary excretion of LTE4 after exercise and attenuation of exercise-induced bronchospasm by montelukast, a cysteinyl leukotriene receptor antagonist. *Thorax* **1997**, *52*, 1030–1035.
120. Singulair. [package insert].: Merck and Co, Inc, West Point, PA, 1999.
121. Altman, L. C., Munk, Z., Seltzer, J., Noonan, N., Shingo, S., Zhang, J. and Reiss. TF. A placebo-controlled, dose-ranging study of montelukast, a cysteinyl leukotriene–receptor antagonist. *J. Allergy Clin. Immunol.* **1998**, *102*, 50–55.
122. Noonan, M. J., Chervinsky, P., Brandon, M., Zhang, J., Kundu, S., McBurney, J., and Reiss, T. J. Montelukast, a potent leukotriene receptor antagonist, causes dose-related improvements in chronic asthma: Montelukast Asthma Study Group. *Eur. Respir. J.* **1998**, *11*, 1232–1239.
123. Bronsky, E. A., Kemp, J. P., Zhan, J., Guerreiro, D., and Reiss, T. F. Dose-related protection of exercise bronchoconstriction by montelukast, a cysteinyl leukotriene–receptor antagonist, at the end of a once-daily dosing interval. *Clin. Pharmacol. Thera.* **1997**, *62*, 556–561.
124. Knorr, B., Holland, S., Rogers, J. D., Nguyen, H. H., and Reiss, T. F. Montelukast adult (10-mg film-coated tablet) and pediatric (5-mg chewable tablet) dose selections J. *Allergy Clin. Immunol.* **2000**, *106*, S172–S178.
125. Reiss, T. F., Knorr, B., Malmstrom, K., Noonan, G., and Lu, S. Clinical efficacy of montelukast in adults and children. *Clin. Exp. Allergy Rev.*, **2001**, *1*, 264–273.
126. Reiss, T. F., Chervinsky, P., Dockhorn, R. J., Shingo, S., Seidenberg, B., and Edwards, T. B. Montelukast, a once-daily leukotriene receptor antagonist, in the treatment of chronic asthma. A multicenter, randomized, double-blind trial. *Arc. Internal Med.* **1998**, *158*, 1213–1220.
127. Malmstrom, K., Rodriguez-Gomez, G., and Guerra, J. Oral montelukast, inhaled beclomethasone, and placebo for chronic asthma: a randomized, controlled trial. *Ann. Internal Med.* **1999**, *130*, 487–495.
128. Knorr, B., Matz, J., Bernstein, J. A., Nguyen, J. H., Seidenberg, B. C., Reiss, T. F., and Becker, A. Montelukast for chronic asthma in 6- to 14-year old children. A randomized, double-blind trial. *J. Am. Med. Assoc.* **1998**, *279*, 1181–1186.
129. Williams, B., Noonan, G., Reiss, T. F., Knorr, B., Guerra, J., White, R., and Matz, J. Long-term asthma control with oral montelukast and inhaled beclomethasone for adults and children 6 years and older. *Clin. Exp. Allergy* **2001**, *31*, 845–854.
130. Knorr, B., Franchi, L. M., Bisgaard, H., Vermeulen, J. H., LeSouef, P., Santanello N., Michele, T. M., Reiss, T. F., Nguyen, H. H., and Bratton, D. L. Montelukast: a leukotriene receptor antagonist, for the treatment of persistent asthma in children aged 2 to 5 years. *Pediatrics* **2001**, *108*, e48.
131. Becker, A. B., Kuznetsova, O., Vermeulen, J., Soto-Quiros, M. E., Young, B., Reiss, T. F., Dass, S. B., and Knorr, B. A. Pediatric Montelukast Linear Growth Study Group. Linear growth in prepubertal asthmatic children treated with montelukast, beclomethasone, or placebo: a 56-week randomized double-blind study. *Ann. Allergy Asthma Immunol.* **2006**, *96*, 800–807.
132. Laviolette, M., Malmstrom, K., Lu, S., Chervinsky, P., Puget, J-P., Perszek, I., Zhang, J. I., and Reiss, T. F. Montelukast added to inhaled beclomethasone in treatment of asthma. *Am. J. Respir. Crit. Care Med.* **1999**, *160*, 1862–1868.
133. Lofdahl, C-G., Reiss, T. F., Leff, J. A., Israel, E., Noonan, M. J., Finn, A. F., Seidenberg, B. C., Capizzi, T., Kundu, S., and Godard, P. Randomised, placebo controlled trial of effect of a leukotriene receptor antagonist, montelukast, on tapering inhaled corticosteroids in asthmatic patients. *Br. Med. J.* **1999**, *319*, 87–90.

134. Leff, J. A., Israel, E., Noonan, M. J., Finn, and Godard, P., et al. Montelukast (MK-0476) allows tapering o of inhaled corticosteroids (ICS) in asthmatic patients while maintaining clinical stability. *Am. J. Respir. Crit. Care Med.* **1997**, *155*, A976 [abstract].
135. Wechsler, M. E., Finn, D., Gunawardena, D., Westlake, R., Barker, A., Haranath, S. P. Pauwels, R. A., Kips, J. C., and Drazen, J. M. Churg-Strauss syndrome in patients receiving montelukast as treatment for asthma. *Chest* **2000**, *117*, 708–713.
136. Bili, A., Condemi, J. J., Bottone, S. M., and Ryan, C. K. Seven cases of complete and incomplete forms of Churg-Strauss syndrome not related to leukotriene receptor antagonists. *J. Allergy Clin. Immunol.* **1999**, *104*, 1060–1065.
137. Wechsler, M. E., Pauwels, R., and Drazen, J. M. Leukotriene modifiers and Churg-Strauss syndrome: adverse effect or response to corticosteroid withdrawal? *Drug Safety* **1999**, *21*, 241–251.
138. Pizzichini, E., Leff, J. A., Reiss, T. F., Hendeles, L., Boulet, L. P., Wei, L. X., Efthimiadis, A. E., Zhang, J., and Hargreave, F. E. Montelukast reduces airway inflammation in asthma: a randomized, controlled trial. *Eur. Respir. J.* **1999**, *14*, 12–18.
139. Bisgaard, H., Loland, L., and Anhùj, J. NO in exhaled air of asthmatic children is reduced by the leukotriene receptor antagonist montelukast. *Am. J. Respir. Crit. Care Med.* **1999**, *160*, 1227–1231.
140. Lagos, J. A., and Marshall, G. D. Montelukast in the management of allergic rhinitis. *J. Thera. Clin. Risk Manag.* **2007**, *3*, 327–332.
141. Nayak, A., and Langdon, R. B. Montelukast in the treatment of allergic rhinitis: an evidence-based review. *Drugs* **2007**, *67*, 887–901.
142. Benfield, T. L., and Lundgren, J. D. PAF receptor antagonists in the treatment of asthma. *Expert Opin. Invest. Drugs.* **1994**, *3*, 733–742.

CHAPTER 9

DISCOVERY AND DEVELOPMENT OF MARAVIROC, A CCR5 ANTAGONIST FOR THE TREATMENT OF HIV INFECTION

Patrick Dorr, Blanda Stammen, and Elna van der Ryst

9.1 BACKGROUND AND RATIONALE

Acquired immunodeficiency syndrome (AIDS) was first described in 1981 [1] with the discovery of the causative viral pathogen, later to be known as the human immunodeficiency virus 1 (HIV-1), shortly afterwards [2,3]. HIV-1 infection and AIDS soon developed into a worldwide pandemic and the major infectious cause of mortality globally. Current estimates of the pandemic indicate 33 million infected individuals, with two million deaths from AIDS last year, and 2.7 million newly infected patients [4].

Initially, HIV infection proved to be almost invariably fatal, with a clinical course characterized by severe opportunistic infections and unusual forms of cancer. Since that time, and starting with the demonstration that zidovudine (azidothymidine, AZT) can improve immunologic function and certain other clinical abnormalities associated with AIDS [5], HIV went from being a fatal disease to a chronic manageable condition. Highly active antiretroviral therapy (HAART) regimens introduced in the mid-1990s profoundly reduced morbidity and mortality due to HIV infection in developed countries. These regimens currently generally include at least three drugs selected from at least two different drug classes [nucleoside/nucleotide reverse transcriptase inhibitors(NRTIs), nonnucleoside reverse transcriptase inhibitors (NNRTIs), protease inhibitors (PIs), integrase inhibitors, and inhibitors of virus entry].

Although effective in reducing plasma viral load, delaying disease progression to AIDS and prolonging survival, HAART has two major limitations. Firstly, drug toxicity and complex dosing schedules can often lead to poor treatment adherence and treatment failure [6]. A further limitation of HAART is the development of viral resistance, which has limited the effectiveness of many antiretroviral drugs [7]. Many individuals were treated with partially effective monotherapy or dual therapy before the advent of HAART, resulting in development of highly resistant virus strains. In one large study of HIV-positive adults who received treatment but had evidence of ongoing viral replication with >500 HIV RNA copies mL^{-1}, it was estimated that approximately 76% had resistance to one or more HIV drugs within 3 years [8]. In addition, HIV-1 resistance to one or more classes of drugs can be transmitted to treatment-naïve patients, limiting treatment options from the outset [9]. These limitations highlight the continuing unmet medical need for anti-HIV agents with novel mechanisms of action.

Case Studies in Modern Drug Discovery and Development, Edited by Xianhai Huang and Robert G. Aslanian.

The first antiretroviral drugs targeted key enzymes involved in the replication of HIV, namely reverse transcriptase (nucleoside/nucleotide reverse transcriptase inhibitors, non-nucleoside reverse transcriptase inhibitors, and protease inhibitors). The demonstration of cross-resistance to other drugs from the same drug class in patients who failed treatment further emphasized the need for drugs acting on different stages of the virus lifecycle and sparked interest in HIV-1 entry as an antiretroviral target.

The first step in the process of HIV-1 entry into the host cell is the specific binding of viral gp120 to CD4, the primary receptor for HIV-1 (Figure 9.1). However, the binding of gp120 to CD4 alone is not sufficient for HIV-1 entry [10]. The observation that human chemokines are capable of inhibiting HIV-1 infection of T-lymphocytes [11], and the identification of polymorphisms in the CCR5 gene that protect some highly exposed individuals from being infected with HIV-1 [12], led to the discovery that a human chemokine receptor is an essential coreceptor for HIV-1 infection [13]. The binding of gp120 to CD4 causes a conformational change in gp120 that exposes the bridging sheet to form a coreceptor binding site [14]. Once this has occurred, coreceptor binding triggers conformational changes in gp41 which drive the remaining steps in fusion and entry of the viral core [15]. The chemokine receptors most commonly utilized by HIV-1 *in vivo* are CC chemokine receptor 5 (CCR5) and/or CX chemokine receptor 4 (CXCR4) [13,16]. The ability of gp120 to bind to either one or both receptors defines the tropism, and HIV-1 strains are categorized as R5 (CCR5-tropic), X4 (CXCR4-tropic), or R5/X4 (strains using both CCR5 and CXCR4; also referred to as "dual-tropic") [17].

A patient plasma sample may also contain a heterogeneous population of viruses with different tropism termed "mixed tropism." The rationale for cell entry as a target was validated by HIV-gp41 binding peptides or fusion inhibitors [18]. The only licensed drug in this class, enfuvirtide (acetyl-YTSLIHSLIEESQNQQEKNE QELLELDKWASLWNWF-amide, Fuzeon®, Trimeris/Roche; formerly known as T-20) acts at the point of virus entry into cells by binding to the viral envelope protein gp41 and prevents a postattachment step of

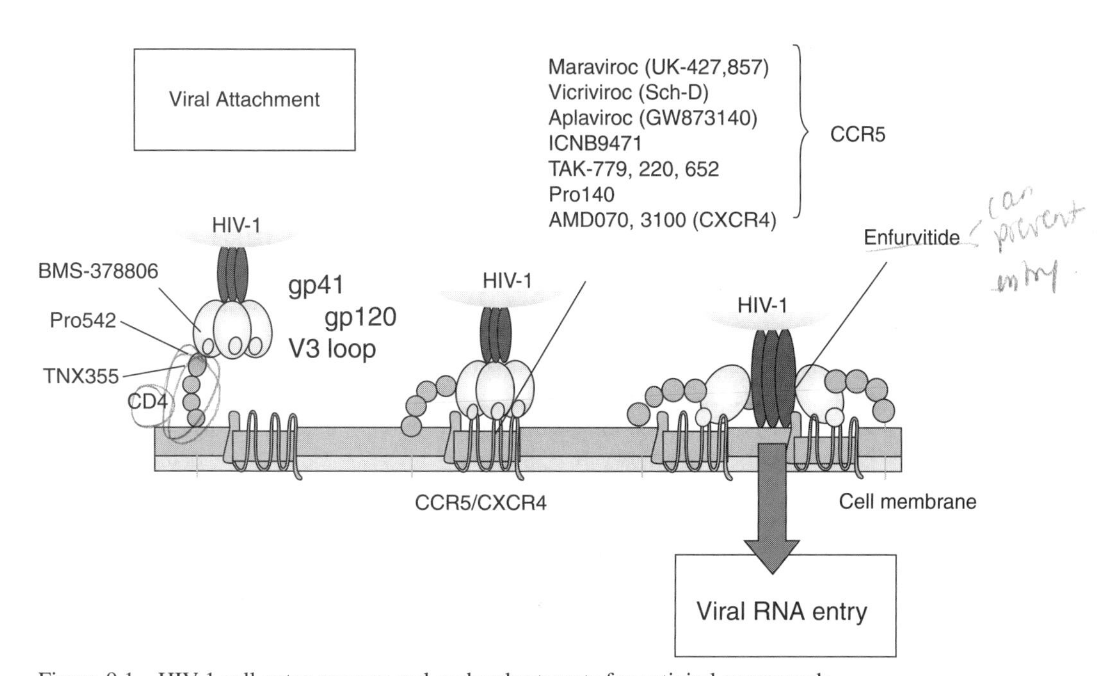

Figure 9.1 HIV-1 cell entry process and molecular targets for antiviral compounds.

the viral entry process [19]. Enfuvirtide demonstrated excellent efficacy in treatment-experienced patients, but the twice daily subcutaneous mode of administration and cost of goods associated with a complex peptide drug have restricted its use [20]. Efforts since have predominantly focused on small molecule HIV-1 entry inhibitors in order to enable oral delivery. Some milestones in this effort have included the discovery of gp120-CD4 binding inhibitors, such as BMS-378806 [21], and blockade of CXCR4 via the antagonists AMD3100 (1,1′-[1,4-phenylenebis(methylene)]bis [1,4,8,11-tetraazacyclotetradecane], plerixafor) and AMD070 [22]. These approaches have met with various challenges in efficacy and potential for significant side effects, respectively. However, the greatest tangible success in targeting HIV-1 entry as a new antiretroviral mechanism has been the discovery, clinical development and approval of the CCR5 antagonist maraviroc for the treatment of HIV-1 infection.

Chemokine receptors are a large family of GPCRs that regulate leukocyte activation and migration to sites of inflammation via interaction with a family of secreted chemoattractant cytokines or "chemokines" [23]. Aminergic GPCRs recognize small molecule ligands and are attractive drug targets as reflected by the success pharmaceutical companies have had in modulating them with small molecules for the successful treatment of many diseases [24]. Chemokine receptors, however, belong to the subfamily of peptidergic GPCRs which have proven far more challenging to develop drugs against and are bound by large peptides.

CCR5 has three extracellular loops (ECL1, ECL2, and ECL3). These together with the extracellular N-terminus enable chemokine binding and interactions with the viral protein gp120 following an initial complex formation with CD4 to enable HIV-1 entry as described above.

The rationale behind the development of CCR5 inhibitors was provided by the discovery of a natural 32-bp deletion (CCR5-Δ32, or Δ32) within the coding sequence of the gene which results in complete absence of CCR5 expression on the cell surface. Subjects (approximately 1% of north European Caucasians and of lower frequencies in other races) who are homozygotes for this deletion are genetically protected from CCR5 tropic HIV-1 infection [25] while heterozygotes have delayed disease progression. Observations that CCR5 promoter polymorphisms also provided considerable resistance to HIV-1 progression following infection also attracted interest [26]. Cognate agonist (endogenous) ligands for CCR5 that caused receptor internalization, thereby making it unavailable for CCR5-tropic (R5) HIV strains, also helped elucidate this receptor as a valid antiviral target [27]. The translation between genetic absence of CCR5 versus "blocked" CCR5 as an antiviral mechanism was born out more recently with the observation from clinical trials that numerous CCR5 antagonists safely reduced viral load in humans [28].

Chemokine interaction with CCR5 initiates several intracellular events culminating in receptor internalization. This is most commonly associated with chemotaxis, although the function of the receptor is not completely understood [29]. A number of cognate/endogenous CC chemokines bind to CCR5 with different affinities and abilities to activate the receptor. Discovery and characterization of novel, noncognate ligands, including quantification of their inhibitory (i.e., antagonistic) potencies can be determined utilizing the various assays used to measure chemokine-induced CCR5 signaling. There is considerable redundancy in the chemokine area of immunology, and it is worth noting that RANTES and MIP-1α can recognize multiple chemokine receptors in addition to CCR5. This is in contrast to CXCR4 that has an exclusive 1:1 association with SDF-1α.

Confidence in safety for the development of a CCR5 antagonist for the treatment of HIV/AIDS was suggested by the observation that there is no overt phenotype associated with CCR5-Δ32 homozygosity (a natural knockout in humans) [25d], although there remained a possibility that inhibition of CCR5 in a fully-matured immune system could have a different effect to the constitutive knock-out that allows an organism to utilize redundancies in order to compensate for the loss of the receptor from conception. Confidence in safety is further supported by the redundancy in the system as discussed earlier.

The complex association between HIV-1 coreceptor tropism, transmission, and pathogenesis which is not yet fully understood provided a further challenge to the development of CCR5 antagonists [30]. Generally, strains that are transmitted and establish new infections in a host are R5 [31]. In some individuals, CXCR4-tropism evolves over time and the emergence of X4 virus has been associated with rapid CD4 T-lymphocyte decline and accelerated disease progression. Although increasing prevalence of X4 virus and decreasing prevalence of R5 virus have been associated with increasing viral load and decreasing CD4 cell counts [32], the emergence of CXCR4-using virus is not a prerequisite for the development of AIDS. Throughout infection, the detection of R5 virus only is most common; dual/mixed-tropic virus is more likely to be detected in advanced patients than early asymptomatic patients, and the detection of X4 virus only is rare [32a,33]. Whether emergence of CXCR4 strains is a marker for disease progression rather than the cause is not known [30b]. It also remains to be determined whether the emergence of CXCR4-using strains during treatment with a CCR5 antagonist is associated with the same clinical outcome as when they emerge during the natural course of HIV-1 infection.

A better understanding of the physiological role of CCR5 may also provide alternative development indications for CCR5 inhibitors, possibly against one or more of the pathologies that have been negatively associated with CCR5 knock-out or inhibition. This is discussed in more detail later (see Section 9.7).

The identification of CCR5 as a putative anti-HIV-1 target prompted widespread discovery activities across academia and industry, which have resulted in many clinical candidates [34]. Antiviral analogs and peptide based mimics of cognate ligands have been reported, [35]. and antibodies against CCR5 continue to progress through clinical trials, for example, HGS004 [36] and PRO-140 [37]. However, the limitations posed by antibodies and peptides, for example, lack of oral delivery, the lack of other known ligands together with breakthroughs in GPCR assays led to high throughput screening approaches to initiate medicinal chemistry for small molecule antagonists. Agonists were not so highly sought due to the perceived risk of triggering inflammatory cascades and coreceptor switch, that is, switch from CCR5 to CXCR-4 usage [35a]. This was the general starting point for a lot of pharmaceutical and biotechnology companies, and indeed a range of antagonists were consequently discovered and some progressed into clinical trials. Many have met with attrition for various reasons (idiosyncratic liver toxicity, QT prolongation, lack of oral bioavailability and inherent polypharmacology [38]. Maraviroc is the first and to date only CCR5 antagonist to meet with formal approval for therapeutic antiretroviral use, having avoided all these attrition factors. The discovery and development of maraviroc by the Pfizer laboratories at Sandwich are specifically described here.

9.2 THE DISCOVERY OF MARAVIROC

9.2.1 HTS and Biological Screening to Guide Medicinal Chemistry

In the absence of convenient high throughput assays mimicking the many events in HIV-1 cell entry at the time of the identification of CCR5 as a coreceptor for HIV-1, radioligand-binding assays using iodinated chemokines adapted from reported techniques [39] were used successfully to identify initial chemical leads [40]. Although these screens/assays have now been supplanted by superior methods (quicker, highly automated, and greater correlation with the coreceptor mediated HIV-1 entry process [29,41].), these radioligand binding approaches were ultimately timely and successfully yielded starting points (hits) for anti-HIV-1 drug discovery. These hits, in turn, were progressed through bespoke screening cascades, that is, screening cascades unique to project and pharmaceutical company with well-defined go-/no-go progression criteria, of virology, primary, and selectivity pharmacology assays followed by pharmacokinetic (PK), toxicological, and clinical evaluation.

The Pfizer CCR5 antagonist program began with a high throughput screen of the corporate screening file (~0.5 million compounds at the time) based on inhibition of the binding of ^{125}I-MIP-1β to human CCR5 as stably integrated and expressed on HEK-293 cells. Several hits emerged from the screen, most prominently UK-107543 (Figure 9.2), which had reasonable inhibitory activity against ^{125}I-MIP-1β binding to the cells ($IC_{50} = 0.6\,\mu M$).

9.2.2 Hit Optimization

UK-107543 was devoid of antiviral activity and proved to be an agonist rather than antagonist of the receptor, as assessed using calcium signaling (FLIPR) assays [40d]. It was also found to be a potent inhibitor of the polymorphic human CYP2D6 enzyme (IC_{50} 40 nM), putatively via coordination of the pyridine N atom to the heme group. Two strategies were adopted to circumvent CYP2D6 inhibition: first, simple replacement of the pyridine N with C retained potent CCR5 receptor binding, but with much reduced CYP inhibition and, second, steric crowding of the piperidine N atom by incorporation into a tropane ring gave further improvements in potency in both the CCR5 binding, see Figure 9.2, and signaling assays, gp120-CD4-CCR5 complex formation screen and HIV fusion assay [40d]. This also effectively ablated CYP inhibition [42]. These screens eventually guided chemistry to further replace one phenyl group from the benzhydryl moiety with an amide function which drove a significant reduction in lead lipophilicity, and, in combination with the tropane ring design, instilled significant and importantly R5-HIV-specific antiviral activity free of cytotoxicity within the series (UK-372673—see Figure 9.2). It was proposed that reducing the conformational flexibility of the propylamino linking group through syn-pentane interactions contributed to the enhanced performance of

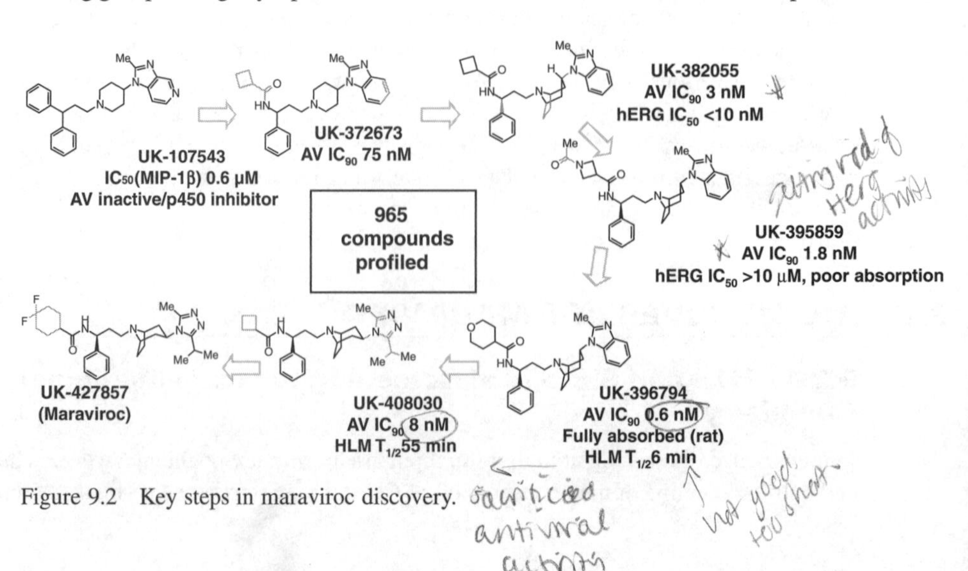

Figure 9.2 Key steps in maraviroc discovery.

the tropane group. SAR studies showed activity in the series to reside within the S-phenyl configuration.

9.2.3 Overcoming Binding to hERG

The Pfizer program then turned to focus on overcoming high and unacceptable affinity for the hERG potassium channel which was not entirely unexpected in light of the series being basic with a positive log*P*. A number of strategies directed toward all locations of the lead structure were deployed, predominantly guided by compound-competition screening against labeled dofetilide binding to hERG-subunit containing cell membranes [43]. The most successful of these sought to introduce polarity in peripheral aromatic regions and optimize substitution patterns for CCR5 binding affinity. The polarity introduced as exemplified by UK-395859 (Figure 9.2) achieved impressive antiviral activity [$IC_{90} \sim 1$ nM HIV-1 (BaL) in peripheral blood lymphocytes (PBL)] and reduced affinity for hERG (IC_{50} $>10\ \mu M$), but showed extremely low penetration of CACO-2 cell layers ($<1\ cm\ s^{-1}$) and no evidence of absorption in rat PK studies (oral dosing and hepatic portal vein and systemic exposure determination). This was presumed to be a consequence of water coating due to hydrogen binding. The tetrahydropyran analogue UK-396794 (Figure 9.2) retained the impressive antiviral/hERG profile and was fully absorbed in rat. However, this compound was quickly metabolized in isolated human liver microsomes (HLMs), suggesting likelihood of a poor PK profile (potential for high peak-trough ratio and unacceptable drug–drug interactions). Synthetic effort led to the triazole UK-408030 (Figure 9.2), a series within which antiviral activity of the exo- and endo-tropanes began to very much favor the exo diastereoisomer and balanced the profile for favorable absorption, stability, hERG, and CCR5-mediated antiviral activity somewhat. Evolution of the cyclobutyl group, powered by parallel chemistry techniques then provided the difluorocyclohexyl group in UK-427857 (later known as maraviroc, Figure 9.2), which showed excellent antiviral potency (R5 HIV-1 cross-clade primary isolate in PBL culture geometric mean $IC_{90} = 1$ nM [40d,44]), with low activity against hERG ($IC_{50} > 10\ \mu M$). Within the triazole series, the 4,4-diflurocyclohexyl group is unique in its antiviral profile and lack of affinity for the hERG channel. Retrospective modeling studies suggest that this group is not tolerated within the hERG channel by virtue of the steric bulk of the cyclohexyl ring, coupled with the dipole created by the difluoro moiety. Profiling *in vitro* highlighted broad anti R5 HIV-1 spectrum in a range of assays and either additive or synergistic properties in combination with other antiretroviral drugs [40d].

9.3 PRECLINICAL STUDIES

9.3.1 Metabolism and Pharmacokinetic Characteristics of Maraviroc

In preclinical ADME studies, maraviroc had high clearance in rat and moderate clearance in dog which appeared to be mediated by a combination of renal, metabolic, and biliary processes [45]. Maraviroc exhibited moderate tissue distribution in keeping with its basic and moderately lipophilic nature. The ratio of cerebro-spinal fluid (CSF) to free plasma concentration is 0.1, indicating limited CSF penetration, as later confirmed in humans [46]. Maraviroc was slowly metabolized by human liver microsomes (HLM). Using expressed human cytochrome p450 enzymes, only CYP2D6 and CYP3A4 metabolized the compound with fivefold higher turnover by CYP3A4. Maraviroc showed only weak inhibition of

TABLE 9.1 Predicted and Measured Human Pharmacokinetic Profile for Maraviroc

Parameter	Maraviroc predicted from rat and dog	Maraviroc measured (30 mg i.v single dose or 100 mg b.i.d. oral)
Clearance (mL min^{-1} kg^{-1})	11	10.5 ± 1.3
V_d (l/kg)	2	2.8 ± 0.9
$t_{1/2}$ (h)	3	13.2 ± 2.8
Absorption (%)	30	55
Bioavailability (%)	20	23 (19.2–27.8)
C_{min} (nM unbound) at 100 mg b.i.d.	1	5.4 ± 1.4

Abbreviations: C_{min}, minimum concentration; V_d, Volume of distribution; $t_{1/2}$, half-life; i.v., intravenous; b.i.d., twice a day.

CYP2D6 ($IC_{50} = 87\ \mu M$) using recombinant CYPs and fluorescent probe substrates. No inhibition of CYP1A2, CYP2C9, CYP2C19, or CYP3A4 (up to 100 μM) was observed.

Maraviroc also showed inherently low membrane permeability in CACO-2 flux studies that predict incomplete absorption in general, with transcellular flux enhanced in the presence of P-glycoprotein inhibitors [45]. It was 20%–30% absorbed in rat, but well absorbed in the dog (50%) and showed nonlinear pharmacokinetics in oral dose escalation studies in human (see Section 9.6.1). Predicting human PK from animal studies and *in vitro* models is challenging. At the time of nomination to clinical evaluation it was estimated that a convenient dosing regime of about 100 mg BID should be well tolerated and maintain unbound compound levels above the geometric mean, cross-clade antiviral IC_{90} in native cell assays [40d]. Retrospectively, the actual absorption and subsequent PK in humans was superior to the predicted profile (Table 9.1). The discovery of the slow physical and functional dissociation of maraviroc and indeed all antagonists reported to date from the CCR5 receptor [44,47] suggested that receptor occupancy might be retained following clearance of free drug, although the turnover of CCR5 and its expressing cells might limit the effectiveness of prolonged receptor occupancy in driving viral load reduction [40d].

9.3.2 Maraviroc Preclinical Pharmacology

Maraviroc was extensively characterized in pharmacology-based assays prior to a regulatory-based preclinical toxicology package to enable evaluation in human phase 1 clinical trials. This included extensive primary pharmacology and virology characterization, selectivity profiling, and *in vitro* immune function evaluation. These studies highlighted the potent and selective CCR5 inhibitory activity of maraviroc, specific anti R5-HIV-1 cross clade activity and inactivity (Table 9.2) against a range of Th1 and Th2 immune functions [40d].

Maraviroc was extensively profiled in hERG-associated assays *in vitro* and *in vivo* (dog hemodynamics), highlighting a low risk of QT prolongation [40d,45]. The overall outcome of these preclinical studies was to conclude that maraviroc showed a profile that was deemed potent enough to enable viral load reduction under a convenient dosing regime without obvious or apparent off-target pharmacology.

9.3.3 Preclinical Investigations into HIV Resistance

Intuitively, CCR5 offers an attractive target for antiviral drug discovery in that targeting a host protein creates an additional hurdle for HIV-1 to gain resistance, as the virus cannot simply rapidly mutate to moderate drug binding to one of its own proteins, as seen for all

TABLE 9.2 ***In Vitro*** **Immune Selectivity Profile of Maraviroc (Methods for assays as reported in Ref. [63])**

Immune function assay	Maraviroc potency
MCP-3 induced intracellular Ca^{2+} release (CCR2)	$IC_{50} > 10\,\mu M$
IL-2-stimulated T-cell proliferation	$IC_{50} > 10\,\mu M$
LPS-stimulated TNF-α release by differentiated THP-1 cell	$IC_{50} > 4\,\mu M$
Antigen-stimulated lymphocyte proliferation	$IC_{50} > 10\,\mu M$
MIP-1α-induced chemotaxis of THP-1 cells (CCR1)	$IC_{50} > 25\,\mu M$
MCP-1-induced chemotaxis of THP-1 cells (CCR2)	$IC_{50} > 25\,\mu M$
ITAC-induced chemotaxis by H9 cells (CCR3)	$IC_{50} > 25\,\mu M$
SLC-induced chemotaxis by H9 cells (CCR7)	$IC_{50} > 25\,\mu M$
IL-8-induced chemotaxis of neutrophils (CXCR1/CXCR2)	$IC_{50} > 25\,\mu M$
Gro-α-induced chemotaxis of neutrophils (CXCR2)	$IC_{50} > 25\,\mu M$
MIP-1α binding to CCR1	$IC_{50} > 10\,\mu M$
Eotaxin binding to CCR3	$IC_{50} > 10\,\mu M$
TARC binding to CCR4	$IC_{50} > 10\,\mu M$
rhMIP-3β binding to CCR7	$IC_{50} > 10\,\mu M$
I309 binding to CCR8	$IC_{50} > 10\,\mu M$
Superoxide production in neutrophils	$IC_{50} > 10\,\mu M$
IL-4-stimulated IgE synthesis in lymphocytes	$IC_{50} \geq 10\,\mu M$ (2 donors) $IC_{50} = 1$ to $10\,\mu M$ (1 donor)

other anti-HIV targets. There are two theoretical ways by which CCR5 virus might escape from a CCR5 antagonist:

1. Selection for virus that uses CXCR4, either through *de novo* acquisition of mutations in the viral envelope allowing the utilization of the CXCR4 coreceptor (true coreceptor "switch"), or expansion of a pre-existing (minor) population of CXCR4-using variants, which is not detected before introduction of the CCR5 antagonist.
2. Selection for virus that continues to use CCR5, either through increased affinity of the virus envelope for unbound CCR5 molecules, or ability of the virus envelope to use compound-bound receptors for entry.

Each of these possible ways of viral escape has been extensively investigated during the development of maraviroc. Preclinical *in vitro* studies have shown that gaining resistance to CCR5 antagonists is relatively difficult [48]. HIV-1 does not mutate to enable entry via the CXCR4 coreceptor switch as observed in animal models, *in vitro* systems, or indeed clinically derived isolates [48,49]. In contrast, CCR5-mediated resistance has been demonstrated in preclinical studies. The pathway to resistance for CCR5 antagonists is characterized by dose–response curves with plateaus at <100% maximal inhibition as is demonstrated in Figure 9.3 for the MVC-resistant CC1/85 virus [48–50]. This phenotype is consistent with the ability of the resistant viruses to use compound-bound receptor for entry. If resistance developed through an increased affinity for unbound CCR5 molecules, it would be characterized phenotypically by a classical shift in IC_{50}.

Phylogenetic analysis of MVC (maraviroc)-resistant viruses demonstrated changes in gp120, concentrated in the V3 loop (but not exclusive to it), accumulating over time. Site-directed mutagenesis of the gp120 envelope from maraviroc-resistant virus confirmed that

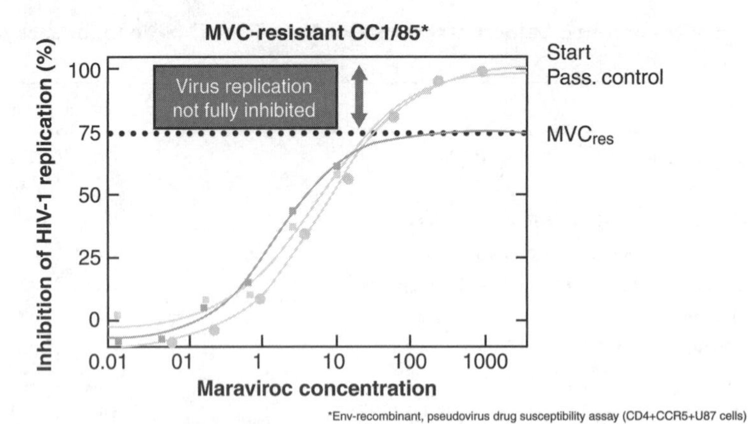

Figure 9.3 Susceptibility of pseudoviruses derived from CC1/85 to maraviroc. CCR5 tropic virus strain CC1/85 was serially passaged in peripheral blood mononuclear cells in the presence or absence of maraviroc. Susceptibility to MVC of resultant viruses was determined using the Phenosense™ HIV Entry Assay. Start = input virus; MVC_{res} = virus passaged in the presence of maraviroc; Pass. control = virus passaged in the absence of maraviroc. Adapted from Ref. [50c]. (See color version of the figure in Color Plate section)

amino acid mutations in the V3 loop conferred the resistant phenotype. However, the gp120 mutations selected in the maraviroc-resistant variants obtained from different HIV-1 strains were different, which suggests that there are multiple genetic pathways to resistance [50c].

Although some of those mutations can confer resistance to chemically-related CCR5 antagonists [50a,50b,51], class resistance is not inevitable [52], and there is a considerable weight of evidence that the resistant strains cannot utilize CCR5 that is occupied by an antagonist that has not been used as the selecting agent for generating the resistant isolate [47a,50c,53]. Indeed, the follow-up clinical candidate to maraviroc, PF-232798 [54], retained full activity against an expanded clone of the B-clade MVC^{RES} HIV-1 isolate CC185 in PBL culture [55]. Partial retention (>50%) of activity was observed against an expanded clone of the G-clade MVC^{RES} HIV-1 isolate RU570, although a lowered plateau effect was observed [38,44,56]. Full retention of activity was also demonstrated against the alternative CCR5 antagonist templates aplaviroc and vicriviroc (data not shown). It remains to be seen if this encouraging trend is observed with clinically derived MVC^{RES} HIV-1, but this is a promising observation for this new class, suggesting that class-resistance may not be as readily achieved as for traditional antiretroviral targets.

9.3.4 Binding of Maraviroc to CCR5

To understand the observations associated with CCR5 antagonist resistance in relationship with maraviroc and other CCR5 antagonists, a bespoke study to investigate the binding mode of these compounds was undertaken. CCR5 antagonists are commonly referred to as allosteric antagonists in that they do not prevent binding by directly blocking the receptor binding site, but rather lead to a conformational change in the binding site. The binding was modeled using the structurally characterized GPCR, rhodopsin [57]. This binding mode is allosteric with respect to the gp120-CD4 complex binding site to CCR5 which binds the extracellular N-terminal and extracellular loop (ECL) regions, especially the second loop [58]. However, the antagonist binding site might be considered as orthosteric with respect to chemokines, part of which bind at sites within the transmembrane "retinol equivalent" site [59]. The basic mechanism of CCR5 antagonist antiviral activity is binding

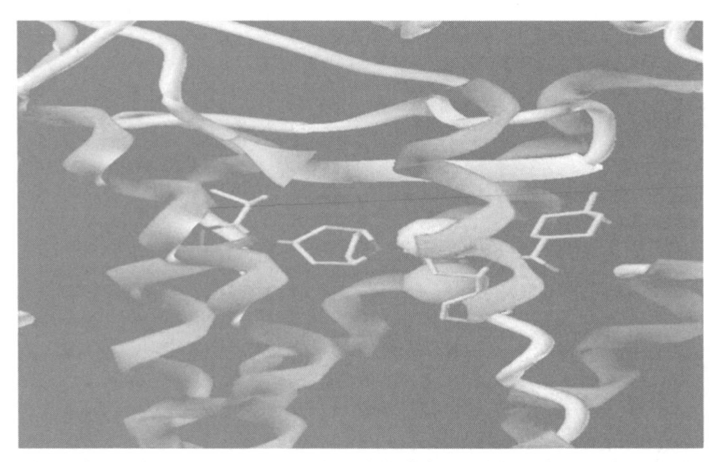

Figure 9.4 Computer-generated model of the docking of maraviroc in the transmembrane pocket of CCR5. Hydrophobic interaction with Y108 (orange residue) and the ionic interaction between the tropane nitrogen with the acidic glutamate (green residue) are highlighted [51].

the receptor to drive re-arrangement of the extracellular loops into a conformation that is no longer recognized by the gp120-CD4 complex. Offset of the antagonist, and in particular the functional recovery of the receptor to enable either chemokine or HIV-1 binding appears to be extremely slow thereafter, as judged by the small reduction in potency in wash and chase experiments [44,56]. CCR5 antagonist resistance seen *in vitro* and observed in clinical practice is underpinned by the mutation of the viral envelope to a form that can recognize the extracellular pattern of the antagonist occupied receptor N-terminus and loops. Different CCR5 antagonists appear to stablize significantly different conformations of the CCR5 ECLs. The SAR for this has been in part characterized through compound screening against MVC^{RES} HIV-1 CC185 coupled with computer-assisted antagonist-receptor docking models (Figure 9.4) based upon data from site-directed mutagenesis mapping of antagonists as previously reported for the maraviroc program [29,38,47a]. These identified the essential hydrophobic interaction between the phenyl moieties of maraviroc with Y108, and the ionic interactions between the basic tropane nitrogen and the acidic residues E283 (also observed independently [57]).

9.4 THE SYNTHESIS OF MARAVIROC

Large-scale preparation of maraviroc as the active ingredient in Celsentri/Selzentry™ relies on four steps (see Figure 9.5 with associated conditions and yields). Improvements over the discovery synthesis have been described by Haycock-Lewandowski et al. [60]. First, ethyl (*S*)-3-[(4,4-difluorocyclohexyl) carboximido]-3-phenylpropanoate, UK-453464, is reduced with sodium borohydride and methanol in tetrahydrofuran to give alcohol UK-453465 which is isolated from either tetrahydrofuran and cyclohexane or from acetone and water. Subsequent oxidization of UK-453465 with aqueous sodium hypochlorite catalyzed by 2,2,6,6-tetramethyl-1-piperidinyloxy free radical in dichloromethane yields aldehyde UK-453453 which is isolated from toluene and/or heptane. In step 3, exo-8-benzyl-3-(3-isopropyl-5-methyl-4H-1,2,4-triazol-4-yl)-8-azabicyclo[3.2.1]octane, UK-408026, is hydrogenolyzed over a palladium on carbon catalyst in the presence of p-toluenesulfonic acid and carbon in methanol or aqueous propan-2-ol to give amine UK-408027-15 which is isolated from

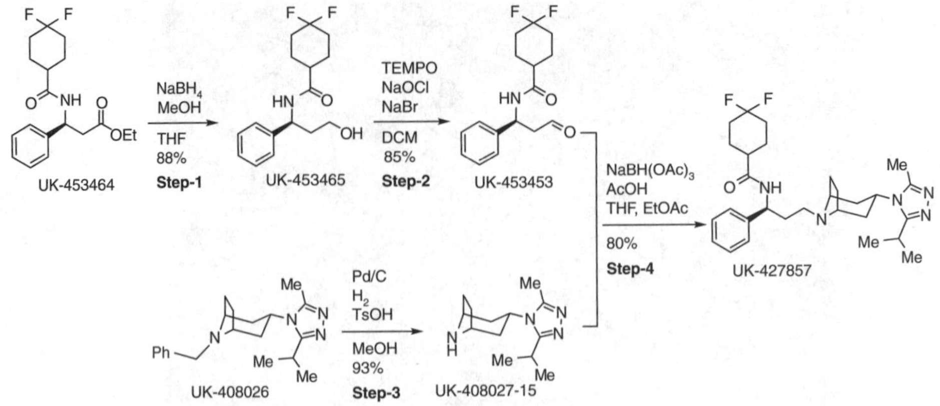

Figure 9.5 Process chemistry synthesis of maraviroc:

propan-2-ol. Lastly, the aldehyde UK-453453 is reductively coupled with the amine UK-408027-15 in the presence of sodium triacetoxyborohydride in tetrahydrofuran and/or ethyl acetate to give maraviroc which is isolated from ethyl acetate.

9.5 NONCLINICAL SAFETY AND TOXICITY STUDIES

9.5.1 Safety Pharmacology

The studies to investigate the toxicity of maraviroc were particularly extensive and rigorous in light of the intention to treat an immune-compromised population through inhibition of a receptor that mediates immune cell signaling with a first-in-class mechanism and structurally completely novel compound. A regulatory-based toxicity/safety pharmacology package involving numerous regulatory toxicity species showed maraviroc to have an extremely well-tolerated profile with no significant adverse findings at systemic free drug exposure levels at high multiples of intended therapeutic exposure levels. Maraviroc had little interaction with physiologically important receptors, binding sites, enzymes, or ion channels apart from weak affinity for the human μ opioid receptor ($K_i = 0.6\,\mu M$) and human α2A adrenergic receptor ($K_i = 10\,\mu M$), which exceeded by >30-fold the measured C_{max}-free drug levels achieved at therapeutic dosing in humans. There were no effects on the central or peripheral nervous, renal, and respiratory systems at relevant exposure levels.

The basic nature and positive log*D* of CCR5 antagonists and, more specifically, the termination of SCH-C, the first compound reported in HIV monotherapy trials, due to QT prolongation has ensured extensive scrutiny of CCR5 antagonists activity at the hERG channel. Results from *in vitro* hERG channel studies showed maraviroc to have very weak binding ($IC_{50} > 10\,\mu M$) and to not affect IKr current and cardiac repolarization *in vivo* at unbound plasma concentrations greater than 3 μM, approximately 10-fold the mean unbound C_{max} in HIV-positive patients at the later established clinical dose of 300 mg BID [40d,45].

9.5.2 Immuno- and Mechanistic Toxicity

Toxicity of single and repeated doses of maraviroc was studied in mouse, rat, dog, and cynomolgous monkey. In terms of metabolism and general pharmacokinetics, these species can all be considered as useful models for humans. While considering pharmacology at the target receptor level the cynomolgous monkey is by far closest to the human in sequence and function. Indeed, maraviroc has similar affinity for this isoform and human CCR5, and achieved complete *in vivo* functional occupancy in this species in short- and long-term toxicity studies. In this study, no CCR5-mediated adverse events were observed [61].

Pivotal toxicity studies after repeated doses including 3 months mouse, 6 months rat, 6 months dog, and a 9-month cynomolgus monkey, at doses shown to yield unbound maraviroc exposure levels at many multiples of expected therapeutic exposure, resulted in an encouraging unremarkable profile.

Detailed immunological and hematology analysis in toxicity studies showed no maraviroc-dependent effects on general hematology or serum globulins; effects or histology changes in bone marrow, lymph nodes, spleen, thymus, and no increase in incidence of infections. Specific immunotoxicology studies in monkeys (at 100% CCR5 functional blockade) showed no changes in lymphocyte subset distribution; NK cell activity; phagocytosis activity/oxidative burst; or humoral response (IgM and IgG). In short, blockade of CCR5 and maraviroc exposure per se were deemed to have a clean profile with no measurable adverse effects on immune function.

9.6 CLINICAL DEVELOPMENT OF MARAVIROC

In addition to demonstrating the safety and efficacy of the compound, the maraviroc clinical development program faced several unique challenges. CCR5 antagonists represent the first class of antiretroviral agent to target a host cellular receptor rather than the virus and in spite of the apparently normal phenotype presented by individual homozygous for the delta 32 deletion, concerns have been raised about the safety of long-term CCR5 blockade. CCR5 is implicated in the immunological response to a variety of pathogens [62] and there is evidence that delta 32 homozygous individuals may have an increased susceptibility to flaviviruses, a family of viruses transmitted by mosquitoes and ticks such as West Nile virus [63] and tickborne encephalitis [64]. In addition, conflicting reports of associations between CCR5-delta32 and various malignancies [65] combined with a cluster of lymphomas observed in the Phase IIb ACTG 5211 study of vicriviroc [66] have also caused concern about potential class-wide toxicity. Similarly, CCR5-delta32 mouse model data indicating increased susceptibility to concanavalin A-induced hepatitis [49,50] which when considered alongside the severe idiosyncratic hepatotoxicity observed during aplaviroc development [67] raised concerns that hepatotoxicity may be a class effect.

Further challenges included evaluating the impact of tropism changes under drug selective pressure, clinically validating a novel assay as part of the phase 2b/3 development program, and elucidating the mechanism by which resistance evolves *in vivo*.

9.6.1 Phase 1 Studies

The aims of the phase 1 program were to characterize the human pharmacokinetic profile of maraviroc, assess safety and tolerability, and to quantify the drug–drug interaction profile.

A range of clinical studies including single and multiple ascending dose studies (including fed and fasted dosing arms), an absolute bioavailability study and radiolabel study were conducted in healthy volunteers to characterize the pharmacokinetic profile of maraviroc. The data demonstrated that maraviroc is rapidly absorbed with T_{max} occurring 4–5 h after dosing with a terminal half-life of 16–23 h following multiple dosing [68]. PK is nonproportional at lower doses (<100 mg) but at the nominal clinical dose of 300 mg, the degree of nonproportionality is small [69]. The most likely reason for this is saturation of certain clearance mechanisms. The predicted absolute bioavailability at 300 mg is 33% [70]. Administration of Maraviroc 300 or 600 mg after a high fat meal resulted in a reduction in exposure of 33%–37% [71]. Doses of $\geq$100 mg BID or higher resulted in unbound exposure levels significantly in excess of the measured antiviral IC_{90} (as derived from the free drug geometric mean cross clade isolate value of 1 nM established *in vitro*) [68,72].

Preclinical pharmacokinetic data indicated that maraviroc was a CYP3A4/Pgp substrate with little potential for CYP3A4 induction or inhibition. Antiretroviral drugs (ARVs) are always used in combination with other ARVs, as part of potent combination regimens. Several of the ARV drug classes have a high drug–drug interaction potential, specifically the protease inhibitors which are potent CYP3A4/Pgp inhibitors and the nonnucleoside reverse transcriptase inhibitors which are potent CYP3A4 inducers. A series of drug–drug interaction studies were therefore conducted in order to characterize the risk for drug–drug interactions with maraviroc and to inform appropriate dose adjustments in the presence of potent CYP3A4/Pgp inhibitors and inducers. These studies demonstrated that, as expected, maraviroc had no effect on other drugs, but that maraviroc exposure was increased in the presence of CYP3A4/Pgp inhibitors and decreased in the presence of inducers [70]. However, these interactions could be managed by either increasing or decreasing the maraviroc dose [73].

To demonstrate proof of pharmacology for maraviroc, CCR5 receptor occupancy was determined using a novel MIP-1β internalization assay on ex vivo blood samples from maraviroc versus placebo-treated subjects [29,74]. High levels of functional occupancy were observed in a dose-dependent manner (Figure 9.6), with a significant degree of occupancy even at subnanomolar-free drug concentrations (EC_{50} for *in vivo* CCR5 functional blockade in humans estimated to be 0.13 nM) [29,75].

Assessment of phase 1 safety data indicated that maraviroc was safe and well tolerated at multiple doses up to 300 mg twice daily (BID) in healthy volunteers. The dose-limiting adverse event in the phase 1 studies was postural hypotension which was seen at a rate higher than placebo at unit doses of $\geq$600 mg [69,76]. A thorough QT study confirmed that maraviroc had no effect on the QTcF interval at single doses of up to 900 mg [77].

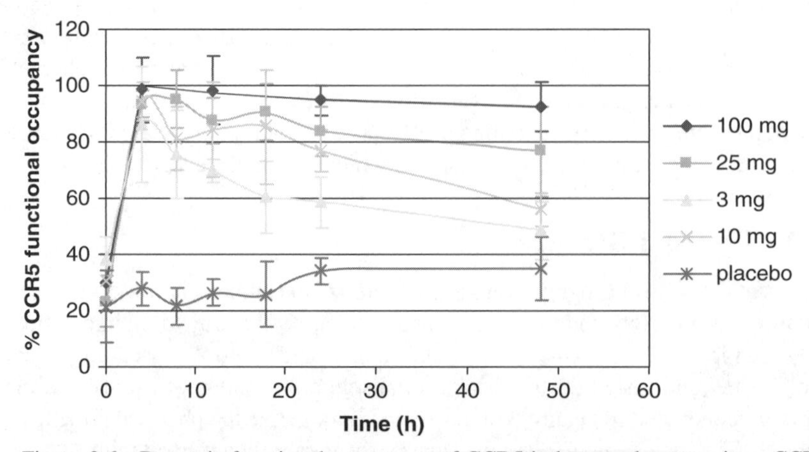

Figure 9.6 Dynamic functional occupancy of CCR5 in humans by maraviroc. CCR5 receptor occupancy was evaluated using an *ex vivo* MIP-1β internalization assay. Peripheral blood mononuclear cells were isolated from blood samples taken at time indicated following single doses to healthy volunteers. Reproduced from Ref. [29]. (See color version of the figure in Color Plate section)

9.6.2 Phase 2a Studies

Following the successful demonstration of proof-of-pharmacology, better than expected PK, and an encouraging safety profile, a phase 2a proof-of-concept program was initiated. Eighty-two patients with HIV RNA >5000 copies mL^{-1}, CD4 >250 cells mm^{-3}, and prescreened for the absence of CXCR4-using virus using a newly developed phenotypic tropism assay were randomized to receive maraviroc monotherapy [25,100, or 300 mg QD or 50, 100, 150 (both fed and fasted) or 300 mg BID] or placebo for 10 days with follow-up until day 40 (Figure 9.7). Maraviroc was well tolerated. Mean viral load change from baseline to day 11 ranged from -0.43 $\log_{10}$ copies mL^{-1} (25 mg QD) to 1.60 $\log_{10}$ copies mL^{-1} (300 mg BID). Maximum viral load reduction occurred between days 10–15 (mean $\geq$1.6 $\log_{10}$ copies mL^{-1} at all doses $\geq$100 mg BID). There was no significant difference in mean viral load reductions at 300 mg QD and 150 mg BID, nor with dosing with food at 150 mg BID [28a].

Since maraviroc does not act on a viral target, but rather is an antagonist of a human cellular receptor, CCR5 receptor occupancy (determined as described above) and pharmacokinetics were examined in parallel. While a relationship could be demonstrated between antiviral efficacy and the plasma AUC of maraviroc, receptor occupancy was not a predictor of virological outcome [28a]. The viral load data was subjected to modeling with the occupancy and PK information. The results demonstrated that 98.5% occupancy was required to achieve the EC_{50} for viral load reduction, with >99.9% required for a maximal response [74b,74c]. The favorable primary pharmacology profile of maraviroc (i.e., potency at the CCR5 receptor and slow offset) enabled potent and prolonged *in vivo* occupancy. However, the inherent replication rate and amplification of HIV-1 means that >99.9% occupancy was required for clinically useful efficacy [74b,74c].

Confirming the safety data obtained from healthy volunteer studies, maraviroc was consistently well tolerated with the only treatment-emergent adverse events occurring more than once in treatment group (including placebo) being headache, asthenia (reduced energy, tiredness), dizziness, gingivitis, and nausea [28a].

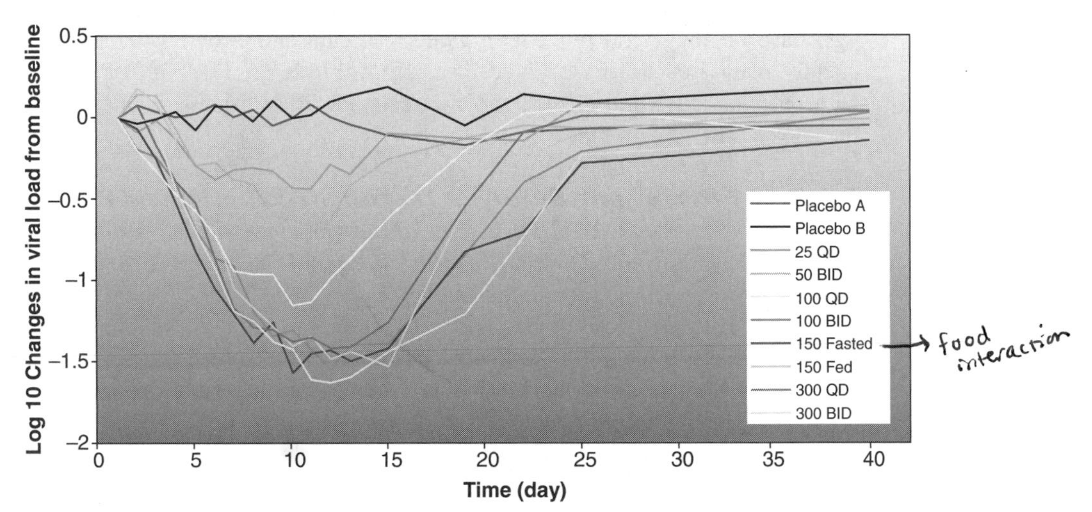

Figure 9.7 Phase 2a dose-ranging studies: dose-dependent reduction in viral load following 10 days of monotherapy. Subjects who were antiretroviral therapy naïve, or have been off therapy for at least 8 weeks, received maraviroc or placebo for 10 days at the doses indicated. HIV-RNA was monitored during dosing and for a 30 day follow-up period after the last dose. QD = once daily; BID = twice daily. Reproduced from Ref. [28]. (See color version of the figure in Color Plate section)

These results provided proof that maraviroc has selective activity against HIV-1 in humans, and demonstrated that it was a safe and viable option for evaluation as part of a combination antiretroviral regimen in a large phase 2b/3 clinical program. Based on assessment of HIV-1 RNA suppression, safety data, pharmacokinetics and modeling and simulation using a PK–PD-disease model, nominal doses of 300 mg QD and 300 mg BID (adjusted to 150 mg in the presence of potent CYP3A4 inhibitors) were selected for testing in a phase 2b/3 program.

9.6.3 Phase 2b/3 Studies

The HIV patient population is extremely heterogeneic, ranging from treatment-naïve to heavily treatment-experienced patients with multiclass resistant virus and very limited or no remaining treatment options. These different patient groups not only represent different challenges, but also have differing needs. In treatment-naïve patients, the key needs are for safe, convenient and well-tolerated drugs in order to improve adherence and prolong efficacy of initial regimens. In contrast, the overwhelming need for heavily treatment-experienced patients is new drugs with activity against multidrug and multi-class resistant virus. As maraviroc represented a new class of antiretroviral therapy with demonstrated *in vitro* activity across a broad range of clinical isolates, including drug-resistant virus, and an excellent safety profile in early clinical studies, evaluation of the long-term safety and efficacy across the entire range of HIV-infected patient populations was merited. The phase 2b/3 program was therefore designed as a book-end program, with studies including patients at the extreme ends of the spectrum, and assuming that demonstration of efficacy and safety at both extremes would translate to the entire population.

The outcome of these studies has been extremely encouraging [78]. Maraviroc (300 mg BID) received approval from the U.S. Food and Drug Administration (FDA) in August 2007, and subsequently from multiple regulatory authorities around the world for use in combination with other antiretroviral agents, in treating adults with R5-HIV-1 infection who have strains that are resistant to multiple other antiretroviral agents and who have ongoing viral replication while receiving antiretroviral therapy [71]. Subsequently, maraviroc 300 mg BID received approval from the FDA for use, in combination with other antiretroviral agents, for the treatment of ART-naïve adults with R5-HIV-1 infection [71b].

9.6.3.1 Efficacy and Safety in Treatment-Experienced Patients Two large phase 3 studies (MOTIVATE 1 and 2) of maraviroc QD or BID plus optimized background therapy (OBT) versus placebo plus OBT in highly treatment-experienced patients with R5 virus at screening visit were conducted [78,79]. A total of 1049 patients received at least one dose of maraviroc across these two studies. Tropism testing was conducted using a laboratory validated phenotypic tropism assay [80]. Individual and pooled 48-week data from the MOTIVATE studies demonstrated a significant virologic benefit for patients receiving an OBT with maraviroc (QD or BID) [79], with >45% of maraviroc treated patients achieving an undetectable viral load (<50 copies mL^{-1}) compared to <20% of those receiving placebo (Figure 9.8).

This benefit was maintained across different subgroups including those with low $CD4^{+}$ cell counts, high baseline viraemia and weak or inactive OBT regimens [78]. Additional MOTIVATE subanalyses assessing the association between OBT activity and maraviroc outcomes have demonstrated that for those patients receiving maraviroc with at least two fully active agents other than NRTIs, a virologic response rate (HIV RNA <50

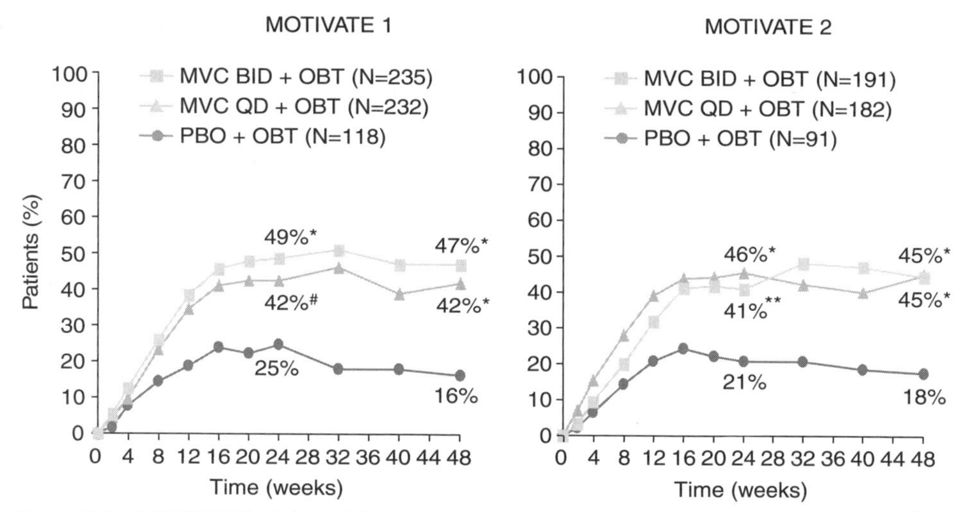

Figure 9.8 MOTIVATE clinical trials: percentage of patients with HIV-1 RNA <50 copies mL^{-1} at week 48 in the MOTIVATE 1 (USA) and MOTIVATE 2 (Europe, Australia and USA) studies. HIV-infected patients with triple class experience and/or triple class resistance were randomised to receive maraviroc once or twice daily, or placebo; all in combination with an optimised background regimen (consisting of 3–6 antiretroviral drugs) selected by the investigator. MVC = maraviroc; OBT = optimised background therapy; PBO = placebo; QD = once daily; BID = twice daily.

copies mL^{-1}) of 70% was observed, rising to 80% in those initiating maraviroc with two active agents and a baseline CD4^{+} count >50 cells mm^{-3} [81].

Maraviroc also demonstrated considerable immunological benefit in the MOTIVATE studies, with consistently greater CD4^{+} cell increases in patients receiving maraviroc compared to those receiving placebo. This benefit was maintained even in patients with very low baseline CD4 counts and high baseline viral load [78,79].

Evaluation of the safety of a CCR5 antagonist in patients infected with a mixture of viruses that may include CXCR4-using variants is important, because such patients could inadvertently receive a CCR5 antagonist. A phase 2b study was therefore conducted to determine the safety and efficacy of maraviroc in combination with optimized background therapy in treatment-experienced patients infected with dual- or mixed-tropic HIV-1. In contrast to the results in treatment-experienced patients with R5 virus, no virological benefit accrued to treatment with maraviroc over placebo when both were given with an OBT to patients with non-R5 virus in the phase 2b 1029 study [82]. However, a significantly greater increase in CD4^{+} cell counts was seen on maraviroc than on placebo in the week 24 primary analysis. This difference was also noted at week 48 but was not statistically significant [82]. Taken together, the results from the MOTIVATE studies in patients with CCR5 tropic virus, together with the lack of virologic benefit demonstrated in this study in patients with non-CCR5 tropic virus validated the clinical predictive value of the tropism assay.

Despite the concerns discussed above regarding the long-term safety of CCR5 antagonists, data from these studies have shown maraviroc to be well tolerated with an adverse event profile similar to placebo and with no evidence of an increased rate of malignancies or hepatotoxicity [79,82]. Although postural hypotension (at unit doses of 600 mg or more) was identified as the dose-limiting adverse event for maraviroc in phase 1 clinical trials, there was no evidence of an excess of adverse events related to postural hypotension in these studies.

9.6.3.2 Efficacy and Safety in Treatment-Naïve Patients Efficacy and safety in treatment-naive patients with R5 virus was demonstrated in the MERIT study, which randomized patients to receive maraviroc QD or BID or efavirenz QD, each with a fixed background of Combivir [83]. Maraviroc QD was discontinued following a week-16 interim analysis on the first 205 patients, as it did not meet predefined noninferiority criteria to efavirenz; randomization to the efavirenz and maraviroc BID arms continued unchanged. In the primary 48-week analysis, 64% of maraviroc-treated patients compared to 69% of efavirenz-treated patients achieved a viral load of <50 copies mL^{-1}; this did not meet the criteria for noninferiority at the 10% threshold level [83]. More maraviroc patients discontinued for lack of efficacy (11.9% vs. 4.2%), but fewer discontinued for adverse events (4.2% vs. 13.6%). Subsequent rescreening of the MERIT patient set with a more sensitive tropism assay [84] identified a 15% incidence of non-R5 screening samples which had been below the limit of detection of the original assay. Exclusion of these patients from a *post-hoc* reanalysis of the main study endpoints resulted in greater response rates in the maraviroc arm at week 48, which fell within the criteria defining noninferiority for the full, prospective patient set at week 48 (Figure 9.9) [83].

With study centers that included sites in both South Africa and South America, this study enrolled a significant proportion of patients with nonclade B infections [including more than 400 patients (~30%) infected with clade C HIV], and therefore provided clinical confirmation of the *in vitro* data showing maraviroc to be active against viruses with envelopes of both B and non-B origin [83].

Consistent with data from the studies in treatment-experienced patients, subjects receiving maraviroc demonstrated greater increases in $CD4^+$ cell count than those receiving efavirenz, with mean changes in $CD4^+$ count from baseline of +170 cells mL^{-1} during maraviroc therapy versus +144 cells mL^{-1} during efavirenz therapy [difference (maraviroc minus efavirenz), +26 cells mL^{-1} (95% CI, +7 to +46 cells mL^{-1})] [83].

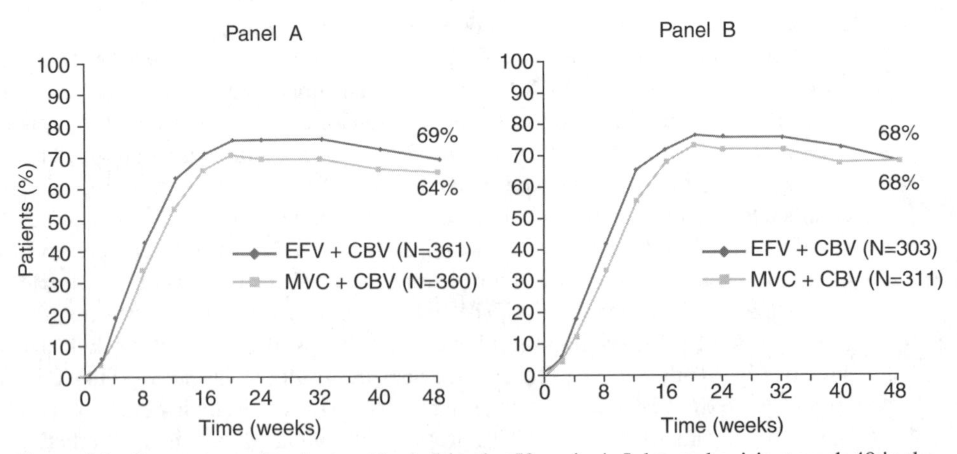

Figure 9.9 Proportions of patients with viral load <50 copies/mL by study visit at week 48 in the primary analysis (Panel A) and in the post hoc reanalysis (Panel B), using the enhanced tropism assay. Treatment-naïve HIV-1 infected patients were randomised to receive maraviroc twice daily or efavirenz once daily, both in combination with combivir. The primary analysis included patients with CCR5 tropic virus as determined using the original Trofile™ (panel A). A post-hoc reanalysis was performed upon release of the enhanced sensitivity Trofile™ assay (panel B). This analysis excluded patients with non-CCR5 tropic virus at screening using the enhanced assay. EFV = efavirenz; MVC = maraviroc; CBV = combivir (lamivudine plus zidovudine fixed dose combination). Adapted from Ref. [83].

A similar proportion of patients on maraviroc and efavirenz experienced adverse events, however, as discussed earlier more patients on efavirenz discontinued therapy due to adverse events. The proportion of patients with grade 3 or 4 adverse events or SAEs were slightly lower in the maraviroc arm. Twice as many patients experienced category C events during efavirenz therapy (3.3% vs. 1.7%). Malignancies were also twice as common in the efavirenz arm [7 vs. 3 events, affecting 7 (1.9%) vs. 2 (0.6%) patients]. The overall incidence of grade 3 or 4 increases in transaminase levels was low, and the incidences were similar in both treatment groups [83]. One patient in the discontinued once-daily maraviroc arm experienced potentially life-threatening hepatotoxicity. The data implicated isoniazid and/or cotrimoxazole toxicity, but maraviroc could not be ruled out as a potential contributor [85].

9.6.4 Development of Resistance to CCR5 Antagonists *In Vivo*

As discussed above (Section 9.3.3), there are two potential pathways of virologic escape from CCR5 antagonists: selection of R5 virus that can use the drug-bound CCR5 receptor to enter host cells; and "un-masking" of pre-existing populations of dual-tropic or CXCR4-tropic (X4) virus (collectively called "CXCR4-using" viruses) during selective drug pressure by a CCR5 antagonist. Viral escape via both of these pathways was assessed in the maraviroc clinical program.

9.6.4.1 Treatment Failure with R5 Virus Plateaus in maximum percentage inhibition (MPI) have been identified as markers of resistance to maraviroc *in vitro* [50c], and are consistent with the drug acting as an allosteric, noncompetitive inhibitor of viral entry [86]. The results of the clinical studies suggest that virologic failure with R5 virus that has reduced susceptibility to maraviroc occurs in <50% of patients. Analysis of isolates from treatment-experienced patients failing maraviroc-containing regimens with R5 virus in the MOTIVATE studies demonstrated that ~40% of patients had maraviroc-resistant virus (MPI value <95%) at virologic failure [87]. For those patients who failed with maraviroc-susceptible R5 virus, virologic failure was accounted for by incomplete adherence to the drug regimen, as evidenced by low or undetectable maraviroc plasma concentrations during periodic pharmacokinetic sampling, or by documented treatment interruption [87]. Virologic failure with maraviroc-resistant R5 virus was primarily observed in patients with persistent detectable viremia who had no fully active drugs present in their OBT at baseline (i.e., who received functional maraviroc monotherapy), or whose only active background drug was an NRTI. No maraviroc resistance was seen in samples from patients receiving maraviroc with the equivalent of at least two fully active background agents (even those who never achieved <50 copies mL^{-1} on study) or among those with virologic rebound following suppression to <50 copies mL^{-1} [88]. Resistance to maraviroc in patients failing with R5 virus was uncommon in the MERIT study (two of 12 patients studied) [89].

9.6.4.2 Treatment Failure with CXCR4-Using Virus Evaluation of tropism data at week 48 in the MOTIVATE studies indicated that ~55% of treatment-experienced patients who failed on a maraviroc-containing regimen had evidence of CXCR4-using virus at the time of virologic failure [78]. Clonal and phylogenetic analyses of a representative subset of these patients found that, in all cases, the CXCR4-using variants observed at virologic failure were the result of unmasking and outgrowth of pre-existing minority populations, present at baseline but at levels too low to be detected by the screening tropism assay [90].

TABLE 9.3 Mean Change from Baseline in CD4$^+$ Count in Patients with Treatment Failure (cells mm^{-3})[120]

	OBT alone $N=209$	MVC QD + OBT $N=414$	MVC BID + OBT $N=426$
All treatment failures[a]	24 ($n=111$)	64 ($n=92$)	74 ($n=96$)
R5 → R5	25 ($n=89$)	77 ($n=3$)	133 ($n=24$)
R5 → D/M or X4	61 ($n=6$)	47 ($n=35$)	51 ($n=41$)

[a]Includes patients with non-R5 tropism result at baseline

Abbreviations: OBT, Optimized background therapy; QD, once daily; BID, twice daily; R5, CCR5 tropic virus; D/M, dual or mixed tropiv virus; X4, CXCR4 tropic virus.

There was a higher mean change in the CD4 cell count in patients in whom maraviroc failed than in patients who received placebo (Table 9.3). Patients with a virus binding to CXCR4 in whom maraviroc failed had a smaller increase in the CD4 cell count from baseline, as compared with patients who had a CCR5 tropism result at the time of failure; however, even in this population, the increase in the CD4 cell count from baseline was still higher than that in the overall placebo group and could be due to the fact that time to virologic failure was approximately 2 months shorter in this group [78].

This finding is further supported by data from the MERIT study, in which patients failing maraviroc, a significant proportion of whom had CXCR4-using virus detected at failure had greater increases in CD4$^+$ cell count at treatment failure than those failing the efavirenz comparator regimen, irrespective of tropism result at failure [89]. Moreover, emergence of CXCR4-using virus on maraviroc treatment does not appear to be associated with an adverse clinical outcome, as evidenced by the lack of any correlation between emergence of CXCR4-using virus and development of CDC category C events (AIDS-defining clinical events) over the course of the MOTIVATE studies [91]. This was also supported by recently published data from the MERIT study demonstrating no adverse clinical or immunological consequence in patients with emergence of CXCR4-using virus [92]. Tropism results showed that the majority of MOTIVATE 1 and 2 patients experiencing treatment failure on maraviroc in the context of CXCR4-using virus with more than 1 month of follow-up had reverted back to R5 after maraviroc withdrawal [91]. Altogether these data indicate that Maraviroc selectively inhibits R5 virus, and if it is administered as part of a suboptimal regimen, pre-existing low (undetected) levels of D/M or X4 virus will emerge as the dominant viral population. Since the dual/mixed or X4 virus is pre-existing, time to failure is shorter than with R5 virus (where maraviroc resistance must be selected *de novo*); this is similar to the rapid outgrowth of pre-existing (archived) drug-resistant virus when failed ARV therapy is reinitiated after treatment interruption. After withdrawal of maraviroc, selective pressure on R5 virus is removed, allowing R5 virus to once more become the dominant population. This reversion to R5 takes approximately 16 weeks, consistent with what has been shown for 3TC [93] and enfuvirtide resistance [94] after withdrawal of these ARVs.

9.7 SUMMARY, FUTURE DIRECTIONS, AND CHALLENGES

Maraviroc is the first host-targeted antiretroviral drug. Its discovery presented multiple challenges. During the discovery process, key challenges were the absence of a convenient high-throughput screening assay and balancing antiviral activity, clearance and hERG activity. In order to arrive at the compound known as maraviroc, more than 900 synthetic analogs were made and a systematic screening cascade was developed to profile the compounds and to select the most appropriate ones for further evaluation. In the clinical development program, extensive use of PK–PD-disease modeling and an aggressive phase 2b/3 development program allowed the demonstration that maraviroc is not only safe and effective in both treatment-naïve and treatment-experienced patient, but that emergence of CXCR4-using virus under selective pressure from maraviroc does not have deleterious consequences, while at the same time validating a novel tropism assay. Additionally the preclinical and clinical mechanism of viral escape from maraviroc was described. In spite of these challenges to the discovery and development program, a new drug application was filed just more than 10 years after the first demonstration of CCR5 as a key HIV-1 coreceptor; which constitutes a remarkable achievement.

The disappointing outcomes to date in HIV vaccine research have resulted in much debate on the use of anti-HIV drugs as prophylactic agents. This follows the phenomenal success in pre-exposure prophylaxis to prevent vertical mother-to-child transmission, and prophylactic strategies have been widely discussed [95]. Although subject to considerable operational challenge, this remains a distinct goal in light of the devastating mortality and morbidity of HIV-1 infection and large numbers of new infections that occur daily. CCR5 antagonists are compelling candidates for either oral or topical prophylactic therapy due to their mechanism of early stage entry inhibition, barrier to resistance, the relative lack of infectivity of CXCR4 utilizing virus and the slow physical and functional offset of CCR5 antagonists yielding a favorable pharmacodynamic effect. The potential for oral prophylaxis, although currently not being evaluated in a clinical setting is an exciting prospect for maraviroc, following encouraging PK data demonstrating high concentrations of maraviroc in the female genital tract and rectal tissue and semen of healthy male volunteers following oral dosing [96]. Encouraging data on CCR5 antagonists [97] and peptide analogs of cognate ligands were also seen in small primate studies [98]. Similar studies have been undertaken with other mechanistic classes [99].

A significant initiative has been the establishment in 2002 of The International Partnership for Microbicides (IPM), aimed at accelerating the development and accessibility of microbicides to prevent HIV-1 transmission in women [100]. By screening compounds, designing optimal formulations, establishing manufacturing capacity, developing trial sites and conducting clinical trials, IPM works to improve the efficiency of all efforts to develop and deliver safe and effective microbicides as soon as possible. The favorable pharmacology of CCR5 antagonists strongly supports the use of these compounds by this approach [101], and many companies have agreed to free licenses to evaluate their respective CCR5 antagonists with respect to prophylactic activity in clinical trials. The IPM has been granted a nonexclusive royalty-free license to develop maraviroc as a vaginal microbicide. Most recently, it has been demonstrated that a maraviroc and dapivirine combination could be effectively incorporated within a single matrix-type silicon vaginal ring device and provide sustained release [102].

The recent demonstration of an important proof of principle that topical antiretroviral drugs could be an effective tool for prevention of HIV-1 infection through the results of the CAPRISA 0004 trial has increased the sense of urgency in this area of HIV research. This double-blind, randomized, controlled study assessed effectiveness and safety of a 1% vaginal gel formulation of tenofovir for the prevention of HIV infection in women. Tenofovir or placebo gel was evaluated in sexually active, HIV-uninfected 18- to 40-year-old women in urban and rural KwaZulu-Natal, South Africa. HIV serostatus was assessed at monthly follow-up visits for 30 months. In high adherers (>80%), HIV incidence was 54% lower ($P = 0.025$) in the tenofovir gel arm. In intermediate adherers (gel adherence 50 to 80%) and low adherers (gel adherence <50%), the HIV incidence reduction was 38% and 28%, respectively. Tenofovir gel, therefore, reduced HIV incidence by an estimated 39% [103].

HIV-1 infection managed through HAART is broadly considered a chronic (indeed life-long) rather than acute disease, and it is the complications of age-related problems that are providing significant new burdens on patients and healthcare systems. This is double-edged as it reflects the overall success of HAART in enabling life expectancy to be near-normal, but the morbidity of liver, kidney, cardiac, and dementia-associated diseases are becoming more prevalent in this population [104]. Importantly, several currently used antiretroviral drug classes are associated with metabolic adverse events which may further increase the risk for cardiovascular disease [105], especially in the context of an aging population. Data from across the phase 2b/3 maraviroc clinical program, which involved >2000 patients exposed to maraviroc over periods in excess of 96 weeks [79,82,83,106], indicate that maraviroc has a tolerability profile similar to that of placebo. Furthermore, analyses of lipid data from the MERIT study have suggested that maraviroc may offer some advantages compared with efavirenz in terms of effects on cholesterol and triglycerides—for example, in patients with elevated levels of low-density lipoprotein cholesterol before treatment, who may be at increased long-term risk for cardiovascular disease [107]. Altogether this may indicate that long-term therapy with maraviroc could result in less metabolic effects than is seen with currently used regimens and merits further study.

Antiretroviral therapy inhibits HIV-1 replication, allowing recovery of $CD4^+$ T-cell numbers and the restoration of immune function; its introduction has led to improved outcomes for individuals with HIV-1 infection. However, it has been observed that some individuals responding to HAART experience a clinical deterioration with symptoms and signs of an inflammatory illness, known as immune reconstitution inflammatory syndrome (IRIS) [108]. This results from pathological immune responses occurring during immune reconstitution. IRIS is best considered a group of disorders with a wide range of clinical manifestations, incorporating disease resulting from pathological inflammation to pathogens, immune-mediated inflammatory disease and autoimmune disease. Clinical effects range from a mild, self-limiting illness to severe morbidity and mortality. Clinicians working in the field of HIV-1 medicine can expect to encounter individuals with IRIS [109]. This is a relatively new area of HIV-1 medicine, and one for which CCR5 antagonists generally could provide utility in treatment (i.e., reduction of IRIS) in light of the mechanism of action involving antagonism of an immune signaling receptor. This remains fairly speculative, but monitoring of inflammatory or indeed cited IRIS biomarkers [110] for retrospective and prospective maraviroc-associated studies has merit.

The high cost and long turnaround times of phenotypic assays for identifying tropism has been a barrier to using maraviroc in some patients, and HIV coreceptor tropism assessment remains an area of active ongoing research. Currently the determination of HIV-1 tropism uses primarily biological phenotypic assays, and this is the only form of tropism testing that has been validated in large scale clinical studies to date. However, there is considerable interest in developing improved genotypic methods to predict tropism [111], which are relatively inexpensive and typically have faster turnaround times compared with the recombinant phenotype methods. Validation of their potential applicability for routine clinical use is underway [112].

Non-HIV indications arguably offer a more compelling and widespread new utility for maraviroc [75]. Discovering drugs for indications other than which they were originally designed for has a very fruitful track record and is associated with low cost R&D

success [113]. This is inherently compelling due to maraviroc being an approved and safe medicine, but also because a host of correlations and supportive data from pharmacogenomic, *ex vivo*, and preclinical studies have directly highlighted, or at least implicated, the use of CCR5 antagonists for many indications [114]. Specifically, these include inflammation [115], multiple sclerosis [116], rheumatoid arthritis [117], graft rejection [118], IBD [119], endometriosis [120], diabetes [115a,121], renal diseases [122], liver fibrosis [123], pancreatitis [119,124], respiratory disease [125], heart disease [126], psoriasis and dermatitis [127], stroke [128], obesity [129], Alzheimer's disease [130], atherosclerosis [131], cancer [119,132], and pain [115b,133].

Evaluation of clinical candidates for efficacy or proof of concept is fraught with high financial risk, so data that provides evidence for the utility of maraviroc in IRIS or non-HIV indications from retrospective and prospective HIV-1 trials by appropriate endpoint analysis and biomarker evaluations is important. Preclinical studies using animal models of disease are challenging and also pose translational risks, especially as maraviroc and other selective CCR5 antagonists to date do not bind rodent CCR5. However, human CCR5 "knock-in" mice (where the human receptor ORF supplants the endogenous murine CCR5 sequence) have been constructed [29,75]. In conclusion, maraviroc and CCR5 antagonists in general represent a significant breakthrough in terms of offering a host-mediated mechanism to combat HIV-1 infection and offer a new therapeutic option for patients. Research to investigate their wider use in HIV-1 infection, prophylaxis, and immunology-associated conditions is merited.

ACKNOWLEDGMENTS

The authors wish to thank all CCR5 and HIV-associated team members at Pfizer, together with collaborators, clinical trial volunteers, and patients for their contributions to the maraviroc project that have provided the substrate for this chapter. Particular thanks are due to Hernan Valdez and Simon Portsmouth for their constructive review of this chapter.

Maraviroc was discovered at Pfizer Sandwich, UK. The legacy of this wonderful site and its talented people will live on.

REFERENCES

1. Masur, H., Michelis, M. A., Greene, J. B., Onorato, I., Stouwe, R. A., Holzman, R. S., Wormser, G., Brettman, L., Lange, M., Murray, H. W., and Cunningham-Rundles, S. An outbreak of community-acquired *Pneumocystis carinii* pneumonia: initial manifestation of cellular immune dysfunction. *N. Engl. J. Med.* **1981**, *305*, 1431–1438.
2. Barre-Sinoussi, F., Chermann, J. C., Rey, F., Nugeyre, M. T., Chamaret, S., Gruest, J., Dauguet, C., Axler-Blin, C., Vezinet-Brun, F., Rouzioux, C., Rozenbaum, W., and Montagnier, L. Isolation of a T-lymphotropic retrovirus from a patient at risk for acquired immune deficiency syndrome (AIDS). *Science*, **1983**, *220*, 868–871.
3. Gallo, R. C., Sarin, P. S., Gelmann, E. P., Robert-Guroff, M., Richardson, E., Kalyanaraman, V. S., Mann, D., Sidhu, G. D., Stahl, R. E., Zolla-Pazner, S., Leibowitch, J., and Popovic, M. Isolation of human T-cell leukemia virus in acquired immune deficiency syndrome (AIDS). *Science*, **1983**, *220*, 865–867.
4. http://www.unaids.org/en/Dataanalysis/Epidemiology/ (**2008**) 2007 AIDS Pandemic Update.
5. Yarchoan, R., and Broder, S. Development of antiretroviral therapy for the acquired immunodeficiency syndrome and related disorders. *N. Engl. J. Med.* **1987**, *316*, 557–564.
6. Carr, A. Toxicity of antiretroviral therapy and implications for drug development. *Nat. Rev. Drug Discov.* **2003**, *2*, 624–634.
7. Martinez-Picado, J., DePasquale, M. P., Kartsonis, N., Hanna, G. J., Wong, J., Finzi, D., Rosenberg, E., Gunthard, H. F., Sutton, L., Savara, A., Petropoulos, C. J., Hellmann, N., Walker, B. D., Richman, D. D., Siliciano, R., and D'Aquila, R. T.

Antiretroviral resistance during successful therapy of HIV type 1 infection. *Proc. Natl. Acad. Sci. USA*. **2000**, *97*, 10948–10953.

8. Richman, D. D., Morton, S. C., Wrin, T., Hellmann, N., Berry, S., Shapiro, M. F., and Bozzette, S. A. The prevalence of antiretroviral drug resistance in the United States. *Aids*, **2004**, *18*, 1393–1401.
9. (a) Little, S. J., Holte, S., Routy, J. P., Daar, E. S., Markowitz, M., Collier, A. C., Koup, R. A., Mellors, J. W., Connick, E., Conway, B., Kilby, M., Wang, L., Whitcomb, J. M., Hellmann, N. S., and Richman, D. D. Antiretroviral-drug resistance among patients recently infected with HIV. *N. Engl. J. Med.* **2002**, *347*, 385–394: (b) Shet, A., Berry, L., Mohri, H., Mehandru, S., Chung, C., Kim, A., Jean-Pierre, P., Hogan, C., Simon, V., Boden, D., and Markowitz, M. Tracking the prevalence of transmitted antiretroviral drug-resistant HIV-1: a decade of experience. *J. Acquir. Immune Defic. Syndr.* **2006**, *41*, 439–446.
10. Maddon P. J., Dalgleish, A. G., McDougal, J. S., Clapham, P. R., Weiss, R. A., and Axel, R. The T4 gene encodes the AIDS virus receptor and is expressed in the immune system and the brain. *Cell*. **1986**, *47*, 333–348.
11. Cocchi, F., DeVico, A. L., Garzino-Demo, A., Arya, S. K., Gallo, R. C., and Lusso P. Identification of RANTES, MIP-1 alpha, and MIP-1 beta as the major HIV-suppressive factors produced by $CD8^+$ T cells. *Science*. **1995**, *270*, 1811–1815.
12. Liu R, Paxton, W. A., Choe, S., Ceradini, D., Martin, S. R., Horuk, R., MacDonald, M.E., Stuhlmann, H., Koup, R. A., and Landau, N. R. Homozygous defect in HIV-1 coreceptor accounts for resistance of some multiply-exposed individuals to HIV-1 infection. *Cell*. **1996**, *86*, 367–377.
13. Feng Y, Broder, C., Kennedy, P. E., and Berger, E. A. HIV-1 entry cofactor: functional cDNA cloning of a seven-transmembrane, *G protein-coupled receptor*. *Science*. **1996**, *272*, 872–877.
14. (a) Kwong, P.D., Wyatt, R., Robinson, J., Sweet, R. W., Sodroski, J., and Hendrickson, W. A. Structure of an HIV gp120 envelope glycoprotein in complex with the CD4 receptor and a neutralizing human antibody. *Nature*. **1998**, *393*, 648–659: (b) Rizzuto, C. D., Wyatt, R., Hernandez-Ramos, N., Sun, Y., Kwong, P. D., Hendrickson, W. A., Sodroski, J. A conserved HIV gp120 glycoprotein structure involved in chemokine receptor binding. *Science*. **1998**, *280*, 1949–1953: (c) Wyatt, R., K. P., Desjardins, E., Sweet, R. W., Robinson, J., Hendrickson, W. A., and Sodroski, J. G. The antigenic structure of the HIV gp120 envelope glycoprotein. *Nature*. **1998**, *393*, 705–711.
15. Chan, D. C., Kim, P. S. HIV entry and its inhibition. *Cell*. **1998**, *93*, 681–684.
16. (a) Dragic, T., Litwin, V., Allaway, G. P., Martin, S. R., Huang, Y., Nagashima, K. A., Cayanan, C., Maddon, P. J., Koup, R. A., Moore, J. P., and Paxton, W. A. HIV-1 entry into $CD4^+$ cells is mediated by the chemokine receptor CC-CKR-5. *Nature*. **1996**, *381*, 667–673: (b) Deng, H., Liu, R., Ellmeier, W., Choe, S., Unutmaz, D., Burkhart, M., Di Marzio, P., Marmon, S., Sutton, R. E., Hill, C. E., Davis, C. B., Peiper, S. C., Schall, T. J., Littman, D. R., and Landau, N. R. Identification of a major co-receptor for primary isolates of HIV-1. *Nature*, **1996**, *381*, 661–666: (c) Choe, H., Farzan, M., Sun, Y., Sullivan, N., Rollins, B., Ponath, P. D., Wu, L., Mackay, C. R., LaRosa, G., Newman, W., Gerard, N., Gerard, C., and Sodroski, J. The beta-chemokine receptors CCR3 and CCR5 facilitate infection by primary HIV-1 isolates. *Cell*. **1996**, *85*, 1135–1148.
17. Berger, E. A., Domas, R. W., Fenyo, E. M., Korber, B. T., Littman, D. R., Moore, J. P., Sattentau, Q. J., Schuitemaker, H., Sodroski, J., and Weiss, R. A. A new classification for HIV-1. *Nature*. **1998**, *391*, 240.
18. (a) Derdeyn, C. A., Decker, J. M., Sfakianos, J. N., Zhang, Z., O'Brien, W. A., Ratner, L., Shaw, G. M., and Hunter, E. Sensitivity of human immunodeficiency virus type 1 to fusion inhibitors targeted to the gp41 first heptad repeat involves distinct regions of gp41 and is consistently modulated by gp120 interactions with the coreceptor *J. Virol.* **2001**, *75*, 8605–8614: (b) Pierson, T. C., Doms, R. W., Pohlmann, S. Prospects of HIV-1 entry inhibitors as novel therapeutics *Rev. Med. Virol.* **2004**, *14*, 255–270.
19. Chen, R. Y., Kilby, J. M., and Saag, M. S. Enfuvirtide. [Review] [27 refs]. *Expert Opin. Invest. Drugs*. **2002**, *11*, 1837–1843.
20. Greenberg, M. L., and Cammack, N. Resistance to enfuvirtide, the first HIV fusion inhibitor. *J. Antimicrob. Chemother.* **2004**, *54*, 333–340.
21. Lin, P. F., Blair, W., Wang, T., Spicer, T., Guo, Q., Zhou, N., Gong, Y. F., Wang, H. G., Rose, R., Yamanaka, G., Robinson, B., Li, C. B., Fridell, R., Deminie, C., Demers, G., Yang, Z., Zadjura, L., Meanwell, N., and Colonno, R. A small molecule HIV-1 inhibitor that targets the HIV-1 envelope and inhibits CD4 receptor binding. [see comment]. *Proc. Natl. Acad. Sci. USA*. **2003**, *100*, 11013–11018.
22. Hendrix, C. W., Collier, A. C., Lederman, M. M., Schols, D., Pollard, R. B., Brown, S., Jackson, J. B., Coombs, R. W., Glesby, M. J., Flexner, C. W., Bridger, G. J., Badel, K., MacFarland, R. T., Henson, G. W., and Calandra, G. Safety, pharmacokinetics, and antiviral activity of AMD3100, a selective CXCR4 receptor inhibitor, in HIV-1 infection *J. Acquir. Immune Defic. Syndr.* **2004**, *37*, 1253–1262.
23. Charo, I. F., and Ransohoff, R. M. The many roles of chemokines and chemokine receptors in inflammation. *N. Engl. J. Med.* **2006**, *354*, 610–621.
24. Wise, A., Gearing, K., and Rees, S. Target validation of G-protein coupled receptors *Drug Discov. Today*. **2002**, *7*, 235–246.
25. (a) Dean, M., Carrington, M., Winkler, C., Huttley, G. A., Smith, M. W., Allikmets, R., Goedert, J. J., Buchbinder, S. P., Vittinghoff, E., Gomperts, E., Donfield, S., Vlahov, D., Kaslow, R., Saah, A., Rinaldo, C., Detels, R., and O'Brien, S. J. Genetic

restriction of HIV-1 infection and progression to AIDS by a deletion allele of the CKR5 structural gene. Hemophilia Growth and Development Study, Multicenter AIDS Cohort Study, Multicenter Hemophilia Cohort Study, San Francisco City Cohort, ALIVE Study. *Science*, **1996** *273*, 1856–1862: (b) Huang, Y., Paxton, W. A., Wolinsky, S. M., Neumann, A. U., Zhang, L., He, T., Kang, S., Ceradini, D., Jin, Z., Yazdanbakhsh, K., Kunstman, K., Erickson, D., Dragon, E., Landau, N. R., Phair, J., Ho, D. D., and Koup, R. A. The role of a mutant CCR5 allele in HIV-1 transmission and disease progression. *Nat. Med.* **1996**, *2*, 1240–1243: (c) Liu, R., Paxton, W. A., Choe, S., Ceradini, D., Martin, S. R., Horuk, R., MacDonald, M. E., Stuhlmann, H., Koup, R. A., and Landau, N. R. Homozygous defect in HIV-1 coreceptor accounts for resistance of some multiply-exposed individuals to HIV-1 infection *Cell*, **1996**, *86*, 367–377: (d) Samson, M., Libert, F., Doranz, B. J., Rucker, J., Liesnard, C., Farber, C. M., Saragosti, S., Lapoumeroulie, C., Cognaux, J., Forceille, C., Muyldermans, G., Verhofstede, C., Burtonboy, G., Georges, M., Imai, T., Rana, S., Yi, Y., Smyth, R. J., Collman, R. G., Doms, R. W., Vassart, G., and Parmentier, M. Resistance to HIV-1 infection in Caucasian individuals bearing mutant alleles of the CCR-5 chemokine receptor gene [see comment]. *Nature*, **1996**, *382*, 722–725.

26. Ometto, L., Bertorelle, R., Mainardi, M., Zanchetta, M., Tognazzo, S., Rampon, O., Ruga, E., Chieco-Bianchi, L., and De Rossi, A. Polymorphisms in the CCR5 promoter region influence disease progression in perinatally human immunodeficiency virus type 1-infected children. *J. Infect. Dis.*, **2001**, *183*, 814–818.
27. (a) Cocchi, F., DeVico, A. L., Garzino-Demo, A., Arya, S. K., Gallo, R. C., and Lusso, P. Identification of RANTES, MIP-1 alpha, and MIP-1 beta as the major HIV-suppressive factors produced by CD8$^+$ T cells. *Science*. **1995**, *270*, 1811–1815: (b) Cocchi, F., DeVico, A. L., Garzino-Demo, A., Cara, A., Gallo, R. C., and Lusso, P. The V3 domain of the HIV-1 gp120 envelope glycoprotein is critical for chemokine-mediated blockade of infection. *Nat. Med.* **1996**, *2*, 1244–1247: (c) Raport, C. J., Gosling, J., Schweickart, V. L., Gray, P. W., and Charo, I. F. Molecular cloning and functional characterization of a novel human CC chemokine receptor (CCR5) for RANTES, MIP-1beta, and MIP-1alpha. *J. Biol. Chem.*, **1996**, *271*, 17161–17166.
28. (a) Fatkenheuer, G., Pozniak, A. L., Johnson, M. A., Plettenberg, A., Staszewski, S., Hoepelman, A. I., Saag, M. S., Goebel, F. D., Rockstroh, J. K., Dezube, B. J., Jenkins, T. M., Medhurst, C., Sullivan, J. F., Ridgway, C., Abel, S., James, I. T., Youle, M., and van der Ryst, E. Efficacy of short-term monotherapy with maraviroc, a new CCR5 antagonist, in patients infected with HIV-1. *Nat. Med.* **2005**, *11*, 1170–1172: (b) Lalezari, J., Goodrich, J., DeJesus, E., Lampiris, H., Gulick, R., Saag, M., Ridgway, C., McHale, M., Van der Ryst. E., and Mayer, H. Efficacy and Safety of Maraviroc plus Optimized Background Therapy in Viremic ART-experienced Patients Infected with CCR5-tropic HIV-1: 24-Week Results of a Phase 2b/3 Study in the US and Canada, *14th Conference on Retroviruses and Opportunistic Infections*, Abstract. **2007**, 104bLB: (c) Lalezari, J., Thompson, M., Kumar, P., Piliero, P., Davey, R., Patterson, K., Shachoy-Clark, A., Adkison, K., Demarest, J., Lou, Y., Berrey, M., and Piscitelli, S. Antiviral activity and safety of 873140, a novel CCR5 antagonist, during short-term monotherapy in HIV-infected adults. *Aids*. **2005**, *19*, 1443–1448: (d) Nelson, M., Fätkenheuer, G., Konourina, I., Lazzarin, A., Clumeck, N., Horban, A., Tawadrous, M., Sullivan, J., Mayer, H., and Van der Ryst, E. Efficacy and Safety of Maraviroc plus Optimized Background Therapy in Viremic, ART-experienced Patients Infected with CCR5-tropic HIV-1 in Europe, Australia, and North America: 24-Week Results. *14th Conference on Retroviruses and Opportunistic Infections. Los Angeles*, **2007**, 104aLB.
29. Mansfield, R., Able, S., Griffin, P., Irvine, R., James, I., Macartney, M., Miller, K., Napier, C., Navratilova, I., Perros, M., Rickett, G., Root, H., Van der Ryst, E., Westby., and Dorr, P. CCR5 pharmacology methodologies and associated applications. *Methods Enzymol.* **2009**, *460*, 17–55.
30. (a) Philpott, S. HIV-1 coreceptor usage, transmission, and disease progression. *Current HIV Res.* **2003**, *1*, 217–227: (b) Moore, J. P., Kitchen. S. G., Pugach, P., Zack, J. A. The CCR5 and CXCR4 coreceptors—central to understanding the transmission and pathogenesis of the human immunodeficiency virus type 1 infection. *AIDS Res. Human Retroviruses.* **2004**, *20*, 111–126.
31. (a) Zhu, T., Mo, H., Wang, N., Nam, D. S., Cao, Y., Koup, R. A., Ho, D. D. Genotypic and phenotypic characterization of HIV-1 patients with primary infection. *Science*. **1993**, *261*, 1179–1181: (b) Shankarappa, R, M. J., Gange, S. J., Rodrigo, A. G., Upchurch, D., Farzadegan, H., Gupta, P., Rinaldo, C. R., Learn, G. H., He, X., Huang, X. L., and Mullins, J. I. Consistent viral evolutionary changes associated with the progression of human immunodeficiency virus type 1 infection. *J. Virol.*, **1999**, *73*, 10489–10502: (c) Schuitemaker, H., K. N., de Goede, R. E., de Wolf, F., Miedema, F., and Tersmette, M. Monocytotropic human immunodeficiency virus type 1 (HIV-1) variants detectable in all stages of HIV-1 infection lack T-cell line tropism and syncytium-inducing ability in primary T-cell culture. *J. Virol.* **1991**, *65*, 356–363.
32. (a) Moyle, G. J., W. A., Mandalia, S., Mayer, H., Goodrich, J., Whitcomb, J., and Gazzard, B. G. Epidemiology and predictive factors for chemokine receptor use in HIV-1 infection. *J. Infect. Dis.* **2005**, *191*, 866–872: (b) Brumme, Z. L., G. J., Mayer, H. B., Brumme, C. J., Henrick, B. M., Wynhoven, B., Asselin, J. J., Cheung, P. K., Hogg, R. S., Montaner, J. S., and

HARRIGAN, P. R. Molecular and clinical epidemiology of CXCR4-using HIV-1 in a large population of antiretroviral-naive individuals. *J. Infect. Dis.* **2005**, *192*, 466–474.

33. WHITCOMB, J. M., H. W., FRANSEN, S., WRIN, T., PAXINOS, E., TOMA, J., GREENBERG, M., SISTA, P., MELBY, T., MATTHEWS, T., DIMASI, R., HEILEK-SNYDER, G., CAMMACK, N., HELLMAN, N., and PETROPOULOS, C. J. in *10th Conference on Retroviruses and Opportunistic Infections*, Vol. 557, Boston, MA, **2003**. Available at http://www.retroconference.org/2003/cd/Abstract/2557.htm.
34. (a) WESTBY, M., and VAN DER RYST, E. CCR5 antagonists: host-targeted antivirals for the treatment of HIV infection. *Antivir. Chem. Chemother.*, **2005**, *16*, 339–354: (b) EMMELKAMP, J. M., and ROCKSTROH, J. K. CCR5 antagonists: comparison of efficacy, side effects, pharmacokinetics and interactions—review of the literature. *Eur. J. Med. Res.*, **2007**, *12*, 409–417.
35. (a) MOSIER, D. E., PICCHIO, G. R., GULIZIA, R. J., SABBE, R., POIGNARD, P., PICARD, L., OFFORD, R. E., THOMPSON, D. A., and WILKEN, J. Highly potent RANTES analogues either prevent CCR5-using human immunodeficiency virus type 1 infection in vivo or rapidly select for CXCR4-using variants. *J. Virol.* **1999**, *73*, 3544–3550: (b) GAERTNER, H., LEBEAU, O., BORLAT, I., CERINI, F., DUFOUR, B., KUENZI, G., MELOTTI, A., FISH, R. J., OFFORD, R., SPRINGAEL, J. Y., PARMENTIER, M., and HARTLEY, O. Highly potent HIV inhibition: engineering a key anti-HIV structure from PSC-RANTES into MIP-1 beta/CCL4. *Protein Eng. Des. Sel.*, **2008**, *21*, 65–72.
36. LALEZARI, J., YADAVALLI, G. K., PARA, M., RICHMOND, G., DEJESUS, E., BROWN, S. J., CAI, W., CHEN, C., ZHONG, J., NOVELLO, L. A., LEDERMAN, M. M., and SUBRAMANIAN, G. M. Safety, pharmacokinetics, and antiviral activity of HGS004, a novel fully human IgG4 monoclonal antibody against CCR5, in HIV-1-infected patients. *J. Infect. Dis.*, **2008**, *197*, 721–727.
37. POLI, G. PRO-140 (Progenics), *I. Drugs.* **2001**, *4*, 1068–1071.
38. DORR, P., PERROS, M. CCR5 inhibitors in HIV therapy. *Expert Opin. Drug Discov.* **2008**, *3*, 1345–1361.
39. COMBADIERE, C., AHUJA, S. K., TIFFANY, H. L., and MURPHY, P. M. Cloning and functional expression of CC CKR5, a human monocyte CC chemokine receptor selective for MIP-1(alpha), MIP-1(beta), and RANTES *J. Leukoc. Biol.* **1996**, *60*, 147–152.
40. (a) ARMOUR, D. R., DE GROOT, M. J., PRICE, D. A., STAMMEN, B. L., WOOD, A., PERROS, M., and BURT, C. The discovery of tropane-derived CCR5 receptor antagonists. *Chem. Biol. Drug Des.* **2006**, *67*, 305–308: (b) BABA, M., NISHIMURA, O., KANZAKI, N., OKAMOTO, M., SAWADA, H., IIZAWA, Y., SHIRAISHI, M., ARAMAKI, Y., OKONOGI, K., OGAWA, Y., MEGURO, K., and FUJINO, M. A small-molecule, nonpeptide CCR5 antagonist with highly potent and selective anti-HIV-1 activity. *Proc. Natl. Acad. Sci. USA.* **1999**, *96*, 5698–5703: (c) CASTONGUAY, L. A., WENG, Y., ADOLFSEN, W., DI SALVO, J., KILBURN, R., CALDWELL, C. G., DAUGHERTY, B. L., FINKE, P. E., HALE, J. J., LYNCH, C. L., MILLS, S. G., MACCOSS, M., SPRINGER, M. S., and DEMARTINO, J. A. Binding of 2-aryl-4-(piperidin-1-yl) butanamines and 1,3 4-trisubstituted pyrrolidines to human CCR5: a molecular modeling-guided mutagenesis study of the binding pocket. *Biochemistry.* **2003**, *42*, 1544–1550: (d) DORR, P., WESTBY, M., DOBBS, S., GRIFFIN, P., IRVINE, B., MACARTNEY, M., MORI, J., RICKETT, G., SMITH-BURCHNELL, C., NAPIER, C., WEBSTER, R., ARMOUR, D., PRICE, D., STAMMEN, B., WOOD, A., and PERROS, M. Maraviroc (UK-427,857), a potent, orally bioavailable, and selective small-molecule inhibitor of chemokine receptor CCR5 with broad-spectrum anti-human immunodeficiency virus type 1 activity. *Antimicrob. Agents Chemother.* **2005**, *49*, 4721–4732: (e) MAEDA, K., YOSHIMURA, K., SHIBAYAMA, S., HABASHITA, H., TADA, H., SAGAWA, K., MIYAKAWA, T., AOKI, M., FUKUSHIMA, D., and MITSUYA, H. Novel low molecular weight spirodiketopiperazine derivatives potently inhibit R5 HIV-1 infection through their antagonistic effects on CCR5. *J. Biologic. Chem.* **2001**, *276*, 35194–35200; (f) SHIRAISHI, M., ARAMAKI, Y., SETO, M., IMOTO, H., NISHIKAWA, Y., KANZAKI, N., OKAMOTO, M., SAWADA, H., NISHIMURA, O., BABA, M., and FUJINO, M. Discovery of novel, potent, and selective small-molecule CCR5 antagonists as anti-HIV-1 agents: synthesis and biological evaluation of anilide derivatives with a quaternary ammonium moiety. *J. Med. Chem.* **2000**, *43*, 2049–2063; (g) STRIZKI, J. M., XU, S., WAGNER, N. E., WOJCIK, L., LIU, J., HOU, Y., ENDRES, M., PALANI, A., SHAPIRO, S., CLADER, J. W., GREENLEE, W. J., TAGAT, J. R., MCCOMBIE, S., COX, K., FAWZI, A. B., CHOU, C. C., PUGLIESE-SIVO, C., DAVIES, L., MORENO, M. E., HO, D. D., TRKOLA, A., STODDART, C. A., MOORE, J. P., REYES, G. R., and BAROUDY, B. M. SCH-C (SCH 351125), an orally bioavailable, small molecule antagonist of the chemokine receptor CCR5, is a potent inhibitor of HIV-1 infection *in vitro* and *in vivo*. *Proc. Natl. Acad. Sci. USA.* **2001**, *98*, 12718–12723.
41. (a) BRADLEY, J., GILL, J., BERTELLI, F., LETAFAT, S., CORBAU, R., HAYTER, P., HARRISON, P., TEE, A., KEIGHLEY, W., PERROS, M., CIARAMELLA, G., SEWING, A., and WILLIAMS, C. Development and automation of a 384-well cell fusion assay to identify inhibitors of CCR5/CD4-mediated HIV virus entry. *J. Biomol. Screen.* **2004**, *9*, 516–524: (b) DORR, P., CORBAU, R., PICKFORD, C., RICKETT, G., MACARTNEY, M., GRIFFIN, P., DOBBS, S., IRVINE, R., WESTBY, M., and PERROS, M. Evaluation of the mechanism underlying the anti-HI activity of a series of experimental CCR5 antagonists. on *43rd Annual Interscience Conference Antimicrobial Agents and Chemotherapy*. September 14-17 **2003**, Chicago, 2003, Poster F1466.
42. ARMOUR, D. R., DE GROOT, M. J., PRICE, D. A., STAMMEN, B. L., WOOD, A., PERROS, M., and BURT, C. The discovery of tropane-derived CCR5 receptor antagonists, *Chem. Biol. Drug Des.* **2006**, *67*, 305–308.

43. Price, D. A., Armour, D., de Groot, M., Leishman, D., Napier, C., Perros, M., Stammen, B. L., and Wood, A. Overcoming HERG affinity in the discovery of the CCR5 antagonist maraviroc *Bioorg. Med. Chem. Lett.* **2006**, *16*, 4633–4637.
44. Dorr, P., Westby, M., McFadyen, L., Mori, J., Davis, J., Perruccio, F., Jones, R., Stupple, P., Middleton, D., and Perros, M. PF-232798, a Second Generation Oral CCR5 Antagonist., *15th Conference on Retroviruses and Opportunistic Infections.* **2008**, 3–6 February, Boston, MA, 2008, p. 737.
45. Napier, C., Dorr P., Gladue, P., Halliday, R., Leishman, D., Machin, I., Mitchell, R., Nedderman, A., Perros, M., Roffey, S., Walker, D., and Webster, R. The preclinical pharmacokinetics and safety Pharmacology of the anti-HIV CCR5 antagonist, UK-427,857 *10th Conference on Retroviruses and Opportunistic Infections*, Boston, MA, 2003.
46. Yilmaz, A. a., Watson, V. b. c., Else, L. b., and Gisslen, M. a. Cerebrospinal fluid maraviroc concentrations in HIV-1 infected patients. AIDS, **2009**, *23*, 2537–2540.
47. (a) Dorr, P., Todd, K., Irvine, B., Robas, N., Thomas, A., Fidock, M., Sultan, H., Mills, J., Perrucio, F., Burt, C., Rickett, G., Perkins, H., Griffin, P., Macartney, M., Hamilton, D., Westby, M., Perros, M.in *45th Interscience Conference on Antimicrobial Agents and Chemotherapy*, Washington DC, **2005**: (b) Napier, C., Sale, H., Mosley, M., Rickett, G., Dorr, P., Mansfield, R., Holbrook, M. Molecular cloning and radioligand binding characterization of the chemokine receptor CCR5 from rhesus macaque and human. *Biochem. Pharmacol.* **2005**, *71*, 163–172.
48. Westby, M., Smith-Burchnell, C., Mori, J., Lewis, M., Whitcomb, J., Petropoulos, C., and Perros, M., in *XIII International HIV Drug Resistance Workshop*, Tenerife, 2004.
49. (a) Stoddart, C., Xu, S., Wojcik, J., Riley, J., Strizki, J. Evaluation of *In Vivo* HIV-1 Escape from SCH-C (SCH 351125) *13th Conference on Retroviruses and Opportunistic Infections*, 2003, p. 614: (b) Trkola, A., Kuhmann, S. E., Strizki, J. M., Maxwell, E., Ketas, T., Morgan, T., Pugach, P., Xu, S., Wojcik, L., Tagat, J., Palani, A., Shapiro, S., Clader, J. W., McCombie, S., Reyes, G. R., Baroudy, B. M., and Moore, J. P. HIV-1 escape from a small molecule, CCR5-specific entry inhibitor does not involve CXCR4 use. *Proc. Natl. Acad. Sci. USA*, **2002**, *99*, 395–400.
50. (a) Marozsan, A. J., Kuhmann, S. E., Morgan, T., Herrera, C., Rivera-Troche, E., Xu, S., Baroudy, B. M., Strizki, J., and Moore, J. P. Generation and properties of a human immunodeficiency virus type 1 isolate resistant to the small molecule CCR5 inhibitor, SCH-417690 (SCH-D). *Virology*. **2005**, *338*, 182–199: (b) Pugach, P., Marozsan, A. J., Ketas, T. J., Landes, E. L., Moore, J. P., and Kuhmann, S. E. HIV-1 clones resistant to a small molecule CCR5 inhibitor use the inhibitor-bound form of CCR5 for entry. *Virology*. **2007**, *361*, 212–228.: (c) Westby, M., Smith-Burchnell, C., Mori, J., Lewis, M., Mosley, M., Stockdale, M., Dorr, P., Ciaramella, G., and Perros, M. Reduced maximal inhibition in phenotypic susceptibility assays indicates that viral strains resistant to the CCR5 antagonist maraviroc utilize inhibitor-bound receptor for entry. *J. Virol.* **2007**, *81*, 2359–2371.
51. Tsibris, A. M., Sagar, M., Gulick, R. M., Su, Z., Hughes, M., Greaves, W., Subramanian, M., Flexner, C., Giguel, F., Leopold, K. E., Coakley, E., and Kuritzkes, D. R. *In vivo* emergence of vicriviroc resistance in a human immunodeficiency virus type 1 subtype C-infected subject. *J. Virol.* **2008**, *82*, 8210–8214.
52. Kuhmann, S. E., and Hartley, O. Targeting chemokine receptors in HIV: a status report. *Annu. Rev. Pharmacol. Toxicol.* **2008**, *48*, 425–461.
53. (a) Kuhmann, S. E., Pugach, P., Kunstman, K. J., Taylor, J., Stanfield, R. L., Snyder, A., Strizki, J. M., Riley, J., Baroudy, B. M., Wilson, I. A., Korber, B. T., Wolinsky, S. M., and Moore, J. P. Genetic and phenotypic analyses of human immunodeficiency virus type 1 escape from a small-molecule CCR5 inhibitor. *J. Virol.* 2004, *78*, 2790–2807: (b) Ogert, R. A., Wojcik, L., Buontempo, C., Ba, L., Buontempo, P., Ralston, R., Strizki, J., and Howe, J. A. Mapping resistance to the CCR5 co-receptor antagonist vicriviroc using heterologous chimeric HIV-1 envelope genes reveals key determinants in the C2-V5 domain of gp120. *Virology*. **2008**, *373*, 387–399: (c) Westby, M., Mori, J., Smith-Burchnell C., Lewis, M., Mosley, M., Perruccio, F., Mansfield, R., Dorr, P., and Perros, M. Maraviroc (UK-427,857)-Resistant HIV-1 Variants are Sensitive to CCR5 Antagonists and Enfuvirtide, *XIV International HIV Drug Resistance Workshop*:. (d) Westby, M., Smith-Burchnell, C., Hamilton, D., Robas, N., Irvine, B., Fidock, M., Mills, J., Perruccio, F., Mori, J., Macartney, M., Barber, C., Dorr, P., and Perros, M.in *12th Conference on Retroviruses and Opportunistic Infections*, Boston, MA, 2005.
54. Stupple, P. A., Batchelor, D. V., Corless, M., Dorr, P. K., Ellis, D., Fenwick, D. R., Galan, S. R., Jones, R. M., Mason, H. J., Middleton, D. S., Perros, M., Perruccio, F., Platts, M. Y., Pryde, D. C., Rodrigues, D., Smith, N. N., Stephenson, P. T., Webster, R., Westby, M., and Wood, A. An Imidazopiperidine Series of CCR5 Antagonists for the Treatment of HIV: The Discovery of *N*-{(1S)-1-(3-Fluorophenyl)-3-[(3-endo)-3-(5-isobutyryl-2-methyl-4,5,6,7-tetrahydr o-1H-imidazo[4,5-c]pyridin-1-yl)-8-azabicyclo[3. 2. 1]oct-8-yl]propyl}acetamide (PF-232798). *J. Med. Chem.* **2011**, *54*, 67–77.
55. Dorr, P., MacFadyen, L., Mori, J., Davis, J., Perruccio, F., Jones, R., Stupple, P., Middleton, D., and Perros, M. in *15th Conference on Retroviruses and Opportunistic Infections*, Boston, MA, 2008, p. 737.
56. Dorr, P. CCR5 pharmacology methodologies and associated applications. in *Methods in Enzymology*

(ed D. Hamel), Elsevier Publishers, Amsterdam, 2009.

57. Kondru, R., Zhang, J., Ji, C., Mirzadegan, T., Rotstein, D., Sankuratri, S., and Dioszegi, M. Molecular interactions of CCR5 with major classes of small-molecule anti-HIV CCR5 antagonists. *Mol. Pharmacol.* **2008**, *73*, 789–800.
58. (a) Liu, S., Fan, S., and Sun, Z. Structural and functional characterization of the human CCR5 receptor in complex with HIV gp120 envelope glycoprotein and CD4 receptor by molecular modeling studies. *J. Mol. Model.* **2003**, *9*, 329–336.: (b) Navenot, J. M., Wang, Z. X., Trent, J. O., Murray, J. L., Hu, Q. X., DeLeeuw, L., Moore, P. S., Chang, Y., and Peiper, S. C. Molecular anatomy of CCR5 engagement by physiologic and viral chemokines and HIV-1 envelope glycoproteins: differences in primary structural requirements for RANTES, MIP-1 alpha, and vMIP-II Binding. *J. Mol. Biol.* **2001**, *313*, 1181–1193: (c) Zhou, N., Luo, Z., Hall, J. W., Luo, J., Han, X., Huang, Z. Molecular modeling and site-directed mutagenesis of CCR5 reveal residues critical for chemokine binding and signal transduction. *Eur. J. Immunol.* **2000**, *30*, 164–173.
59. Blanpain, C., Doranz, B. J., Bondue, A., Govaerts, C., De Leener, A., Vassart, G., Doms, R. W., Proudfoot, A., and Parmentier, M. The core domain of chemokines binds CCR5 extracellular domains while their amino terminus interacts with the transmembrane helix bundle. *J. Biol. Chem.*, **2003**, *278*, 5179–5187.
60. Haycock-Lewandowski, S. J., Wilder, A., and Ahman, J. Development of a bulk enabling route to maraviroc (UK-427,857), a CCR-5 receptor antagonist, *Org. Proc. Res. & Dev.* **2008**, *12*, 1094–1103.
61. Peters, C. *ICAAC*, **2005**, *H1100.*
62. Telenti, A. Safety concerns about CCR5 as an antiviral target. *Curr. Opin. HIV AIDS*, **2009**, *4*, 131–135.
63. Lim, J. K., Louie, C. Y., Glaser, C., Jean, C., Johnson, B., Johnson, H., McDermott, D. H., and Murphy, P. M. Genetic deficiency of chemokine receptor CCR5 is a strong risk factor for symptomatic West Nile virus infection: a meta-analysis of 4 cohorts in the US epidemic. *J. Infect Dis.* **2008**, *197*, 262–265.
64. Kindberg, E., Mickiene, A., Ax, C., Akerlind, B., Vene, S., Lindquist, L., Lundkvist, A., and Svensson, L. A deletion in the chemokine receptor 5 (CCR5) gene is associated with tickborne encephalitis. *J. Infect Dis.* **2008**, *197*, 266–269.
65. McNiff, T., and Dezube, B. J. CCR5 antagonists in the treatment of HIV-infected persons: is their cancer risk increased, decreased, or unchanged. *AIDS Read.* **2009**, *19*, 218-222, 224.
66. Gulick, R. M., Su, Z., Flexner, C., Hughes, M. D., Skolnik, P. R., Wilkin, T. J., Gross, R., Krambrink, A., Coakley, E., Greaves, W. L., Zolopa, A., Reichman, R., Godfrey, C., Hirsch, M., and Kuritzkes, D. R. Phase 2 study of the safety and efficacy of vicriviroc, a CCR5 inhibitor, in HIV-1-Infected, treatment-experienced patients: AIDS clinical trials group 5211. *J. Infect Dis.* **2007**, *196*, 304–312.
67. Nichols, W. G., Steel, H. M., Bonny, T., Adkison, K., Curtis, L., Millard, J., Kabeya, K., and Clumeck, N. Hepatotoxicity observed in clinical trials of aplaviroc (GW873140). *Antimicrob. Agents Chemother.* **2008**, *52*, 858–865.
68. (a) Abel, S., Van der Ryst, E., Muihead, G. J., Rosario, A., Edgington, A., and Weissgerber, G.,in *10th Conference on Retroviruses and Opportunistic Infections*, Boston, MA, **2003**, p. 547: (b) Walker, D. K., Abel, S., Comby, P., Muirhead, G. J., Nedderman, A. N., and Smith, D. A. Species differences in the disposition of the CCR5 antagonist, UK-427,857, a new potential treatment for HIV. *Drug Metab. Dispos.* **2005**, *33*, 587–595.
69. Abel, S., Van der Ryst, E., Rosario, M. C., Ridgway, C. E., Medhurst, C. G., Taylor-Worth, R. J., and Muirhead, G. J. Assessment of the pharmacokinetics, safety and tolerability of maraviroc, a novel CCR5 antagonist, in healthy volunteers. *Br. J. Clin. Pharmacol.* **2008**, 65 Suppl *1*, 5–18.
70. Abel, S., Back, D. J., and Vourvahis, M. Maraviroc: pharmacokinetics and drug interactions. *Antivir. Ther.* **2009**, *14*, 607–618.
71. (a) Available at: http://www.medicines.org.uk/EMC/medicine/20386/SPC/Celsentri+150mg+film-coated+tablets/Celsentri Summary of Product Characte-ristics: (b) Available at: http://www.viivhealthcare.com/en/products/~/media/Files/G/GlaxoSmithKline-Plc/Attachments/pdfs/products/selzentry_maraviroc_tablets_5 May, 2010.pdf Selzentry US Prescribing information.
72. Russell, D., Bakhtyari, A., Jazrawi, R. P., Whitlock, L., Ridgway, C., McHale, M., and Abel, S., in *43rd Interscience Conference on Antimicrobial Agents and Chemotherapy*, Chicago, IL, USA, 2003.
73. (a) Abel, S., Jenkins, T. M., Whitlock, L. A., Ridgway, C. E., and Muirhead, G. J. Effects of CYP3A4 inducers with and without CYP3A4 inhibitors on the pharmacokinetics of maraviroc in healthy volunteers. *Br. J. Clin. Pharmacol.* **2008**, *65*, 38–46: (b) Abel, S., Russell, D., Whitlock, L. A., Ridgway, C. E., and Muirhead, G. J. Effect of maraviroc on the pharmacokinetics of midazolam, lamivudine/zidovudine, and ethinyloestradiol/levonorgestrel in healthy volunteers. *Br. J. Clin. Pharmacol.* **2008**, *65*, 19–26: (c) Abel, S., Russell, D., Whitlock, L. A., Ridgway, C. E., and Muirhead, G. J. The effects of cotrimoxazole or tenofovir co-administration on the pharmacokinetics of maraviroc in healthy volunteers. *Br. J. Clin. Pharmacol.* **2008**, *65*, 47–53: (d) Abel, S., Russell, D., Whitlock, L. A., Ridgway, C. E., Nedderman, A. N., and Walker, D. K. Assessment of the absorption, metabolism and absolute bioavailability of maraviroc in healthy male subjects. *Br. J. Clin. Pharmacol.* **2008**, *65*, 60–67.
74. (a) Dorr, P., Rickett, G., and Perros, M. Method for identifying CCR5 receptor antagonists by measuring residency time. US Patent Appl. 20040023845, 2004: (b) Rosario, M. C., Jacqmin, P., Dorr, P., James, I., Jenkins, T. M., Abel, S., and Van der Ryst, E.

Population pharmacokinetic/pharmacodynamic analysis of CCR5 receptor occupancy by maraviroc in healthy subjects and HIV-positive patients. *Br. J. Clin. Pharmacol.* **2008**, *65*, 86–94: (c) Rosario, M. C., Jacqmin, P., Dorr, P., Van der Ryst, E., and Hitchcock, C. A pharmacokinetic–pharmacodynamic disease model to predict *in vivo* antiviral activity of maraviroc. *Clin. Pharmacol. Ther.* **2005**, *78*, 508–519.
75. Dorr., P. Maraviroc outlook in HIV and non-HIV diseases. *in HIV-Infection and Organ Transplantation Symposium*, University Medical Center Hamburg-Eppendorf Hamburg, Germany, 2008.
76. McHale, M., A. S., Russell, D., Gallagher, J., and Van der Ryst, E.,in *3rd International AIDS Conference*, Brazil, 2005.
77. Davis, J. D., Hackman, F., Layton, G., Higgins, T., Sudworth, D., and Weissgerber, G. Effect of single doses of maraviroc on the QT/QTc interval in healthy subjects. *Br. J. Clin. Pharmacol.* **2008**, 65 Suppl *1*, 68–75.
78. Fatkenheuer, G., Nelson, M., Lazzarin, A., Konourina, I., Hoepelman, A. I., Lampiris, H., Hirschel, B., Tebas, P., Raffi, F., Trottier, B., Bellos, N., Saag, M., Cooper, D. A., Westby, M., Tawadrous, M., Sullivan, J. F., Ridgway, C., Dunne, M. W., Felstead, S., Mayer, H., and Van der Ryst, E. Subgroup analyses of maraviroc in previously treated R5 HIV-1 infection. *N. Engl. J. Med.* **2008**, *359*, 1442–1455.
79. Gulick, R. M., Lalezari, J., Goodrich, J., Clumeck, N., DeJesus, E., Horban, A., Nadler, J., Clotet, B., Karlsson, A., Wohlfeiler, M., Montana, J. B., McHale, M., Sullivan, J., Ridgway, C., Felstead, S., Dunne, M. W., Van der Ryst, E., and Mayer, H. Maraviroc for previously treated patients with R5 HIV-1 infection. *N. Engl. J. Med.* **2008**, *359*, 1429–1441.
80. Whitcomb, J. M., Huang, W., Fransen, S., Limoli, K., Toma, J., Wrin, T., Chappey, C., Kiss, L. D., Paxinos, E. E., and Petropoulos, C. J. Development and characterization of a novel single-cycle recombinant-virus assay to determine human immunodeficiency virus type 1 coreceptor tropism. *Antimicrob. Agents Chemother.* **2007**, *51*, 566–575.
81. Boucher, C., S. J., Kuritzkes, D., Llibre, J. M., Lewis, M., Simpson, P., Delogne, C., Sharma, V., Parliyan, A., Chapman, D., Perros, M., Valdez, H., and Westby, M., Genotypic- and phenotypic-weighted OBT susceptibility scores are similarly strong predictors of virologic response <50 copies/ml at week 48 in Motivate 1 and 2, Vol. *Abstract* 48, Fort Myers, FL, 2009.
82. Saag, M., Goodrich, J., Fatkenheuer, G., Clotet, B., Clumeck, N., Sullivan, J., Westby, M., Van der Ryst, E., and Mayer, H. A double-blind, placebo-controlled trial of maraviroc in treatment-experienced patients infected with non-R5 HIV-1. *J. Infect Dis.* **2009**, *199*, 1638–1647.
83. Cooper, D. A., Heera, J., Goodrich, J., Tawadrous, M., Saag, M., DeJesus, E., Clumeck, N., Walmsley, S., Ting, N., Coakley, E., Reeves, J. D., Reyes-Teran, G., Westby, M., Van der Ryst, E., Ive, P., Mohapi, L., Mingrone, H., Horban, A., Hackman, F., Sullivan, J., and Mayer, H. Maraviroc versus efavirenz, both in combination with zidovudine-lamivudine, for the treatment of antiretroviral-naive subjects with CCR5-tropic HIV-1 infection. *J. Infect Dis.* **2010**, *201*, 803–813.
84. Reeves, J. D., C. E., Petropoulos, C. J., and Whitcomb, J. M. An enhanced-sensitivity Trofile HIV coreceptor tropism assay for selecting patients for therapy with entry inhibitors targeting CCR5: a review of analytical and clinical studies. *J. Viral Entry.* **2009**, *3*, 94–102.
85. Hoepelman, I., Ayoub, A., and Heera, J.The Incidence of Severe Liver Enzyme Abnormalities and Hepatic Adverse Events in the Maraviroc Clinical Development Programme., *11th European AIDS Conference (EACS)*, 2007.
86. Watson, C., Jenkinson, S., Kazmierski, W., and Kenakin, T. The CCR5 receptor-based mechanism of action of 873140, a potent allosteric noncompetitive HIV entry inhibitor. *Mol. Pharmacol.* **2005**, *67*, 1268–1282.
87. Mori, J., Lewis, M., Simpson, P., Whitcomb, J., Perros, M., van der Ryst, R., in *European HIV Drug Resistance Workshop, Vol. Abstract 51* Budapest, 2008
88. Jubb, B., Lewis, M., Simpson, P., Craig, C., Haddrick, M., Perros, M., and Westby M., in *16th Conference on Retroviruses and Opportunistic Infections*, Montreal, Canada, 2009.
89. Heera, J., Saag, M., Ive, P., Whitcomb, J., Lewis, M., McFadyen, L., Goodrich, J., Mayer, H., Van der Ryst, E., and Westby, M. Virological Correlates Associated with Treatment Failure at Week 48 in the Phase 3 Study of Maraviroc in Treatment-naive Patients. in *15th Conference on Retroviruses and Opportunistic Infections*, 2008, 40LB.
90. Lewis, M., Simpson, P., Fransen, S., and Westby, M. CXCR4-using virus detected in patients receiving maraviroc in the phase III studies MOTIVATE 1 and 2 originates from a pre-existing minority of CXCR4-using virus. in *XVI International HIV Drug Resistance Workshop*, Abstract 56 2007.
91. Van der Ryst E, W. M., in *47th Interscience Conference on Antimicrobial Agents and Chemotherapy (ICAAC), Vol. Abstract H-715*, Chicago, USA, 2007.
92. Portsmouth, S. D., L. M., Carig, C., Chapman, D., Swenson, L. C., Heera, J., in *International HIV and Hepatitis Drug Resistance Workshop*, June 8–12, 2010, Dubrovnic, Croatia, 2010.
93. Zaccarelli, M., Perno, C. F., Forbici, F., Cingolani, A., Liuzzi, G., Bertoli, A., Trotta, M. P., Bellocchi, M. C., Di Giambenedetto, S., Tozzi, V., Gori, C., D'Arrigo, R., De Longis, P., Noto, P., Girardi, E., De Luca, A., and Antinori, A. Using a database of HIV patients undergoing genotypic resistance test after HAART failure to understand the dynamics of M184V mutation. *Antivir. Ther.* **2003**, *8*, 51–56.
94. Deeks, S. G., Lu, J., Hoh, R., Neilands, T. B., Beatty, G., Huang, W., Liegler, T., Hunt, P., Martin, J. N., and

KURITZKES, D. R. Interruption of enfuvirtide in HIV-1 infected adults with incomplete viral suppression on an enfuvirtide-based regimen. *J. Infect Dis.* **2007**, *195*, 387–391.
95. BUCHBINDER, S. HIV testing and prevention strategies. *Top HIV Med.* **2008**, *16*, 9–14.
96. (a) DUMOND, J., PATTERSON, K., PECHA, A., WERNER, R., ANDREWS, E., DAMLE, B., TRESSLER, R., WORSLEY, J., BOGGESS, K., and KASHUBA, A. Maraviroc (MVC) Pharmacokinetics (PK) in Blood Plasma (BP), Genital Tract (GT) Fluid and Tissue in Healthy Female Volunteers. in *15th Conference on Retroviruses and Opportunistic Infections.* Abstract 135LB, 2008:. (b) BROWN, K. C., P. K., MALONE, S. A., SHAHEEN, N. J., PRINCE, H. M. A., DUMOND, J. B., SPACEK, M., HEIDT, P. E., COHEN, M. S., KASHUBA, A. D. M.in *17th CROI Conference on Retroviruses and Opportunistic Infections*, San Francisco, CA, 2010.
97. (a) VEAZEY, R. S., KLASSE, P. J., SCHADER, S. M., HU, Q., KETAS, T. J., LU, M., MARX, P. A., DUFOUR, J., COLONNO, R. J., SHATTOCK, R. J., SPRINGER, M. S., and MOORE, J. P. Protection of macaques from vaginal SHIV challenge by vaginally delivered inhibitors of virus-cell fusion. *Nature*, **2005**, *438*, 99–102: (b) VEAZEY, R. S., SPRINGER, M. S., MARX, P. A., DUFOUR, J., KLASSE, P. J., and MOORE, J. P. Protection of macaques from vaginal SHIV challenge by an orally delivered CCR5 inhibitor. *Nat. Med.* **2005**, *11*, 1293–1294.
98. LEDERMAN, M. M., VEAZEY, R. S., OFFORD, R., MOSIER, D. E., DUFOUR, J., MEFFORD, M., PIATAK, M., JR., LIFSON, J. D., SALKOWITZ, J. R., RODRIGUEZ, B., BLAUVELT, A., and HARTLEY, O. Prevention of vaginal SHIV transmission in rhesus macaques through inhibition of CCR5. *Science.* **2004**, *306*, 485–487.
99. DUMOND, J. B., YEH, R. F., PATTERSON, K. B., CORBETT, A. H., JUNG, B. H., REZK, N. L., BRIDGES, A. S., STEWART, P. W., COHEN, M. S., and KASHUBA, A. D. Antiretroviral drug exposure in the female genital tract: implications for oral pre- and post-exposure prophylaxis. *Aids.* **2007**, *21*, 1899–1907.
100. Available at: http://www.ipmglobal.org/Inter-national Partnership for Microbicides, 2008.
101. VEAZEY, R. S., KETAS, T. J., DUFOUR, J., MORONEY-RASMUSSEN, T., GREEN, L. C., KLASSE, P. J., and MOORE, J. P. Protection of rhesus macaques from vaginal infection by vaginally delivered maraviroc, an inhibitor of HIV-1 entry via the CCR5 co-receptor. *J. Infect Dis.* **2010**, *202*, 739–744.
102. FAHEEM, A., M. C., MCBRIDE, M., MALCOLM, K., WOOLFSON, D., SPARKS, M., in *16th Conference on Retroviruses and Opportunistic Infections*, **2009**, p. Poster 1069.
103. KARIM, Q. A., KARIM, S. S., FROHLICH, J. A., GROBLER, A. C., BAXTER, C., MANSOOR, L. E., KHARSANY, A. B., SIBEKO, S., MLISANA, K. P., OMAR, Z., GENGIAH, T. N., MAARSCHALK, S., ARULAPPAN, N., MLOTSHWA, M., MORRIS, L., and TAYLOR, D. Effectiveness and safety of tenofovir gel, an antiretroviral microbicide, for the prevention of HIV infection in women. *Science.* **2010**, *329*, 1168–1174.
104. (a) LUNZEN, J. Treatment of heavily antiretroviral-experienced HIV-infected patients. *AIDS Rev.* **2007**, *9*, 246–253: (b) LUNZEN, J. State of the ART 2008. in *HIV-Infection and Organ Transplantation Symposium University Medical Center Hamburg-Eppendorf Hamburg, Germany*, **2008**: (c) SELIK, R. M., BYERS, R. H., JR., and DWORKIN, M. S. Trends in diseases reported on U.S. death certificates that mentioned HIV infection, 1987-1999. *J. Acquir. Immune Defic. Syndr.* **2002**, *29*, 378–387.
105. MARTINEZ, E., LARROUSSE, M., and GATELL, J. M. Cardiovascular disease and HIV infection: host, virus, or drugs? *Curr. Opin. Infect. Dis.* **2009**, *22*, 28–34.
106. AYOUB, A., G. J., VAN DER RYST, E., HEERA, J., and MAYER, H., in *Program and abstracts of the 48th Interscience Conference on Antimicrobial Agents and Chemotherapy/46th Annual Meeting of the Infectious Diseases Society of America, Vol. Abstract H-1264* Washington, DC, 2008.
107. DEJESUS, E., W. S., COHEN, C., COOPER, D., HIRSCHEL, B., GOODRICH, J., VALDEZ, H., HEERA, J., RAJICIC, N., and MAYER, H.,in *15th Conference on Retroviruses and Opportunistic Infections, Vol. Abstract 929* Boston, MA, **2008**.
108. LEDERMAN, M. M., and ESTE, J. Targeting a host element as a strategy to block HIV replication: is it nice to fool with Mother Nature? *Curr. Opin. HIV AIDS.* **2009**, *4*, 79–81.
109. (a) CROTHERS, K., and HUANG, L. Pulmonary complications of immune reconstitution inflammatory syndromes in HIV-infected patients. *Respirology.* **2009**. *23*, 23: (b) CRUM-CIANFLONE, N. F. Immune reconstitution inflammatory syndromes: what's new? *AIDS Read.*, **2006**, *16*, 199-206, 213, 216-217;discussion 214–197: (c) ELSTON, J. W., and THAKER, H. Immune reconstitution inflammatory syndrome. *Int. J. STD AIDS.* **2009**, *20*, 221–224.
110. BONHAM, S., MEYA, D. B., BOHJANEN, P. R., and BOULWARE, D. R. Biomarkers of HIV immune reconstitution inflammatory syndrome. *Biomark. Med.* **2008**, *2*, 349–361.
111. LOW, A. J., SWENSON, L. C., and HARRIGAN, P. R. HIV coreceptor phenotyping in the clinical setting. *AIDS Rev.* **2008**, *10*, 143–151.
112. HARRIGAN, P. R., M. R., DONG, W., et al., in *XVIII International HIV Drug Resistance Workshop, Vol. Abstract 15*, Fort Myers, USA, 2009.
113. CHONG, C. R., SULLIVAN, D. J. JR. New uses for old drugs. *Nature.* **2007**, *448*, 645–646.
114. (a) RIBEIRO, S., and HORUK, R. The clinical potential of chemokine receptor antagonists. *Pharmacol. Ther.* **2005**, *107*, 44–58: (b) WELLS, T. N., POWER, C. A., SHAW, J. P., and PROUDFOOT, A. E. Chemokine blockers–therapeutics in the making? *Trends Pharmacol. Sci.* **2006**, *27*, 41–47.
115. (a) NAVRATILOVA, Z. Polymorphisms in CCL2&CCL5 chemokines/chemokine receptors genes and their

association with diseases. *Biomed. Pap. Med. Fac. Univ. Palacky. Olomouc. Czech Repub.* **2006**, *150*, 191–204: (b) Schroder, C., Pierson, R. N., 3rd, Nguyen, B. N., Kawka, D. W., Peterson, L. B., Wu, G., Zhang, T., Springer, M. S., Siciliano, S. J., Iliff, S., Ayala, J. M., Lu, M., Mudgett, J. S., Lyons, K., Mills, S. G., Miller, G. G., Singer, II, Azimzadeh, A. M., and DeMartino, J. A. CCR5 blockade modulates inflammation and alloimmunity in primates. *J. Immunol.* **2007**, *179*, 2289–2299.

116. (a) Eikelenboom, M. J., Killestein, J., Izeboud, T., Kalkers, N. F., Van Lier, R. A., Barkhof, F., Uitdehaag, B. M., and Polman, C. H. Chemokine receptor expression on T cells is related to new lesion development in multiple sclerosis. *J. Neuroimmunol.* **2002**, *133*, 225–232: (b) Otaegui, D., Ruiz-Martinez, J., Olaskoaga, J., Emparanza, J. I., and Lopez de Munain, A. Influence of CCR5-Delta32 genotype in Spanish population with multiple sclerosis. *Neurogenetics.* **2007**, *8*, 201–205; (c) Sellebjerg, F., Madsen, H. O., Jensen, C. V., Jensen, J., and Garred, P. CCR5 delta32, matrix metalloproteinase-9 and disease activity in multiple sclerosis. *J. Neuroimmunol.* **2000**, *102*, 98–106: (d) Szczucinski, A., and Losy, J. Chemokines and chemokine receptors in multiple sclerosis. Potential targets for new therapies. *Acta. Neurol. Scand.* **2007**, *115*, 137–146.

117. (a) Aggarwal, A., Agarwal, S., and Misra, R. Chemokine and chemokine receptor analysis reveals elevated interferon-inducible protein-10 (IP)-10/CXCL10 levels and increased number of CCR5$^+$ and CXCR3$^+$ CD4 T cells in synovial fluid of patients with enthesitis-related arthritis (ERA). *Clin. Exp. Immunol.* **2007**, *148*, 515–519.; (b) Prahalad, S. Negative association between the chemokine receptor CCR5-Delta32 polymorphism and rheumatoid arthritis: a meta-analysis. *Genes Immun.* **2006**, *7*, 264–268; (c) Wheeler, J., McHale, M., Jackson, V., and Penny, M. Assessing theoretical risk and benefit suggested by genetic association studies of CCR5: experience in a drug development programme for maraviroc. *Antivir. Ther.* **2007**, *12*, 233–245.

118. (a) Bogunia-Kubik, K., Duda, D., Suchnicki, K., and Lange, A. CCR5 deletion mutation and its association with the risk of developing acute graft-versus-host disease after allogeneic hematopoietic stem cell transplantation. *Haematologica.* **2006**, *91*, 1628–1634; (b) Fischereder, M., Luckow, B., Hocher, B., Wuthrich, R. P., Rothenpieler, U., Schneeberger, H., Panzer, U., Stahl, R. A., Hauser, I. A., Budde, K., Neumayer, H., Kramer, B. K., Land, W., and Schlondorff, D. CC chemokine receptor 5 and renal-transplant survival. *Lancet.*, **2001**, *357*, 1758–1761; (c) Panzer, U., Reinking, R. R., Steinmetz, O. M., Zahner, G., Sudbeck, U., Fehr, S., Pfalzer, B., Schneider, A., Thaiss, F., Mack, M., Conrad, S., Huland, H., Helmchen, U., and Stahl, R. A. CXCR3 and CCR5 positive T-cell recruitment in acute human renal allograft rejection. *Transplantation.* **2004**, *78*, 1341–1350.

119. Maggs, J. R., and Chapman, R. W. Sclerosing cholangitis. *Curr. Opin. Gastroenterol.* **2007**, *23*, 310–316.

120. Hornung, D., Bentzien, F., Wallwiener, D., Kiesel, L., and Taylor, R. N. Chemokine bioactivity of RANTES in endometriotic and normal endometrial stromal cells and peritoneal fluid. *Mol. Hum. Reprod.* **2001**, *7*, 163–168.

121. Kalev, I., Oselin, K., Parlist, P., Zilmer, M., Rajasalu, T., Podar, T., and Mikelsaar, A. V. CC-chemokine receptor CCR5-del32 mutation as a modifying pathogenetic factor in type I diabetes. *J. Diabetes Complications.* **2003**, *17*, 387–391.

122. (a) Panzer, U., Schneider, A., Steinmetz, O. M., Wenzel, U., Barth, P., Reinking, R., Becker, J. U., Harendza, S., Zahner, G., Fischereder, M., Kramer, B. K., Schlondorff, D., Ostendorf, T., Floege, J., Helmchen, U., and Stahl, R. A. The chemokine receptor 5 Delta32 mutation is associated with increased renal survival in patients with IgA nephropathy. *Kidney Int.* **2005**, *67*, 75–81; (b) Stasikowska, O., Danilewicz, M., and Wagrowska-Danilewicz, M. The significant role of RANTES and CCR5 in progressive tubulointerstitial lesions in lupus nephropathy. *Pol. J. Pathol.* **2007**, *58*, 35–40;(c) Teramoto, K., Negoro, N., Kitamoto, K., Iwai, T., Iwao, H., Okamura, M., and Miura, K. Microarray analysis of glomerular gene expression in murine lupus nephritis. *J. Pharmacol. Sci.* **2008**, *106*, 56–67.

123. (a) Hellier, S., Frodsham, A. J., Hennig, B. J., Klenerman, P., Knapp, S., Ramaley, P., Satsangi, J., Wright, M., Zhang, L., Thomas, H. C., Thursz, M., and Hill, A. V. Association of genetic variants of the chemokine receptor CCR5 and its ligands, RANTES and MCP-2, with outcome of HCV infection. *Hepatology.* **2003**, *38*, 1468–1476;(b) Schwabe, R. F., Bataller, R., and Brenner, D. A. Human hepatic stellate cells express CCR5 and RANTES to induce proliferation and migration. *Am. J. Physiol. Gastrointest. Liver Physiol.* **2003**, *285*, G949–G958.

124. Goecke, H., Forssmann, U., Uguccioni, M., Friess, H., Conejo-Garcia, J. R., Zimmermann, A., Baggiolini, M., and Buchler, M. W. Macrophages infiltrating the tissue in chronic pancreatitis express the chemokine receptor CCR5. *Surgery.* **2000**, *128*, 806–814.

125. (a) Chvatchko, Y., Proudfoot, A. E., Buser, R., Juillard, P., Alouani, S., Kosco-Vilbois, M., Coyle, A. J., Nibbs, R. J., Graham, G., Offord, R. E., and Wells, T. N. Inhibition of airway inflammation by amino-terminally modified RANTES/CC chemokine ligand 5 analogues is not mediated through CCR3. *J. Immunol.* **2003**, *171*, 5498–5506; (b) Kallinich, T., Schmidt, S., Hamelmann, E., Fischer, A., Qin, S., Luttmann, W., Virchow, J. C., and Kroczek, R. A. Chemokine-receptor expression on T cells in lung

compartments of challenged asthmatic patients. *Clin. Exp. Allergy*. **2005**, *35*, 26–33; (c) Lun, S. W., Wong, C. K., Ko, F. W., Ip, W. K., Hui, D. S., and Lam, C. W. Aberrant expression of CC and CXC chemokines and their receptors in patients with asthma. *J. Clin. Immunol.* **2006**, *26*, 145–152; (d) Srivastava, P., Helms, P. J., Stewart, D., Main, M., and Russell, G. Association of CCR5Delta32 with reduced risk of childhood but not adult asthma. *Thorax*. **2003**, *58*, 222–226.

126. (a) Candore, G., Balistreri, C. R., Caruso, M., Grimaldi, M. P., Incalcaterra, E., Listi, F., Vasto, S., and Caruso, C. Pharmacogenomics: a tool to prevent and cure coronary heart disease. *Curr. Pharm. Des.* **2007**, *13*, 3726–3734; (b) Damas, J. K., Eiken, H. G., Oie, E., Bjerkeli, V., Yndestad, A., Ueland, T., Tonnessen, T., Geiran, O. R., Aass, H., Simonsen, S., Christensen, G., Froland, S. S., Attramadal, H., Gullestad, L., and Aukrust, P. Myocardial expression of CC- and CXC-chemokines and their receptors in human end-stage heart failure. *Cardiovasc. Res.*, **2000**, *47*, 778–787: (c) Kraaijeveld, A. O., de Jager, S. C., de Jager, W. J., Prakken, B. J., McColl, S. R., Haspels, I., Putter, H., Van Berkel, T. J., Nagelkerken, L., Jukema, J. W., and Biessen, E. A. CC chemokine ligand-5 (CCL5/RANTES) and CC chemokine ligand-18 (CCL18/PARC) are specific markers of refractory unstable angina pectoris and are transiently raised during severe ischemic symptoms, *Circulation.*, **2007**, *116*, 1931–1941.

127. (a) Kato, Y., Pawankar, R., Kimura, Y., and Kawana, S. Increased expression of RANTES, CCR3 and CCR5 in the lesional skin of patients with atopic eczema. *Int. Arch. Allergy Immunol.* **2006**, *139*, 245–257; (b) Ottaviani, C., Nasorri, F., Bedini, C., de Pita, O., Girolomoni, G., and Cavani, A. CD56 bright CD16 (−) NK cells accumulate in psoriatic skin in response to CXCL10 and CCL5 and exacerbate skin inflammation. *Eur. J. Immunol.* **2006**, *36*, 118–128.

128. Jiang, L., Newman, M., Saporta, S., Chen, N., Sanberg, C., Sanberg, P. R., and Willing, A. E. MIP-1alpha and MCP-1 induce migration of human umbilical cord blood cells in models of stroke. *Curr. Neurovasc. Res.* **2008**, *5*, 118–124.

129. Huber, J., Kiefer, F. W., Zeyda, M., Ludvik, B., Silberhumer, G. R., Prager, G., Zlabinger, G. J., and Stulnig, T. M. CC chemokine and CC chemokine receptor profiles in visceral and subcutaneous adipose tissue are altered in human obesity. *J. Clin. Endocrinol. Metab.* **2008**, *93*, 3215–3221.

130. Reale, M., Iarlori, C., Feliciani, C., and Gambi, D. Peripheral chemokine receptors, their ligands, cytokines and Alzheimer's disease. *J. Alzheimers Dis.* **2008**, *14*, 147–159.

131. (a) Afzal, A. R., Kiechl, S., Daryani, Y. P., Weerasinghe, A., Zhang, Y., Reindl, M., Mayr, A., Weger, S., Xu, Q., and Willeit, J. Common CCR5-del32 frameshift mutation associated with serum levels of inflammatory markers and cardiovascular disease risk in the Bruneck population. *Stroke*. **2008**, *39*, 1972–1978; (b) Braunersreuther, V., Steffens, S., Arnaud, C., Pelli, G., Burger, F., Proudfoot, A., and Mach, F. A novel RANTES antagonist prevents progression of established atherosclerotic lesions in mice. *Arterioscler. Thromb. Vasc. Biol.* **2008**, *28*, 1090–1096; (c) Braunersreuther, V., Zernecke, A., Arnaud, C., Liehn, E. A., Steffens, S., Shagdarsuren, E., Bidzhekov, K., Burger, F., Pelli, G., Luckow, B., Mach, F., and Weber, C. CCR5 but not CCR1 deficiency reduces development of diet-induced atherosclerosis in mice. *Arterioscler. Thromb. Vasc. Biol.* **2007**, *27*, 373–379; (d) Van Wanrooij, E. J., Happe, H., Hauer, A. D., de Vos, P., Imanishi, T., Fujiwara, H., Van Berkel, T. J., and Kuiper, J. HIV entry inhibitor TAK-779 attenuates atherogenesis in low-density lipoprotein receptor-deficient mice. *Arterioscler. Thromb. Vasc. Biol.* **2005**, *25*, 2642–2647; (e) Zernecke, A., Shagdarsuren, E., and Weber, C. Chemokines in atherosclerosis: an update. *Arterioscler. Thromb. Vasc. Biol.* **2008**, *19*, 19.

132. Wu, Y., Li, Y. Y., Matsushima, K., Baba, T., and Mukaida, N. CCL3–CCR5 axis regulates intratumoral accumulation of leukocytes and fibroblasts and promotes angiogenesis in murine lung metastasis process. *J. Immunol.* **2008**, *181*, 6384–6393.

133. Bhangoo, S., Ren, D., Miller, R. J., Henry, K. J., Lineswala, J., Hamdouchi, C., Li, B., Monahan, P. E., Chan, D. M., Ripsch, M. S., and White, F. A. Delayed functional expression of neuronal chemokine receptors following focal nerve demyelination in the rat: a mechanism for the development of chronic sensitization of peripheral nociceptors. *Mol. Pain.* **2007**, *3*, 38.

CHAPTER 10

DISCOVERY OF ANTIMALARIAL DRUG ARTEMISININ AND BEYOND

Weiwei Mao, Yu Zhang, and Ao Zhang

10.1 INTRODUCTION: NATURAL PRODUCTS IN DRUG DISCOVERY

Throughout the history of the development of mankind, nature has played a central role providing food and medicines. Plants, in particular, have made a significant contribution in the development of traditional medicines for the treatment of a wide spectrum of abnormal symptoms and diseases. In earlier time periods, medicines were directly prepared from natural sources as a crude complex. The use of natural substances as medicines can be dated back to Egyptian medicine as early as 2900 BCE, but especially in the "The Erbers Papyrus" in 1550 BCE which contains 700 formulas and remedies. All these substances were used on the basis of a long tradition of empirical practice and observations. The discovery that natural substances can be purified, isolated, and used as a single component in a precise dosage form occurred only about 200 years ago, by a young pharmacist's apprentice, Friedrich SertÜmer, who isolated the first pharmacologically active chemical compound morphine in pure form from the opium poppy, Papaver somniferum [1]. This may represent one of the earliest examples of modern drug discovery from natural resources, and prompted further efforts to isolate more natural products.

Morphine, aspirin, digitoxin, quinine, and pilocarpine are among the earliest modern natural medicines. The discovery of the antibacterial drug penicillin in 1928 led to a revolution in drug discovery, and a number of antibacterial drugs including streptomycin, chloramphenicol, chlortetracycline, cephalosporin C, erythromycin, and vancomycin were developed subsequently [2]. Following this, additional natural products useful for treating a variety of diseases were isolated including anticancer agents (taxol, doxorubicin, and camptothecin), lipid control drugs of which lovastatin, atorvastatin, fluvastatin, and simvastatin were derived from, immunosuppressants (cyclosporine, rapamycin) and so on. It is roughly estimated that more than 65% of currently used medicines are natural products or natural product-inspired derivatives. In several therapeutic areas including anticancer drugs and antibiotics, this percentage is up to 85% [3]. Given the modern improvements in the isolation, purification, characterization and identification of novel natural products, and with advances in modern synthetic and medicinal chemistry, the use of natural products in the discovery of new medicines has a bright future.

10.2 NATURAL PRODUCT DRUG DISCOVERY IN CHINA

Although China was not involved as early as Egypt or India in using natural substances as medicines, it is the country where the preparation of natural or herbal medicines was most

Case Studies in Modern Drug Discovery and Development, Edited by Xianhai Huang and Robert G. Aslanian.

thoroughly documented and utilized. In ancient times, medicines in China were called "Ben Cao" (materia medica). The earliest written record exclusively devoted to disease treatment was the "*Wu Shi Er Bing Fang Lun*" from the Dynasty between 1065 and 771 BC describing *Prescriptions and formulations for fifty-two diseases.* The "*Shen Nong Ben Cao Jing" (Shennong Herbal)*, compiled sometime between the first century BC and the second century AD, describing 365 drugs, and the "*Ben Cao Gang Mu*," compiled in 1596 by the great Ming Dynasty physician Shi-Zhen Li, are the two classical Chinese pharmacopoeia with detailed descriptions. The latter one was considered the Bible for Chinese physicians in ancient times and is still widely referred to even now for modern drug researchers and doctors. It took Li 38 years to complete, mostly based on his own medical and herbal practices. It describes a total of 1892 drugs with 11,096 prescriptions, for treating hundreds of illnesses, ranging from the common cold to drunkenness and food poisoning. The most recent compilation of Chinese herbal medicine is the "Zhong Yao Da Ci Dian" (Encyclopedia of Chinese Materia Medica) published in 1977. It is the most extensive work ever in the field of materia medica, describing a total of 5767 drugs mostly from plant origin (over 4800) with 900 derived from animal or mineral sources [3,4].

One major feature that distinguishes Traditional Chinese Medicines (TCM) from those of most other countries is the specific and often complicated procedures for their preparation and use in patients. Over the centuries, specific methods were applied to the crude natural drugs to yield the desired therapeutic effects, including boiling or heating in water or mixing with other herbs such as licorice, ginger, or black beans. The major objective of these procedures was to extract the active components from the crude drug into water.

Since the beginning of the modern drug discovery era early in the 20th century, China has made tremendous progress bringing traditional medicines into a modern environment. Although the insistence in using crude TCM may have contributed to China's lag behind the Western world in drug discovery, China has made great progress in scrutinizing traditional medicines with modern chromatographic and spectroscopic methods. It has been roughly estimated that over 13,000 chemical substances from natural sources have been recorded in China, over 11,000 of which are originated from plants, 1600 from animals and a small portion (less than 100) from minerals [3,4]. The pharmacological activity of many of these has been validated through bioassay-guided technology, and a number of bioactive components have been identified and subjected to further scrutiny. Representative examples include the well-known antimalarial drug Artemisinin and its derivative artemether, the anti-Alzheimer drug Huperzine A and its analog Schiperine and so on. It should be pointed out that although many of these drugs were developed early in China, their acceptance to the rest of the world was limited due to cultural barriers and more importantly to the late realization of the importance of intellectual property.

10.3 DISCOVERY OF ARTEMISININ: BACKGROUND, STRUCTURAL ELUCIDATION AND PHARMACOLOGICAL EVALUATION

10.3.1 Background and Biological Rationale

Malaria is the most common parasitic disease and is widespread in tropical and subtropical regions. It continues to be one of the major causes of mortality and morbidity in the world. It is estimated that over 40% of the population of the world lives in areas endemic with malaria. Its emergence, fast spread and resistance to existing drugs contributes to the short life-expectancy in undeveloped countries, developing countries, and the rural areas of the developed countries as well. The UN WHO recently announced that malaria still remains one of the largest global health care problems in the 21st century, and more than 380 million cases of malaria occur annually and account for over 1 million deaths overall [5]. Although several small molecule drugs are available now to treat this disease, the battle against malaria is far from over.

10.3.1.1 Biological Rationale To identify efficient medication to treat malaria, tremendous effort has been made to explore the pathology of this disease and the mechanism of action of many antimalarial drugs. This led to the recognition of heme as the trigger and target of malaria [6]. It has been found that heme is not only the active site for oxygen-binding hemoglobin, but also the prosthetic group of many different heme-containing enzymes, cytochromes P450 [7], peroxidases [8], catalase [9], and several heme-containing proteins involved in electron transfer [10]. All these metalloproteins or metalloenzymes have the same flat iron-tetrapyrrolic motif, namely, heme as the active site with a fast interaction with molecular oxygen when the central iron is reduced to the oxidation state +II.

It was further proposed that heme plays an essential role in the mechanism of action of many different antimalarial drugs. *Plasmodium* is a hematophagous parasite responsible for deadly forms of malaria disease. During the infection of erythrocytes, it was found that the parasite can digest up to 80% of the hemoglobin to collect amino-acids for its own protein production. The released heme is then efficiently polymerized by the parasite to hemozoin, the malaria pigment that is easily recognized by optical microscopy within infected erythrocytes [11]. Hemozoin is the result of the aggregation of heme dimers [12] mediated by different parasitic proteins including HRP (histidine-rich protein) and the recently characterized HDP (heme detoxification protein) [13,14]. A lipidic environment has also been proposed to play a role in the nucleation of hemozoin crystals [15].

10.3.2 The Discovery of Artemisinin through Nontraditional Drug Discovery Process

Quinine (**1**), the earliest natural antimalarial drug, was isolated by French researchers in 1817 from the bark of the cinchona tree which grows at high altitudes in the mountains of South America [16]. Over the last two centuries, it has held a central role among natural products as the first drug effective for treating malaria caused by *Plasmodium falciparum*. However, drug-resistance was unexpectedly observed during the Vietnam War in the early 1960s. The mutation of *P. falciparum* and resistance to other existing antimalarial drugs, for example, chloroquine (**2**) was a major problem for both American and Vietnamese soldiers. It was reported that appropriately 800,000 American soldiers were infected during 1967–1970. Under such urgent circumstance, immediate efforts were undertaken by the Walter Reed Army Institute of Research (WRAIR) in the United States to develop new drugs effective against multidrug-resistant malaria [17]. This program eventually led to two new drugs, Mefloquine (**3**) and Halofantrine (**4**) (Figure 10.1) which were produced by two contractors, Hoffmann La Roche and Smith Kline & French. However, on the opposite side, North Vietnam did not have a drug discovery program, especially given the circumstances at the time. Therefore, after a request from the North Vietnamese government, China launched a bioassay-guided program to search for new drugs to help North Vietnam fight against multidrug-resistant malaria., The program, launched by the Chinese government and Military on May 23, 1967 (called "Project 523"), was aimed at discovering new antimalarial therapies to overcome drug resistance and provide much needed relief to both the North Vietnamese and the populations in the southern parts of China [18]. It leads to the discovery of the well-known drug Artemisinin (**5**) and its derivatives (Figure 10.2).

It is also noteworthly that during that period of time, China was enduring a particularly difficult time, with endemic poverty and the disastrous culture revolution. Despite these

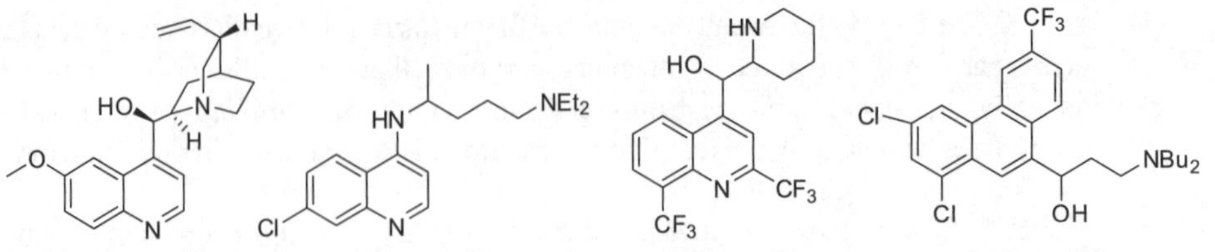

Quinine (**1**) Chloroquine (**2**) Mefloquine (**3**) Halofantrine (**4**)

Figure 10.1 Earlier antimalarial drugs.

hardships, the office of "Project 523" (also called "Office 523") rapidly gathered the best medical research scientists nationwide, including both synthetic and natural product chemists, pharmacologists, biologists, and clinical doctors, and set up a drug discovery effort, including both traditional and modern approaches, that would be considered modern even today. The traditional approach included temporary isolation of the infected individuals to prevent further spread, use of new insect repellents, gametocytocides, tissue or blood schizontocides, and acupuncture therapy, whereas the modern approach was to combine a bioassay-guided drug discovery strategy with TCM, especially those well-known or well-recorded folk medicines known to be useful for treating malaria. Therefore, in a very short time frame, they identified several folk plants or their extracts (*Agrimonia pilosa, Artabotrys hexapetalus, Artemisia annua, Polyalthia nemoralis, Hypericum juponicum, Brucea javanica, Nandina domestica*) with antimalarial activity, among which the extracts of *Artemisia annua* stood out with significant activity against both severe and uncomplicated malaria [19].

The plant "Qin hao" has been widely used to treat various diseases in China and was recorded in ancient Chinese herb books, including *Wu Shi Er Bing Fang Lu, Shen Nong Ben Cao Jing,* and *Ben Cao Gang Mu*. However, due to different origins of this plant and the various extraction strategies, validation of the active components of "Qin Hao" was not easy. It was found that only one species, *Artemisia annua* Linnaeu (also called "Huang hua hao" in Chinese) contains the active component, especially in the leaves and flowers. Extracts from other species were either inactive or active but with very low abundance. A high content (>1.0% of dry weight) of the active component was found only in the plants isolated from the Yunnan and Shandong provences of China [20]. Further, the antimalarial

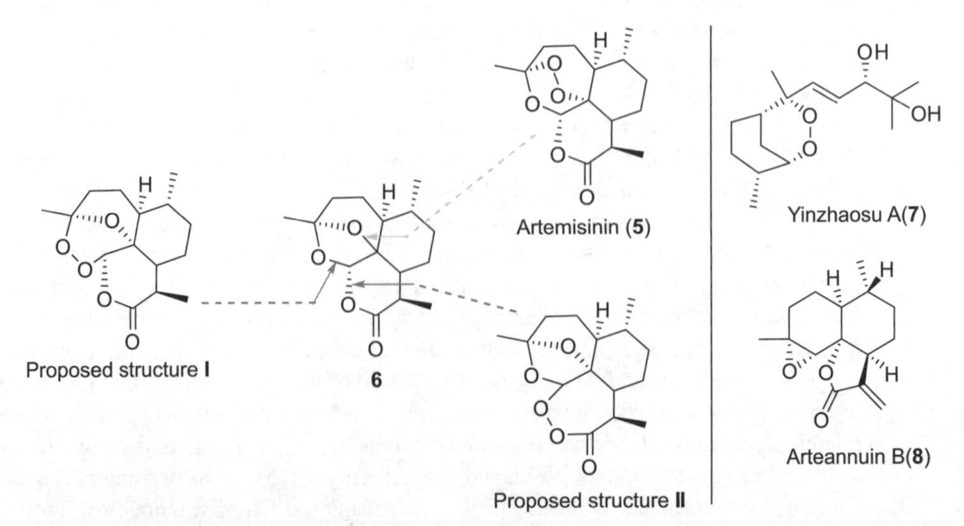

Figure 10.2 Assignment of the structure of Artemisinin.

component could only be extracted by diethyl ether, petroleum ether or acetone, while extracts isolated using other solvents, including warm water, alcohol or benzene, were inactive [20,21]. Quite fortuitously, the active compound crystallized from diethyl ether as a single component, which was named "Qin Hao Su" (Artemisinin) later.

10.3.3 Structural Determination of Artemisinin

In addition to the breakthrough of establishing a stable extraction strategy to access the active component of *Artemisia annua L.*, the structural elucidation of Artemisinin turns out to be the second milestone in the long history of the discovery of this antimalarial drug [20b]. With the broad usage of artemisinin, it was essential to identify the structure of this drug which would provide bases for potential chemical synthesis to increase supply.

Artemisinin has a unique sesquiterpene trioxane lactone structural core, with a molecular weight of 282 and molecular formula $C_{15}H_{22}O_5$. It is poorly soluble in water and has a melting point of 151–154°C. The initial difficulty in elucidating the chemical structure of Artemisinin was how to assign the five oxygen atoms to the 15 carbon atoms when only one can be identified as a carbonyl group based on its ^{13}C-NMR spectrum. From ^{1}H-NMR spectra, the existence of a singlet peak for one proton with a chemical shift of 5.68 ppm implied that Artemisinin should have an O–CH–O structural unit so the structure **6** was proposed in which one oxygen atom was excluded. The remainder of the structural assignment of Artemisinin, reduced to identifying where the remaining oxygen atom belonged.

Generally, compounds containing a peroxide fragment are not considered stable. Therefore a peroxide structure was not considered for Artemisinin since the compound was found to be very stable up to its melting point of 150°C. A significant breakthrough came from the structural determination of another TCM, Yinzhaosu A(**7**) [22] containing a peroxide structural unit, by another group of Chinese scientists in 1975. Encouraged by this result, organic chemists from Shanghai Institute of Organic Chemistry (SIOC) in China conducted both NaI/AcOH qualitative analysis and PPh_3-quantitative analysis experiments and confirmed the existence of a peroxide substructure in Artemisinin. Nevertheless, determination of the exact location of the peroxide subunit was not easy since there are three possible ways to insert the oxygen atom in **6** resulting in three different peroxide structures, Artemisinin (**5**), and compounds **I** and **II** as outlined in Figure 10.2. It was not until late in the 1970s, based on the identification of another component of *Artemisia annua L.*, arteannuin B (**8**), and the success in obtaining a single crystal X-ray structure, that the absolute structure of Artemisinin (**5**) was finally determined by scientists from SIOC and Institute of Biophysics of Chinese Academy of Sciences [23].

10.3.4 Pharmacological Evaluation and Clinical Trial Summary of Artemisinin

10.3.4.1 DMPK Evaluation Due to the difficulty in determining its structure, the therapeutic evaluation of Artemisinin was not initiated till the end of 1969 in Jiangsu providence of China using crude extracts to validate the therapeutic effects in malaria-infected rats or directly in local malarial patients with various dosages. The inconsistent efficacy and variable cardiac toxicity observed with different extracts and from plants from different locations prompted the scientists to identify a way to standardize the substance. After identification of the active plant, *Artemisia annua L.*, and isolation of the active principle—a needlelike crystal of unknown structure, pharmacologists, and physicians were able to evaluate this drug more precisely. Since 1973, under the organization of "Office 523," a systematic evaluation of Artemisinin was conducted in several malaria-endemic areas, especially in the southern regions of China adjacent to Vietnam and Cambodia. Therefore, an increasing amount of data on efficacy, toxicity, recrudescence rate, duration of action, formulation, resistance to chloroquine and so on, was collected on different cohorts of patients in a very short time. It is noteworthy that this progress was made with a multidisciplinary team working in a collaborative manner in much the same way that modern drug discovery is performed in today's major pharmaceutical companies. Although information on the therapeutic effect, safety index, and mechanism of action was very limited at that time, free radical intermediates may be involved in view of the peroxide structural unit. Meanwhile, activity against other parasitic diseases was also reported especially *Schistosoma japonicum*, *Toxoplasma gondii*, *Theileria annulatan*, and *Clonorchis Sinensis*. The potential to prevent the development of mature female worms was also observed in several animal models. Later on, activity against many viruses such as hepatitis B and C, human cytomegaloviruses, and herpes simplex was also claimed.

10.3.4.2 Clinical Trial Summary By 1975, over 900 clinical trials on malarial patients had completed confirming the outstanding parasiticidal effects of Artemisinin on *plasmodium* in the erythrocytic stage with rapid action, low toxicity, and high effects on both drug-sensitive and chloroquine-resistant *falciparum* malaria, although several concerns on the poor bioavailability and higher recrudescence ratio were raised. Artemisinin was launched as a new antimalarial therapy throughout China. At the same time, additional work was initiated to identify structural analogs of aremisinin with an improved biological and pharmacokinetic profile and to improve the formulation.

The discovery of Artemisinin as a antimalarial drug was a great success and milestone in Chinese research, although many details behind its discovery were restricted and not disclosed during the time of cold war [19,20]. It was not until 1977 and 1979, respectively, that the chemical structure and comprehensive pharmacology of Artemisinin were first reported [24]. The official disclosure of the Artemisinin project was at "The Fourth Meeting of the Scientific Working Group on the Chemotherapy of Malaria" sponsored by WHO in Beijing in 1981 [25]. After that, the details of the clinical trials were disclosed. In the final official report of "Project 523" in 1982, it was stated that Artemisinin (Qinghaosu) is a quick-acting and effective antimalarial drug against the asexual forms of the erythrocytic stage of *P. falciparum* and *P. vivax* [26]. It cannot kill the gametocytes of *P. falciparum*. The therapeutic effects of its oil solution (total dose 900 mg), oil suspension (900 mg), or water suspension (1.2 gm) in a 3-day course of treatment were also found to be quite satisfactory in several clinical studies. The cure rate in *falciparum* malaria is around 90%. It is effective against chloroquine-resistance and can be considered as the drug of first choice for the treatment of malaria in areas where chloroquine-resistant *falciparum* malaria is endemic. Since no toxic side-effects or adverse reactions on the heart, liver, or kidney have been observed when treating malaria, it can be used for patients with cardiac, liver, or renal disorders [27].

Since their introduction, the oil- and water-formulations of Artemisinin have been widely used by millions of patients in many South Asian countries, including Vietnam, Thailand, and Cambodia.

10.4 THE SYNTHESIS OF ARTEMISININ

Due to differences in the strains and geographical locations, the general content of Artemisinin in the plant *Artemisia annua L.* ranges from 0.1% to 1.5% of the dried leaves. Therefore, the availability of Artemisinin and its analogs is heavily dependent on extensive harvesting of the

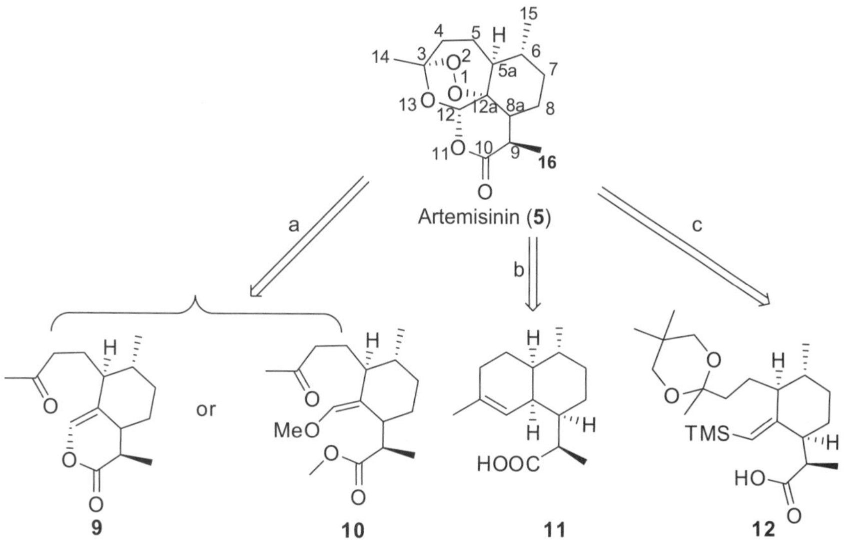

Figure 10.3 Synthetic approaches to access Artemisinin.

plant which makes the cost of Artemisinin very high. To address this issue, numerous biosynthetic, semisynthetic, and total synthetic strategies were studied in an attempt to achieve a significant increase of overall Artemisinin production [28]. Compared to the progress made on the biosynthesis of artemisinin, including the identification of the catalytic enzymes and genes along with their clones and expression, the total synthesis of Artemisinin has not proven to be practical, although it may be useful for the preparation of labeled samples for analytical and biodistribution studies. Therefore, semisynthetic pathways have been well developed during the past two decades. Since current supply of artemisinin is still from natural product extraction which limits its availability, it is therefore important to identify routes to prepare this natural product through chemical synthesis. This effort will help to increase the supply of this drug, and provide the possibility of synthesizing artemisinin analogs which may serve as next generation antimalarial drugs. Different synthetic routes at discovery stage are summarized here to showcase the challenges that scientists have to face in the preparation of this complex natural product in bulk quantity.

The most striking structural feature of Artemisinin is the existence of a trioxane ring, which was reported to be crucial for its antimalarial action [29]. Therefore, the key strategy to access this molecule is to establish a practical methodology to construct the trioxane core. Since its structure was released publicly in 1977 [23b], Artemisinin has been a popular synthetic target for both synthetic and medicinal chemists, and so far more than 10 synthetic approaches have been reported. Based on the differences in constructing the trioxane unit, these reported syntheses can be classified into path a–c, where the trioxane core was established by photooxidation of ketoenol ethers **9** and **10** (*path a*), ozonolysis of dihydroarteannuic acid **11** (*path b*) and ozonolysis of vinyl silane **12** (Figure 10.3).

10.4.1 Synthesis of Artemisinin using Photooxidation of Cyclic or Acyclic Enol Ether as the Key Step

Starting from natural product, (−)-isopulegol, Hofheinz and his colleagues from *F. Hoffmann-La Roche and Co.* reported the first total synthesis of Artemisinin in 1983 [30]. As outlined in Scheme 10.1, (−)-isopulegol was converted to ether **13** in five

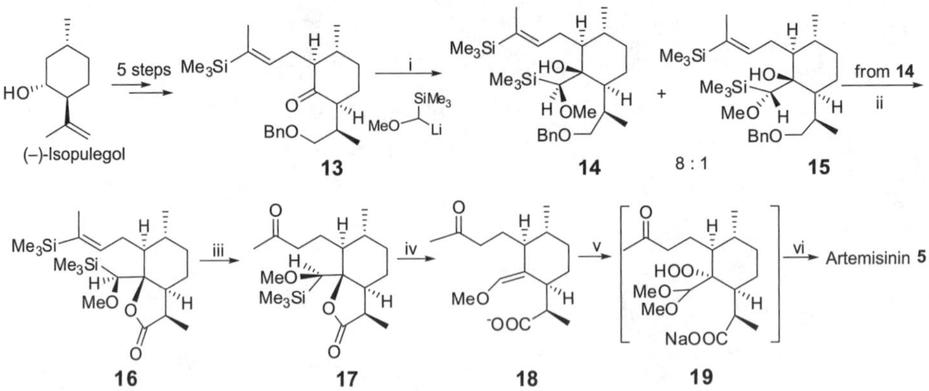

Scheme 10.1 Hofheinz's total synthesis of Artemisinin. Reagents and conditions: (i) THF, −78°C, ~100%; (ii) (a) Li, NH_3 (l); (b) PCC, CH_2Cl_2, 15 h, 75%; (iii) m-CPBA, CH_2Cl_2; TFA, CH_2Cl_2, 0°C, 3 min, 72%; (iv) TBAF, THF, r.t., 2 h, 95%; (v) Na salt, O_2, methylene blue, hν, MeOH, −78°C; (vi) HCO_2H, DCM, 0°C, 24 h, 30% (two steps).

steps with an overall yields of 28%. Treating ketone **13** with a large excess of trimethylsilyl methoxymethyl lithium yielded nucleophilic adduct **14** as the major product in 89% yield. Removal of benzyl group with lithium in ammonia followed by oxidation (PCC) afforded lactone **16** in 67% overall yield. Further oxidation of vinylsilane **16** with *m*-CPBA provided ketone **17** in 72% yield. Desilylation was realized by treating with TBAF accompanied by simultaneous generation of enol ether **18** in 95% yield. Photooxidation of enol ether **18** using singlet oxygen occurred in an ene-like reaction giving intermediate **19**, which was then treated with HCOOH leading to the formation of Artemisinin (**5**) in 30% overall yield. Although the absolute configures of compounds **14**–**17** were not established during the synthetic sequence, the correct structure of the final compound **5** confirmed the proposed stereochemistry. The synthesis included 12 liner steps from (−)-isopulegol and offered Artemisinin (**5**) in 3.8% overall yield.

In the same year, Zhou et al. from the Shanghai Institute of Organic Chemistry also reported a synthetic approach to assemble Artemisinin with arteannuic acid as the starting material [31]. Since artemisinic acid is another chemical component isolated from the plant *Artemisia annua L.* with higher abundance than that of Artemisinin, it was believed to be a biogenetic precursor for the plant to biosynthesize Artemisinin. Therefore, it was more attractive for synthetic chemists to explore useful methods to convert arteannuic acid to Artemisinin. As described in Scheme 10.2, esterification of arteannuic acid followed by $NaBH_4/NiCl_2$-reduction yielded dihydro arteannuic acid ester. Treating this ester with O_3 provided keto-aldehyde **20**. Selective protection of the keto group as the dithiane followed by conversion of the aldehyde function to the enol ether with $HC(OMe)_3$ provided **23** after deprotection of the ketone. The key intermediate **23** was obtained in 20% overall yield in seven steps. Photooxidation with O_2 followed by acidic hydrolysis ($HClO_4/H_2O$) led to the formation of Artemisinin (**5**) in 28% yield (two steps). Therefore, from arteannuic acid, Zhou et al. completed the synthesis of Artemisinin in nine steps with 5.6% overall yield. Although the reaction conditions were further investigated later, the overall yield was not improved. In addition, a synthesis of dihydroarteannuic acid from commercially available (+)-citronellal was also established later by the same group, therefore facilitating a second total synthesis of Artemisinin which did not rely on a starting material derived from *Artemisia annua L.*

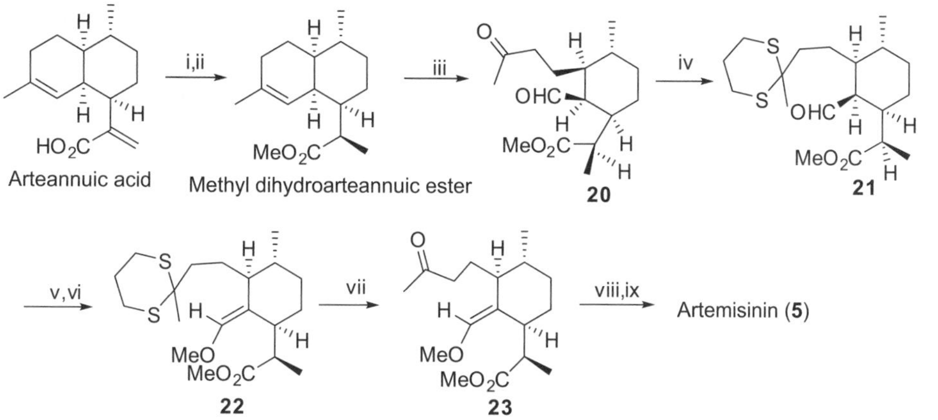

Arteannuic acid → (i,ii) → Methyl dihydroarteannuic ester → (iii) → 20 → (iv) → 21 → (v,vi) → 22 → (vii) → 23 → (viii,ix) → Artemisinin (5)

Scheme 10.2 Zhou's total synthesis of Artemisinin. Reagents and conditions: (i) CH_2N_2-Et_2O; (ii) $NaBH_4$, $NiCl_2$, MeOH, −15°C; (iii) O_3, CH_2Cl_2-MeOH, Me_2S; (iv) $HS(CH_2)_2SH$, BF_3Et_2O; (v) $HC(OMe)_3$, TsOH; (vi) heat, xylene; (vii) $HgCl_2$, $CaCO_3$, aq.CH_3CN, 33% (four steps); (viii) O_2, MeOH, Rose Bengal, hν, −78°C; (ix) 70% $HClO_4$-THF-H_2O, 28%.

In 1990, Wu and his colleagues from SIOC reported an improved synthesis of Artemisinin from arteannuic acid (Scheme 10.3) [32]. With this improved procedure, Artemisinin (**5**) was synthesized from arteannuic acid in eight steps with 38% overall yield, which was a significant enhancement compared to the earlier synthesis.

In 1992 and 1998, Nowak et al. at New York State University reported the first synthesis of Artemisinin (**5**) from arteannuin B (**8**), another constituent of *A. annua* with twice the natural abundance of Artemisinin (Scheme 10.4) [33]. This strategy was also used to synthesize Artemisinin from arteannuic acid. In this process, from arteannuin B, Nowak et al. established a synthesis of Artemisinin in 10 steps with an overall yield of 9.6%.

Similar strategies using singlet oxygen-oxidation of enol ethers as the key step were also reported by Hiremath and Sabitha [34].

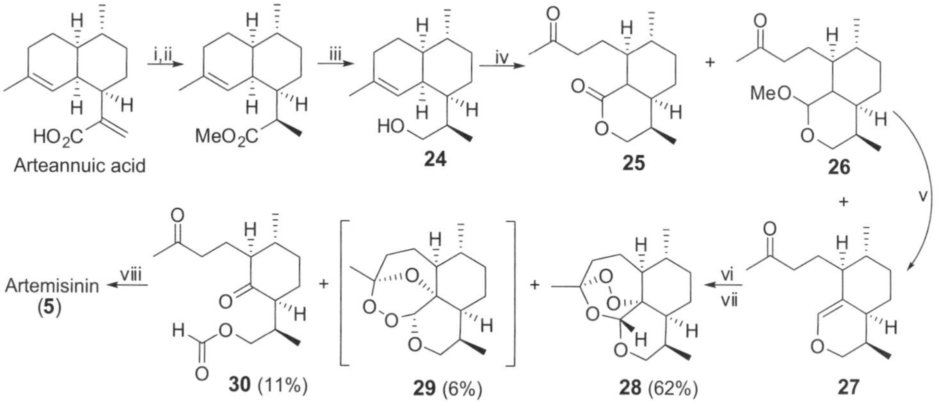

Arteannuic acid → (i,ii) → → (iii) → 24 → (iv) → 25 + 26 → (v) → 27 → (vi, vii) → 28 (62%) + 29 (6%) + 30 (11%) → (viii) → Artemisinin (5)

Scheme 10.3 Wu's total synthesis of Artemisinin. Reagents and conditions: (i) CH_2N_2-Et_2O; (ii) $NaBH_4$, $NiCl_2.6H_2O$, MeOH, −15°C; (iii) $LiAlH_4$, Et_2O, reflux, 85.2%; (iv) O_3, MeOH, CH_2Cl_2, −78°C, Me_2S; (v) cat. TsOH, xylene, reflux, 98%; (vi) O_2, methylene blue, hν, CH_2Cl_2, −70 ∼−78°C; (vii) TMSOTf; (viii) $RuCl_3$-$NaIO_4$, MeCN-H_2O-CCl_4, 96%.

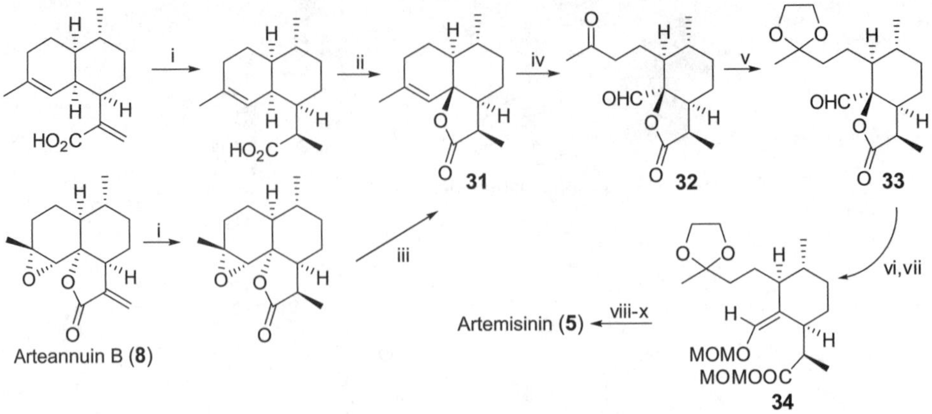

Scheme 10.4 Nowak's total synthesis of Artemisinin. Reagents and conditions: (i) H_2, $(PPh_3)_3RhCl$, 1:1 PhH/EtOH; (ii) CrO_3-3,5-dimethylpyrazol, CH_2Cl_2, −20 to −10°C, 59%; (iii) WCl_6, BuLi (2 eq), THF, −78°C, 59%; (iv) O_3, 1:1 $MeOH/CH_2Cl_2$, −78°C; Me_2S, 93%; (v) $(TMSOCH_2)_2$, TMSOTf, CH_2Cl_2, −78°C, 96%; (vi) NaNaph, −25°C; (vii) MOMCl, Et_3N, −25°C -rt, 82%; (viii) O_2, CD_3OD, Rose Bengal, hv, −78°C; (ix) TMSOTf, CH_2Cl_2, −78°C; (x) CSA, CH_2Cl_2, H_2O, rt, 32%.

10.4.2 Synthesis of Artemisinin by Photooxidation of Dihydroarteannuic Acid

Researchers from George Mason University and the Walter Reed Army Institute of Research's (WRAIR) were the first to investigate the direct conversion of arteannium B or arteannuic acid or other components isolated from the plant *A. annua* to antimalarial drug Artemisinin (**5**) [35].

In 1989, they first reported a successful low-temperature photooxidation of arteannuic acid to Artemisinin (**5**) in an overall yield of 17% [35a]. This procedure involved a reduction of the exocyclic methylene group in arteannuic acid to dihydroarteannuic acid followed by treating with O_2 and methylene blue with irradiation by a Westinghouse Ceramalux high intensity C400S51 electric discharge street lamp for 90 min, and then standing in the air for 4 days. The mechanism of this approach involves an ENE reaction of dihydroarteannuic acid with singlet oxygen yielding hydroperoxide **35**, which was then oxidized with triplet oxygen (air) leading to the final product, Artemisinin (**5**) via several intermediate steps as delineated in Scheme 10.5 [35b]. Jung also reported a similar conversion of arteannuic acid to deoxoartemisinin (**28**), a key intermediate to Artemisinin. They first converted arteannuic acid to alcohol **24**, which was then photooxidized by singlet oxygen followed by treating with strongly acidic Dowex-resin facilitating the formation of deoxoartemisinin (**28**) in 18% overall yield.

Several other procedures were also reported by Haynes [36], Liu [37], and Constantino [38], but the overall yields were still low.

10.4.3 Synthesis of Artemisinin by Ozonolysis of a Vinylsilane Intermediate

In 1987 and 1992, Avery et al. [39] reported a total synthesis of Artemisinin (**5**) through oxidation of a vinylsilane intermediate involving addition of O_2 to the vinyl bond following by cyclic cleavage, a similar strategy described by Buchi in 1978. They started from (*R*)-(+)-pulegone by converting it to sulfoxide **37** in three steps with 70% overall

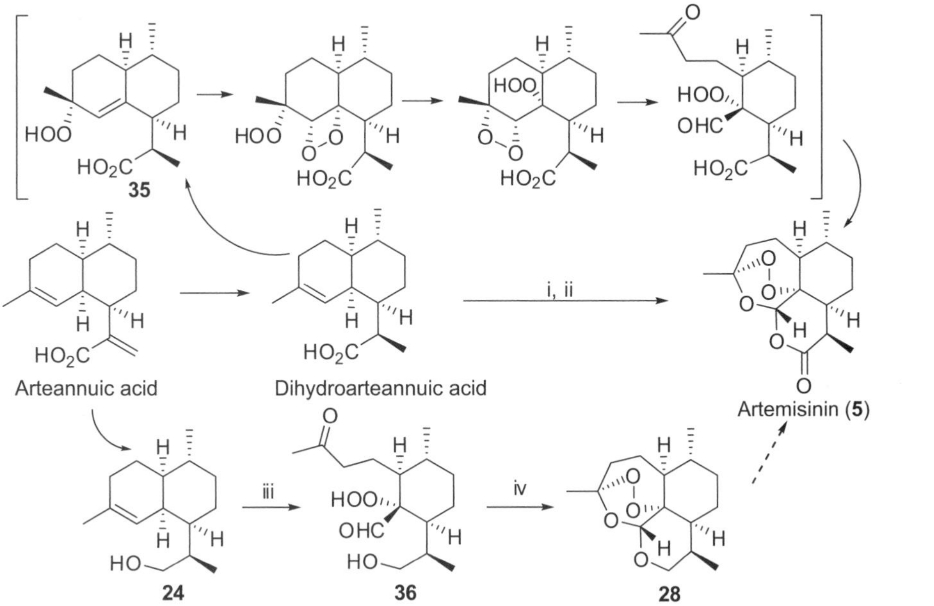

Scheme 10.5 WRAIR's total synthesis of Artemisinin. Reagents and conditions: (i) O_2, methylene blue, hv, CH_2Cl_2, $-78°C$, 90 min; (ii) petroleum ether, rt, 4d, air, 17%; (iii) O_2, methylene blue, $-78°C$; (iv) Dowex-resin (strongly acidic), rt.

yield (Scheme 10.6). Dianion alkylation of sulfoxide **37** followed by desulfurization with Al/Hg generated *trans* 2,3-disubstituted cyclohexanone **39** in 43% average overall yield (two steps). Treating cyclohexanone **39** with $TsNHNH_2$ provided hydrazone **40** in 86% yield, which was then treated with excess *n*-BuLi in TMEDA and quenched with DMF region selectively afforded unsaturated aldehyde **41** in 70% yield. Silyl anion addition to aldehyde **41** with $(Me_3Si)_3Al$ followed by quenching with Ac_2O yielded a single diastereomer **42** in 88% yield. Tandem Claisen ester-enolate rearrangement and dianion alkylation with a diastereoselective silyl anion addition afforded the key intermediate,

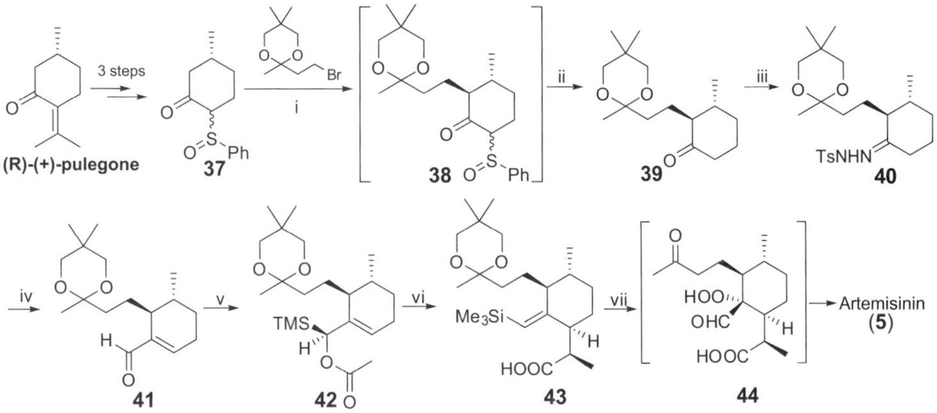

Scheme 10.6 Avery's total synthesis of Artemisinin. Reagents and conditions: (i) 2 eq. LDA, HMPT or DMTP, THF, $-35°C$; (ii) Al/Hg, wet. THF, ~43% (two steps); (iii) $TsNHNH_2$, neat, 1 mmHg, 86%; (iv) 4 eq. BuLi, TMEDA, 0°C; DMF, 70%; (v) $(Me_3Si)_3Al.Et_2O$, Et_2O, $-78°C$; Ac_2O, DMAP, then 23°C, 88%; (vi) 2 eq. LDEA, THF, $-78°C$ to 23°C; 2.0 eq. LDA, 0 to 45°C; MeI, $-78°C$ to r.t., 61%; (vii) O_3/O_2, CH_2Cl_2, $-78°C$; SiO_2; 3M H_2SO_4, 35%.

fully functionalized vinylsilane **43** in 61% overall yield. The final cyclization was completed by ozonolysis of **43** with O_3 in CH_2Cl_2 followed by successive addition of aqueous H_2SO_4 (3M) and silica gel, generating Artemisinin (**5**) in 35% overall yield. Therefore, using (*R*)-(+)-pulegon as the starting material, Avery et al. furnished a total synthesis of Artemisinin (**5**) in 10 steps with 3.4% overall yield.

As summarized above, the total synthesis studies of artemisinin could only provide small amount of this compound which severely limited their application in large-scale preparation of this drug. However, on the other hand, these studies did provide pathways for extensive analog preparation of artemisinin which resulted in the discovery of next generation of antimalarial drugs such as artemether and artesunate.

10.5 SAR STUDIES OF STRUCTURAL DERIVATIVES OF ARTEMISININ: THE DISCOVERY OF ARTEMETHER

Artemisinin (**5**) is among the most potent antimalarial drugs, effectively combating most sexual and asexual parasite stages. It has a fast onset of action and a high parasite reducing ratio of over 10,000 per erythrocytic cycle. Nevertheless, it suffers from both poor aqueous and oil solubility that limit its use. Therefore, the search for artemisinin analogs with better solubility but retaining antimalarial potency was conducted very early, and also by others later after the absolute structure of artemisinin was settled. Many reactions on the structure of Artemisinin were investigated, including reduction, acidic or basic hydrolysis (degradation), pyrolysis and even biotransformations. As outlined in Figure 10.4, reduction of Artemisinin with Pd/C under H_2 atmosphere removed one oxygen atom from the peroxide bridge yielding desoxoartemisinin **45**, which was inactive toward malarial parasites indicating the critical role of the peroxide function [40]. It was found that the lactone function can be reduced with $NaBH_4$ to afford dihydroartemisinin (**46**, DHA), an even more potent antimalarial analog and an important intermediate for further development of new derivatives [41]. In addition, reduction with $NaBH_4$ in the presence of $BF_3.Et_2O$ led to removal of the carbonyl moiety and afforded the synthetic intermediate deoxoartemisinin **28** [42]. However, strong reducing agents such as $LiAlH_4$ yielded complex mixtures. Treating artemisinin with $AcOH/H_2SO_4$

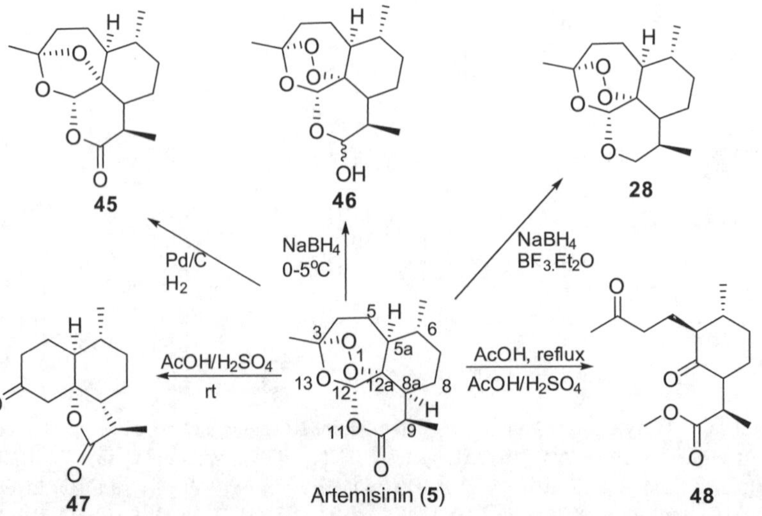

Figure 10.4 Typical reactions of Artemisinin.

generated several compounds, with keto-lactone **47** (and its diastereomers) as the major product. Refluxing Artemisinin in AcOH produced a mixture which upon further treating with AcOH/H_2SO_4 provided keto-ester **48** as the major product [43].

Meanwhile, synthetic analogs with additional modifications at either C-9, or C-10, or both, as well as C-11, C-14 to C-16 also become readily available through chemical synthesis. For convenient comparison, all the biological data were included in Table 10.1, and the research details were summarized in the following sections.

TABLE 10.1 Antimalarial Activity of Artemisinin Analogues

Compound	Antimalarial activity	Ref.
1	$IC_{50} = 159.61$ ng mL^{-1} (D6); 149.88 ng mL^{-1} (W2)	85
2	$IC_{50} = 7.58$ ng mL^{-1} (D6); 118.04 ng mL^{-1} (W2)	85
3	$IC_{50} = 45.55$ ng/mL (D6); 34.06 ng/mL (W2)	85
5	$SD_{90} = 6.20$ mg kg^{-1}	40(b)
46	$SD_{90} = 3.65$ mg kg^{-1}	40(b)
49	$IC_{50} = 1.90$ (W2)	45
50	$IC_{50} = 2.18$ (W2)	45
51	$IC_{50} = 4.07$ ng mL^{-1} (D6); 1.38 ng mL^{-1} (W2)	50
56	$IC_{50} = 4.628 \pm 0.1$ nm	55
57	$IC_{50} = 3.8 \pm 0.1$ nm	57b
58	$IC_{50} = 121.5$ ng mL^{-1} (D6); 34.07 ng mL^{-1} (W2)	58
59	$IC_{50} = 13.13$ ng mL^{-1} (D6); 35.60 ng mL^{-1} (W2)	58
60	$IC_{50} = 2.57$ ng mL^{-1} (D6); 0.82 ng ml^{-1} (W2)	58
61	$IC_{50} = 710$ ng mL^{-1} (D6); 171 ng mL^{-1} (W2)	58
63	$IC_{50} = 0.15$ng mL^{-1} (K1); 0.44 ng mL^{-1} (NF54)	60
64	$IC_{50} = 6.19 \pm 2.68$ nm	62
68	$ED_{50} = 0.58$ mg kg^{-1}; $ED_{90} = 1.73$ mg kg^{-1}	67
69	$ED_{50} = 7.08$ mg kg^{-1}; $ED_{90} = 60.99$ mg kg^{-1}	67
71	$IC_{50} = 24$ nm	68b
72	$IC_{50} = 0.87$ nm	68b
73	$IC_{50} = 0.59$ nm	68b
74	$IC_{50} = 0.91$ nm	68b
75	$EC_{50} = 2.4$ nm	69
76	$IC_{50} = 0.2 \pm 0.3$ nm (K1); 0.09 ± 0.1 (BH3)	70b
77	$IC_{50} = 0.5 \pm 0.1$ nm (K1); 0.18 ± 0.2 (BH3)	70b
78a	$IC_{50} = 0.61$ ng mL^{-1} (D6); 0.0.64 ng ml^{-1} (W2)	75a
80	$ED_{90} = 0.78$ mg kg^{-1}	75b
81	$ED_{90} = 0.46$ mg kg^{-1}	75b
82	$ED_{90} = 0.18$ mg kg^{-1}	75b
87	$IC_{50} = 31$ nm (W2)	78
88	$IC_{50} = 3.8$ ng mL^{-1} (D6); 1.1 ng mL^{-1} (W2)	76
89	$IC_{50} = 2.6$ nm (W2)	78
90	$ED_{50} = 1.25$ mg kg^{-1}; $ED_{90} = 6.4$ mg kg^{-1}	79
91	$IC_{50} = 5.30$ ng mL^{-1} (D6); 7.44 ng mL^{-1} (W2)	80a
92a + **93a**	$SD_{50} = 2.38$ mg kg^{-1}; $SD_{90} = 6.52$ mg kg^{-1}	82
92b	$SD_{50} = 5.48$ mg kg^{-1}; $SD_{90} = 11.41$ mg kg^{-1}	82
92c	$SD_{50} = 3.94$ mg kg^{-1}; $SD_{90} = 10.05$ mg kg^{-1}	82
93c	$SD_{50} = 1.59$ mg kg^{-1}; $SD_{90} = 56.03$ mg kg^{-1}	82

(continued)

TABLE 10.1 (*Continued*)

Compound	Antimalarial activity	Ref.
94	$IC_{50} = 1.9\,\mu m$	83
95e	$IC_{50} = 11.6\,\mu m$	83
95f	$IC_{50} = 44.7\,\mu m$	83
100	$ED_{50} = 15.0\,mg\,kg^{-1}$; $ED_{90} = 51.0\,mg\,kg^{-1}$	64a
101	$IC_{50} = 1.3$ nm	64a
102	$IC_{50} = 1.2$ nm (D6); 1.4 nm (W2)	88
103	$IC_{50} = 0.5$ nm (D6); 1.2 nm (W2)	88
104	$IC_{50} = 1$ nm (D6); 2 nm (W2)	88
105	$IC_{50} = 1.4$ nm (D6); 1.2 nm (W2)	88
106	$IC_{50} = 0.6$ nm (D6); 0.5 nm (W2)	88

10.5.1 C-10-Derived Artemisinin Analogs

10.5.1.1 Ethers, Ester, and Carbonates DHA (**46**) is one of the most widely used precursors to prepare various C-10 substituted analogs through generation of an oxonium ion intermediate. DHA can interact with alkyl alcohols, phenols, electron-rich aromatic compounds, silyl enol ethers, functionalized silanes, and alkynes to afford a large number of C-10 *O*-, *C*-, or *N*-substituted artemisinin analogs [44]. Typical examples include ether derivatives artemether (**49**), arteether (**50**), and ester derivative sodium artesunate (**52**) (Figure 10.5), which were obtained by simple etherization or esterification of DHA, and are clinically useful drugs, especially in Southeast Asian countries [45]. However, there is strong evidence that some of the artemisinin derivatives, such as DHA or its ether or ester derivatives, might be neurotoxic in chronically infected rats or dogs [46]. Therefore, new derivatives with better safety and pharmacokinetic profiles are still highly needed.

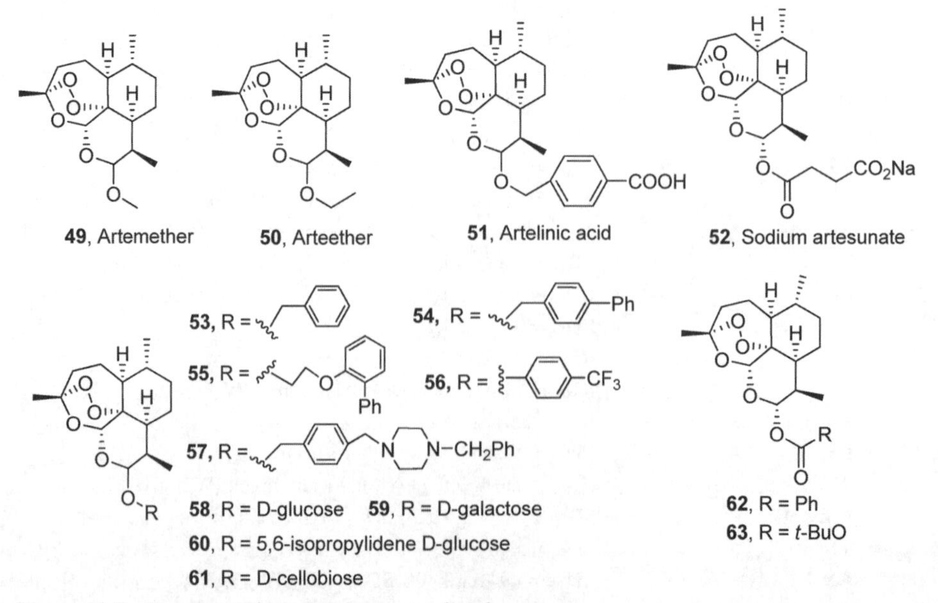

Figure 10.5 Representative ethers, ester, and carbonates.

In fact, the above-mentioned ethers, esters and carbonates, especially compounds **49–52** have long been considered to be the first generation of antimalarial drugs, and are currently still the drugs of choice for the treatment of malaria caused by multidrug-resistant *P. falciparum* [45]. The oil-soluble artemether (**49**) was first synthesized and purified early in the 1970s as the β-epimer by Li et al. from DHA (**46**) in a mixed solution of methanol–benzene containing BF_3 etherate [47,48]. Similarly, the oil-soluble arteether (**50**), along with many other ethers, was also synthesized by the same group. The preparation of the water-soluble artesunate **52** is much more straightforward than that of artemether and arteether. It was synthesized from DHA and succinic anhydride in the presence of pyridine as base and solvent with yields up to 65%. The ester compounds were found to be much more potent than the parent compound Artemisinin. The relative overall antimalarial potencies can be arranged in the following order: Artemisinin < ethers < ester < carbonates. In spite of the high potency, these first-generation semisynthetic Artemisinin analogs are generally cleared from blood within a short time ($t_{1/2}$, 30 min), and the parasites that are not eliminated within this time can re-emerge, resulting in parasite recrudescence. To prevent recrudescence, these Artemisinin derivatives are generally used as combination therapies with drugs that have longer half-lives (e.g., amodiaquine, mefloquine, piperaquine, and lumefantrine) [49]. To treat advanced cases of *P. falciparum* malaria, a water-soluble derivative of Artemisinin is required, which can be delivered quickly by intramuscular injection [50]. The water-soluble sodium artesunate (**52**) is currently prescribed as a clinical antimalarial drug [51] and is administered in combination most often with mefloquine [52].

Meanwhile, many other C-10 etheric Artemisinin derivatives, in addition to compounds **49–51**, were also reported. Benzyl ether **53**, reported by Kingston [53], showed IC_{50} values in the range of 0.25–250 ng mL^{-1} against chloroquine-resistant *P. falciparum* strain W2. Singh and coworkers [54] recently reported a new series of orally active Artemisinin derivatives with high efficacy against multidrug-resistant malaria in mice. They found that among most of the ether derivatives, α-isomers are generally more active than the β-isomers. Ether derivatives **54** and **55**, the most active compounds in this series, provided 100% protection to infected mice at 12 mg kg^{-1} × 4 days. In addition, many substituted phenyl ethers of DHA, such as compound **56** also exhibited appreciable *in vitro* and *in vivo* antimalarial activity [55]. Moreover, compound **56** showed better *in vivo* activity than artemether, DHA and sodium artesunate with a half maximal effective dose (ED) value of 2.12 mg kg^{-1} in a *Plasmodium berghei* mouse model [56]. Incorporation of an *N*-phenylpiperazinyl moiety-yielded compound **57** [57] possessing remarkedly enhanced *in vitro* antimalarial activity. In order to elevate further the water solubility along with antimalarial activity, Lin and coworkers [58] synthesized several carbohydrate-associated etheric derivatives. These compounds (**58–61**) were found to be more effective against W2 and D6 clones and were not cross-resistant with existing antimalarials in an *in vitro* antimalarial bioassay against *P. falciparum*. An *in vivo* study indicated that the increase in polarity and water solubility of these compounds led to decreased antimalarial activity. In addition to sodium artesunate **52**, the C-10 ester derivative **62** also displayed high potency with IC_{50} values in the range of 0.07–119 ng mL^{-1}, and proved to be most active against both W2 and the chloroquine-sensitive strain D6 [59]. Other substituted esters of DHA, such as compound **63** exhibited significant *in vitro* antimalarial activity against *P. falciparum* K1 and *P. falciparum* FN54 with IC_{50} values of 0.15 and 0.44 ng mL^{-1}, respectively. In the mouse antimalarial test, mice subcutaneously injected with 10 mg kg^{-1} of compound **63** showed *plasmodium* decreases of 99.97%. Thirty days after injection the mice remained *plasmodium* negative in contrast to artemether [60].

10.5.1.2 C-10 Alkyl and Aryl Derivatives Improved stability could be achieved by replacing the exocyclic oxygen atom with an alkyl or aryl group. Consequently, several groups have developed synthetic and semisynthetic approaches to C-10 carba-analogs. By direct substitution of the DHA ester with diversified alkylating reagents, a large number of C-10 alkyl derivatives have been developed and pharmacologically evaluated [61]. In the antimalarial bioassay, the C-10 alkyl analog **64** demonstrated superior activity to artemether and artesunate both *in vitro* and *in vivo* [62]. The synthesis of metabolically more stable C-10 aryl analogs of DHA has been the focus of new antimalarial drug development for many years. Representative C-10 aryl or heteroaryl derivatives included **65–67**, which were synthesized by Haynes's [63] and Posner's [64] groups. Compound **66**, 10-(phenyl)-DHA has been reported to exhibit an IC_{50} value of 0.31 and 0.73 ng mL^{-1} against *P. falciparum* strain W2 and D6, respectively [65]. *para*-F or *para*-Cl-substituted analogs **67** were highly potent against either chloroquine-sensitive (D6 or 3D7) or chloroquine-resistant (W2 or K1) strains of *P. falciparum* [66].

Wang et al. [67] reported that treating the C-10-α–acetate of DHA with 2-naphthol in the presence of $BF_3 \cdot$ etherate yielded a 1:1 mixture of the C-10-arylated derivatives **68** and **69**. The *9R,10R*-diastereoisomer **68** which has the "correct" configuration (i.e., same configuration as in Artemisinin) at C-9 showed high antimalarial activity in the preliminary *in vivo* test in mice against *P. berghei* IC173 strain. The *9S,10S* isomer **69** bearing the "abnormal" configuration in C-9 was found to be much less potent than **68**.

Recently, a new series of trioxane dimers including compounds **70** and **71** were reported [68]. These compounds are generally prepared by combining two Artemisinin or DHA core structures through a functionalized alkyl linker. Further modification of the functionalized linker provided additional dimeric analogs **72–77** as shown in Figure 10.6. Alcohols **72**, **73** and ketone **74** showed enhanced potencies compared to compound **71**. These compounds were 10-fold more potent than Artemisinin possessing IC_{50} values of 0.87, 0.59, and 0.91 nM, respectively [68b].

In addition, several dimeric Artemisinin analogs bearing carboxylic acid-containing linkers were prepared with the aim to improve the low water solubility of the corresponding dimers. The isobutyric acid analog **75** was safer and displayed a therapeutic index six times higher than that of sodium artesunate (**52**) [69]. Phosphates **76** and **77** represented another interesting example of orally active, Artemisinin-derived dimeric trioxane derivatives. In these cases, the C-10 position was replaced by a methylene unit, offering greater metabolic stability than the original acetal analogs with longer half-lives and less toxicity [70]. Phosphate **76** showed an IC_{50} value of 0.2 nM against the chloroquine-resistant K1 strain of *P. falciparum*, while compound **77** presented an IC_{50} value of 0.5 nM, which is almost 50-fold more potent than Artemisinin ($IC_{50} = 12.3$ nM) and 15-fold more effective than the acetal artemether. Moreover, these drugs were 400- to 900-fold more potent than chloroquine ($IC_{50} = 190$ nM). In addition, phosphates **76** and **77** were much more potent against the chloroquine-sensitive HB_3 strain as well, with IC_{50} values of 0.09 and 0.18 nM, respectively [71b].

10.5.1.3 C-10 Amino Derivatives Mono- or di-substituted cyclic or acyclic amino groups have been attached to the C-10 position of DHA to replace the hydroxyl group for the purpose of preparing water soluble salts [63e,71]. It was found that arylamine derivatives bearing halogen at C-9 instead of the original methyl group were inactive *in vivo* indicating the importance of the C-9-methyl group due to either its electronic character or stereochemical effect, or both [72]. The C-10 arylamino derivatives were synthesized by treating DHA with arylamines in the presence of pyridinium sulfate in pyridine, however, this method is unsuccessful for the synthesis of C-10 alkylamino derivatives [73]. In general,

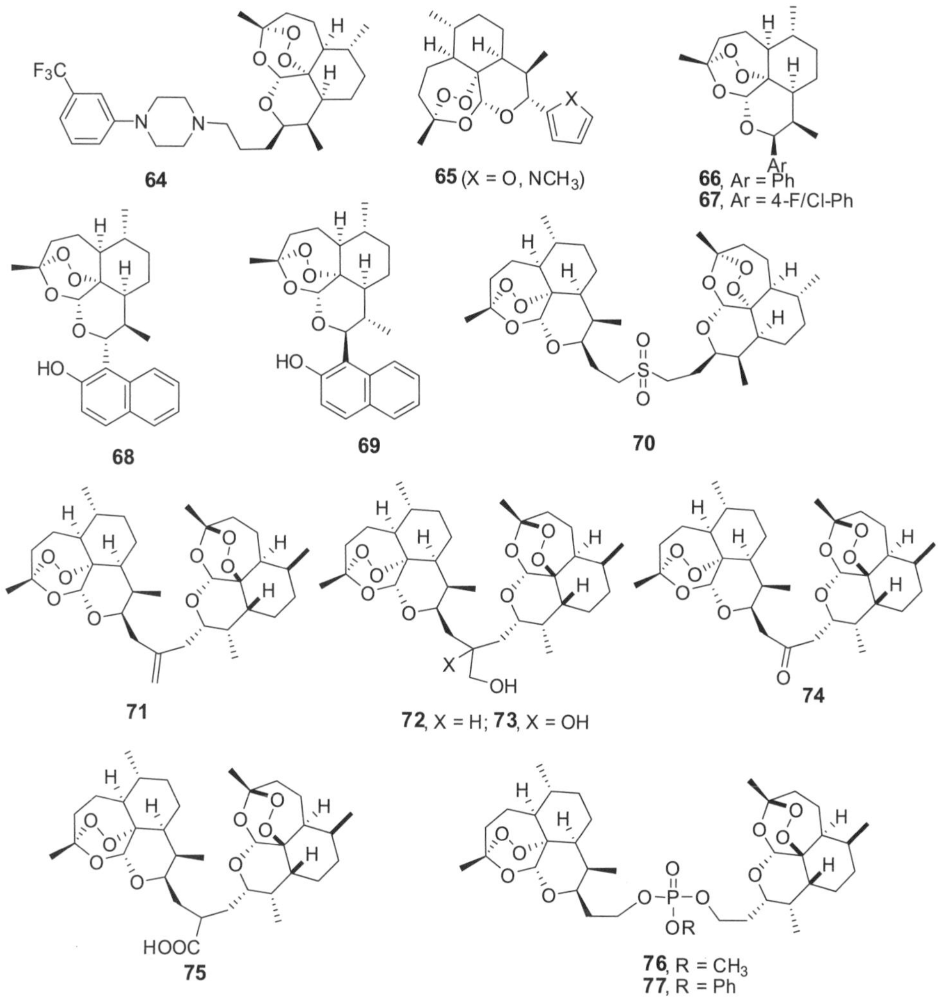

Figure 10.6 Representative C-10 alkyl and aryl derivatives.

the C-10 alkylamino derivatives were obtained by simple conversion of the hydroxyl group in DHA to active esters (e.g., OAc, OTs, and OMs) followed by nucleophilic substitution with a primary or secondary alkylamine.

Haynes and coworkers have prepared a number of new C-10 aryl- or alkyl-amino–derived DHA derivatives [63c,74]. Representative compounds **78–86** (Figure 10.7) were very potent against either chloroquine-sensitive (D6 or 3D7) or chloroquine-resistant (W2 or K1) strains of *P. falciparum*. All the compounds were substantially more active than artesunate **52**, especially compound **79**, which is active in the picograms per milliliter range against *P. falciparum*. *In vivo* screenings against chloroquine sensitive *P. berghei* and chloroquine-resistant *Plasmodium yoelii* in mice were conducted and [75] the amino derivatives were generally 3–26 times more active than artesunate *via* the subcutaneous route, or three to seven times more active by the po route in the *P. berghei* assays. In the *P. yoelii* assays, these compounds were 2–81 times more active by the subcutaneous route. The activities of these compounds in the murine malaria models appeared to be superior to those of any other artemisinins, and are

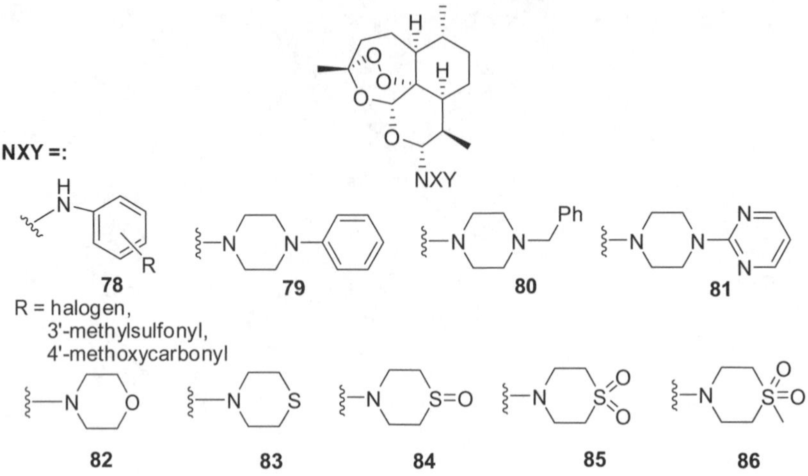

Figure 10.7 Representative C-10 amino derivatives.

comparable to the most potent synthetic trioxolane peroxidic antimalarials reported today. Piperazinyl compounds **80** and **81** were 20-fold more potent than artesunate **52**, however, they showed neurotoxic effects in many tests.

Artemisone (**85**) was obtained in only three steps from DHA. This compound was significantly more potent than Artemisinin, chloroquine and pyrimethamine against both drug-resistance and drug-sensitive strains of *P. falciparum* exhibiting IC_{50} values at the very low nanomolar range in all cases studied [76]. Later, recrudescence was observed on *P. falciparum* Vietnam-Oak Knoll (FVO) isolate infected-Aotus monkeys treated with **85**. Moreover, an important synergistic effect was observed when compound **85** was used together with mefloquine or amodiaquine. Complete cure was accomplished in infected monkeys when treated orally with **85** ($10\,mg\ kg^{-1}$) plus mefloquine ($5\,mg\ kg^{-1}$) or **85** ($10\,mg\ kg^{-1}$) plus amodiaquine ($20\,mg\ kg^{-1}$). In conclusion, the C-10 aminoalkyl derivative **85** has proven to be a promising antimalarial agent possessing enhanced potency over the current artemisinins with minor neurotoxicity [76].

10.5.1.4 C-10 Fluoro Derivatives In the search for more stable antimalarial artemisinins, Ziffer et al. reported several fluorinated derivatives **87–90**, prepared by fluorination of the corresponding acetal and ketal derivatives (Figure 10.8) [76]. These compounds exhibited good *in vitro* IC_{50} values. However, possibly due to the difficulty in preparing sufficient quantities of these compounds, data on *in vivo* activity was seldom disclosed [77]. The C-10 trifluoromethyl derivative **89** is more potent than artemether and artesunate against D6 and W2 drug-resistant strains of *P. falciparum* (D6: $IC_{50} = 2.6$ nM; W2: $IC_{50} = 0.9$ nM). Moreover, it is also active against wild isolates from African patients

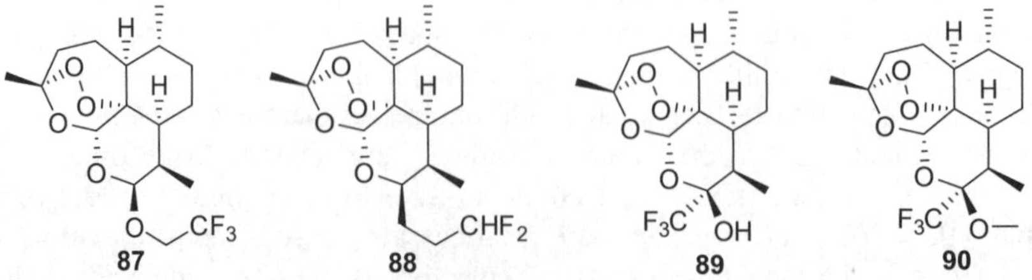

Figure 10.8 Representative C-10 fluoro derivatives

(with Senegalese isolates, $IC_{50} = 3.3$ nM) [78]. Compound **89** is also more active *in vivo* (i.p, s.c., or oral administration) than artesunate **52** in mice infected with murine *P. berghei.*

Magueur et al. [79] have explored the possibility of introducing a C-10-trifluoromethyl group to improve the hydrolytic stability of the acetal functionality in DHA. Impressively, the lead compound **90** from this group was about 33-fold more stable than artemether in simulated stomach acid, and showed an ED_{50} value of 1.25 mg kg^{-1} when tested intraperitonially in mice infected with *P. berghei* (cf. artemether = 2.5 mg kg^{-1}).

10.5.2 C-9 and C-9,10 Double Substituted Analogs

Compared to the large number of C-10-substituted artemisinin derivatives, only a few C-9 substituted or C-9,10 double substituted derivatives were reported [75]. Representative compounds (**91–99**) are listed in Figure 10.9. The synthesis of these compounds involved the conversion of artemisinin to artemisitene **91** followed by Michael addition of various donor synthons. Artemisitene **91** is also a natural substance existing in the same plant but with much lower abundance and has less antimalarial activity than artemisinin [80a,81].

Li et al. reported a small series of C-9-heterocyclic alkyl substituted analogs **92a–c** and **93a–c** bearing a 1,2,4-triazolo, benzotriazolo, or benzimidazolo substituent. In *in vivo* antimalarial tests against K173 strain of *P. bergei,* the diastereomeric mixture of **92a** and **93a** showed ninefold [SD_{50} (mg kg^{-1} day^{-1}) = 2.38, $SD_{90} = 6.52$] more potent than

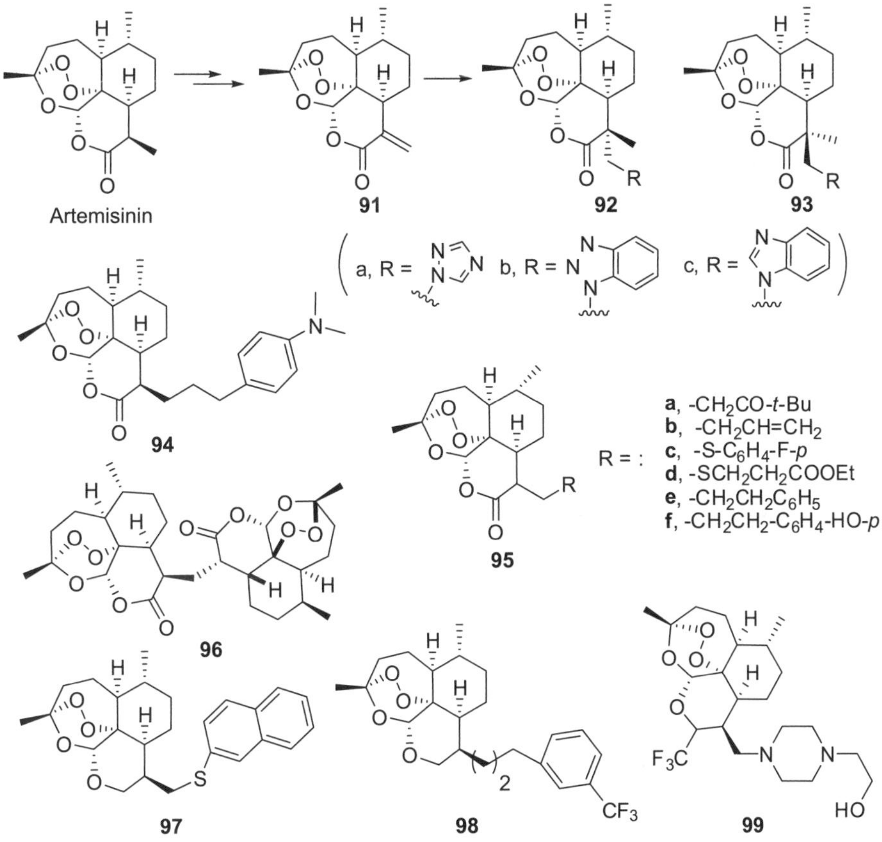

Figure 10.9 Representative C-9 substituted and C-9,10 double substituted analogues.

artemisinin [SD_{50} (mg kg^{-1} day^{-1}) = 18.75, SD_{90} = 56.66]. Compound **92b** showed activity comparable to that of artemisinin. Benzoimidazole **92c** and **93c** were also more active than artemisinin, and compound **92c** had higher activity than its diastereomer **93c** [82].

Other interesting C-9 substituted and C-9,10 double substituted derivatives included compounds **95–99** as listed in Figure 10.9. Replacement of the C-9 methyl in artemisinin with an aryl substituted propyl group led to compound **94** exhibiting IC_{50} values of 7.6–21.6 ng mL^{-1} against different strains of *P. falciparum* [83]. Compounds **95a–f** represent a different subseries of C-9-substituted analogs with dual action as antimalarial and antileishmaniasis drugs. Most of these compounds were more potent than artemisinin against the chloroquine-resistant *P. falciparum* strain (W2) and mefloquine-resistant *P. falciparum* strain (D6). For example, **95e** ($R = CH_2CH_2C_6H_5$) exhibited IC_{50} values of 4.7 and 1.3 nM against D6 and W2 strains, respectively, while **95f** ($R = CH_2CH_2$-Ph-*p*-OH) showed IC_{50} values of 7.9 and 4.7 nM against D6 and W2 strains, respectively [83]. The naphthalen-2-ylthio compound **97**, without a functional group in C10 position was claimed with an *in vitro* IC_{50} value of 2.7 ng mL^{-1} against the W2 strain [84]. Further replacement of the naphthalenylthio moiety with an arylethyl group yielded compound **98** showing an ED_{50} value of 1.25 mg kg^{-1} (cf. sodium artesunate = 2.4 mg kg^{-1}) when tested orally in mice infected with *P. berghei* (N) [85]. A number of C9β arylethyl analogs of artemisinin were found to be remarkably active, but their solubility needed to be optimized to address concerns associated with formulation and drug absorption [85]. In a related study, Grellepois et al. reported the preparation of a number of C-9 analogs directly derived from 16-bromo-10-trifluoromethyl anhydrodihydroartemisinin, which was accessible readily from artemisinin [86]. Among these compounds, 10-trifluoromethyl-9-(4-hydroxyethyl-piperazin-1-yl)methyl analog **99** [87] produced 100% inhibition of parasitemia by day 4 (on oral as well as s.c. administration of a 10 mg kg^{-1} dose) when tested in mice infected with *P. berghei.* It was remarkably more potent than artesunate **52**, and showed an ED_{90} value below 10 mg kg^{-1}, and 25-fold higher oral bioavailability than artemether (**49**).

10.5.3 C-3 Substituted Analogs

C-3 Substituted artemisinin analogs are rare due to the difficulty in preparation, mostly through total synthesis. Aryl substituted compounds **100** and **101** are two examples of this category of derivatives (Figure 10.10). Compound **100** was found to possess good thermal stability and aqueous solubility and showed an ED_{50} value of 15 mg kg^{-1} when tested orally in *P. berghei* infected mice [64a]. Removal of the carboxylic acid function in compound **100** afforded compound **101**, showing an *in vitro* antimalarial IC_{50} value of 1.3 nM. Although 3-phenyltrioxane **101** displayed high *in vitro* antimalarial activity, it could not be easily administered *in vivo* intravenously or orally because of its insolubility in water.

10.5.4 C-6 or C-7 Substituted Derivatives

Compounds **102–106** as illustrated in Figure 10.11 can be classified as C-6 or C-7 substituted analogs of arteether (**50**). Ziffer and coworkers reported the synthesis of

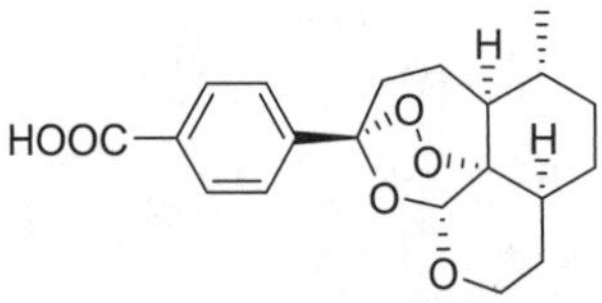

100 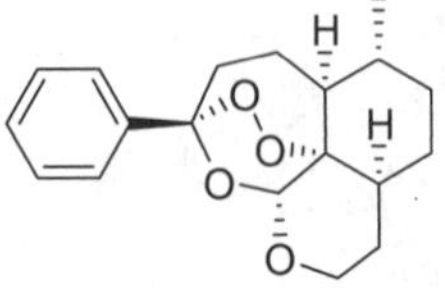 **101**

Figure 10.10 Representative C-3 substituted analogues.

TABLE 10.2 ***In Vitro*** **Data of Compounds against Two Drug-Resistant Strains of** ***P. falciparum*** **(nM)**

	W-2		D-6	
Compound	IC_{50} 1/cpd	IC_{50} 4/cpd	IC_{50} 1/cpd	IC_{50} 4/cpd
102	1.4	0.8	1.2	0.1
103	1.2	0.6	0.5	0.05
104	2	1.5	1	0.3
105	1.2	0.8	1.4	0.5
106	0.5	0.3	0.6	0.2

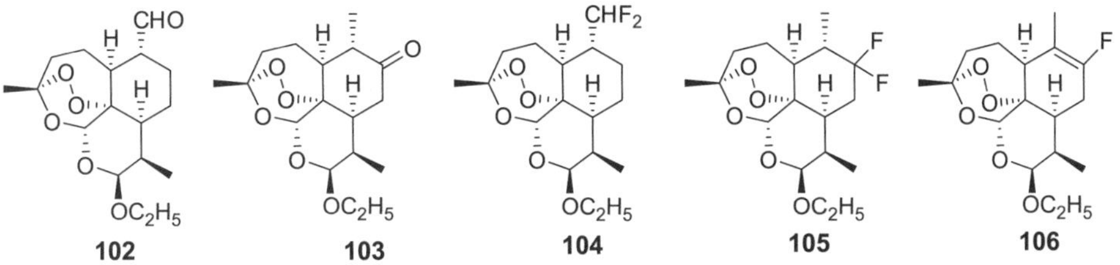

Figure 10.11 Representative C-6 or C-7 substituted analogues.

aldehyde **102** and ketone **103** by using corresponding hydroxyl precursors as the key intermediates. Treating aldehyde **102** and ketone **103** with DAST provided corresponding germinal difluoro derivatives **104** and **105**. In addition to **105**, a monofluoro olefin **106** was also obtained [88]. The *in vitro* assays of these compounds against two drug-resistant strains of *P. falciparum* were listed in Table 10.2.

A comparison of the activities of the carbonyl derivatives **102** and **103** (Table 10.2) with the corresponding germinal difluoro derivatives **104–106** showed that the latter compounds were slightly more active. The increase in activity is consistent with earlier observations that lipophilic derivatives are more active than their more polar counterparts, for example, esteric and etheric artemisinin derivatives are more active than the corresponding alcohols or acids.

10.5.5 C-11-Substituted Analogs

It has been found that the endocyclic lactone moiety in artemisinin can be converted into a lactam and retain antimalarial activity [89]. 11-Aza-artemisinin (**108**), was first made by Ziffer and coworkers [90] through directly treating artemisinin with an appropriate amine agent as shown in Figure 10.12. This compound has an IC_{50} value of 1.73 and 2.60 ng mL^{-1}, against the W2 and D6 strains, respectively [91].

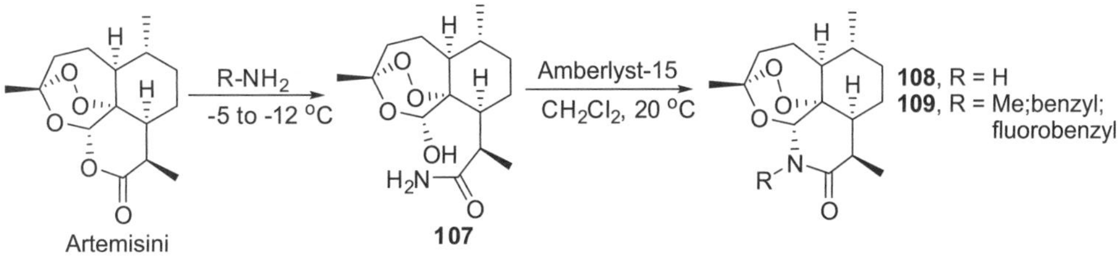

Figure 10.12 11-Aza derivatives.

Since the NH- moiety in the lactam **108** is relatively acidic, deprotonation can be readily realized by treating with a base such as NaH in the presence of Michael acceptors [92]. *N*-Alkylation with an appropriate alkylating reagents was also developed therefore facilitating a series of *N*-substituted lactams **109**, as shown in Figure 10.12 [93]. However, this reaction does not work when aromatic amines, or primary amines bearing other functional groups, for example, hydroxyl or thiol, are used in which case the 2-deoxy aza-artemisinin product is generally obtained as the major product [94].

Compared to artemisinin's lactone component, 11-aza-analogs **109**, possess better chemical stability and lack the potential to be metabolized to DHA, and therefore, have longer half-lives and an elevated therapeutic index. These compounds were found to be more active against the malaria parasite than artemisinin, and no neurotoxicity has been reported so far. Therefore, this class of compounds is worthy of further evaluation.

As discussed above, extensive SAR studies of artemisinin analogs were carried out and many potent compounds were identified. Among these analogs, artemether stood out as one of the lead compounds with an improved profile compared to artemisinin and became one of the next generation of antimalarial drugs.

10.6 DEVELOPMENT OF ARTEMETHER

10.6.1 Profile and Synthesis of Artemether

In patients with severe malaria, oral treatment is often impossible and a parenteral formulation of the drug artemisinin is necessary. Therefore, the oil-soluble artemether (**49**) was developed for intravenous and intramuscular administration, respectively. This semisynthetic derivative of artemisinin is effective against both chloroquine-sensitive and chloroquine-resistant *P. falciparum,* and is clinically used for the treatment of cerebral malaria. Artemether is now also used as an oral formulation (artemether–lumefantrine). It is the WHO's policy to promote the use of these drugs (artemether) intrarectally as an emergency treatment in primary healthcare situations in developing countries. However, delays in treatment, often caused by the long travel distance for the patients to the hospital, play a significant factor in the high mortality in children. Artemether and artesunate also exert their actions through formation of dihydroartemisinin (**46**, DHA) *in vivo*. This metabolite is often present in higher concentrations than the parent drugs, and exhibits higher activity *in vitro*.

Artemether has potent parasite killing activity *in vitro* with IC_{50} values of 0.1–10 ng mL^{-1} [95], which is more potent *in vitro* than artemisinin itself. All the etheric artemisinin derivatives including artemether are active against *P. falciparum strains*, which are resistant to a broad spectrum of other antimalarials [96].

Being much more oil soluble, artemether was administered as an oil solution by intramuscular injection. The total dosage was 0.24–0.64 g given over a 3-day period. It is noteworthy that fever subsidence and parasitemia clearance were independent of the dosages given, although certain positive correlations did exist in the radical cure rates. It was estimated that a 480 mg dose of artemether was similar in therapeutic efficacy to 900 mg of artemisinin in oil solution or suspension. However, a 600 mg/3-day treatment was suggested for artemether as the preferred regimen.

After oral intake of artemether, high concentrations of dihydroartemisinin were observed which paralleled the artemether concentrations [97]. The relative bioavailability of oral artemether compared to intramuscular administration was 43% [98].

Less dihydroartemisinin was observed after intramuscular administration than from the oral route, suggesting that some dihydroartemisinin formation may be due to metabolism by the gut lumen.

Although demethylation of artemether is probably mediated by cytochrome *P* (CYP) 450 enzymes, no effect was observed from specific CYP 2D6- and CYP 2C19-inhibition on the pharmacokinetics of artemether [99]. It was concluded that artemether is not a substrate of these enzymes and thus not subject to the genetic polymorphisms of these enzymes *in vivo*. From *in vitro* results, a major role for CYP 3A4 was proposed to be responsible for the conversion of artemether to dihydroartemisinin [100]. This enzyme is probably also important in the primary metabolism of artemether to dihydroartemisinin. In interaction studies with grapefruit juice, a strong inhibitor of CYP3A4, there was a more than twofold increase in artemether bioavailability, which suggests a role for CYP3A4 in the first-pass elimination of artemether.

There are several factors influencing the pharmacokinetics of the artemisinin drugs. In patients with uncomplicated malaria, a higher C_{max} was observed than in healthy subjects [101]. A reduced volume of distribution due to malaria or nonlinear (saturable) pharmacokinetics of artemether is believed to be involved. Food has no effect on the pharmacokinetics of artemether [102]. Although it is thought that drugs, like artemisinin and artemether, are predominantly metabolized through hepatic transformations, liver cirrhosis does not influence bioavailability, nor delay the elimination [103]. In acute renal failure, artemether levels after intramuscular administration were increased, possibly related to the reduced volume of distribution as renal elimination of this drug is negligible [104].

In multiple dosage studies with artemether both in healthy subjects and in patients, peak plasma artemether concentrations on day 6 were reduced to only 20% of those on day one, whereas the half-life was unchanged [105]. It was suggested that auto-induction of enzymes in the liver or gut is responsible for this time-dependent increase in first-pass effect. It is possible that these decreasing plasma concentrations over time contribute to the recrudescences observed in treatment trials with this group of compounds [106]. Time dependent pharmacokinetics has also been observed in studies with artemether [107].

Artemether (**49**) and related etheric derivatives are currently prepared in two steps. In the first step, artemisinin is reduced with $NaBH_4$ in MeOH to furnish DHA as described in Figure 10.4. However, this step generally suffers from certain major drawbacks [94], especially that the reaction conditions are highly basic which can lead to rapid degradation of artemisinin and dihydroartemisinin, while stringent low temperature conditions (0°C) are not maintained. In the second step, dihydroartemisinin is reacted with an appropriate alcohol in the presence of an acid catalyst such as $BF_3{\cdot}Et_2O$, HCl, Me_3SiCl or PTSA [108]. This step again requires aqueous work-up. Thus, conversion of artemisinin to its etheric derivatives requires two independent steps, both of which require aqueous work-up. Singh and coworkers reported an improved one-pot conversion of artemisinin to its etheric derivatives, which does not suffer from the above-mentioned drawbacks. This process consists of reducing artemisinin with the combination of $NaBH_4$/Amberlyst-15 to dihydroartemisinin following by *in situ* conversion to the final etheric derivatives by adding an appropriate alcohol.

10.6.2 Clinical Studies Aspects of Artemether

The Effectiveness of artemether in the treatment of severe malaria has been demonstrated by a number of uncontrolled and controlled but nonrandomized studies [109–113]. Uncontrolled studies cannot differentiate between nonspecific effects such as the natural course of disease and specific therapeutic effects [114], while nonrandomization may lead to substantial overestimation of the effect and thus introduce bias [115]. Pittler and Ernst [116] utilized randomized controlled trials (RCTs) to estimate the true clinical effectiveness of artemether for severe malaria. This meta-analysis is aimed at assessing the evidence from RCTs regarding the clinical effectiveness of artemether for severe malaria. Computerized literature searches identified all randomized clinical trials of artemether in comparison with quinine. Standardized data extraction was independently performed by both authors. Results of nine trials, entered in the meta-analysis, demonstrate the absence of a significant difference between artemether and quinine in terms of mortality rate [odds ratio (OR), 0.76; 95% confidence interval (CI), 0.50–1.14]. Statistical pooling of data from trials in Southeast Asia showed a trend toward enhanced reduction of mortality (OR, 0.38; 95% CI, 0.14–1.02). These data demonstrate the equality of artemether and quinine for severe malaria and indicate a trend toward greater effectiveness of artemether in regions where there is recognized quinine resistance.

10.7 CONCLUSION AND PERSPECTIVE

The discovery of artemisinin as a novel antimalarial drug is a great success and a milestone for the Chinese pharmaceutical industry and to the scientists who were involved in this project. It is also a miracle to the rest of the world, even though many details behind were restricted and not disclosed due to a number of reasons. This drug, along with several derivatives (artemether, artesunate, etc.) has served as the first-line treatment to combat severe malaria, and saved millions of lives all over the world.

Artemisinin, also known as qinghaosu, is a novel sesquiterpene lactone, extracted from the leaves of the shrub *Artemisia annua* and possesses an endoperoxide bridge which is a rare structural feature in natural products, and is essential for its antimalarial activity.

It has to be mentioned that although artemisinin (**5**) is effective against both chloroquine-sensitive and chloroquine-resistant *P. falciparum,* and is clinically used for the treatment of cerebral malaria in early China and other Asian countries, its usage as a monotherapy is explicitly discouraged by the WHO. Therefore, combination therapies with artemisinin partnered with other drugs are the preferred treatment and are both effective and well tolerated in most patients.

Artemether (**49**) is a lipid soluble methyl ether derivative of artemisinin, also known as dihydroartemisinin methyl ether. Artemether is highly effective against the blood schizonts of both malarial parasites *P. falciparum* and *P. vivax*. Artemether is active against all Plasmodia including those which may be resistant to other antimalarials, therefore is approved and widely prescribed in many countries.

It has to be mentioned that in 2007, artesunate injection (**52**) (60 mg of artesunic acid with a separate ampoule of 5% sodium bicarbonate solution) was enrolled in the 15th *List* for use in the management of severe malaria, and artesunate tablet (50 mg $tablet^{-1}$) was used in combination with amodiaquine, mefloquine, or sulfadoxine–pyrimethamine [99].

ACKNOWLEDGMENT

The authors are grateful to the Shanghai Commission of Science and Technology (10410702600, 10JC1417100, and 10dz1910104). Valuable suggestion on the historical retrospect on the development of artemisinin and its analogs from Professor Ying Li was also highly appreciated.

REFERENCES

1. Hamilton, G. R., and Baskett, T. F. In the arms of Morpheus: the development of morphine for postoperative pain relief. *Can. J. Anaesth.* **2000**, *47*, 367–374.
2. Butler, M. S. The role of natural product chemistry in drug discovery, *J. Nat. Prod.* **2004**, *67*, 2141–2153.
3. Wang, M. W., Hao, X. J., and Chen K. X. Biological screening of natural products and drug innovation in China. *Phil. Trans. R. Soc. B.* **2007**, *362*, 1093–1105.
4. Haynes, R. K., and Vonwiller, S. C. From qinghao, marvelous herb of antiquity, to the antimalarial trioxane qinghaosu—and some remarkable new chemistry. *Acc. Chem. Res.* **1997**, *30*, 73–79.
5. Available at: http://www.unicef.org/health/index_malaria.html accessed on December 20, 2011.
6. Bernard M., and Anne, R. Heme as trigger and target for trioxane-containing antimalarial drugs. *Acc. Chem. Res.* **2010**, *43*, 1444–1451.
7. Meunier, B., de Visser, S. P., and Shaik, S. Oxidation reactions catalyzed by cytochrome P450 enzymes. *Chem. Rev.* **2004**, *104*, 3947–3980.
8. Dawson, J. H. Probing structure-function relations in heme-containing oxygenases and peroxidases. *Science* **1988**, *240*, 433–439.
9. Fita, I., and Rossmann, M. G. The active center of catalase. *J. Mol. Biol.* **1985**, *185*, 21–37.
10. Edwards, S. L., and Kraut, J. Crystal structure of nitric oxide inhibited cytochrome *c* peroxidase. *Biochemistry* **1988**, *27*, 8074–8081.
11. Francis, S. E., Sullivan, D. J., and Goldberg, D. E. Hemoglobin metabolism in the malariaparasite, *Plasmodium falciparum. Annu. Rev. Microbiol.* **1997**, *51*, 97–123.
12. Pagola, S., Stephens, P. W., Bohle, D. S., Kosar, A. D., and Madsen, S. K. The structureof malaria pigment beta-hematin. *Nature* **2000**, *404*, 307–310.
13. Sullivan, D. J., Gluzman, I. Y., and Goldberg, D. E. *Plasmodium* hemozoin formation mediated by histidine-rich proteins. *Science* **1996**, *271*, 219–222.
14. Jani, D., Nagarkatti, R., Beatty, W., Angel, R., Slebodnick, C., Andersen, J., Kumar, S., and Rathore, D. HDP—a novel heme detoxification protein from the malaria parasite. *PLoS Pathog.* **2008**, *4*(e1000053)1–15.
15. Egan, T. G. Recent advances in understanding the mechanism of hemozoin (malariapigment) formation. *J. Inorg. Biochem.* **2008**, *102*, 1288–1299.
16. Kyle, R. A., and Shampe M. A. Discoverers of quinine. *JAMA.* **1974**, *229*, 462.
17. Plowe, C. V. Antimalarial drug resistance in Africa: strategies for monitoring and deterrence. *Curr. Top. Microbiol. Immunol.* **2005**, *295*, 55–79.
18. Zhang, J. F. *Late Report–Record of Project 523 and the Research and Development of Qinghaosu*, Yangcheng Evening News Publisher, Guangzhou, **2007**.
19. Bai, D. L., and Chen, K. X. *Advances in Pharmaceutical Chemistry* **2004**, Chemical Industry Press Publisher, Beijing.
20. (a) Li, Y. *Discovery and Development of New Antimalarial Durg Qinghaosu (Artemisinin)* **2007**, Shanghai Scientific & Technical Publisher, Shanghai; (b) Klayman, D. L. Qinghaosu (artemisinin): an antimalarial drug from China. *Science* **1985**, *228*, 1049–1055.
21. (a) Lusha, X.-M. A new drug for malaria. *China Reconstructs* **1979**, 48–49; (b) Li, Y., and Wu, Y.-L. An over four millennium story behind qinghaosu (artemisinin—a fantastic antimalarial drug from a traditional Chinese herb). *Curr. Med. Chem.* **2003**, *47*, 2197–2230–2964; (c) Wei, Z.-X.Faming Zhuanli Shenqing Gongkai Shuomingshu CN 1047503 A 5 Dec **1990** (Chem. Abs. 115:15580); (d) Klayman, D. L., Lin, A.- J., Acton, N., Scovill, J. P., Hoch, J. M., Milhous, W. K., Theoharides, A. D., and Dobek, A. S. Isolation of artemisinin (qinghaosu) from Artemisia annua growing in the United States. *J. Nat. Prod.* **1984**, *47*, 715–717; (e) ElSohly, H. N., Croom, E. M., El-Feraly, F. S., and El-Sherei, M. M. A large-scale extraction technique of artemisinin from artemisia annua *J. Nat. Prod.* **1990**, *53*, 1560–1564; (f) Zhang, J.-S., Fan, D.-W., and Ma, X.-B. Method for Extraction of Artemisinin. CN 1092073 14 September **1994** (Priority Date 9 March 1993).
22. Liang, X. T., Yu, D. Q., Wu, W. L., and Deng, H. C. The structure of Yingzhaosu A. *Acta Chim. Sin.* **1979**, *37*, 215–230.
23. (a) Qinghaosu Antimalaria Coordinating Research, Group. Antimalaria studies on qinghao-su. *Chinese Med. J.* **1979**, *92*, 811–816; (b) Co-Operative Research Group on Qinghaosu. Absolute crystal structure of qinghaosu. *Kuo Xue Tong Bao* **1977**, *22*, 142; (c) Qinghaosu Research Group, Institute of Biophysics, Academia. Sinica. Qinghaosu Research Group of Institute of Biophysic, crystal structure and absolute configuration of qinghaosu, *Scientia Sinica* **1980**, *23*, 380–396.
24. (a) Coordinating Research Group for the structure of Artemisinin, a new type of sesquiterpene lactone-artemisinin. *Kexue Tongbao*, **1977** *22*, 142; (b) Liu, J. M., Ni, M. Y., Fan, J. F., Tu, Y. Y., Wu, Z. H., Wu, Y. L., and Zhou, W. S. The structure and reaction of arteannuin. *Acta Chim. Sin.* **1979**, *37*, 129–141.
25. UNDP/World Bank/WHO. Fourth meeting of the Scientific Working Group on the Chemotherapy of Malaria, Beijing (6–10 October, 1981). Geneva: UNDP/World Bank/WHO, **1981**.
26. White, N. J. Assessment of the pharmacodynamic properties of antimalarial drugs *in vivo. Antimicrob. Agents Chemother.* **1997**, *41*, 1413–1422.
27. (a) Vugt, M. V., Wilairatana, P., Gemperli, B., Gathmann, I., Phaipun, L., Brockman, A., Luxemburger, C., White, N. J., Nosten, F., and Looareesuwan, S. Efficacy of six doses of artemether-lumefantrine (benflumetol) in multidrug-resistant *Plasmodium falciparum* malaria. *Am. J. Trop. Med.*

Hyg. **1999**, *60*, 936–42; (b) LEFÈVRE, G., LOOAREESUWAN, S., TREEPRASERTSUK, S., KRUDSOOD, S., SILACHAMROON, U., GATHMANN, I., MULL, R., and BAKSHI, R. Doses of artemether-lumefantrine for multidrug-resistant *Plasmodium falciparum* malaria in Thailand. *Am. J. Trop. Med. Hyg.* **2001** *64*, 247–56.

28. BOUWMEESTER, H. J., WALLAART, T. E., JANSSEN, M. H., VAN LOO, B., JANSEN, B. J., POSTHUMUS, M. A., SCHMIDT, C. O., DE KRAKER, J. W., KNIG, W. A., and FRANSSEN, M. C. Amorpha-4,11-diene synthase catalyses the first probable step in artemisinin biosynthesis. *Phytochemistry* **1999**, *52*, 843–854.
29. JEFFORD, C. W. New developments in synthetic peroxidic drugs as artemisinin mimics. *Drug Discov. Today* **2007**, *12*, 487.
30. SCHMID, G., and HOFHEINZ, W. Total synthesis of qinghaosu *J. Am. Chem. Soc.* **1983**, *105*, 624.
31. XU, X. X., ZHU, J., HUANG, D. Z., and ZHOU, W. S. The stereocontrolled syntheses of arteannuin and deoxyarteannuin from arteannuic acid. *Acta. Chim. Sin.* **1983**, *41*, 574–576.
32. YE, B., and WU, Y. L. An efficient synthesis of qinghaosu and deoxoginghaosu from arteannuic acid. *Chem. Commun.* **1990**, *10*, 726–727.
33. (a) LANSBURY, P. T., and NOWAK, D. M. An efficient partial synthesis of (+) artemisinin and (+) deoxoartemisinin. *Tetrahedron Lett.* **1992**, *33*, 1029–1032; (b) NOWAK, D. M., and LANSBURY, P. T. Synthesis of (+). Artemisinin and (+) Deoxoartemisinin from arteannuina B and arteannuic acid. *Tetrahedron* **1998** *54*, 319–336.
34. (a) RAVINDRANATHAN, T., ANIL KUMAR, M., MENON, R. B., and HIREMATH, S. V. Stereoselective synthesis of artemisinin+. *Tetrahedron Lett.* **1990**, *31*, 755–758; (b) YADAV, J. S., SATHEESH BABU, R., and SABITHA, G. Stereoselective total synthesis of (+)-artemisinin. *Tetrahedron Lett.* **2003** *44*, 387–389.
35. (a) ROTH, R. J., and ACTON, N. A simple conversion of artemisinic acid into artemisinin. *J. Nat. Prod.* **1989**, *52*, 1183–1185; (b) ACTON, N., and ROTH, R. J. On the conversion of dihydroartemisinic acid into artemisinin *J. Org. Chem.* **1992**, *57*, 3610–3614; (c) ACTON, N., and ROTH, R. J. Acid decomposition of the antimalarial beta-arteether. *Heterocycles* **1995** *41*, 95–102.
36. HAYNES, R. K. Artemisinin in traditional tea preparations of Artemisia annua. *Curr. Top. Med. Chem.* **2006**, *6*, 509–537.
37. LIU, H. J., YEH, W. L., and CHEW, S. Y. A total synthesis of the antimalarial natural product (+)- quinghaosu. *Tetrahedron Lett.* **1993**, *34*, 4435–4438.
38. CONSTANTINO, M. G., BELTRAME, M., and DASILVA, G. V. J. A novel asymmetric total synthesis of (+)-artemisinin. *Synthetic Commun.* **1996**, *26*, 321–329.
39. (a) AVERY, M. A., JENNINGSWHITE, C., and CHONG, W. K. M. The total synthesis of (+)-artemisinin and (+)-9-desmethyltemesinin *Tetrahedron Lett.* **1987**, *28*, 4629–4623; (b) AVERY, M. A., CHONG, W. K. M., and JENNINGSWHITE, C. Stereoselective total synthesis of (+)-artemisinine, the antimalarial constituent of Artemisia annua L. *J. Am. Chem. Soc.* **1992** *114*, 974–979.
40. (a) LI, Y., YU, P. L., CHEN, Y. X., LI, L. Q., GAI, Y. Z., WANG, D. S., and ZHENG, Y. P. Synthesis of some artemisinin derivatives. *Chinese Sci. Bull.* **1979**, *24*, 667–669; (b) LI, Y., YU, P. L., CHEN, Y. X., LI, L. Q., GAI, Y. Z., WANG, D. S., and ZHENG, Y. P., Studies of analogs of artemisinine I. The synthesis of ethers, carboxylic esters and carbonates of dihydroartemisinine. *Acta Pharmaceutica Sinica*, **1981** *16*, 429–439.
41. LIU, J. M., NI, M. Y., FAN, J. F., and TU, Y. Y. Structure and reaction of arteannuin *Acta. Chimica. Sinica.* **1979**, *37*, 129–140.
42. JUNG, M., LI, X., BUSTOS, D. A., EISOHLY, H. N., MCCHESNEY, J. D. A short and stereospecific synthesis of (+)-deoxoartemisinin and (−)-deoxodesoxyartemisinin *Tetrahedron Lett.* **1989**, *30*, 5973–5976.
43. LI, Y., YU, P. L., and CHEN, Y. X. Studies on analoges of qinghaosu—some acidic degradations of qinghaosu. *Kexue Tong bao*, **1986**, *31*, 1038–1040.
44. (a) VAN AGTMAEL, M. A., EGGELTE, T. A., and VAN BOXTEL, C. J. Artemisinin drugs in the Treatment of Malaria: from Medicinal Herb to Registered Medication. *Trends Pharmacol. Sci.* **1999**, *20*, 199; (b) PLOYPRADITH, P. Development of artemisinin and its structurally simplified trioxane derivatives as antimalarial drugs. *Acta. Trop.* **2004**, *89*, 329.
45. VROMAN, J. A., ALVIM-GASTON, M., and AVERY, M. A. Current progress in the chemistry, medicinal chemistry and drug design of artemisinin based antimalarials. *Curr. Pharm. Des.* **1999**, *5*, 101–138.
46. BREWER, T. G., GRATE, S. J., PEGGINS, J. O., WEINA, P. J., PETRAS, J. M., LEVINE, B. S., HEIFFER, M. H., and SCHUSTER, B. G. Fatal neurotoxicity of arteether and artemether. *Am. J. TRcp. Med. Hyg.*, **1994**, *51*, 251–259.
47. LI, Y., YU, P.-L., CHEN, Y.-X., LI, L.-Q., GAI, Y.-Z., WANG, D.-S., and ZHENG, Y.- P. Synthesis of some derivatives of artimisinin. *Ke Xue Tong Bao* **1979**, *24*, 667–669.
48. LI, Y., YU, P.-L., CHEN, Y.-X., and JI, R.-Y. Studies on analogs of arteannuin. II. Synthesis of some carboxylic esters and carbonates of dihydroarteannuin by using 4-(*N,N*-dimethylamino)pyridine as an active acylation catalyst. *Acta. Chimica. Sinica* **1982**, *40*, 557–561.
49. (a) BUKIRWA, H. Artemisinin combination therapies for treatment of uncomplicated malaria in Uganda. *PLoS Clin. Trials.* **2006**, *1*, e7; (b) DANIS, M., and BRICAIRE, F. The new drug combinations: their place in the treatment of uncomplicated *Plasmodium falciparum* malaria. *Fundam. Clin. Pharmacol.* **2003**, *17*, 155–160; (c) OLLIARO, P. L., and TAYLOR, W. R. J. Developing artemisinin based drug combinations for the treatment of drug resistant *falciparum* malaria: a review. *J. Postgrad. Med.* (Bombay) **2004**, *50*, 40–44; (d) ADJEI, G. O., KURTZHALS, J. A. L., RODRIGUES, O. P., ALIFRANGIS, M., HOEGBERG, L. C. G., KITCHER, E. D., BADOE, E. V., LAMPTEY, R., and GOKA, B. Q. Amodiaquine-artesunate vs. artemether-lumefantrine for uncomplicated malaria in Ghanaian children: a randomized efficacy and safety trial with one year follow-up. *Malar. J.* **2008**, *7*, 127; (e) PENALI, L. K., and JANSEN, F. H. Single day, three dose treatment with fixed dose to cure *Plasmodium*

falciparum malaria. *Int. J. Infect. Dis.* **2008**, *12*, 430–437.
50. Lin, A. J., Lee, M., and Klayman, D. L. Antimalarial activity of new water-soluble dihydroartemisinin derivatives. 2. Stereospecificity of the ether side chain. *J. Med. Chem.* **1989**, *32*, 1249–1252.
51. Awad, M. I., Alkadru, A. M., Berhens, R. H., Baraka, O. Z., and Eltayeb, I. B. Descriptive study on the efficacy and safety of ar-tesunate suppository in combination with other antimalarials in the treatment of severe malaria in Sudan. *Am. J. Trop. Med. Hyg.* **2003**, *68*, 153–158.
52. Barradell, L. B., and Fitton, A. Artesunate: a review of its pharmacology and therapeutic efficacy in the treatment of malaria. *Drugs* **1995**, *50*, 714–741.
53. Kingston, H.R., Wai-Lun, L., Ho-Wai, C., and Hing-Wo, T. Artemisinin derivatives EP0974354 2000.
54. Singh, C., Chaudhary, S., and Puri, S. K. New orally active derivatives of artemisinin with high efficacy against multidrug-resistant. *J. Med. Chem.* **2006**, *49*, 7227–7233.
55. O'Neill, P. M., and Ward, S. A.Peroxide-based antimalarial compounds. WO0104123 2001.
56. O'Neill, P. M., Miller, A., Bishop, L. P. D., Hindley, S., Maggs, J. L., Ward, S. A., Roberts, S. M., Scheinmann, F., Andrew V. Stachulski, A. V., Posner, G.H., and Park, B. K. Synthesis, antimalarial activity, biomimetic iron(II) chemistry, and the *in vitro* metabolism of novel, potent C-10-phenoxy derivatives of dihydroartemisinin *J. Med. Chem.* **2001**, *44*, 58.
57. (a) O'Neill, P. M., Higson, A. P., Taylor, S., and Irving, E. WO03048167 **2003**; (b) Hindley, S., Ward, S. A., Storr, R. C., Searle, N. L., Bray, P. G., Park, B. K., Davies, J., and O'Neill, P. M. Mechanism-based design of parasite-targeted artemisinin derivatives: synthesis and antimalarial activity of new diamine containing analogues. *J. Med. Chem.*, **2002**, *45*, 1052.
58. Lin, A. J., Li, L.-Q., Andersen, S. L., and Klayman, D. L. Antimalarial activity of new dihydroartemisinin derivatives. 5. Sugar analogs. *J. Med. Chem.* **1992**, *35*, 1639–1642.
59. Kingston, H. R., Wai-Lun, L., Ho-Wai, C., and Hing-Wo, T. Artemisinin derivatives as anti-infective agent. EP0974594 2000.
60. Li, Y., Wang, F. D., Zhang, Y., and Sui, Y. Synthesis and Preliminary Antitumor Activity of New Artemisinin Derivatives. Chinese Patent ZL02128494. 2001.
61. (a) Haynes, R. K., and Vonwiller, S. C. Cyclic Peroxy Acetal Lactone and Ether Compounds, WO 91/04970 18 April **1991**; (b) Haynes, R. K., and Vonwiller, S. C. Catalyzed oxygenation of allylic hydroperoxides derived from Qinghaosu (Artemisinic) acid. *J. Chem. Soc., Chem. Commun.* **1990**, 451–453; (c) Vonwiller, S. C., Warner, J. A., Mann, S. T., and Haynes, R. K. Copper(II) trifluoromethanesulfonate-induced cleavage oxygenation of allylic hydroperoxides derived from qinghao acid in the synthesis of qinghaosu derivatives: evidence for the intermediacy of enols *J. Am. Chem. Soc.* **1995**, *117*, 11098–11105; (d) Haynes, R. K., and Vonwiller, S. C. From qinghao, marvelous herb of antiquity, to the antimalarial trioxane qinghaosu-and some remarkable new chemistry. *Acc. Chem. Res.*, **1997**, *30*, 73–79; (e) Jung, M., Bustos, D. A., El Sohly, H. N., and McChesney, J. D. A concise and stereoselective synthesis of (+)-12-n-butyldeoxoartemisinin. *Synlett.* **1990**, 743–744; (f) Jung, M., Yu, D., Bustos, D. A., ElSohly, H. N., McChesney, J. D., Jung, M., Yu, D., Bustos, D. A., ElSohly, H. N., and McChesney, J. D. A concise synthesis of 12-(3′-hydroxy-*n*-propyl)-deoxoartemisinin). *Bioorg. Med. Chem. Lett.* **1991**, *1*, 741–744; (g) Haynes, R. K., and Vonwiller, S. C. Efficient preparation of novel qinghaosu artemisinin derivatives. *Synlett* **1992**, 481–483. (h) Jung, M., Freitas, A. C. C., McChesney, J. D., and El Sohly, H. N. A practical and general synthesis of (+)-carboxyalkyldeoxoartemisinins. *Heterocycles* **1994**, *39*, 23–29. (i) Jung, M., and Schinazi, R. F. Synthesis and in vitro anti-human immunodeficiency virus activity of artemisinin (qinghaosu)-related trioxanes. *Bioorg. Med. Chem. Lett.* **1994**, *4*, 931–934 (j) Jung, M., and Lee, S. A concise synthesis of novel aromatic analogues of artemisinin. *Heterocycles* **1997**, *45*, 1055–1058. (k) Jung, M. Synthesis and cytotoxicity of novel artemisinin analogues. *Biorg. Med. Chem. Lett.* **1997**, *7*, 1091–1094.
62. Hindley, S., Ward, S. A., Storr, R. C., Searle, N. L., Bray, P. G., A. J. Park, B. K., Davies, J., and O'Neill, P. M. Mechanism-based design of parasite-targeted artemisinin derivatives: synthesis and antimalarial activity of new diamine containing analogues. *J. Med. Chem.*, **2002**, *45*, 1052.
63. (a) Haynes, R. K. Artemisinin and its derivatives: the future for malaria treatment? *Curr. Opin. Infect. Dis.* **2001**, *14*, 719–726; (b) Haynes, R. K., Fugmann, B., Stetter, J., Rieckmann, K., Heilmann, H.–D. Chan, H.–W., Cheung, M.–K., Lam, W.–L., Wong, H.–N., Croft, S. L., Vivas, L., Rattray, L., Stewart, L., Peters, W., Robinson, B. L., Edstein, M. D., Kotecka, B., Kyle, D. E., Beckermann, B., Gerisch, M., Radtke, M., Schmuck, G., Steinke, W., Wollborn, U., Schmeer, K., and Römer, A. Artemisone—a highly active antimalarial drug of the artemisinin class. *Angew. Chem. Int. Ed.* **2006**, *45*, 2082–2088; (c) Haynes, R. K., Ho, W.–Y., Chan, H.–W., Fugmann, B., Stetter, J., Croft, S. L., Vivas, L., Peters, W., and Robinson, B. L. Highly antimalaria-active artemisinin derivatives: biological activity does not correlate with chemical reactivity. *Angew. Chem. Int. Ed.* **2004**, *43*, 1381–1385; (d) Haynes, R. K. Reply to comments on "highly antimalaria-active artemisinin derivatives: biological activity does not correlate with chemical reactivity." *Angew. Chem. Int. Ed.* **2005**, *44*, 2064–2065; (e) Haynes, R. K., Chan, H.–W., Cheung, M.–K., Chung, S.–K., Lam, W.–L., Tsang, H.–W., Voerste, A., Williams, I. D. Stereoselective preparation of 10α- and 10β-aryl derivatives of dihydroartemisinin. *Eur. J. Org. Chem.* **2003**, 2098–2114.
64. (a) Posner, G. H., Jeon, H. B., Ploypradith, P., Paik, I.-H., Borstnik, K., Xie, S.-J., and Shapiro, T. A. Orally

active, water-soluble antimalarial 3-aryltrioxanes: short synthesis and preclinical efficacy testing in rodents. *J. Med. Chem.* **2002**, *45*, 3824–3828; (b) Woodard, L., Chang, E. W., Chen, X.-C., Liu, J. O., Shapiro, T. A., and Posner, G. H. Malaria-infected mice live until at least day 30 after a new monomeric trioxane combined with mefloquine are administered together as a single low oral dose *J. Med. Chem.*, **2009**, *52*, 7458–7462.

65. Haynes, R. K., Chan, H. W., Lam, W. L., Tsang, H. W., and Cheung, M. K. WO0004024 2000.

66. Haynes, R. K., Fugmann, B., Stetter, J., Rieckmann, K., Heilmann, H.-D., Chan, H.-W., Cheung, M.-K., Lam, W.-L., Wong, H.-N., Croft, S. L., Vivas, L., Rattray, L., Stewart, L., Peters, W., Robinson, B. L., Edstein, M. D., Kotecka, B., Kyle, D. E., Beckermann, B., Gerisch, M., Radtke, M., Schmuck, G., Steinke, W., Wollborn, U., Schmeer, K., and Römer, A. Artemisone—a highly active antimalarial drug of the artemisinin class. *Angew. Chem. Int. Ed.* **2006**, *45*, 2082–2088.

67. Wang, D.-Y., Wu, Y.-K., Wu, Y.-L., Li, Y., and Shan, F. Synthesis, iron(II)-induced cleavage and *in vivo* antimalarial efficacy of 10-(2- hydroxy-1-naph-thyl)-deoxoqinghaosu (-deoxoartemi-sinin) *J. Chem. Soc. Perkin Trans. I* **1999**, 1827–1831.

68. (a) Jung, M., Lee, S., Ham, J., Lee, K., Kim, H., and Kim, S. K. Antitumor activity of novel deoxoartemisinin monomers, dimers, and trimer. *J. Med. Chem.*, **2003**, *46*, 987; (b) Posner, G. H., Paik, I.–H., Sur, S., McRiner, A. J., Borstnik, K., Xie, S., and Shapiro, T. A. Orally active, antimalarial, anticancer, artemisinin-derived trioxane dimers with high stability and efficacy. *J. Med. Chem.* **2003**, *46*, 1060–1065.

69. Posner, G.H., McRiner, A. J., Paik, I. H., Sur, S., Borstnik, K., Xie, S., Shapiro, T. A., Alagbala, A., and Foster, B. Anticancer and antimalarial efficacy and safety of artemisinin-derived trioxane dimers in rodents. *J. Med. Chem.*, **2004**, *47*, 1299.

70. (a) Hindley, S., Ward, S. A., Storr, R. C., Searle, N. L., Bray, P. G., Park, B. K., Davies, J., and O'Neill, P. M. Mechanism-based design of parasite-targeted artemisinin derivatives: synthesis and antimalarial activity of new diamine containing analogues. *J. Med. Chem.* **2002**, *45*, 1052–1063; (b) Jeyadevan, J. P., Bray, P. G., Chadwick, J., Mercer, A. E., Byrne, A. E., Ward, S. A., Park, B. K., Williams, D. P., Cosstick, R., Davies, J., Higson, A. P., Irving, E., Posner, G. H., and O'Neill, P. M. Antimalarial and antitumor evaluation of novel C-10 non-acetal dimers of 10beta-(2-hydroxyethyl) deoxoartemisinin. *J. Med. Chem.* **2004**, *47*, 1290–1298.

71. (a) Yu, P.-L., Chen, Y.-X., Li, Y., and Ji, R.-Y. Analogs of qing hao Su (artemisinin, arteannuin). IV. Synthesis of derivatives of qing hao su contaiing halogen, nitrogen, and sulfur heteroatoms. *Acta. Pharmac. Sinica* **1985**, *20*, 357–365; (b) Li, Y., Zhu, Y.-M., Jiang, H.-J., Pan, J.-P., Wu, G.-S., Wu, J.-M., Shi, Y.-L., Yang, J.-D., and Wu, B.-A. Synthesis and antimalarial activity of artemisinin derivatives containing an amino group. *J. Med. Chem.* **2000**, *43*, 1635–1640; (c) Hindley, S., Ward, S. A., Storr, R. C., Searle, N. L., Bray, P. G., Park, B. K., Davies, J., and O'Neill, P. M. Mechanism-based design of parasite-targeted artemisinin derivatives: synthesis and antimalarial activity of new diamine containing analogues. *J. Med. Chem.* **2002**, *45*, 1052–1063.

72. (a) Lin, A. J., Li, L.-Q., Klayman, D. L., George, C. F., and Flippen-Anderson, J. L. Antimalarial activity of new water-soluble dihydroartemisinin derivatives. 3. Aromatic amine analogues. *J. Med. Chem.* **1990**, *33*, 2610–2614; (b) Capon, B., and Connett, B. E. The mechanism of the hydrolysis of *N*-aryl-D-ghcosylamines *J. Chem. Soc.* **1965**, 4497–4502.

73. Yang, Y.-H., Li, Y., Shi, Y.-L., Yang, J.-D., and Wu, B.-A. Artemisinin derivatives with 12-aniline substitution: synthesis and antimalarial activity. *Bioorg. Med. Chem. Lett.* **1995**, *5*, 1791–1794.

74. Haynes, R. K. Artemisinin and derivatives: the future of malaria treatment. *Curr. Opin. Infect. Dis.* **2001**, *14*, 719–726.

75. (a) Haynes, R. K., Chan, H.-W., Ho, W.-Y., Ko, C. K-. F., Gerena, L., Kyle, D. E., Peters, W., and Robinson, B. L. Convenient access both to highly antimalaria-active 10-arylaminoartemisinins, and to 10-alkyl ethers including artemether, arteether, and artelinate. *Chem. Bio. Chem.* **2005**, *6*, 659–667; (b) Haynes, R. K., Ho, W.-Y., Chan, H.- W., Fugmann, B., Stetter, J., Croft, S. L., Vivas, L., Peters, W., and Robinson, B. L. Highly antimalaria-active artemisinin derivatives: biological activity does not correlate with chemical reactivity. *Angew. Chem. Int. Ed.* **2004**, *43*, 1381–1385.

76. Pu, Y. M., Torok, D. S., Ziffer, H., Pan, F X. Q., and Meshnick, S. R. Synthesis and antimalarial activities of several fluorinated artemisinin, derivatives. *J. Med. Chem.* **1995**, *38*, 4120-L 4124.

77. Parshikov, I. A., Muraleedharan, K. M., Avery, M. A., and Williamson, J. S. Transformation of artemisinin by *Cunninghamella elegans. Appl. Microbiol. Biotechnol.* **2004**, *64*, 782–786.

78. Thanh Nga, T. T., Ménage, C., Bégué, J. P., Bonnet-Delpon, D., Gantier, J. C., and Pradines, B., Doury, J. C., Truong, T. D. Synthesis and antimalarial activities of fluoroalkyl derivatives of dihydroartemisinin. *J. Med. Chem.* **1998**, *41*, 4101–4108.

79. Magueur, G., Crousse, B., Charneau, S., Grellier, P., Bégué, J.-P., and Bonnet-Delpon, D. Fluoroartemisinin: trifluoromethyl analogues of artemether and artesunate *J. Med. Chem.* **2004**, *47*, 2694–2699.

80. (a) Acton, N., Karle, J. M., and Miller, R. E. Synthesis and antimalarial activity of some 9-substituted artemisinin derivatives *J. Med. Chem.* **1993**, *36*, 2552; (b) Jung, M., ElSoholy, H. N., and McChesney, J. D. A concise synthesis of novel c-13 functionalized deoxoartemisinins synlett **1993**, 43; (c) Avery, M. A., Gao, F., Chong, W. K. M., Mehrotra, S., and Mihous, W. K. Synthesis and comparative molecular field analysis of C-9 analogs of artemisinin and 10-deoxoartemisinin. *J. Med. Chem.* **1993**, *36*, 4264; (d) Avery, M. A., Mehrotra, S., Johnson, T. L., Bonk, J. D., Vroman, J. A., and Miller, R. structure–activity relationships of the antimalarial agent artemisinin. 5. Analogs of

10-deoxoartemisinin substituted at C-3 and C-9. *J. Med. Chem.* **1996**, *39*, 4149.

81. Acton, N., and Klayman, D. Artemisitene, a new sesquiterpene lactone endoperoxide from Artemisia annua. *Planta Med.* **1985**, *51*, 441.
82. Liao X. B., Han, J. Y., and Li, Y. Michael addition of artemisitene. *Tetrahedron Lett.* **2001**, *42*, 2843.
83. Avery, M. A., Muraleedharan, K. M., Desai, P. V., Bandyopadhyaya, A. K., Furtado, M. M., and Tekwani, B. L. Structure–activity relationships of the antimalarial agent artemisinin. 8. Design, synthesis, and CoMFA studies toward the development of artemisinin-based drugs against leishmaniasis and malaria. *J. Med. Chem.* **2003**, *46*, 4244–4258.
84. Haynes, R. K., Chan, H. W., Lam, W. L., and Tsang, H. W. WO0004025 2000.
85. Avery, M. A., Alvim-Gaston, M., Vroman, J. A., Wu, B., Ager, A., Peters, W., Robinson, B. L., and Charman, W. Structure–activity relationships of the antimalarial agent artemisinin. 7. Direct modification of (+)-artemisinin and *in vivo* antimalarial screening of new, potential preclinical antimalarial Candidates. *J. Med. Chem.* **2002**, *45*, 4321–4335.
86. Grellepois, F., Chorki, F., Ourévitch, M., Charneau, S., Grellier, P. McIntosh, K. A., Charman, W. N., Pradines, B., Crousse, B., Bonnet-Delpon, D., and BéguéOrallyl, J.-P. Active antimalarials: hydrolytically stable derivatives of 10-trifluoromethyl anhydrodihydroartemisinin. *J. Med. Chem.* **2004**, *47*, 1423–1433.
87. Hindley, S., Ward, S. A., Storr, R. C., Searle, N. L., Bray, P. G., Park, B. K., Davies, J., and O'Neill, P. M. Mechanism-based design of parasite-targeted artemisinin derivatives: synthesis and antimalarial activity of new diamine containing analogues *J. Med. Chem.* **2002**, *45*, 1052–1063.
88. Pu, Y. M., Torok, D. S., and Ziffer, H. Synthesis and antimalarial activities of several fluorinated artemisinin derivatives *J. Med. Chem.* **1995**, *38*, 4120–4124.
89. Wright, C.W. Traditional antimalarials and the development of novel antimalarial drugs. *J. Ethnopharmacol.*, **2005**, *100*, 67.
90. (a) Torok, D. S., and Ziffer, H. Synthesis and reactions of 11-azaartemisinin and derivatives *Tetrahedron Lett.* **1995**, *36*, 829–832; (b) Torok, D. S., and Ziffer, H. Syntheses and antimalarial activities of *N*-substituted 11-azaartemisinins *J. Med. Chem*, **1995**, *38*, 5045–5050.
91. Haynes, R. K., Pai, H.-O., and Voerste, A. Ring opening of artemisinin (qinghaosu) and dihydroartemisinin and interception of the open hydroperoxides with formation of *N*-oxides— a chemical model for antimalarial mode of action. *Tetrahedron Lett.* **1999**, *40*, 4715–4718.
92. Mekonnen, B., Weiss, E., Katz, E., Ma, J., Ziffer, H., and Kyle, D. E. Synthesis and antimalarial activities of base-catalyzed adducts of 11-azaartemisinin. *Bioorg. Med. Chem.* **2000**, *8*, 1111–1116.
93. Al-Oqail, M. M., Galal, A. M., Ahmad, M. S., Al-Fishawi, A. M., and El-Feraly, F. S. New bioactive azaartemisinin derivatives. *Molecules* **2003**, *8*, 901–909.
94. Singh, C., and Tiwari, P. New bioactive azaartemisinin derivatives. *Tetrahedron Lett.* **2002**, *43*, 7235–7237.
95. Trigg, P. I. Qinghaosu (artemisinin) as an antimalarial drug. *Econ. Med. Plant Res.* **1989**, *3*, 19–55.
96. Lin, A. J., Klayman, D. L., and Mlihouse, W. K. Antimalarial activity of new water-soluble dihydroartemisinin derivatives. *J. Med. Chem.* **1987**, *30*, 2147–2150.
97. Mordi, M. N., Mansor, S. M., Navaratnam, V., and Wernsdorfer, W. H. Single dose pharmacokinetics of oral artemether in healthy Malaysian volunteers. *Br. J. Clin. Pharmacol.* **1997**, *43*, 363–365.
98. Karbwang, J., Na-Bangchang, K., Congpuong, K., Molunto, P., and Thanavibul, A. Pharmacokinetics and bioavailability of oral and intramuscular artemether. *Eur. J. Clin. Pharmacol.* **1997**, *52*, 307–310.
99. Van Agtmael, M. A., Van der Graaf, C. A. A., Dien, T. K., Koopmans, R. P., and Van Boxtel, C. J. The contribution of the enzymes CYP2D6 and CYP2C19 in the demethylation of artemether in healthy subjects. *Eur. J. Drug Metab. Pharmacokinet.* **1998**, *23*, 429–436.
100. Baker, J. K., McChesney, J. D., and Chi, H. T. Decomposition of arteether in simulated stomach acid yielding compounds retaining antimalarial activity. *Pharmacol. Res.* **1993**, *10*, 662–666.
101. Na-Bangchang, K., Karbwang, J., Thomas, C. G., Thanavibul, A., Sukontason, K., Ward, S. A., and Edwards, G. Pharmacokinetics of artemether after oral administration to healthy Thai males and patients with acute, uncomplicated *falciparum* malaria. *Br. J. Clin. Pharmacol.* **1994**, *37*, 249–252.
102. Dien, T. K., de Vries, P. J., Nguyen, X. K., Koopmans, R., Le Nguyen, B., Dao D. D., Kager, P. A., and van Boxtel, C. J. Effect of food intake on pharmacokinetics of oral artemisinin in healthy Vietnamese subjects. *Antimicrob. Agents Chemother.* **1997**, *41*, 1069–1072.
103. De Vries, P. J., Khanh, N. X., Died, T. K., Binh, L. N., ThiYen, N., Duc, D. D., van Boxtel, C. J., and Kage, P. A. The pharmacokinetics of a single dose of artemisinin in subjects with liver cirrhosis. *Trop. Med. Int. Health* **1997**, *2*, 957–962.
104. Karbwang, J., Na-Bangchang, K., Sukontason, T. Tin, K., Rimchala, W., and Harinasuta, T. Pharmacokinetics of intramuscular artemether in patients with severe *falciparum* malaria with or without acute renal failure. *Br. J. Clin. Pharmacol.* **1998**, *45*, 597–600.
105. (a) Ashton, M., Hai, T. N., Sy, N. D., Huong, D. X., Van Huong, N., Niêu, N. T., and Công, L. D. Artemisinin pharmacokinetics is time-dependent in healthy subjects. *Drug Metab. Dispos.* **1998**, *26*, 25–27; (b) Hassan, A. M., Ashton, M., Kihamia, C. M., Mtey, G. J., and Bjorkman, A. Multiple dose pharmacokinetics of oral artemisinin and comparison of its efficacy with that of oral artesunate in *falciparum* malaria patients. *Trans. R. Soc. Trop. Med. Hyg.* **1996**, *90*, 61–65; (c) Svensson, U. S. H., Ashton, M., Hai, T. N., Bertilsson, L., Huong, D. X., Van Huong, N., Nieu, N. T., Sy, N. D., Lykkesfeldt, J., and Cong, L. D. Artemisinin induces

omeprazole metabolism in human beings. *Clin. Pharmacol. Ther.* **1998**, *64*, 160–167.

106. Ashton, M., Sy, N. D., Huong, N. V., Gordi, T., Hai, T. N., Huong, D. X., Nieu, N. T., and Cong, L. D. Artemisinin kinetics and dynamics during oral and rectal treatment of uncomplicated malaria. *Clin. Pharmacol. Ther.* **1998**, *63*, 482–493.
107. van Agtmael, M. A. Shan, C. Q., Jiao, X. Q., Mull, R., and van Boxtel, C. J. Multiple dose pharmacokinetics of artemether in Chinese patients treated for *falciparum* malaria. *Int. J. Antimicrob. Agents.* **1999**, *12*, 151–158.
108. (a) Lin, A. J., Klayman, D. L., and Milhous, W. K. Antimalarial activity of a new water soluble dihydroartemisinin derivative. *J. Med. Chem.* **1987**, *30*, 2147; (b) Yun, R. J. Artemether. *Drugs Future* **1982**, VII, 716; (c) Bhakuni, R. S., Jain, D. C., and Sharma, R. P. An improved procedure for the synthesis of ethers of dihydroartemisinin. *Ind. J. Chem.* **1995**, *34B*, 529; (d) El-Feraly, F. S., Al-Vahya, M. A., Oribi, K. V., McPhail, D. R., and McPhail, A. T. A new method for the preparation of arteether and its C-9 epimer *J. Nat. Prod.* **1992**, *55*, 878.
109. Sowunmi, A., and Oduola, A. M. J. Efficacy of artemether in severe *falciparum* malaria in African children. *Acta Trop.* **1996**, *61*, 57–63.
110. Bunnag, D., Karbwang, J., and Harinasuta T. Artemether in the treatment of multiple drug resistant *falciparum* malaria. *Southeast Asian J. Trop. Med. Public. Health.* **1992**, *23*, 762–767.
111. Myint, P.T., Shwe, T., Soe, L., Htut, Y., and Myint, W. Clinical study of the treatment of cerebral malaria with artemether (qinghaosu derivative). *Trans. R Soc. Trop. Med. Hyg.* **1989**, *83*, 72.
112. Myint, P. T., and Shwe T. A controlled clinical trial of artemether (qinghaosu-derivative) versus quinine in complicated and severe *falciparum* malaria. *Trans. R Soc. Trop. Med. Hyg.* **1987**, *81*, 559–561.
113. Pe Than Myint, Tin Shwe. The efficacy of artemether (qinghaosu) in *Plasmodium falciparum* and *P. vivax* in Burma. *Southeast Asian J. Trop. Med. Public Health* **1986**, *17*, 19–22.
114. Resch, K. L., and Ernst, E. Research methodologies in complementary medicine: making sure it works. in *Complementary Medicine* (ed. E. Ernst), Butterworth, London, 1996.
115. Schulz, K. F., Chalmers, J., Hyes, R. J., and Altman, D. G. Empirical evidence of bias. *JAMA* **1995**, *273*, 408–12.
116. Pittler, M. H., and Ernst, E. Artemether for severe malaria: a meta-analysis of randomised clinical trials. *Clin. Infect. Dis.* **1999**, *28*, 597–601.

CHAPTER 11

DISCOVERY AND PROCESS DEVELOPMENT OF MK-4965, A POTENT NONNUCLEOSIDE REVERSE TRANSCRIPTASE INHIBITOR

Yong-Li Zhong, Thomas J. Tucker, and Jingjun Yin

11.1 INTRODUCTION

Since their discovery in the early 1990s, nonnucleoside reverse transcriptase inhibitors (NNRTIs) have become an important component of highly active antiretroviral therapy (HAART). These drugs have become an integral part of the treatment of HIV-positive patients, and as part of combination therapy have been shown to suppress viral replication to undetectable levels [1]. There are three commercially available first-generation NNRTIs that have been approved for clinical practice: Efavirenz, Nevirapine, and Delavirdine (Figure 11.1, **1–3**). Both Efavirenz and Nevirapine are commonly used as first line therapy in naïve patients, and the clinical use of Delavirdine is limited by its somewhat lower levels of antiviral potency. Numerous reviews of the first-generation agents have been published in the past 10 years [2–4]. All these compounds target an allosteric binding site on the reverse transcriptase (RT) enzyme that is adjacent to the active site, and their binding is noncompetitive with respect to dNTPs and template/primer [5]. The compounds appear to act by locking the RT enzyme in an unfavorable conformation, thereby preventing motions in the RT enzyme that are necessary for successful processing of genetic material [6]. The structure and function of RT has been reviewed, and numerous co-crystal structures of a variety of inhibitors bound to the allosteric binding site have been published [7].

Although these first-generation compounds are reasonably well tolerated and have been shown to produce robust antiviral effects, viral breakthrough still occurs in a growing number of patients largely due to the presence of resistant viral mutations.

When the viral breakthrough is observed with Efavirenz and Nevirapine, the K103N mutation is almost always observed [8]. This mutation is highly resistant to all the first-generation NNRTIs, occurs from a single-point mutation, and is observed in almost 20% of newly infected patients [8]. The Y181C mutation, which is highly resistant to Nevirapine, is also commonly observed in clinical practice, along with a growing number of other resistant mutations [8]. The low genetic barrier to mutation observed with the first-generation NNRTIs is a characteristic of this entire group of compounds, and is caused by the extraordinarily high rate of error of the RT enzyme. In an untreated, newly infected individual, it is estimated that every possible mutation in the genome occurs at least once

Case Studies in Modern Drug Discovery and Development, Edited by Xianhai Huang and Robert G. Aslanian.

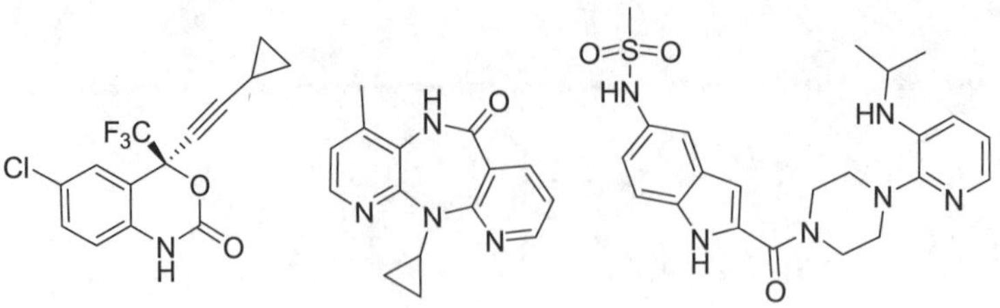

Figure 11.1 Structures of compounds **1–3**.

on a daily basis. This creates a huge pool of preexisting viral mutants, and all that is needed to produce large-scale resistance is the selection pressure of a chemotherapeutic agent. The first-generation NNRTIs preferentially shut down the replication of susceptible viruses, while allowing more resistant and more robust viruses to take over and flourish. Most of the observed resistant variants are in the region of the enzyme immediately surrounding the allosteric binding site. The RT binding site is interesting in that it is not observed as a distinct pocket in the native enzyme and is only observable once an inhibitor has bound to the site [6]. The bound crystal structure of Efavirenz (Figure 11.2) shows many of the critical residues in the NNRTI binding site, and it is readily apparent that most of the commonly mutated residues lie close to the bound inhibitor or are in direct contact with it [9]. It is likely that most of the resistant mutations occur because of close contacts between the inhibitors and the side chains of the mutated residues. The K103N mutation is particularly difficult in that it not only lies central in the NNRTI binding site and is in direct contact with the inhibitor in most published co-crystal structures, but also in the unbound K103N enzyme the side chain of the asparagine appears to make a hydrogen bonding interaction with the phenolic OH of Y188 [9,10]. This interaction may act as a gating mechanism, helping to keep the active site inaccessible, and making the accessibility of inhibitors more difficult [9,10].

Given the inevitability of resistance in most long-term patients, researchers have more recently focused on the design of novel NNRTIs that would be less susceptible to resistance. This work has led to the recent approval of the initial representative of this next generation of NNRTIs, Etravirine (TMC-125/Intelence^{TM}, **4**, Figure 11.3). This compound is the first

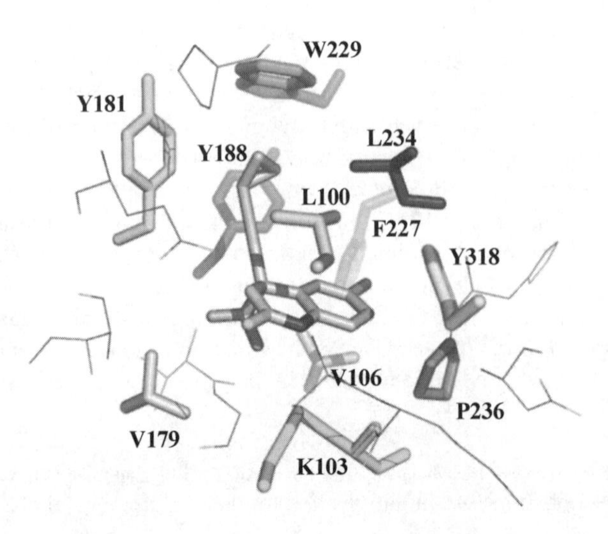

Figure 11.2 Crystal structure of Efavirenz bound in the WT-RT binding site. (See color version of the figure in Color Plate section)

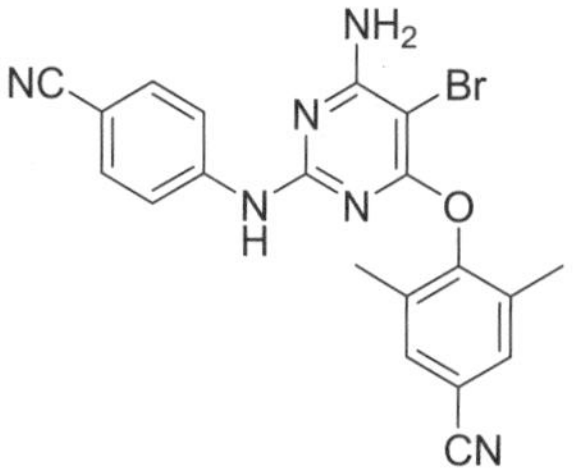

Figure 11.3 Structures of compounds **4** and **5**.

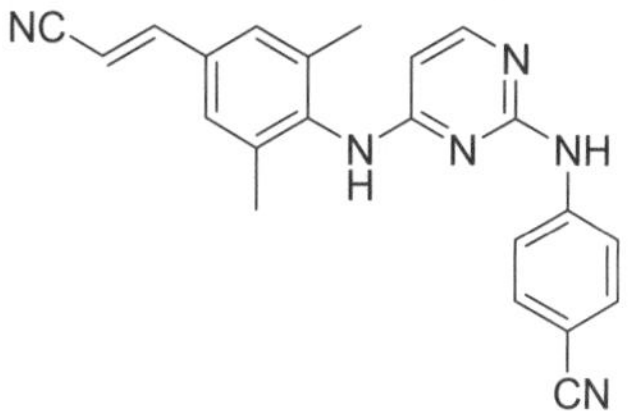

approved NNRTI to offer a higher barrier to resistance than the first-generation compounds, and the development and properties of these compounds and related analogs have been reviewed extensively [11–13]. While the compound retains good potency versus key RT mutations, it is compromised somewhat by its requirement for twice a day dosing, as well as for the occurrence of severe skin and hypersensitivity reactions such as Stevens–Johnson syndrome (as detailed in the prescribing information), and a high propensity for drug–drug interactions based on its metabolic profile [12,13]. A second compound in this series, Rilpivirine (TMC-278, **5**, Figure 11.3) is also undergoing clinical trials and has advanced to Phase III trials [13]. This compound offers the potential advantage of once a day dosing as well as a generally reduced adverse effect profile; however, no extensive data regarding the outcome of Phase II trials with the compound has yet been published or presented. Rilpivirine is a substrate and a mild inducer of CYP3A4, and as such, combinations with known inhibitors of this enzyme should be made with caution as Rilpivirine concentrations may be elevated, potentially increasing the risk of some toxicities including possible QTc prolongation [13]. Interestingly, despite the high lipophilicity and moderate solubility of Rilpivirine, excellent oral bioavailability is observed clinically with the compound, likely because of a complex mechanism involving the formation of spherical nanoparticles in a surfactant-independent fashion at low pH [14].

There continues to be extensive work ongoing to design novel next-generation NNRTIs. Theoretically if one were able to optimize interactions with the side chains of residues that cannot be productively mutated by the virus (such as W229), or if one were able to maximize hydrogen bonding interactions with the amino acid backbone, it may be possible to minimize the impact of some resistance mutations. Such an approach has become the key to the design and synthesis of next-generation NNRTIs. There are a number of characteristics that are desirable in an ideal next generation NNRTI which are critical for the successful development of such a compound. Ideally, the compound should be highly potent against the wild type (WT) RT enzyme and should also have high levels of inherent inhibitory potency toward key RT mutations such as K103N, Y181C, and the double mutant K103N/Y181C. These mutant enzymes along with other common mutant enzymes are commonly chosen for counterscreening of next-generation compounds. These compounds should also demonstrate high levels of antiviral potency in cell-based assays, against the WT virus as well as key mutant viruses such as those previously mentioned. Antiviral activity in cell-based assays in the presence of serum is critical, as assays of this type provide feedback that is directly applicable to clinical situations. Once compounds are identified with excellent inhibitory and antiviral potency against the WT and key mutants, a broader screening of RT mutations can be used to identify the subgroup of compounds showing broad activity against numerous RT mutations, thus suggesting a higher general genetic barrier to resistance. These studies can be confirmed by serial passage experiments in cell culture which also address potential new mutations that might emerge to novel classes of compounds. Good physical properties allowing broad and flexible formulation of compounds is also a critical characteristic of the best compounds, and good pharmacokinetics that allow for both IV and oral dosing of the compounds is among the most important of all properties. The most viable agents will have good IV/PO pharmacokinetics, with high levels of oral bioavailability, low clearance, long half life, and excellent exposure. Especially critical for the development of all HIV therapeutics is the trough concentration after dosing. This concentration needs to remain at a level that will fully suppress the replication of the WT virus as well as all key mutations. Inability to maintain adequate trough levels is a sure path to the rapid induction of resistance, and the importance of this parameter to development potential cannot be overemphasized. Since most HIV-positive patients are on multiple drug regimens, it is critically important that the potential for drug–drug interactions is well understood and minimized in potential candidate compounds. Finally, major side effects and toxicities must also be minimized in any potential HIV therapeutic, as these compounds will likely be long term, chronic therapy that a patient will need to take for a lifetime. Viable candidate compounds should have high margins of safety and selectivity, and should be well tolerated and easy and practical for patients to dose. A once a day oral compound that is safe, well tolerated, and lacks major side effects and drug–drug interactions would be an ideal therapeutic for further development.

11.2 THE DISCOVERY OF MK-4965

11.2.1 Background Information

In the period of time just after the approval of the initial first-generation NNRTIs (the mid/late-1990s), some initial work began in an attempt to address the resistance issues that were becoming apparent with the first-generation compounds. Lead structures for this initial work were either the first-generation structures themselves, or novel leads were developed from the reliable approach of general screening (which had given rise to all of the first-generation compounds as well). Structural information on the binding of first-generation compounds was just beginning to become commonplace in the literature, so some of this initial work was guided by empirical data or molecular modeling without the benefit of extensive crystallographic data. These compounds served as a bridge from the first-generation compounds to the second-generation agents, and clinical information and structural data eventually obtained with these compounds provided valuable insight for the design and optimization of the next generation of inhibitors, including the Merck compound that is the subject of this review chapter. These compounds are directly relevant to the development of our in-house program and as such provide an excellent starting point for this discussion.

In the late 1990s, researchers at Shionogi reported that the imidazole-based compound Capravirine (S-1153, Figure 11.4, **6**) was a potent NNRTI with high levels of activity versus WT-RT and key resistant mutants (WT EC_{50} = 0.31 nM; K103N = 0.31 nM; Y181C = 4.2 nM; G190A = 0.34 nM) [15]. Analysis of cell culture passage experiments with Capravirine showed that at least two mutations (K103N/V106A/L234I; V106A/F227L) were necessary for resistance [15]. The resiliency of Capravirine to common RT resistance mutations is a likely function of its enhanced binding interactions with the NNRTI site. Crystallographic studies [16] with the compound show direct hydrogen bonding interactions with the backbone of K101, K103, and P236; therefore, side-chain mutations at these or other positions would not be likely to disturb these interactions. The compound was licensed by Pfizer, and was moved into clinical

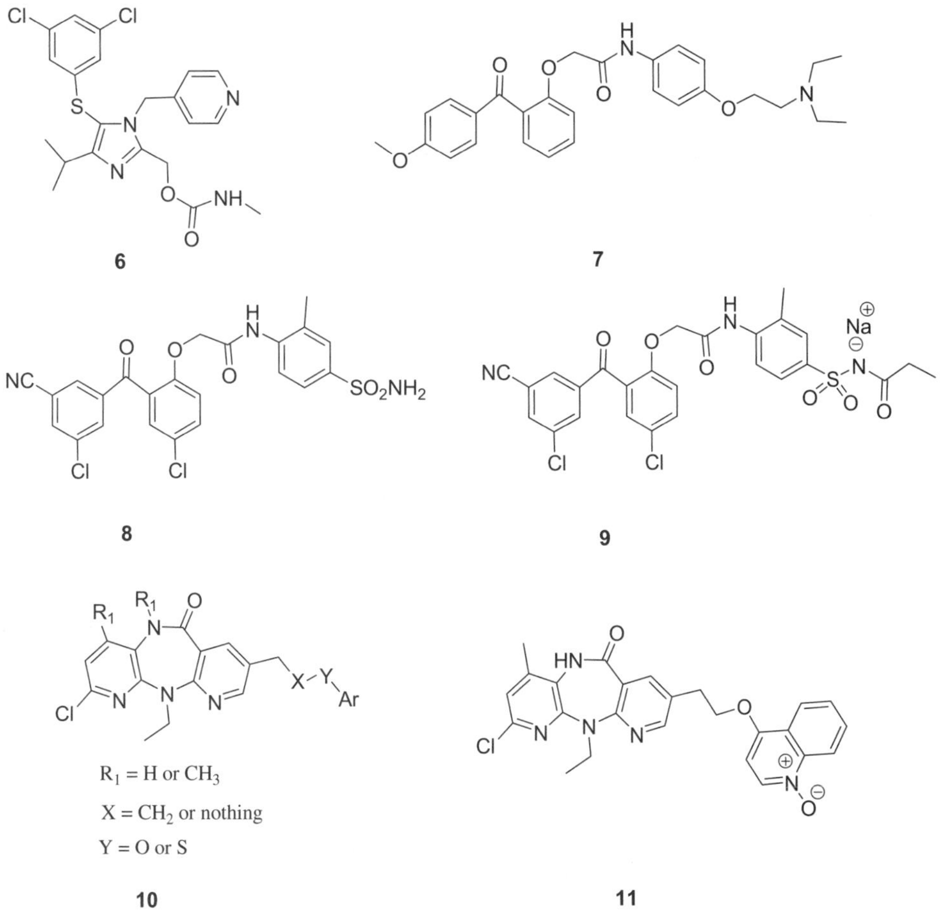

6

7

8

9

R_1 = H or CH_3

X = CH_2 or nothing

Y = O or S

10

11

Figure 11.4 Structures of compounds **6–11**.

development. Early clinical trials demonstrated good efficacy in both treatment naïve and treatment experienced patients [17]. Unfortunately, the compound exhibited a complex metabolism profile in humans along with moderate pharmacokinetics, resulting in the need for high dosing levels [18]. Development of the compound was halted after a Phase II study in which the compound was dosed with two nucleosides along with the HIV-Protease inhibitor Nelfinavir (which boosts the exposure of Capravirine by twofold due to p450 inhibition), which failed to show any advantage from adding Capravirine to the drug cocktail [19]. Nonetheless, the compound had clearly demonstrated that inhibitors that made direct hydrogen bonding interactions with the amino acid backbone could provide some level of activity versus key clinical mutant viruses.

In 1995, scientists at GSK disclosed the discovery of a novel series of benzophenone-based NNRTIs [20]. Initial lead compounds were derived from a high-throughput screening approach, and **7** (Figure 11.4) [20] was identified as an early compound of interest. Further optimization [21,22] of compounds in this series led to the discovery of **8** (Figure 11.4, GW-8248), which was shown to possess potent antiviral activity versus WT and key mutant enzymes (WT $IC_{50} = 0.5$ nM; K103N = 1.0 nM; Y181C = 0.7 nM; V106A = 3.4 nM) [22]. Moderate pharmacokinetics observed preclinically and clinically with **8** led to the development of the prodrug **9** (Figure 11.4, GW-695634), which was moved forward into clinical development [23]. Published results from Phase IIa studies with **9** demonstrated a potent antiviral effect after twice a day oral dosing. Once again, crystallographic studies [24] indicate that favorable hydrogen bonding interactions between the amide carbonyl and the backbone N–H of K103 as well as direct interactions with immutable residue W229 likely contribute to the favorable profile observed with the compound. The crystal structure also shows that Y181 is rotated forward by 90° away from the inhibitor, thus minimizing interactions with this residue and likely contributing to the excellent potency seen against the Y181C mutant. This characteristic rotation of the Y181 residue is seen in many similar series of compounds that bind in an analogous manner. The compounds bind in an elongated version of the NNRTI binding site, in which the P236 residue is rotated upward by several angstroms allowing the aryl anilide/sulfonamide functionality to occupy the space under the residue, with the polar sulfonamide tail lying along the enzyme–solvent interface. This elongated binding mode was a key discovery and has become critical for the design of a number of subsequent series of inhibitors including the Merck inhibitors that will be described in more depth later in this chapter. Despite these encouraging findings, development of the compound was discontinued in Phase II due to elevated liver enzymes/ potential liver toxicity, as well as the development of severe rash in a number of patients [25]. This compound also clearly demonstrated the potential for the development of effective second-generation agents by designing interactions into the compounds that favor activity against a wider variety of viral mutants.

Finally, the Nevirapine molecule itself became the starting platform for a series of 8-substituted dipyridodiazepineones disclosed by Boeringer Ingelheim (Figure 11.4, **10**) [26–29]. A member of this class, BILR-355 BS (Figure 11.4, **11**) is reported to have good potency versus WT and key mutant viruses (WT $IC_{50} = 17$ nM; K103N = 44 nM; Y181C = 51 nM; G190A = 25 nM), and has been moved forward into clinical development [30]. The compound appears to retain activity versus some clinically relevant mutations, but V106A and Y188L appear to confer some level of resistance, and the K103N/V106A double mutant is highly resistant. Limited clinical data has been published on this compound; however, it appears that co-dosing with Ritonavir (HIV-Protease inhibitor with potent P450 inhibitory activity) is necessary to achieve and sustain trough levels suitable to suppress WT and the most sensitive mutants [30]. The co-crystal structure of the compound with WT-RT has been described [31], and it appears that the dipyridodiazepinone core binds in a manner essentially identical to that observed for Nevirapine. However, the side chain in the 8-position appears to bind in a similar region to that described above for the anilide/aryl sulfonamide of the GSK compounds (as mentioned earlier), and this may indicate that this binding mode helps to enhance the genetic barrier of the compounds to resistance by providing increased interactions with the active site. In general, the compounds were reported to be more flexible and to have greater ability to modify their orientation in the active site of various mutant RTs [31].

The above-detailed bridge compounds set the stage for the development of many novel NNRTIs, and were a key foundation upon which our in-house program evolved. The key insights such as an elongated and more flexible binding mode, the ability to design direct interactions with important mutated binding site backbone residues, and the ability to use the solvent–enzyme interface to install polar residues with potential to enhance physical properties were all important contributors to our compound design as we began the task of developing novel, next-generation NNRTIs.

11.2.2 SAR Studies Leading to the Discovery of MK-4965

NNRTI research at Merck has focused on a series of novel compounds known as diaryl ethers. Program goals were focused on the design and synthesis of novel and patentable

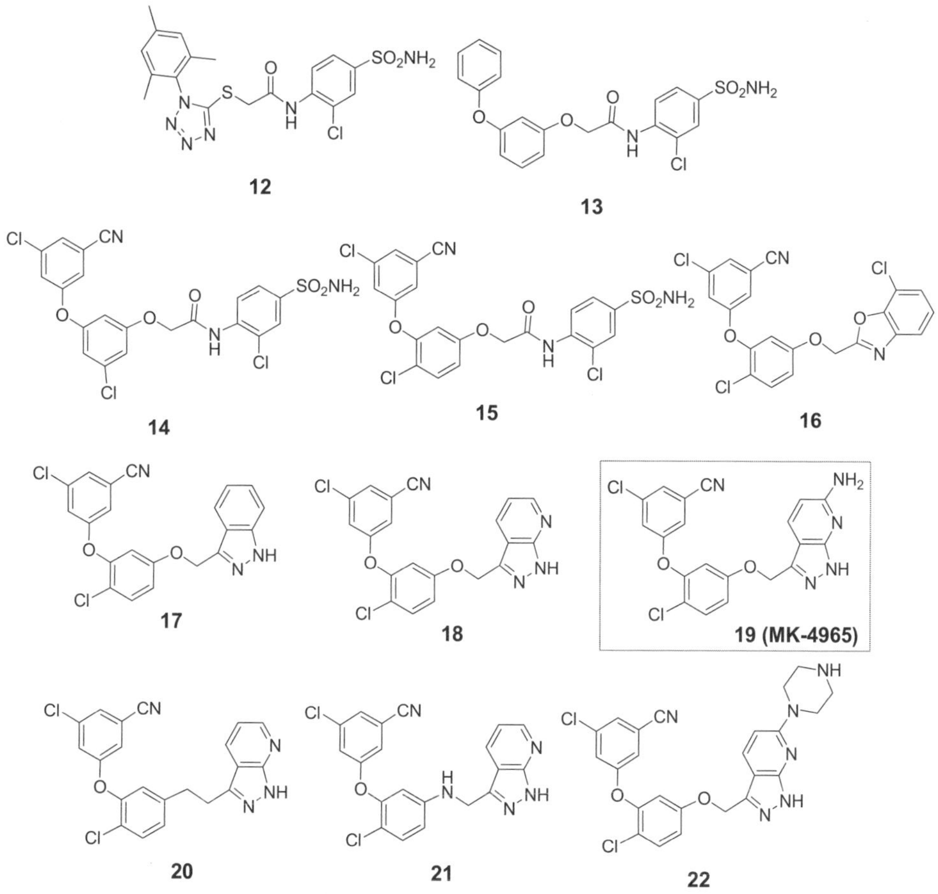

Figure 11.5 Structures of compounds **12–22**.

NNRTIs that exhibited potent antiviral activity versus WT and key mutant viruses in the presence of plasma, while demonstrating a pharmacokinetic profile suitable for once a day oral dosing clinically. Early efforts in this series centered on the synthesis of analogs of **12** (Figure 11.5) which were derived from high-throughput screening [32].

Disappointing pharmacokinetic results from this structural class forced a retargeting of efforts toward more novel compounds, and efforts were refocused on replacing the phenyl tetrazole of **12**. A direct molecular modeling comparison of **12** with the previously described GSK compound **8** suggested that the eastern acetanilide functionality on each molecule was likely to bind in a similar region, thereby also suggesting that the biaryl western regions were likely to bind in a similar region as well [32]. Modeling studies suggested that the biaryl portions of both of these compounds likely filled the large lipophillic pocket formed by the Y181–Y188–W229 residues. This pocket is well characterized and utilized by all the known first-generation NNRTIs. This hypothesis led to a synthetic strategy in which the oxyacetanilide substructure was held constant and the biaryl region was modified via a rapid analog approach [32]. From this effort, a simple diphenyl ether analog **13** quickly emerged as a novel lead structure. Further molecular modeling comparisons between **8** and **13** suggested that the compounds bound to the NNRTI site in a very similar manner, with the anilide carbonyl of both compounds making a direct hydrogen bonding interaction with the backbone of K103, the aryl sulfonamide lying under P236 with the sulfonamide group

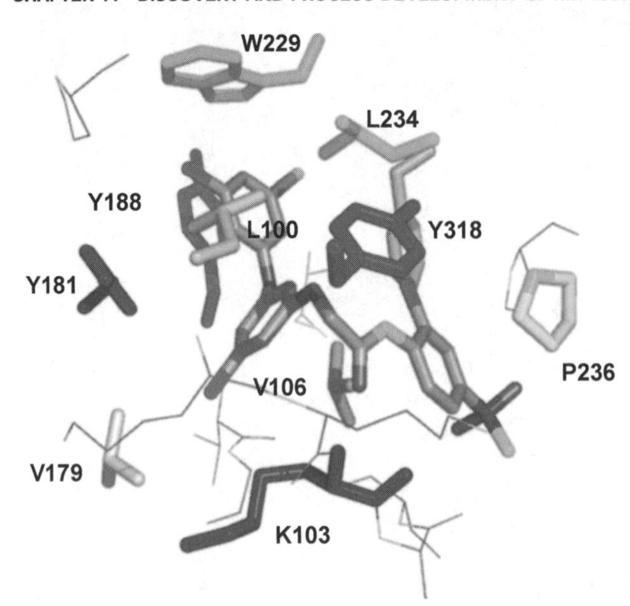

Figure 11.6 The X-ray crystal structure of compound **14** (salmon with blue nitrogen, red oxygen, green chlorine, and orange sulfur) bound to the NNRTI binding site (2.5 Angstrom resolution) [32].

solvent exposed, and the easternmost phenyl ring of the diaryl ether moiety making a pi–pi stacking interaction with Y188 and an edge on interaction with W229 [32]. The overlay of the two compounds suggested that the distal phenyl ring could be modified by the addition of two meta substituents, and the central aryl ring could be modified by the addition of a chlorine or other similar group to either the 2 or 3 position. Addition of an m-chloro and m-cyano substituent to the distal phenyl ring, and a 3-chloro group to the central aromatic ring provided **14**, which had nanomolar potency against the WT, K103N, and Y181C enzymes (WT IC_{50} = 2.1 nM; K103N = 3.5 nM; Y181C = 2.7 nM) but exhibited poor pharmacokinetics after oral dosing to animals [33]. Crystallographic studies with **14** confirmed the predictions suggested by the earlier molecular modeling studies (Figure 11.6). The carbonyl oxygen of the acetanilide moiety makes a direct hydrogen bonding interaction with the backbone N-H of K103, while the phenyl ring of the acetanilide lies under P236, with the sulfonamide moiety solvent exposed. The diaryl ether substructure fills the large lipophilic pocket created by Y181–Y188–W229, with the distal aromatic ring making a direct pi-stacking interaction with Y188 and an edge on interaction with the immutable W229 residue. Interestingly, the Y181 side chain is rotated forward approximately 90° away from the inhibitor, minimizing contacts that the compounds have with this residue and likely contributing to the excellent activity seen against mutations at this position; this is a characteristic of all co-crystal structures in this series and is similar to what was observed with the previously described GSK compound **9** [24]. The chlorine atom on the central aromatic ring fills the front of the large lipophilic pocket and interacts directly with V179. Moving the chlorine atom on the central phenyl ring from the 3-position to the 2-position provided **15,** which demonstrated a 10-fold increase in potency versus WT, K103N, and Y181C RTs (WT IC_{50} = 0.14 nM; K103N = 0.21 nM; Y181C = 0.28 nM) [32]. This change in position of the chlorine atom causes the compound to make somewhat less direct contact with V179, allowing the molecule to relax and fit the entire site in a more relaxed manner [32]. Unfortunately, the pharmacokinetics of the compound remained poor, and an analysis of the metabolism of this compound and others in the series suggested that metabolic hydrolysis of the acetanilide amide bond was a major route of metabolism. Attempts to block this amide hydrolysis by cyclizing from the 2-position of the acetanilide phenyl ring back onto the nitrogen of the amide were successful and high levels of potency were maintained, but the oral bioavailability of the compounds remained quite low [32]. Attempts at replacing the acetanilide region with a fused heterocyclic system provided a series of novel analogs represented by **16**. While some of these compounds maintained good levels of potency versus WT and key mutant enzymes and obviated the metabolism issues observed with the amides, no single compound possessed the combination of potency, antiviral activity, and pharmacokinetics necessary to warrant further interest [32]. Further analysis of crystallographic results from this series, along with molecular modeling analysis/comparison of potential new templates, led to the hypothesis that an indazole moiety might be a reasonable replacement for the acetanilide region [32]. The indazole ring system had the potential to replace most of the lipophilic interactions provided by the earlier acetanilides, while the cyclic hydrazino moiety of the indazole appeared capable of making two hydrogen bonding interactions with the N-H and the carbonyl of K103. This novel binding mode presented the potential for excellent potency in a small, synthetically accessible heterocyclic system. Synthesis of this novel template provided **17**, which demonstrated excellent inhibitory potency (WT $IC_{50} = 1.4$ nM; K103N = 1.1 nM; Y181C = 2.6 nM) and good antiviral activity (WT CIC_{95}(10% FBS) = 22.6 nM; K103N = 33.4 nM; Y181C = 101.5 nM; WT(50% NHS) = 114 nM) versus WT and the K103N and Y181C mutants [32]. The antiviral potency of the compound is shifted upward in the presence of normal human serum (NHS), indicating the critical role of plasma protein binding in determining antiviral activity. Crystallographic studies with **17** demonstrated the unique binding mode of the molecule. The diaryl ether portion of the molecule fits the NNRTI site in an almost identical manner as the previously described amide analogs; however, the indazole ring provided novel hydrogen bonding interactions with both the N–H and the carbonyl of K103 as had been suggested by earlier modeling studies. The bottom edge of the phenyl ring of the indazole moiety lies along the solvent–enzyme interface and is directly solvent exposed, suggesting that this region would be an area for further exploration with polar substituents. Despite the successful removal of the amide moiety from the molecules, the pharmacokinetics and oral bioavailability in the series remained poor, and the shift in antiviral activity in the presence of serum remained an issue. These issues largely appeared to be a function of the solubility, physical properties, and high lipophilicity of the compounds. As such, a focused effort was undertaken to improve these properties. Systematic rotation of a pyridine nitrogen around the indazole aromatic ring led to the discovery of **18**, which retained excellent enzyme (WT $IC_{50} = 0.4$ nM; K103N = 0.5 nM; Y181C = 0.2 nM) and antiviral potency (WT CIC_{95}(10% FBS) = 10.3 nM; K103N = 14.6 nM; Y181C = 22.0 nM; WT(50% NHS) = 34.0 nM) versus WT, K103N, and Y181C, and also demonstrated good oral bioavailability and pharmacokinetics in animals after IV/PO dosing [33]. Crystallographic studies with **18** bound in the K103N mutant RT demonstrated that the compound fits the mutant enzyme site in essentially a similar manner as seen with **17** in the WT site, indicating that the binding of the compound is completely unaffected by the K103N mutation [32,33]. Broad screening of **18** versus a library of RT mutants showed that the compound maintained a high genetic barrier and was largely unaffected by most mutations with the exception of Y188L. This mutation did appear to be somewhat resistant to the compound, likely due to the direct pi-stacking interaction that the compound makes with Y188. The consequences of this are unknown, but studies with the compounds suggest that this may not be a major issue as Y188L is a rare and difficult to derive mutation, and the compounds do not appear to select for this mutation in cell culture experiments [32,33]. Given its excellent overall profile, **18** was selected for further development and was designated as MK-1107 [33]. During the workup of this compound, major difficulty was encountered producing an oral formulation that could provide the high levels of exposure necessary to support full safety assessment studies [33]. Further studies demonstrated that the compound was only orally bioavailable when dosed as a solution, and the limited solubility of the compound did not allow oral dosing at higher levels. This finding led to the suspension of development of **18**, and to further analog preparation in the series in an effort to design compounds with even better solubility and physical properties. After an extensive examination of the SAR of the pyrazolopyridine moiety, the installation of an amino group in the 6-position of the pyrazolopyridine adjacent to the pyridyl nitrogen gave **19**, which showed excellent enzyme (WT $IC_{50} = 0.2$ nM; K103N = 0.5 nM; Y181C = 0.4 nM) and cell-based (WT CIC_{95}(10% FBS) = 8.4 nM; K103N = 11.4 nM; Y181C = 19.0 nM; WT (50% NHS) = 34.0 nM) potency versus WT, K103N, and Y181C [33]. The compound demonstrated approximately 10-fold higher solubility, and good IV/PO pharmacokinetics and excellent oral bioavailability in animals, and showed broad antiviral activity versus a panel of clinically derived RT mutations [33]. As in the case of **18**, the potency of **19** was compromised by the Y188L mutation. Crystallographic data for the compound bound to the WT and Y181C confirmed a similar fit for both enzymes that was almost identical to the fit observed earlier for co-crystal structures of **17** and **18** and either WT or K103N RT. The newly installed amino group does not appear to interact in any direct way with the NNRTI site, and lies along the enzyme–solvent interface and is directly solvent exposed. Given its excellent overall properties and enhanced solubility, **19** was moved forward as a development candidate and was designated as MK-4965.

11.3 PRECLINICAL AND CLINICAL STUDIES OF MK-4965 (19)

Safety and ancillary studies with MK-4965 (**19**) showed that the compound had no major safety issues, and its potential for drug–drug interactions was low [33]. Metabolism studies with the compound showed a balanced metabolism via P450-mediated oxidation and also glucuronidation [33,34]. Cell-based resistance selection experiments showed a high barrier to the selection of mutations. At low multiples of infection (MOI) conditions of 1–5X, the CIC_{95}, Y181C, P236L, and V106A were observed within a 2-week window [33,34]. At higher MOI, the mutations became less prevalent, and at 1000 nM, no resistant mutants emerged even after multiple months of exposure [33,34]. Based on the excellent overall preclinical profile demonstrated for the compound, **19** was positioned to move forward into Phase I clinical trials for the treatment of HIV infection. Detailed results of the clinical studies with **19** have not been published to date and will not be discussed in this chapter.

11.4 SUMMARY OF BACK-UP SAR STUDIES OF MK-4965 SERIES

More generic SAR on this series has been detailed in a series of presentations [35,36]. The SAR surrounding the distal ring of the diaryl ether substructure has been described [36]. In general, 3,5-disubstitution on this ring is optimal, with electron withdrawing substituents such as chloro or cyano favored over donating substituents. Polar groups or polar heterocycles are not well tolerated and cause reductions in potency, and the addition of any substitution at the 4-position of this ring is not well tolerated [36]. The linker between the central phenyl ring and the pyrazolopyridine ring has also been extensively investigated [35]. Replacement of the oxymethylene linker of compounds like **18** and **19** with a two-carbon linker provides compounds such as **20**, which show similar levels of enzyme potency versus WT and key mutants, but in general exhibit somewhat diminished antiviral activity and generally less optimal pharmacokinetics [35]. The diminished antiviral activity is presumed to be due to the enhanced lipophilicity and higher levels of protein binding observed with these compounds [35]. Replacement of the oxymethylene linker with an aminomethylene linker provides analogs such as **21**, which also retain potent enzyme inhibitory activity and antiviral activity versus WT and key mutant RTs. These compounds also show somewhat less optimal pharmacokinetic profiles [35]. Finally, the SAR surrounding the amino substitution at the 6-position of the pyrazolopyridine moiety has been described [35]. Various basic groups are well tolerated at this position, and even larger substituents such as the piperazine ring of **22** are tolerated with retention of subnanomolar inhibitory potency and nanomolar antiviral potency versus WT and key mutants [35]. This is presumably possible because this region is solvent exposed, and these groups do not make direct interactions with any residues in the NNRTI binding site. In general, the rat pharmacokinetics of these analogs are similar to that seen with the parent compounds; however, a trend toward increased clearance is observed as the molecules become larger [35].

11.5 PROCESS DEVELOPMENT OF MK-4965 (19)

A key element to the success of moving a drug candidate from discovery stage to full development is the process chemistry development. Once a candidate is selected for development, a large amount of material is required to support the preclinical and clinical studies. An efficient manufacturing process needs to be developed whether the drug will ultimately reach the market or not. In the following sections, a detailed showcase of the complexity and challenges of the process chemistry development is demonstrated using the MK-4965 development as an example.

11.5.1 Medicinal Chemistry Route

The medicinal chemistry route for the synthesis of MK-4965 (**19**) was carried out in eight linear steps in approximately 0.8% overall yield [32,33]. In order to support all preclinical and clinical studies, an efficient, practical and cost-effective synthetic route to MK-4965 (**19**) was required. The retrosynthetic analysis of **19** by the medicinal chemistry group led to three components: biaryl ether **23**, pyrazolo[3,4-b]pyrimidine **24,** and *p*-methoxybenzylamine (PMBA) (Scheme 11.1). S_N2 replacement of **24** with **23**, followed by S_NAr replacement of the floride with PMBA and deprotection would give MK-4965 (**19**).

The synthesis of the key intermediate **24** began with 2,6-difluoropyridine **25** (Scheme 11.2). Ortho lithiation with LDA followed by quenching with *N*-methoxy-*N*-methylacetamide afforded ketone **26** in 25% yield. The yield was hard to improve despite numerous attempts. Treatment of the ketone **26** with 2 equiv of hydrazine and 2 equiv of titanium(IV) isoproxide in dichloromethane gave the corresponding hydrazones ***27Z*/*27E***

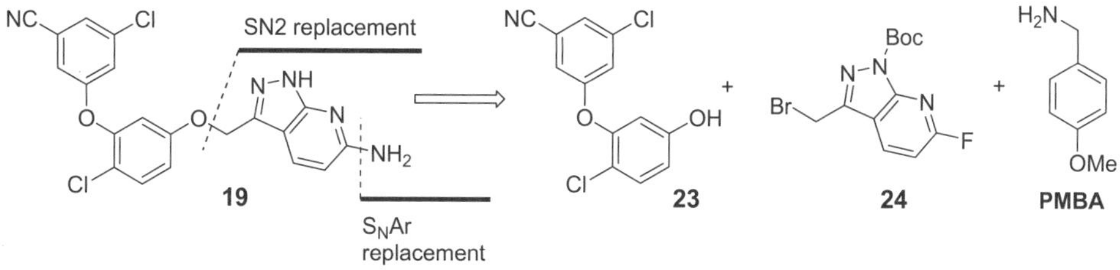

SN2 replacement

19

S_NAr replacement

23

24

PMBA

Scheme 11.1 Retrosynthetic analysis of **19**.

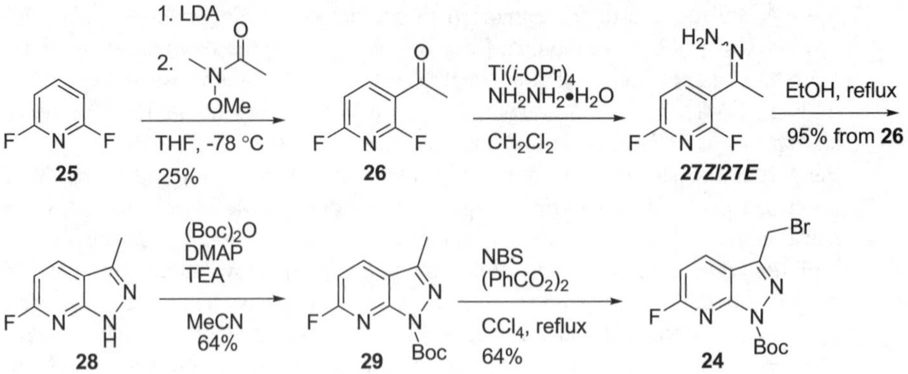

Scheme 11.2 Synthesis of pyrazolo[3,4-b]pyridine **24**.

as a *cis/trans* mixture, which was cyclized in refluxing ethanol to give the pyrazolo[3,4-b] pyridine **28** in 95% yield from **26**. Boc protection of the pyrazole nitrogen **28** gave the protected pyrazole **29** in 64% yield, which was converted to bromide **24** in 64% yield by treatment with NBS in the presence of catalytic amount of benzoyl peroxide in carbon tetrachloride.

The phenol **23** was prepared as shown in Scheme 11.3. S_NAr replacement of the fluoride **30** with phenol **31** in the presence of potassium carbonate in NMP afforded biaryl ether **32** in 75% yield. Removal of the methyl protecting group with 1.25 equiv of boron tribromide in dichloromethane afforded phenol **23** in 95% yield.

With the two key intermediate **23** and **24** in hand, S_N2 replacement of the bromide **24** with phenol **23** in the presence of Cs_2CO_3 in NMP afforded compound **33** in 86% yield (Scheme 11.4). S_NAr displacement of the fluoride **33** with PMBA gave the protected MK-4965 (**34**) in 31% yield. Global deprotection of **34** in the presence of a large excess of TFA furnished the synthesis of MK-4965 (**19**) in 30% yield, an overall 0.8% yield over eight linear steps.

The medicinal chemistry route described above proved only suitable for the generation of milligram to gram quantities of **19**. To provide large quantities of MK-4965, a new synthetic process was clearly needed to address several key problems of the original route:

1. Several low yielding steps including formation of the ketone **26**, the amidation, and the final global deprotection.
2. Use of undesirable halogenated solvents such as dichloromethane and carbon tetrachloride in multiple steps.
3. Chromatographic purification in seven steps.
4. Low yields of many steps.

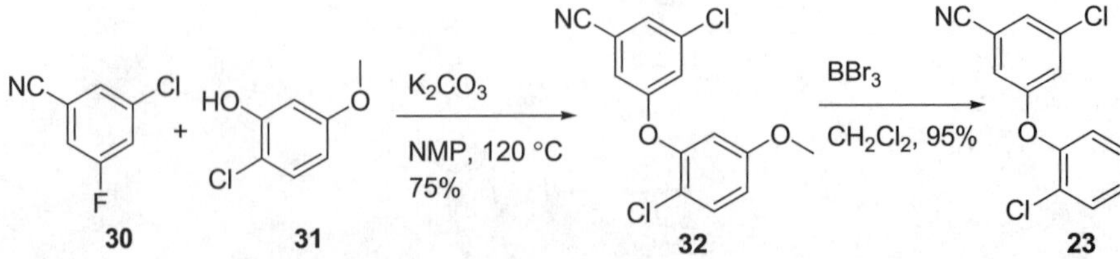

Scheme 11.3 Synthesis of phenol **23**.

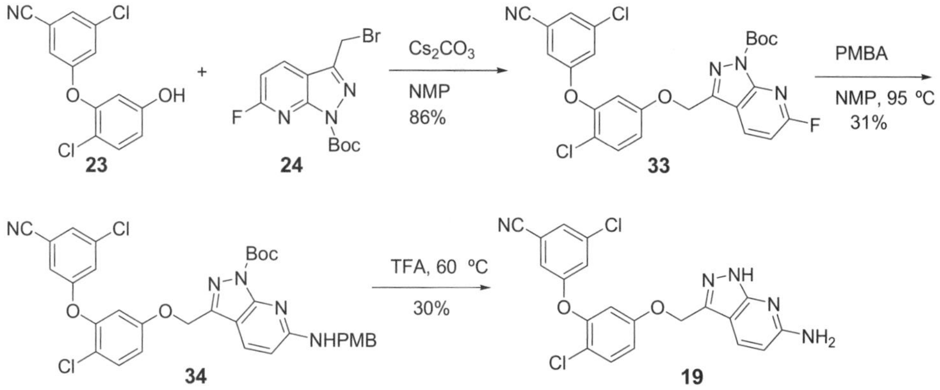

Scheme 11.4 End game for the synthesis of MK-4965 (**19**).

11.5.2 Process Development

11.5.2.1 First-Generation Process for the Synthesis of MK-4965

Retrosynthetic Analysis of First-Generation Process In order to prepare multikilogram quantities of **19**, a scalable and high-yielding process was required. The first-generation retrosynthetic process approach is shown in Scheme 11.5. MK-4965 (**19**) could be derived from **18**, the second-generation NNRTI from Merck, by amination. This was a particularly attractive approach because **18** was in development and multikilogram quantities were available. Further disassembly of the intermediate **18** by cleavage of the ether bond led to two key fragments, **23** and **35**, which in turn could be derived in two steps from pyrazole **36** through an N–H protection and an allylic bromination.

Synthesis of Ether 24 The synthesis of **18** closely paralleled the Medicinal Chemistry synthesis and started from the known 3-methyl-pyrazolo[3,4-b]pyridine **36**

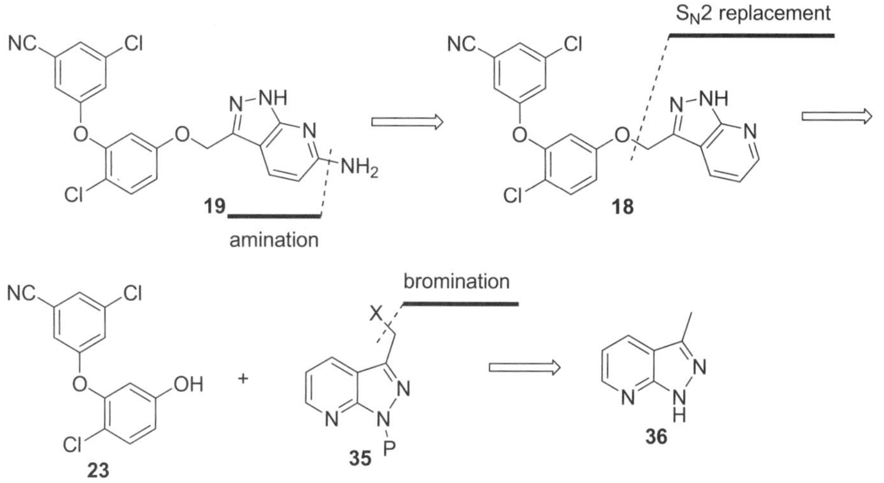

Scheme 11.5 Retrosynthetic analysis of **19**.

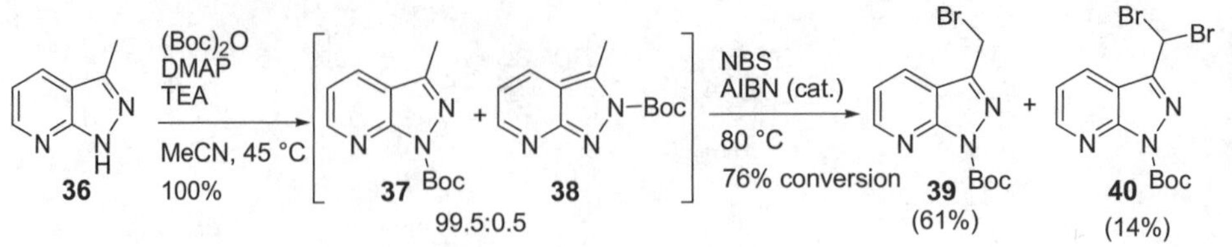

Scheme 11.6 Synthesis of bromide **39**.

(Scheme 11.6) [37]. N-H protection of **36** with Boc_2O in the presence of 20 mol% DMAP in MeCN at 45°C initially gave a mixture of **37** and **38**. However, prolonged heating led to nearly complete conversion of **38** to **37** (99.5:0.5). The crude product **37** was carried forward in the next step without further purification. After changing the solvent to trifluorotoluene, crude **37** was treated with NBS in the presence of a catalytic amount of AIBN at 80°C to give a statistical mixture of the desired bromide **39** (61%), dibromide **40** (14%), and starting material **36** (24%). Numerous attempts to drive the reaction to completion failed to improve the yield of **39**. However, bromide **39** could be isolated in 42% yield from **36** after purification by silica–gel chromatography followed by recrystallization from MTBE/heptane. It was worth noting that storage of bromide **39** at room temperature for prolonged periods of time led to significant degradation, but it was stable for up to 2 years at 0–5°C.

The Medicinal Chemistry route for the synthesis of phenol **23** was used in our first-generation process without further optimization [33]. The initial route for the preparation of **18** involved alkylation of phenol **23** with bromide **39** in the presence of sodium hydride in DMF. Subsequent Boc deprotection with TFA afforded **18** in 67% yield for the two-step sequence. However, the use of sodium hydride in conjunction with DMF raised serious safety concerns for a large-scale process, so safer conditions for the alkylation reaction were required. Our initial experiments showed that treatment of 1 equiv of **23** with 1 equiv of **39** in the presence of 6 equiv of CsF as the base and 1.5 equiv of KI as an additive afforded **41** in 70–78% yield (Scheme 11.7), but with a significant amount of over-alkylated by-product **42**. The addition of KI to the reaction mixture can dramatically increase the rate of reaction where the rapid formation of iodide intermediate **43** could be observed by HPLC. Further

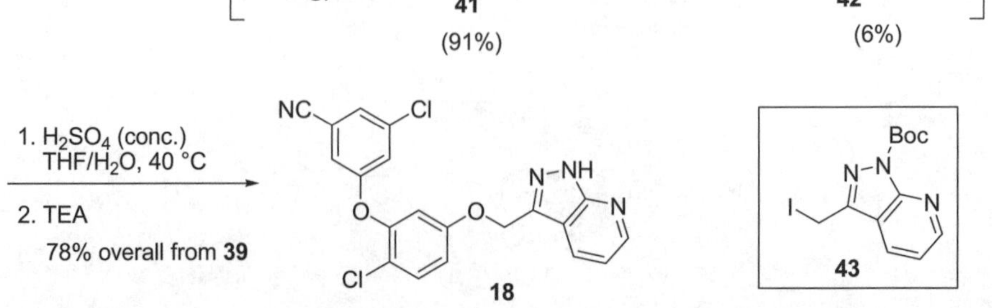

Scheme 11.7 Synthesis of ether **18**.

optimization of the reaction conditions led to portion-wise addition of 1.08 equiv of bromide **39** to a preformed mixture of 1 equiv of **23** and 3 equiv of CsF in DMF at room temperature. After workup, the crude product **41** was obtained in 91% HPLC yield. Compound **41** was directly used in the deprotection step without further purification.

The Boc protecting group of **41** was effectively removed using 2.5 equiv of concentrated sulfuric acid at 35–40°C in aqueous THF. A crystalline hemisulfate salt of **18** was directly isolated from the reaction mixture. The freebase of **18** was obtained by neutralization with triethylamine to pH = 8–9. Analytically pure **18** was obtained in 78% overall yield from **23** by recrystallization of the crude **18** from 1:1 MeOH/MeCN.

Conversion of 18 to 19 With the key compound **18** in hand, we believed that direct amination of the compound would provide MK-4965 (**19**). A few methods for introducing a 2-amino group on the pyridine moiety have been reported. One reported method is substitution of 2-halopyridines and analogs with ammonia or an ammonia equivalent at high temperature (150–250°C) and high pressure or using transition metal catalyzed conditions. For this approach, a halogen atom must be installed at the 2-position first, but this approach typically gives poor 2,4-regioselectivity and low yields [38]. When we attempted 2-chlorination of the *N*-oxide **45**, the 4-chloro product was observed as the major isomer. An alternative amidation approach involved the use of the Chichibabin reaction, which gives 2-aminopyridines directly from sodium amide and pyridines [39]. This method was found to be very limited in scope, with unsatisfactory yields and poor functional group tolerance, most likely due to the strongly basic conditions and high temperatures. The harsh conditions rendered this approach unsuitable for our substrate. We instead chose to investigate a milder reaction to introduce the amine group directly at the 2-pyridine position via the *N*-oxide.

Development for the 2-Amination of Pyridines Pyridine *N*-oxides such as **45** can be prepared by oxidation of the corresponding pyridines (Scheme 11.8). The 2-position of compound **46** is highly activated, and the rearrangement products can be formed by reaction of the *N*-oxide with electrophiles. When ammonia or an amine is used as an

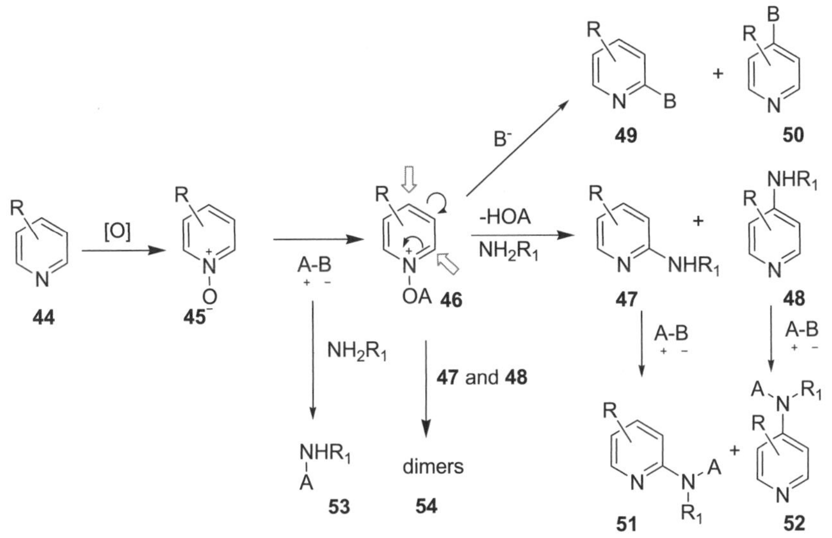

Scheme 11.8 Amination of pyridines.

electrophile, 2-aminopyridines **47** (as the major component) along with the by-product 4-aminopyridine **48** (as the minor component) could be obtained. However, this process is generally not efficient due to multiple side reactions that form various by-products (**49–54**) as shown in Scheme 11.8. Most notably, the amine can react with the activating agent or highly unstable intermediate **46** to form byproduct **54**. The intermediate **46** itself is susceptible to the attack of the counterion of the activating agent to form byproducts **49** and **50**. In addition, the product itself can react with the activated intermediate **44** to form dimers. Only a few examples of the conversion of (iso)quinoline *N*-oxides to 2-amino(iso) quinolines have been reported with yields in the 60–70% range [40]. The corresponding reaction has consistently failed with pyridine *N*-oxides.

In the first attempt, the amination of pyridine *N*-oxide with TsCl–NH_4OH gave a 10% yield of the desired product **47** ($R_1 = H$) while a large amount of $TsNH_2$ and Py_2NTs was generated due to dimerization and further tosylation of the product **47** as detailed in Scheme 11.8. We envisioned that the use of a bulky *tert*-butylamine as an ammonia equivalent might prevent the formation of such undesired by-products **49–54**. In addition, other reaction parameters such as the activating reagents and solvents were screened (Table 11.1) [41].

When pyridine *N*-oxide **55** was treated with 1.75 equiv of TsCl and 4.5 equiv of tBuNH_2 (which served both as the reagent and the base for the reaction) a 61% conversion was observed with little dimerization or tosylation by-product generated. Most importantly, good regioselectivity was observed for this amination. Since reaction of the activating reagent with *tert*-butylamine to form **58** was the only major side reaction, it was reasonable to monitor the efficiency of the reaction under different conditions using the ratio of the desired product **57** to undesired products **58** and **59**.

A screen of the activating agent found that both TsCl and Ts_2O gave comparable results, while AcCl, MsCl, or Ms_2O were ineffective (entries 1–9). A solvent screen showed that both EtOAc and trifluorotoluene gave the best overall reaction profile in terms of the conversion (ratio of **57**/**58**) and the selectivity (ratio of **57**/**59**) (Table 11.1, entries 10–19). Further optimization using Ts_2O as activating agent and trifluorotoluene as solvent gave the best results. With an excess of reagents, the highest selectivity (ratio of **57**/**59**) and conversion were achieved at 0°C (Table 11.1, entry 21). The slightly lower conversion ratio was likely due to the higher concentration (Table 11.1, entry 19 vs. 20). Although compound **57** could be isolated at this point in 92% yield and the corresponding 2-aminopyridine was obtained by deprotection of **57** in neat TFA, a more robust one-pot process was realized by adding TFA (2.5 mL $mmol^{-1}$) to the reaction mixture after completion of *tert*-butylamination followed by heating at 70°C to provide 2-aminopyridine in 84% yield.

Using the above optimized one-pot conditions, a variety of substituted pyridine *N*-oxides, quinoline *N*-oxides, and isoquinoline *N*-oxides were directly aminated at the 2-position in high yields (Table 11.2). The amination step was typically completed within a few minutes, while the *in situ* deprotection with TFA required 2–6 h. The one-pot process showed good functional group compatibility and gave excellent overall yields.

End Game of the First-Generation Synthesis of MK-4965 With sufficient quantities of compound **18** and the robust one-pot direct amination at the 2-position of pyridine *N*-oxide in hand, conversion of **18** to MK-4965 (**19**) was investigated. Initially, the pyridine nitrogen of **18** was oxidized with 1.7 equiv of MCPBA in acetic acid at 55°C to provide *N*-oxide intermediate **63** in 98% isolated yield (Scheme 11.9).

The next step was the installation of the amino substituent on the pyridine ring. Attempts to directly install the *tert*-butylamine group on **63** failed due to competitive

TABLE 11.1 Optimization for the Amination of Pyrimidine *N*-Oxide

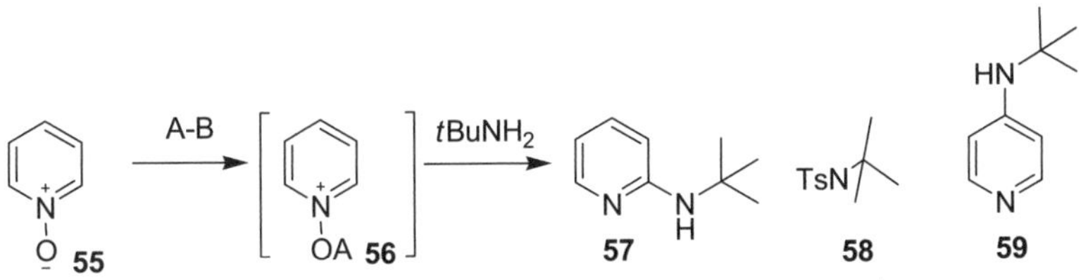

Entry	A-B	Solvent	Conversion	**57/58**	**57/59**
1	TsCL	CH_2CL_2	61	0.46	19
2	Ts_2O	CH_2CL_2	60	0.48	14
3[b]	TsCL	CH_2CL_2	61	0.46	12
4[b]	Ts_2O	CH_2CL_2	25	0.17	3.8
5[c]	Ts_2O	CH_2CL_2	27	0.18	4.5
6[b]	AcCL	CH_2CL_2	0	0	–
7	AcCL	CH_2CL_2	0	0	–
8	MsCL	CH_2CL_2	0	0	–
9	Ms_2O	CH_2CL_2	16	–	8.6
10	Ts_2O	THF	68	0.58	12
11	Ts_2O	MeCN	5	0.02	–
12	Ts_2O	DMF	8	0.05	–
13	Ts_2O	EtOAc	87	0.80	18
14[d]	Ts_2O	EtOAc	74	0.76	43
15[d]	TsCL	EtOAc	20	0.15	48
16	TsCL	$CHCL_3$	79	0.80	14
17	TsCL	DCE	55	0.38	16
18	TsCL	$PhCF_3$	74	0.61	30
19	Ts_2O	$PhCF_3$	84	1.3	22
20[e]	Ts_2O	$PhCF_3$	60	0.66	25
21[d,e,f]	Ts_2O	$PhCF_3$	100	0.83	59

[a]Reaction conditions: To a solution of 0.25 mmol of **55** and 4.5 eq of *t*$BuNH_2$ in 2.5 mL solvent was added 1.75 equiv of activating reagent A–B at room temperature. Most reactions gave no further conversion after 15 min (those with TsCl took a few hours).

[b]Activating reagent was added before *t*$BuNH_2$.

[c]Ts_2O was aged with **55** for 30 min before adding *t*$BuNH_2$.

[d]Run at 0°C.

[e]5 mL solvent/mmol **55**.

[f]6 equiv of *t*$BuNH_2$ and 2.5 equiv Ts_2O were used.

tosylation of the pyrazole nitrogen atom. After evaluation of several common protecting groups, we found that tetrahydropyranyl (THP) was a suitable protecting group for pyrazole **63**. Thus, treatment of **63** with 4.7 equiv. of 3,4-dihydro-2*H*-pyran (DHP) in the presence of a catalytic amount of TsOH afforded **64** in 80% yield. Because of its low solubility in trifluorotoluene and ethyl acetate, dichloromethane was selected as the solvent for the amination. A preformed mixture of **64** and 4 equiv of *tert*-butylamine in CH_2Cl_2 was added to a solution of 2.1 equiv of Ts_2O in CH_2Cl_2 at 0–5°C to give **65** and the by-product

TABLE 11.2 Direct 2-Amination of Pyridine and (iso)quinoline *N*-Oxides

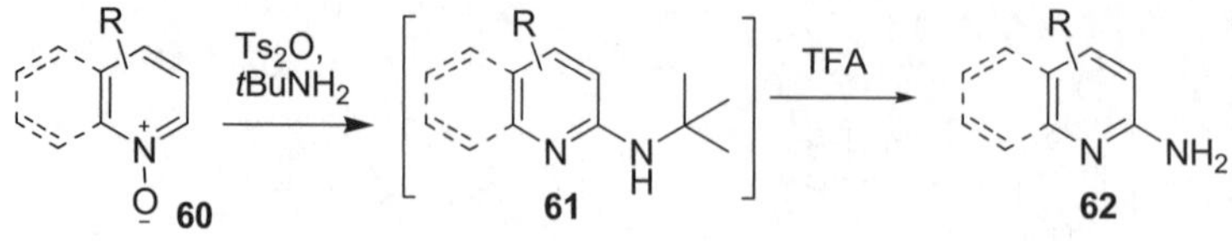

R, **60** —(Ts_2O, tBuNH$_2$)→ [R, N, N, H, **61**] —(TFA)→ R, N, NH_2, **62**

Entry	*N*-Oxides	Product	Yld(%)
1	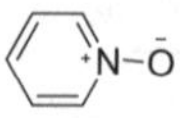 N–O	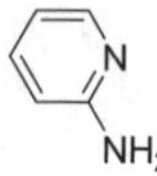 N, NH_2	84
2	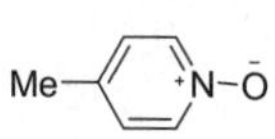 Me, N–O	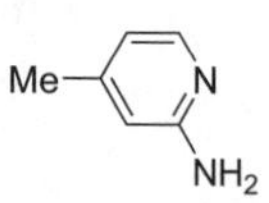 Me, N, NH_2	88
3	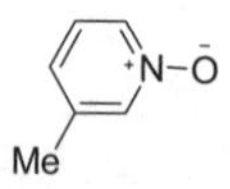 N–O, Me	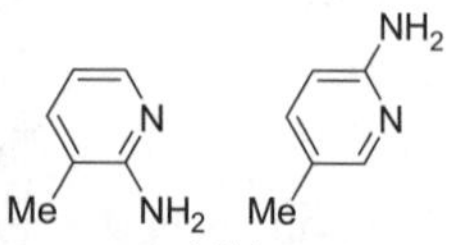 N, Me, NH_2; NH_2, N, Me; 1.7:1	83[b]
4	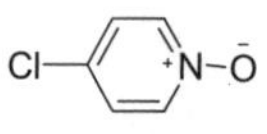 Cl, N–O	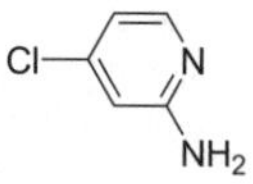 Cl, N, NH_2	71
5	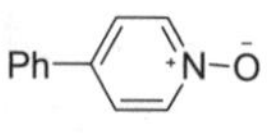 Ph, N–O	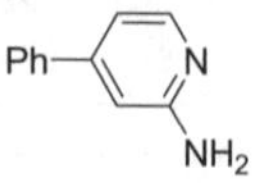 Ph, N, NH_2	92
6	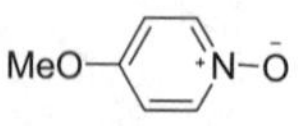 MeO, N–O	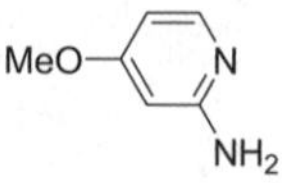 MeO, N, NH_2	90
7	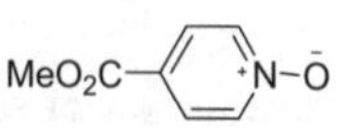 MeO_2C, N–O	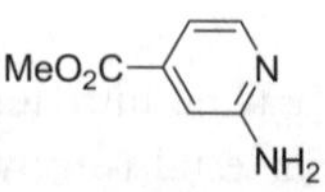 MeO_2C, N, NH_2	92
8	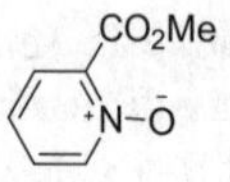 CO_2Me, N–O	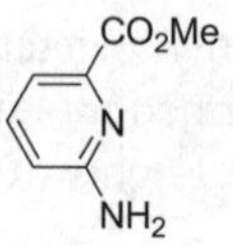 CO_2Me, N, NH_2	80

TABLE 11.2 (Continued)

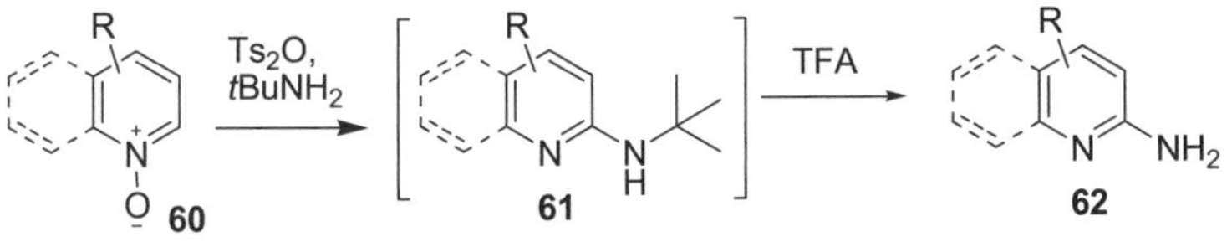

60 → (Ts_2O, tBuNH$_2$) → [61] → (TFA) → 62

Entry	*N*-Oxides	Product	Yld(%)
9	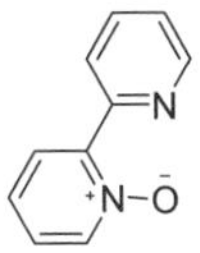	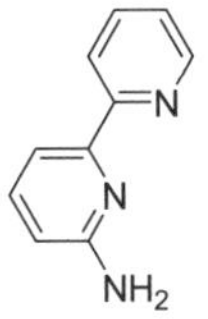 NH_2	81
10	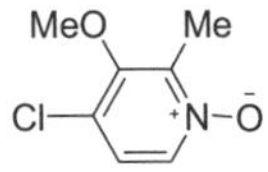 MeO, Me, Cl, N–O	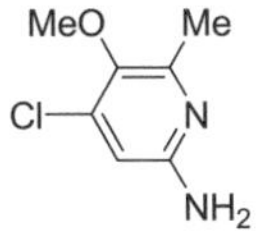 MeO, Me, Cl, N, NH_2	82
11	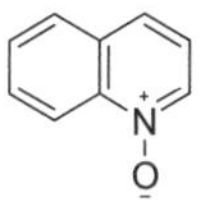	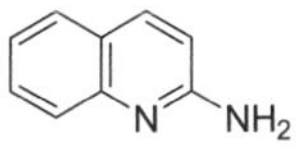 NH_2	91
12	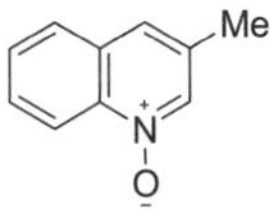 Me	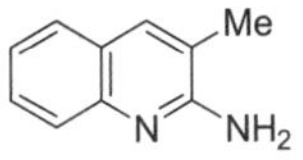 Me, NH_2	92
13	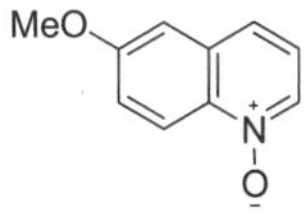 MeO	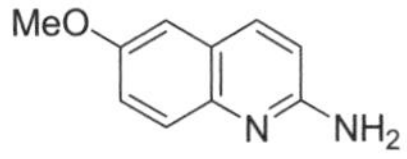 MeO, NH_2	83
14	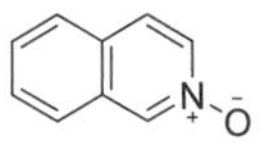	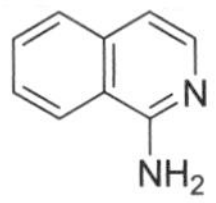 NH_2	75

tert-butylsulfonamide **58**. Compound **58** was easily removed by filtration. The crude **65** in acetonitrile was directly deprotected to remove both the THP and *tert*-butyl groups.

Initially, the global deprotection of **65** required rather harsh conditions. Treatment of **65** with 5 equiv of anhydrous TsOH and 25 equiv of TFA in MeCN at 70°C for 3 h afforded

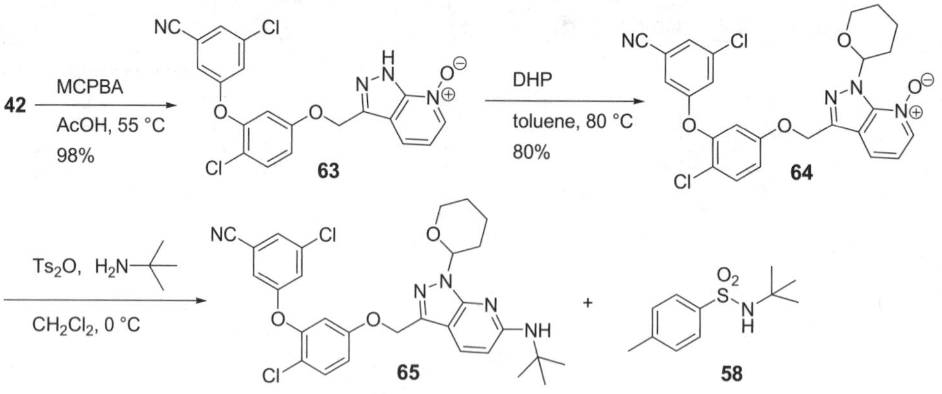

Scheme 11.9 Synthesis of **65**.

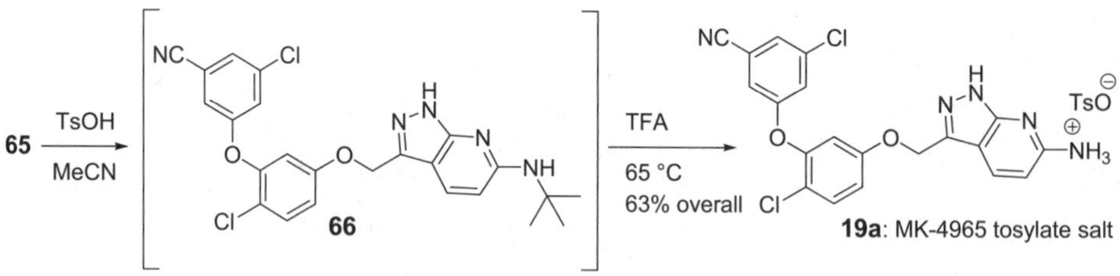

Scheme 11.10 Synthesis of MK-4965 tosylate salt (**19a**).

tosylate salt **19a**, which crystallized from the crude reaction mixture in 55–60% yield (Scheme 11.9). It is worth noting that the product **19a** appeared to be decomposing with prolonged reaction time. The cyano group of **65** was potentially hydrolyzed under the extremely acidic reaction conditions and at high temperature. Commercial TsOH is typically a monohydrate, necessitating azeotropic removal of water from the TsOH prior to the addition of **65** and TFA. After further optimization (Scheme 11.10), global deprotection of **65** was accomplished by addition of 4 equiv of dry TsOH in MeCN to a solution of **65** in MeCN, followed by the addition of 25 equiv of TFA. The reaction mixture was stirred at 65°C for 4 h to give 90% conversion and 80% HPLC yield. Prolonged reaction did not improve the conversion but decreased the assay yield. The reaction mixture was cooled to room temperature and was seeded with pure tosylate salt **19a**. A crystalline slurry was formed, water was added, and **19a** was isolated in 63% overall yield from **64**. The first-generation process for the synthesis of MK-4965 tosylate salt (**19a**), which included the preparation of **18**, required nine linear steps in 13% overall yield.

11.5.2.2 Second-Generation Process for the Synthesis of MK-4965

The first-generation route described above was suitable for generation of gram to multi-kilogram quantities of **19**. Several key problems with this route were still unsolved and had to be addressed for the long term approach:

1. The statistical bromination step provided intermediate **39** in moderate yield and still required chromatographic purification.
2. Multiple steps still required undesirable, environmentally unfriendly halogenated solvents.
3. Volume productivity was still limited in several steps.

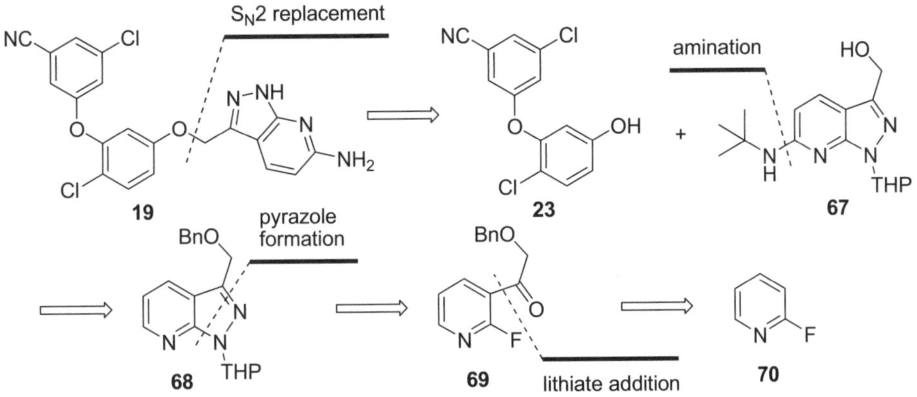

Scheme 11.11 Retrosynthetic analysis of **19**.

4. Moderate yields in a few steps.
5. Use of an undesirable oxidation process.

Retrosynthetic Analysis of Second-Generation Synthesis Our second-generation retrosynthetic approach is shown in Scheme 11.11 [37]. **19** would be derived from **23** and **67** by cleavage of the ether bond. Further disassembly of the key intermediate **67** by cleavage of the C–N bond would furnish **68**, which in turn could be prepared in two steps from 2-fluoropyridine **70** through a lithiate addition and pyrazole formation.

Construction of the Pyrazolo[3,4-b]pyridine Core We started our second-generation synthesis by developing an efficient synthesis of the pyrazololpyridine core **68**. Two common routes to access pyrazolo[3,4-b]pyridines **71** have been reported in the literature: construction of the pyridine ring from a 5-aminopyrazole **72** (Scheme 11.12 route-I) [42], or building the pyrazole ring from a 3-acetyl, 3-carboxy, or 3-cyanopyridine **73** bearing a leaving group at the 2-position (Scheme 11.12 route-II) [43]. After evaluation of these two routes for our target compound **68**, route-II was further investigated for the preparation of intermediate **68**.

Lithiation of 1.3 equiv of 2-fluoropyridine **70** with 1.3 equiv of LDA followed by addition of 1 equiv of Weinreb amide **74** at less than −50°C gave pure **75** in 61% yield after column chromatography (Scheme 11.13) [44]. Treatment of **75** with 5 equiv of 35 wt% hydrazine at 80°C in isopropanol provided the desired product **76**. Monitoring the process for the pyrazole formation showed that a mixture of the hydrazones **77*E*** and **77*Z*** was quickly formed within 1 h, while the ring closure to pyrazole **76** required 10–15 h. The use of less than 5 equiv of hydrazine resulted in incomplete conversion, likely due to the formation of azines. When the reaction was completed, pure **76** was directly crystallized in 80% isolated yield after diluting with water.

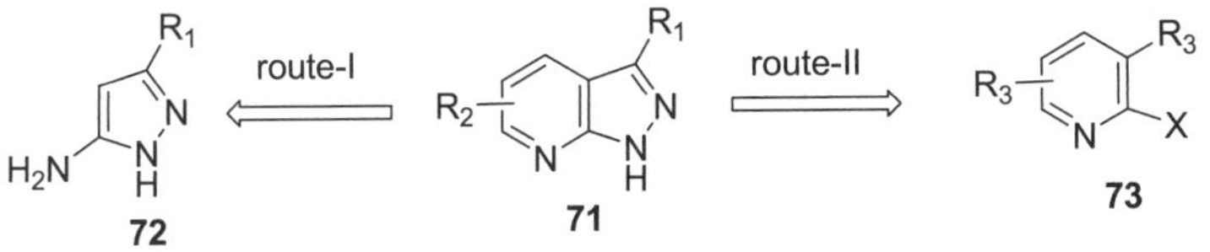

R_1 = Me, Ar, OH, NH_2
R_3 = COMe, COAr, CO_2Me, CN
X = leaving group

Scheme 11.12 Synthetic route to pyrazolo[3,4-b]pyridines **71**.

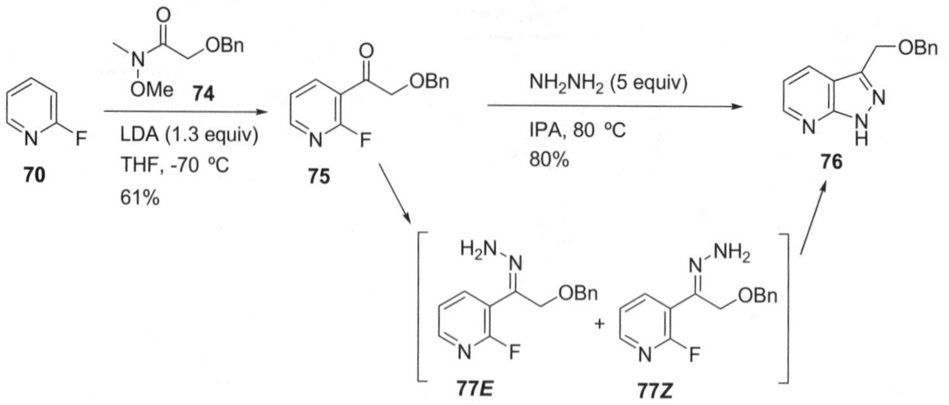

Scheme 11.13 Synthesis of the pyrazolo[3,4-b]pyridine **76**.

This method proved to be general for preparing a variety of functionalized 3-alkoxymethyl pyrazolo[3,4-b]pyridines (Table 11.3). Both the ketone formation and pyrazole formation gave good to excellent yields when X is a proton and R is methyl, 2-THP, *p*-methoxybenzyl (PMB), and *p*-methoxyphenyl (entries 1–4). Interestingly, during the cyclization of phenoxy ketone to pyrazole (entry 5), about 5% of the phenol was identified as a by-product obtained by cleavage of the ether bond. If the benzene ring of the phenoxy group was substituted with electron withdrawing groups such as 4-chloro- and 3,4-dichloro-, the corresponding by-products 4-chlorophenol and 3,4-dichlorophenol were isolated in 45% and >99% yield, respectively, while the reaction gave a very low yield of the

TABLE 11.3 Synthesis of Pyrazolo[3,4-b]pyridines

78 + 79 → (LDA (1.3 equiv), THF, -70 °C, *step-1*) → 80 → (NH_2NH_2, IPA, 80 °C, *step-2*) → 81

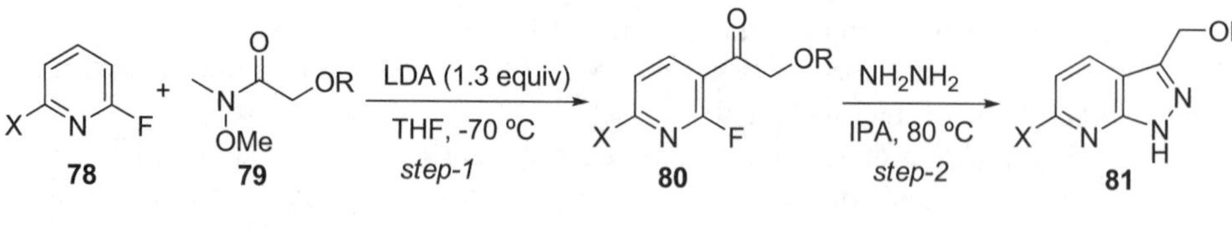

Entry	X	R	pKa(H_2O)	ROH(%)	Step-1, yield (%)	Step-2, yield (%)
1	H	Me	15.54	ND	66	90
2	H	THP	13.34	ND	65	74
3	H	PMB	14.43	ND	74	81
4	H	*p*-$MeOC_6H_4$	10.50	ND	69	91
5	H	C_6H_5	9.99	5	71	89
6	H	*p*-ClC_6H_4	9.37	45	73	48
7	H	3,4-Cl_2-C_6H_3	8.56	>99	27	0
8	Cl	Bn	–	–	73	90
9	Cl	*p*-$MeOC_6H_4$	–	–	31	97
10	Cl	C_6H_5	–	–	42	96
11	Cl	*p*-ClC_6H_4	–	–	34	81
12	Cl	3,4-Cl_2-C_6H_3	–	–	38	52

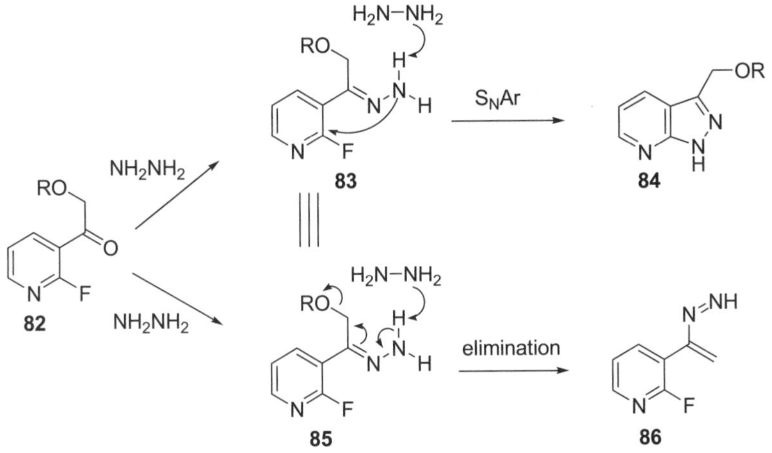

Scheme 11.14 A plausible mechanism.

desired product (48%, entry 6) or no desired product at all (entry 7). In all cases where X is chloride, no phenol formation was observed (entries 8–12).

The difference between the productive S_NAr cyclization in most cases and the phenol elimination in entries 5–7 is likely due to the electronic nature of the phenoxy groups. A plausible mechanism for these two competitive reactions is proposed in Scheme 11.14. As soon as the hydrazone intermediate **83/85** was formed, it can either proceed with the productive S_NAr cyclization by attack of the terminal hydrazone nitrogen on the pyridyl fluoride (S_NAr path) or with the elimination of the phenoxy moiety to form a vinyl azine (elimination path). In the case of entries 1–5, the S_NAr path for an alkoxy or electron rich/neutral phenoxy groups ($pK_a > 10$) is facile, and good yields of the desired pyrazoles are expected. In contrast, the elimination path is favored for more acidic phenols, such as 3,4-dichlorophenol ($pK_a = 8.56$) (entries 6–7).

Synthesis of the Key Intermediate 67 With the intermediate pyrazolo[3,4-b]pyridine **76** in hand, *N*-oxidation was accomplished by treating **76** with 1.3 equiv of MCPBA in isopropyl acetate (IPAc) at 35°C (Scheme 11.15). The resulting product **87** precipitated from the reaction mixture during the oxidation and was isolated by direct filtration of the crude reaction mixture in 82% yield. THP protection of **87**, followed by amination of the resulting compound **88** to **89,** was initially conducted in a one-pot process. Treatment of **87** with 5 equiv of DHP in the presence of a catalytic amount of pyridine *p*-toluenesulfonate (PPTS) in trifluorotoluene gave THP-protected *N*-oxide **88** in nearly quantitative yield. Direct amination of the reaction mixture of **88** under our typical conditions gave a mixture of **89** and **90** in ~6.5:1 as determined by NMR. The desired regioisomer **89** was purified by silica gel chromatography and was obtained in 65–67% yield.

The amination was further optimized in terms of the solvent, temperature, and order of addition of reagents. It was found that the amination of **88** was best performed in THF. Thus, after THP-protection in trifluorotoluene, the reaction solvent was switched to THF followed by addition of 10 equiv of *tert*-butylamine. The resulting solution was then added dropwise to a cold slurry (−10 to −15°C) of 5 equiv of Ts_2O in THF to give a 10.5:1 mixture of **89:90**. All attempts to crystallize **89** from the reaction mixture failed. Direct hydrogenation of the reaction mixture to cleave the benzyl group of **89** was unsuccessful. Further investigation of the hydrogenation reaction indicated that up to 8% residual **58** did

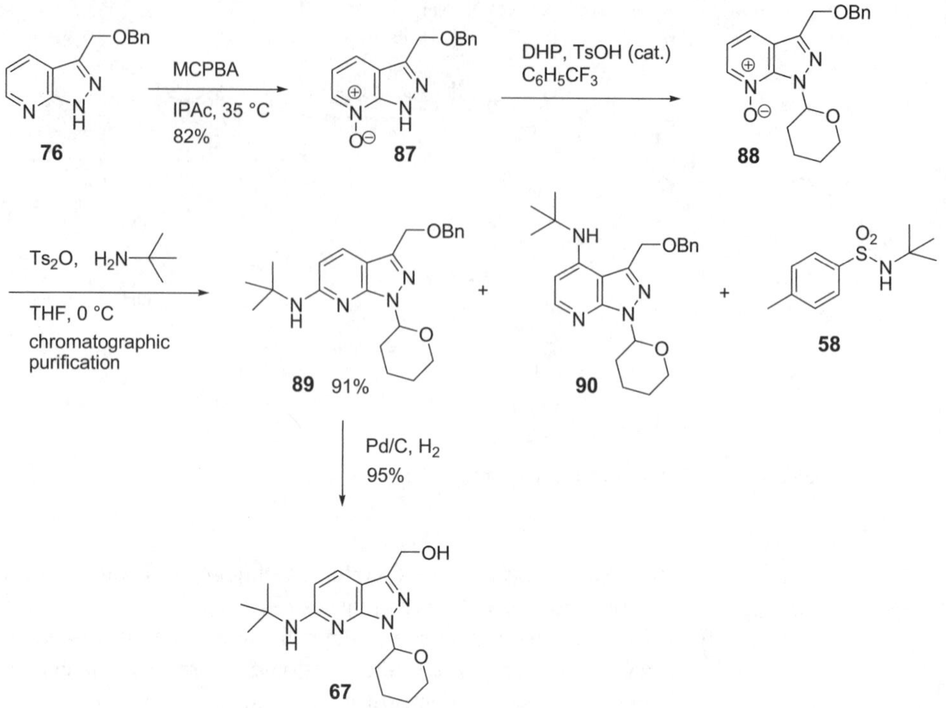

Scheme 11.15 Synthesis of the key intermediate **67**.

not affect the hydrogenation. However, a trace amount of regioisomer **90** could completely shut down the hydrogenation, likely due to **90** acting as a catalyst poison in the hydrogenation. All traces of this isomer had to be removed prior to the hydrogenation. Unfortunately, all attempts to completely remove the regioisomer **90** without recourse to chromatography were unsuccessful. Thus, the reaction mixture was purified by silica–gel chromatography to provide **89** in 91% yield. Removal of the benzyl protecting group of **89** in the presence of 5% Pd/C-afforded alcohol **67** in 95% yield. The process for the synthesis of **67** from commercial 2-fluoropyridine proceeded in six linear steps and 34% overall yield. The conversion of **67** to **19** will be discussed in detail in the section detailing third-generation synthesis.

11.5.2.3 Third-Generation Process (Manufacturing Route) for the Synthesis of MK-4965

The second-generation route for the synthesis of **19** addressed several unsolved problems from the first generation such as the statistical bromination step, use of undesirable halogenated solvents, and low volume productive steps.

However, for the development of a manufacturing route, several issues and a new safety concern were raised:

1. The regioisomer **90** was acting as a catalyst poison in the hydrogenation, and its removal still required chromatographic purification.
2. The pyrazole formation required heating excess (5 equiv) hydrazine at 80°C, which raised a safety concern on large scale.
3. Moderate yield (61%) in the Weinreb addition step.
4. The undesired oxidation process was still required.

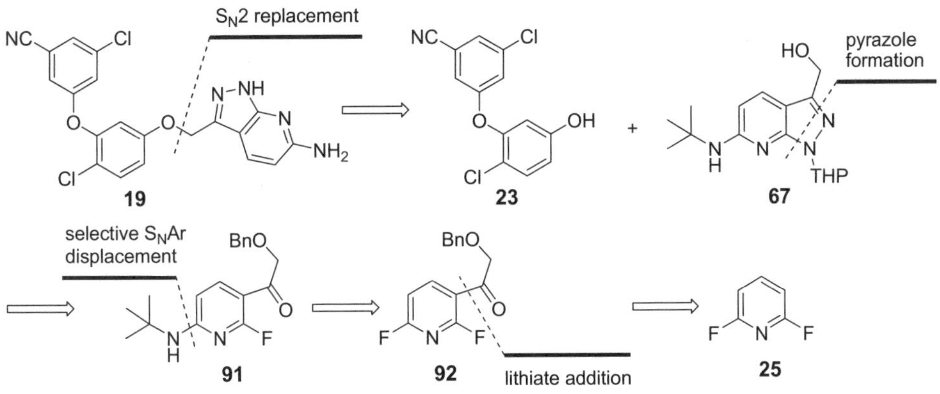

Scheme 11.16 Retrosynthetic analysis of **19**.

Retrosynthetic Analysis of the Third-Generation Synthesis Benzylic alcohol **67** was identified as the key intermediate for the second-generation synthesis of **19**. To address all the issues faced in the second-generation synthesis, our third-generation retrosynthetic approach focused on a more efficient and practical synthesis of the key intermediate **67**, which is indefinitely stable at room temperature (Scheme 11.16). Disassembly of the key intermediate **67** by cleavage the C–N and C=C bonds would furnish fragment **91**. Instead of going through the *N*-oxide chemistry for amination that created a few issues, the amino group would be introduced via an S_NAr reaction on the 6-fluoropyridine. Therefore, cleavage of the C–N bond of intermediate **91** led to the difluoroketone **92**, which in turn could be derived from 2,6-difluoropyridine **25** through a lithiate addition to a Weinreb amide.

Methodology Development for the Construction of 6-Aminopyrazolo [3,4-b]pyridine Core To date only a few methods for the synthesis of 3,6-disubstituted-1*H*-pyrazolo[3,4-b]pyridines have been reported. However, the known syntheses required harsh conditions and a 4-step sequence starting from 2,6-difluoropyridine in a very low overall yield [45]. We proposed that the desired compounds **94** could be assembled in a one-pot protocol from 2,6-difluoro-3-ketopyridines **93** via a selective double S_NAr reaction followed by pyrazole formation (Scheme 11.17) [46].

The new approach began with the generation of lithiated 2,6-difluoropyridine **25** followed by addition of Weinreb amides to give a variety of 2,6-difluoro-3-ketopyridines **93** (Table 11.4). Medicinal chemistry efforts showed that 2,6-difluoro-3-methylketopyridine **26** could be prepared in 25% yield via LDA-mediated lithiation of 2,6-difluoropyridine **25** followed by Weinreb amide addition [32,33]. *Ortho* lithiation of 2-fluoropyridine and 2,6-difluoropyridine using stronger bases such as *n*-BuLi is well known to be complicated by the addition of the base to the pyridine ring, even at very low temperatures. However, given the cost benefit and convenience of using *n*-BuLi alone, it was worth reexamining the deprotonation of 2,6-difluoropyridine with *n*-BuLi. To our delight,

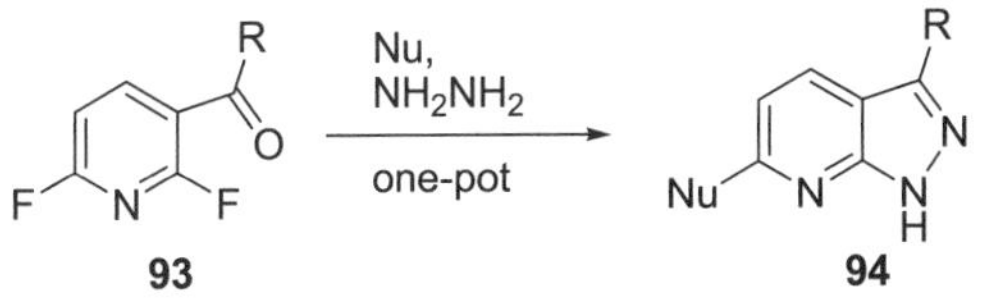

Scheme 11.17 Proposed one-pot synthesis of **94**.

TABLE 11.4 Synthesis of 2,6-Difluoropyridine Ketones

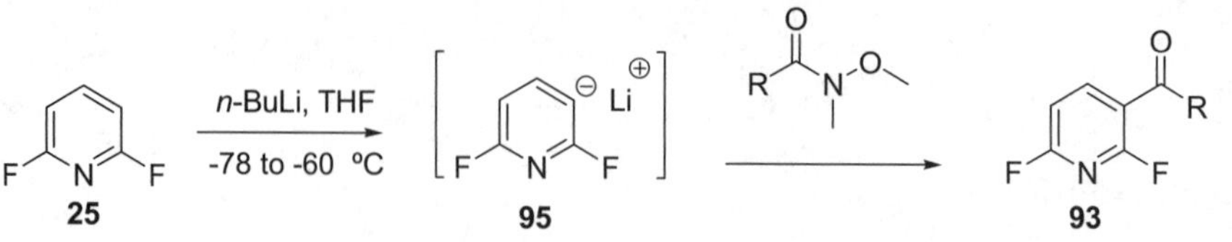

25 → (n-BuLi, THF, -78 to -60 °C) → [95] → 93

Entries	Substrates	Products	Isolated yields(%)
1	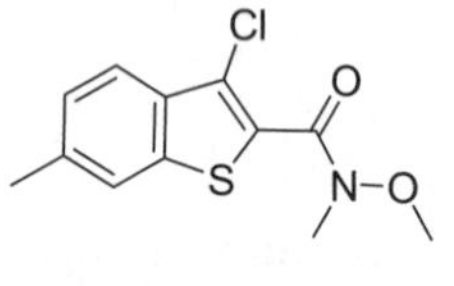	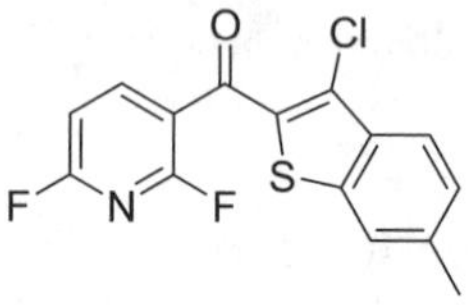	95
2	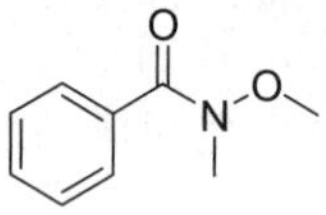	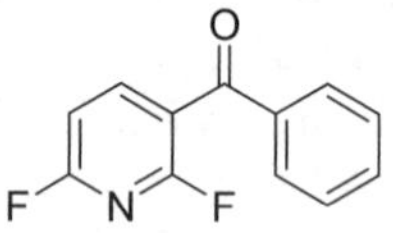	93
3	R = Br	R = Br	92
4	R = OMe	R = OMe	97
5	R = NO_2	R = NO_2	96
6	R = Br	R = Br	98
7	R = OMe	R = OMe	92
8	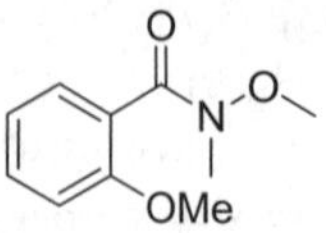	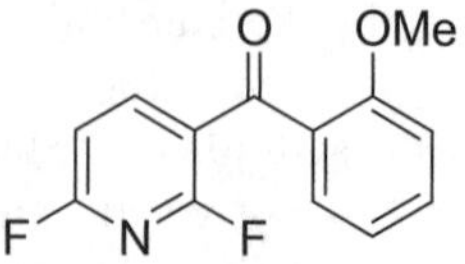	93
9	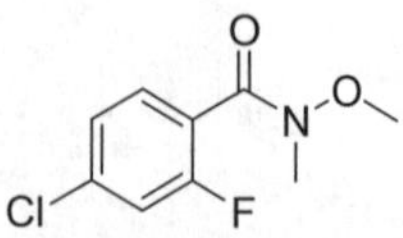	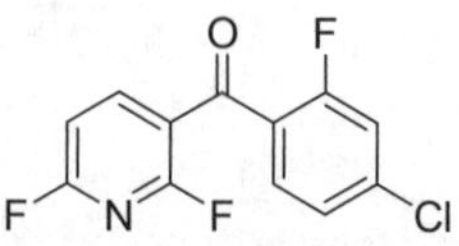	70

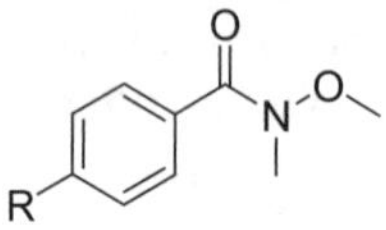

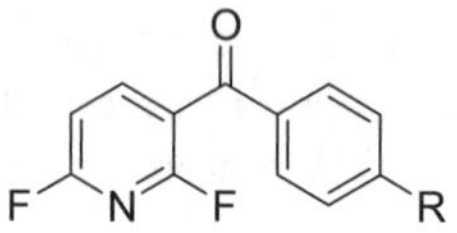

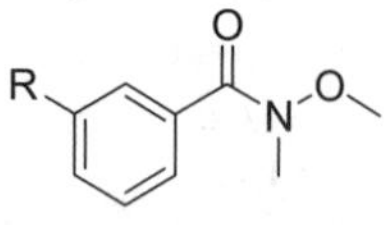

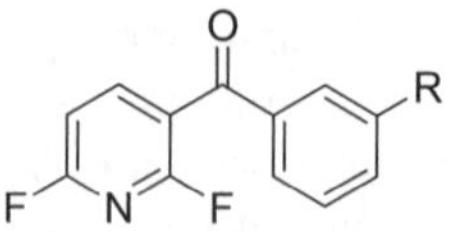

TABLE 11.4 *(Continued)*

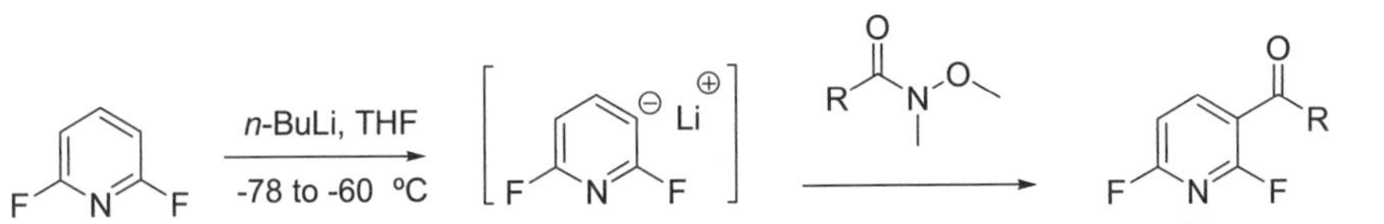

Entries	Substrates	Products	Isolated yields(%)
10	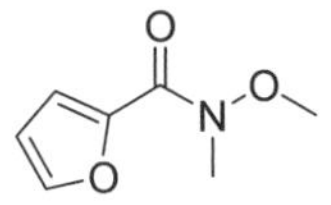	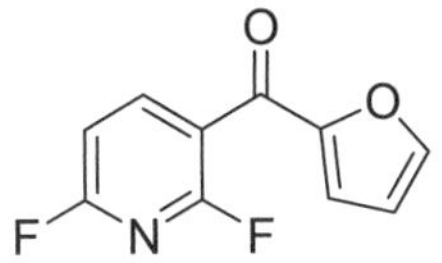	83
11	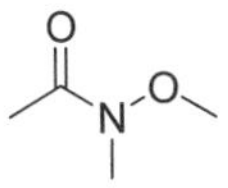	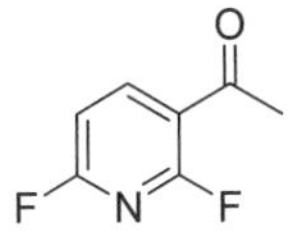	50

lithiation of **25** by slowly addition of 1.1 equiv of 1.6 M *n*-BuLi in hexane at less than −60°C, followed by addition of a precooled (−55°C) solution of a variety of Weinreb amides gave the desired product 2,6-difluoro-3-benzoyl-pyridines in good to excellent yield (Table 11.4, entries 1–11).

With the desired 2,6-difluoro-3-keto-pyridines in hand, a one-pot synthesis of 3,6-substituted-1*H*-pyrazolo[3,4-b]pyridines was investigated. Selective replacement of the 6-fluoride with nucleophiles, such as *tert*-butylamine, followed by displacement of the 2-fluoride by hydrazine and closure of the pyrazole ring would lead to the desired 3,6-disubstituted-1*H*-pyrazolo[3,4-b]pyridines. Initial studies began with selective S_NAr substitution of the 6-fluorine of compound **93** with *tert*-butylamine. It was found that treatment of the ketone with *tert*-butylamine in *N,N*-dimethylacetamide (DMA) at 0–5°C afforded a clean reaction, but as a mixture of 6-*tert*-butylamino-2-fluoro-3-pyridine and 2-*tert*-butylamino-6-fluoro-pyridine in a 4:1 ratio (Table 11.5, entry 1). Running the reaction in aprotic solvents, such as DMF, NMP, and DMSO, provided a similar outcome. However, the reaction gave a reversal of selectivity in EtOAc, MTBE, and THF. A highly selective formation of the undesired 2-*tert*-butylamino-6-fluoro-pyridine was found in toluene (6-*t*BuNH:2-*t*BuNH = 1:16.7). Solvent effects observed for the S_NAr displacement can be explained based on hydrogen bonding effects. A lower ratio of desired product/undesired product was observed at higher temperatures as well.

After the 2,6-difluoroketones were fully converted into the *tert*-butylamino-monofluoroketone, hydrazine monohydrate was slowly added to the reaction mixture at 0–5°C, and the reaction was warmed to room temperature to afford 6-*tert*-butylamino-3-aryl-1*H*-pyrazolo[3,4-b]pyridines **96** in 51–84% overall yield as an one-pot protocol starting from ketones **93** (Table 11.5).

TABLE 11.5 One-Pot Synthesis of 6-Aminopyrazolo[3,4-b]pyridines 96

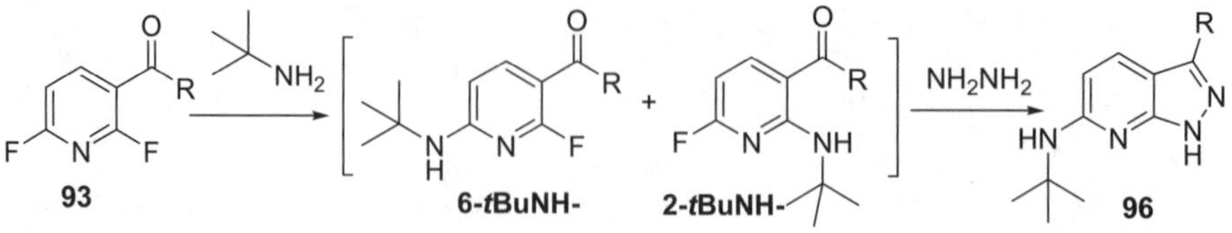

93 → (t-BuNH$_2$) → [6-*t*BuNH- + 2-*t*BuNH-] → (NH_2NH_2) → 96

Entries	Substrates	6-/2-*t*BuNH-ratio	Products	Isolated yields(%)
1	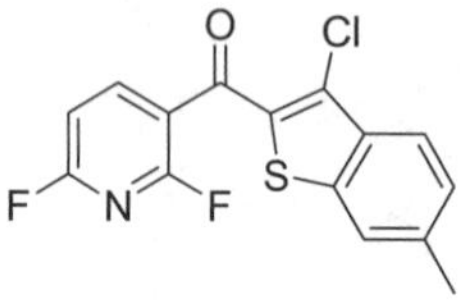	4.0:1	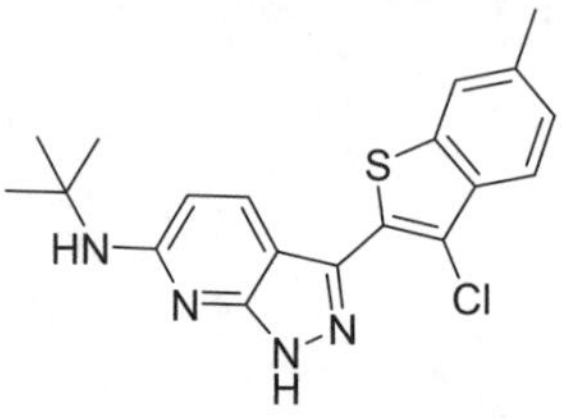	77
2	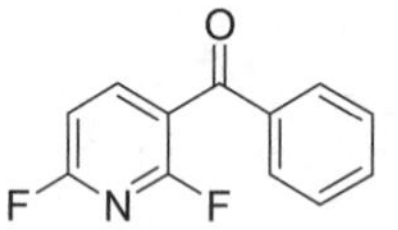	2.0:1	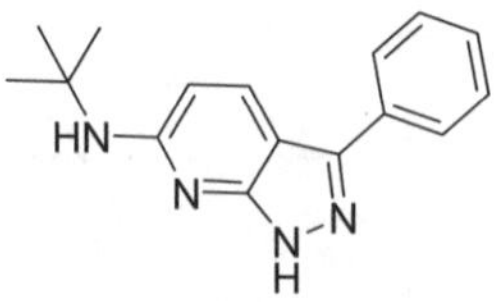	67
3	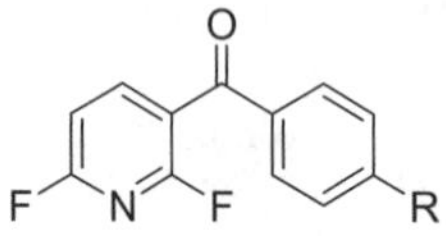 R = Br	2.3:1	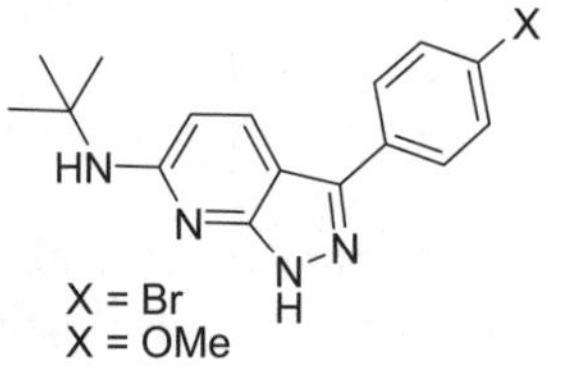 X = Br	70
4	R = OMe	1.1:1	X = OMe	51
5	R = NO_2	4.1:1	X = NO_2	80
6	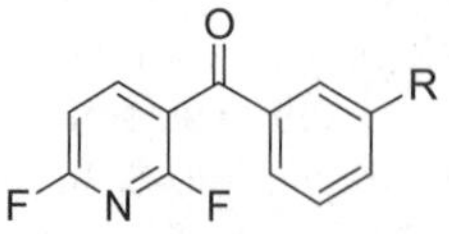 R = Br	2.9:1	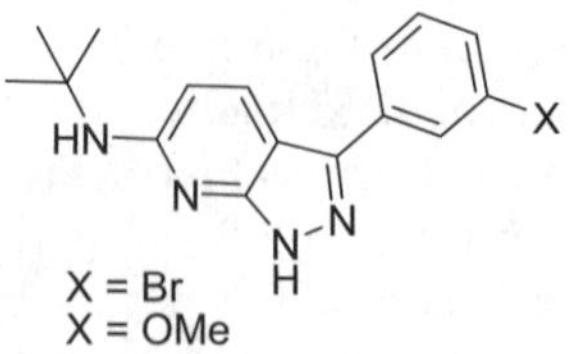 X = Br	73
7	R = OMe	2.0:1	X = OMe	61
8	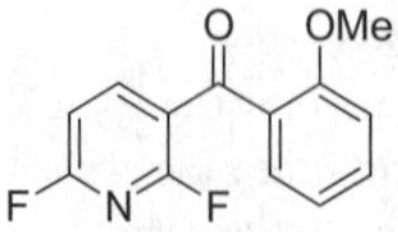	3.2:1	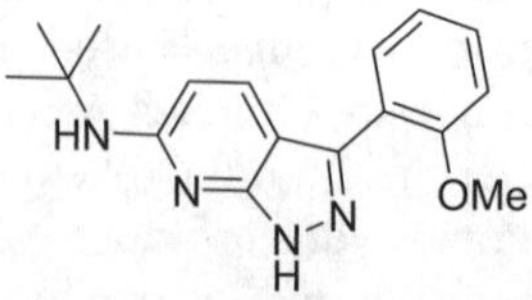	75

TABLE 11.5 (Continued)

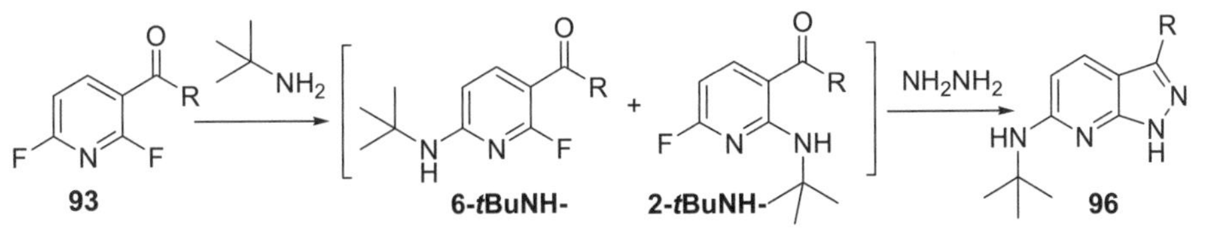

Entries	Substrates	6-/2-*t*BuNH-ratio	Products	Isolated yields(%)
9	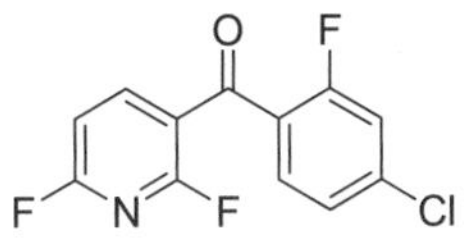	5.3:1	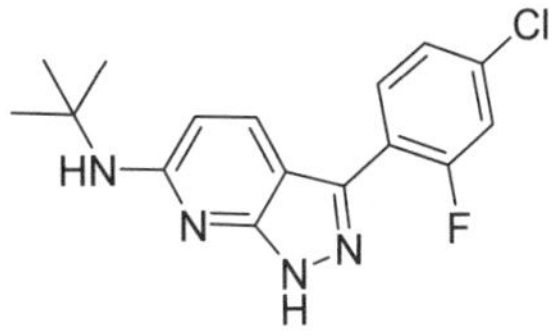	84
10	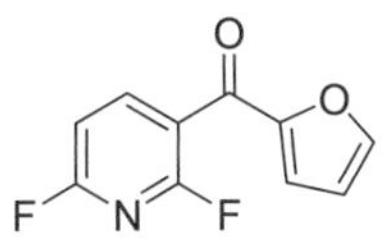	2.0:1	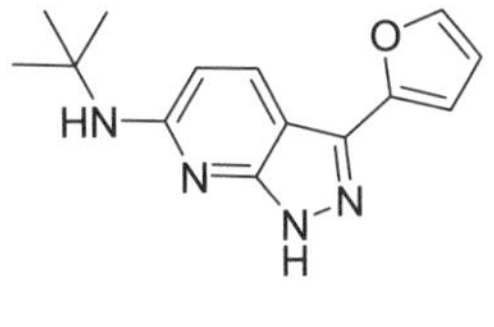	65
11	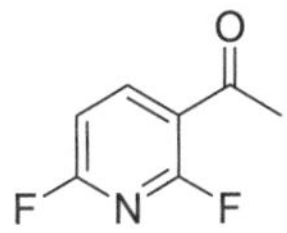	8.6:1	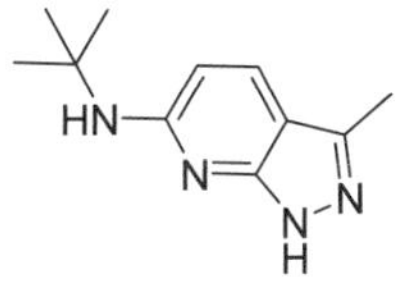	69

The use of other nucleophiles for the selective substitution of the 6-fluorine of 2,6-difluoro-3-substitutedaryl-pyridines **97**, followed by hydrazine substitution of the 2-fluorine and pyrazole formation was also investigated. Reaction of ketone **97** with *tert*-butyl thiol (entry 1), a secondary amine (entry 2), an aniline (entry 3), phenol (entry 4), or amino acids (entries 5, 6) proceeded smoothly and proved efficiently generating the corresponding pyrazoles **98** in moderate-to-excellent yields (Table 11.6).

Process Development for the Synthesis of Key Intermediate 67 and Phenol 23 Employing the new protocol for the construction of 6-amino-pyrazolo [3,4-b]pyridines described above, the third-generation synthesis of **19** started from the lithiation of 2,6-difluoropyridine **25** (Scheme 11.18) [37] followed by addition of Weinreb amide **74**. An aqueous workup gave crude ketone **92** in 81% HPLC assay yield. Although ketone **92** could be isolated in analytically pure white crystals by crystallization from EtOAc/heptane, it was found that purification of this intermediate was unnecessary. A one-pot process for conversion of crude **92** to pyrazole **101** was developed where the presence of impurities **25**, **99**, and other small impurities was found to be inconsequential to the reaction outcome. Treatment of crude **92** with 5 equiv of *tert*-butylamine in NMP at 0–5°C afforded a

TABLE 11.6 A One-Pot Synthesis of 6-Substituted-Pyrazolo[3,4-b]pyridines 98

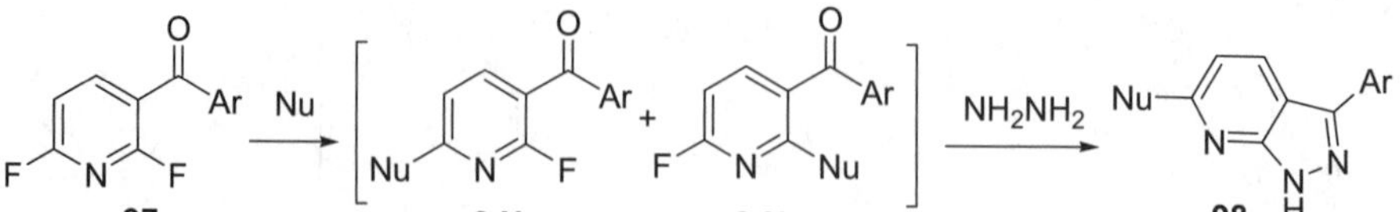

97 (Ar = 4-bromo-phenyl) → Nu → [6-Nu- + 2-Nu-] → NH_2NH_2 → 98

Entries	Nu	**6-Nu-/2-Nu**-ratio	Products	Isolated yields(%)
1	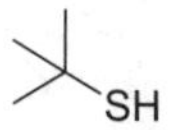 t-BuSH	19:1	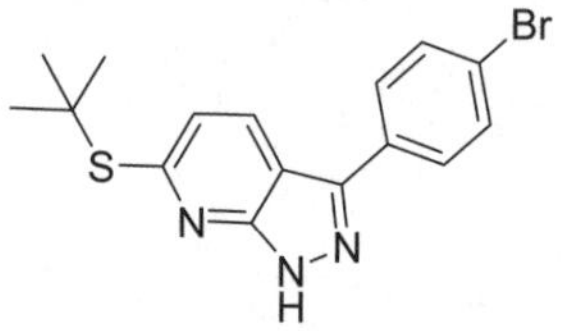	91
2	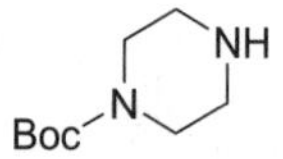 Boc-piperazine	3.2:1	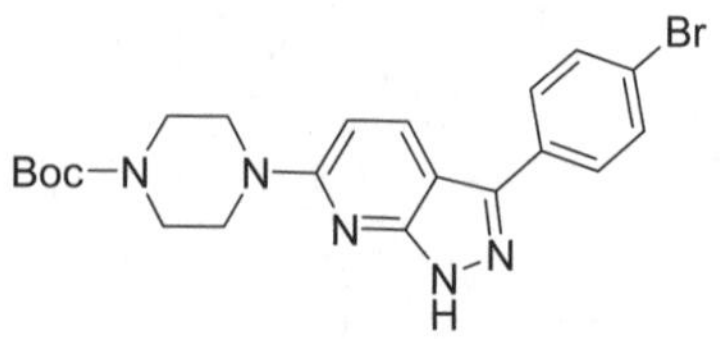	75
3	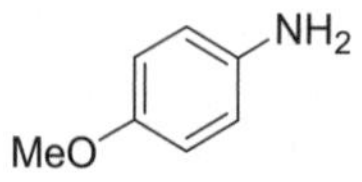 4-MeO-aniline	1.5:1	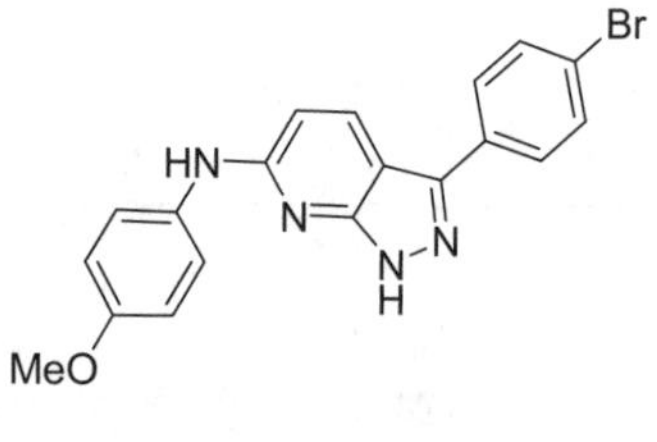	59
4	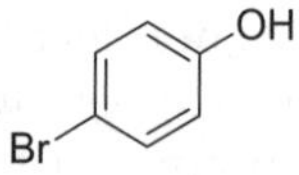 4-Br-phenol	20:1	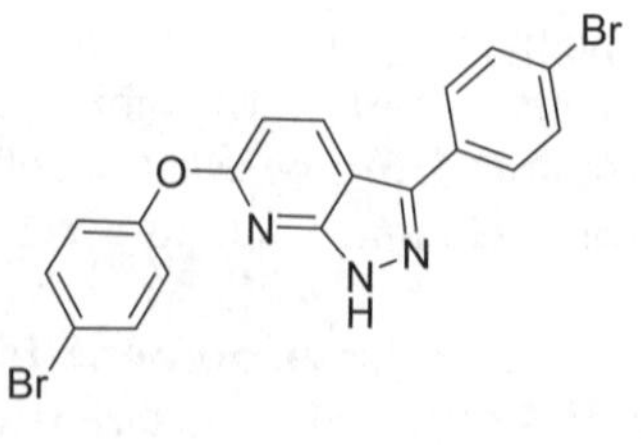	84
5	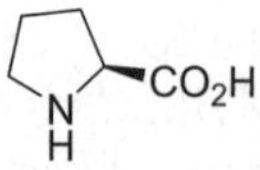 L-proline	1.2:1	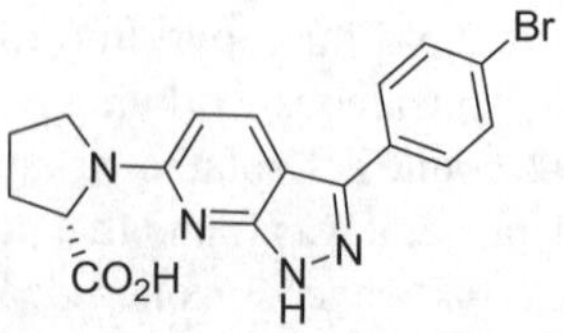	43

TABLE 11.6 ***(Continued)***

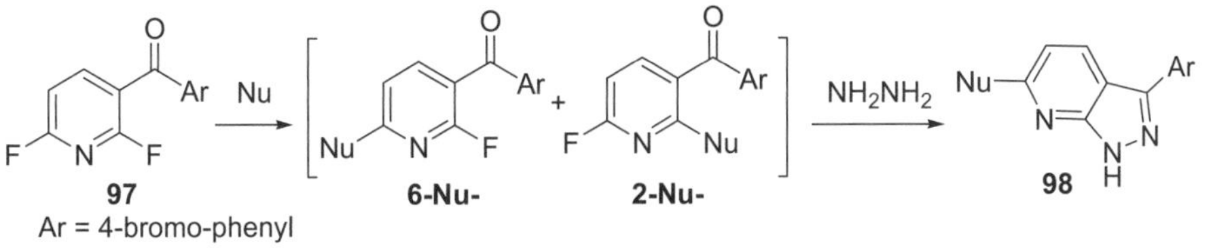

97 Ar = 4-bromo-phenyl; 6-Nu-; 2-Nu-; NH_2NH_2; 98

Entries	Nu	**6-Nu-/2-Nu**-ratio	Products	Isolated yields(%)
6	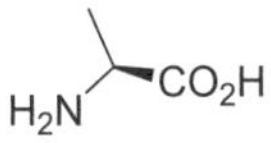	1.7:1	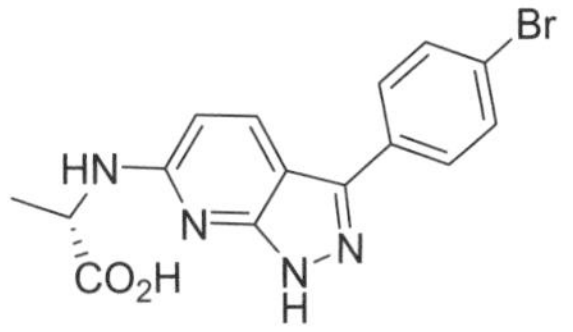	55

10:1 mixture of the desired addition product **91** and the undesired regioisomer **100**. After complete consumption of **92**, 5 equiv of 64 wt% or 35 wt% of an aqueous solution of hydrazine was added to the reaction mixture, and the reaction was stirred at room temperature until complete conversion of **91** to pyrazole **101** was observed. The pH of the reaction mixture was adjusted to 5 with 5 N sulfuric acid and **101** was extracted into MTBE. The solvent was then switched to toluene, providing pyrazole **101** in 81% HPLC

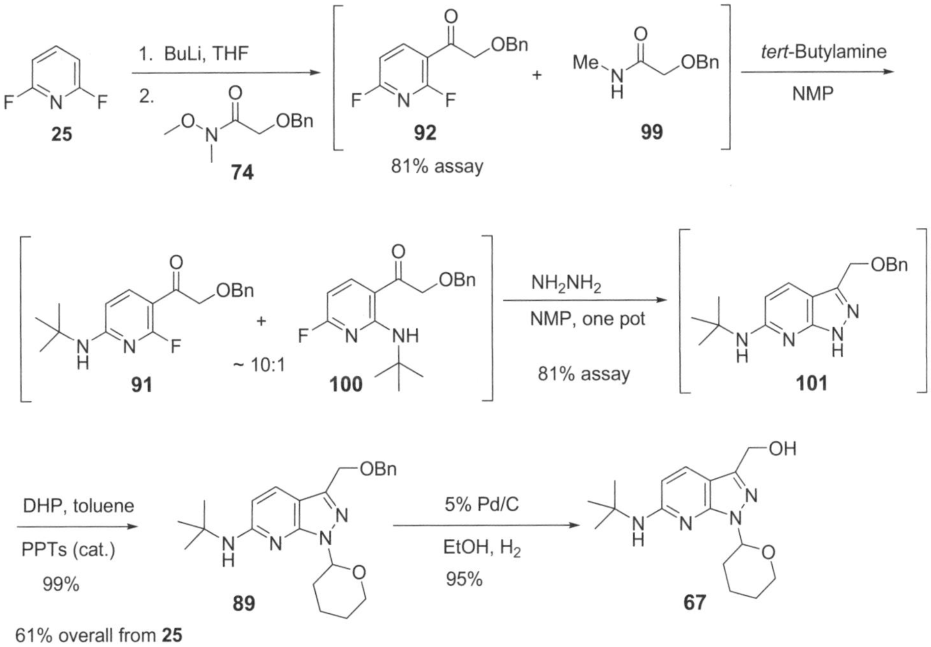

Scheme 11.18 Synthesis of key intermediate **67**.

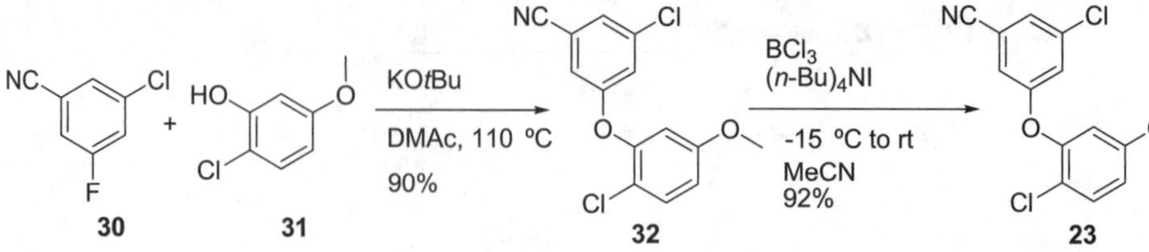

Scheme 11.19 Optimization for the synthesis of phenol **23**.

yield from **92**. The material was used in the next reaction without further purification. The solution was treated with 5 equiv of DHP and 5 mol% of PPTS to give nearly quantitative conversion to THP-pyrazole **89**, which was isolated from cyclohexane as an off-white crystalline solid in 61% overall yield from difluoropyridine **25**. Hydrogenation of **89** in the presence of 5 mol% of Pd/C in EtOH at 20 psi of H_2 provided **67** in quantitative yield. Compound **67** was isolated as a white crystalline solid from EtOH/water in 95% yield and an overall yield of 58% from 2,6-difluoropyridine **25**.

The synthesis of phenol **23** was the next reaction that required optimization (Scheme 11.19) [47]. Displacement of the fluoride **30** with phenol **31** was investigated through screening different bases (Cs_2CO_3, K_2CO_3, KF, KO*t*Bu, NaO*t*Bu, K_3PO_4, and DBU), solvents (NMP, DMF, DMA, and toluene), and different temperatures. It was found that treatment of **30** with **31** in DMA in the presence of KO*t*Bu at 110°C gave biaryl ether **32** in 90% isolated yield. The original conditions for the removal of the methyl protecting group required 1.25 equiv of expensive boron tribromide and a halogenated solvent, dichloromethane. After optimization, we found that a combination of 3 equiv of inexpensive boron trichloride and 1.1 equiv of $(n\text{-}Bu)_4NI$ can replace boron tribromide for the demethylation. When the reaction was complete, a solvent switch from acetonitrile to IPA followed by addition of water gave crystalline **23** in 92% isolated yield.

Synthesis of Protected MK-4965 (65) With the alcohol **67** and phenol **23** in hand, the conversion of **67** to intermediate **65** was extensively optimized. Activation of alcohol **67** with 1.05 equiv of MsCl in 2-MeTHF in the presence of 1.10 equiv of Hünig's base at 0–8°C (Scheme 11.20) provided mesylate **102** as the major product with chloride

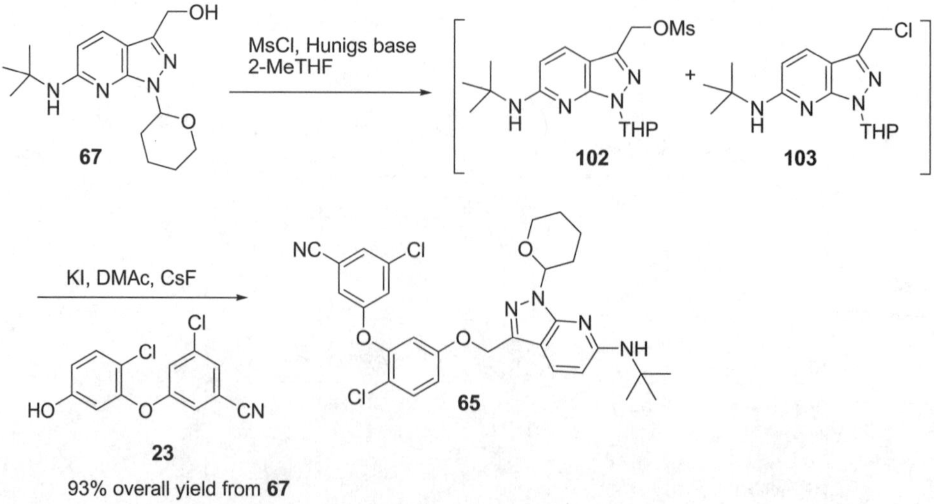

Scheme 11.20 Synthesis of protected MK-4965 (**65**) via mesylate (**102**).

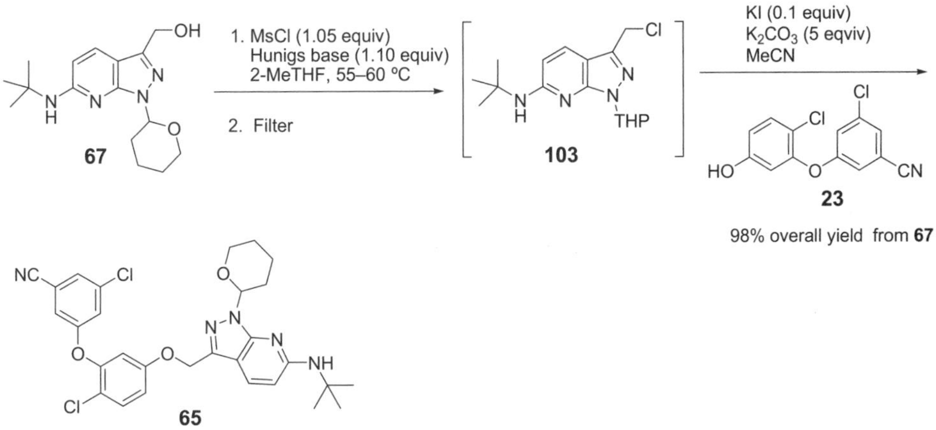

Scheme 11.21 Synthesis of protected MK-4965 (**65**) via chloride (**103**).

103 as a minor by-product (3–5%). When the reaction mixture was allowed to warm up to room temperature, the chloride **103** increased to 20–25%. Because mesylate **102** was sensitive to moisture and readily hydrolyzed back to alcohol **67** when exposed to water, an aqueous workup was avoided and the crude reaction mixture was instead filtered to remove the precipitated ammonium salts. The crude mesylate in 2-MeTHF was concentrated and redissolved in DMA, and the solution was treated with 1.7 equiv of KI, 0.93 equiv of phenol **23**, and 5 equiv of CsF. The mixture was stirred at room temperature for 12 h to give **65** in 93% HPLC assay yield.

Although the conditions shown in Scheme 11.20 were successfully used for the preparation of **65**, the unstable mesylate **102** was a concern for the large-scale process. In order to obtain a more robust process, further optimization was required. Because chloride **103** is a relatively stable intermediate, it is ideal to completely form **103** prior to reaction with phenol **23** (Scheme 11.21). Thus, chloride **103** was obtained in quantitative yield by reaction of **102** with 1.05 equiv of MsCl in the presence of 1.10 equiv of Hunig's base in 2-MeTHF at room temperature followed by heating the reaction mixture at 55–60°C for 3–3.5 h. After screening solvents, bases, temperatures, and amounts of KI using the crude **103** in 2-MeTHF solution, the optimal alkylation conditions were found to be 1 equiv of chloride **103** reacting with 1 equiv of phenol **23**, 5 equiv of K_2CO_3, and 0.1 equiv of KI in MeCN at 55–60°C. The reaction was complete in 7–8 h and gave **65** in 98% HPLC yield after aqueous workup. Compound **65** was used in the final deprotection without further purification.

End Game of the Third-Generation Synthesis for the Synthesis of MK-4965 Salt (19b) and MK-4965 Free Base (19) As mentioned above in the first-generation synthesis, the global deprotection of **65** involved addition of 4 equiv of dry TsOH and 25 equiv of TFA to provide MK-4965 salt (**19a**) in 63% overall yield. Further optimization of the global deprotection of **65** was carried out using high-throughput experiments (HTE) and design of experiments (DOE) [48]. Screening results found that it could be achieved in a one-pot procedure employing sulfuric acid in MeCN at 70°C instead of the original combination of TsOH and TFA. However, the HPLC assay yields of **17** remained <70%. Careful analysis of the reaction found that the by-products of the THP cleavage were the cause of the low yields for the global deprotection. To overcome the problem, we employed 1-octanethiol as a scavenging reagent to trap the THP

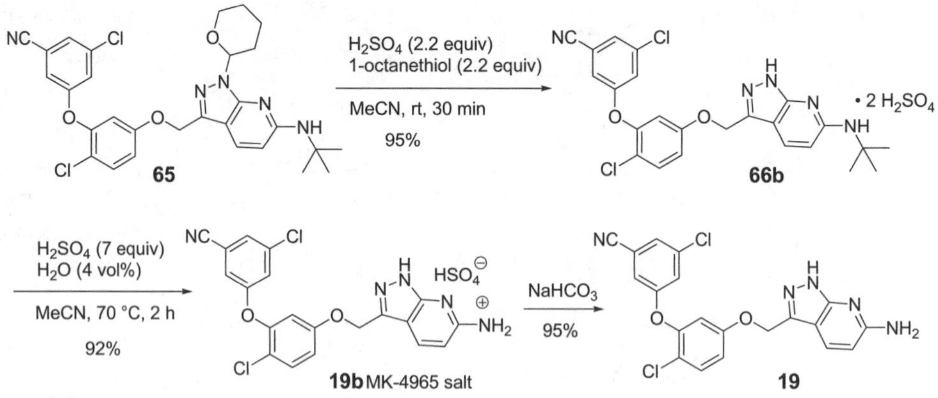

Scheme 11.22 Synthesis of MK-4965 salt (**19b**) and MK-4965 free base (**19**).

by-products associated with THP removal after treatment of **65** at room temperature with 2.2 equiv of conc. sulfuric acid in MeCN. The des-THP intermediate **66b** crystallized from the reaction mixture as the bis-sulfate salt in 95% isolated yield. The *tert*-butyl group of **66b** was removed by treatment with 7 equiv of concentrated sulfuric acid in MeCN in the presence of 4 vol% of water at 70°C for 2 h, and the sulfate salt **19b** crystallized from the reaction mixture in 92% isolated yield. The crystalline-free base of **19** was obtained in >95% yield by neutralization of **19b** with $NaHCO_3$ in EtOAc at 50°C and subsequent crystallization from EtOH. The third-generation process for the chromatography-free synthesis of MK-4965 (**19**) was accomplished in nine linear steps and 47% overall yield (Scheme 11.22) [37].

11.6 CONCLUSION

11.6.1 Lessons Learned from the Medicinal Chemistry Effort of MK-4965 Discovery

The Merck series of diaryl ethers has clearly demonstrated that a combination of traditional medicinal chemistry/SAR analysis and structural (crystallography and molecular modeling) information can be used to enhance the WT and mutant potency profiles of NNRTIs. A systematic approach to modifying first the diaryl region of the molecules, followed by replacement of the difficult amide bond with heterocycles that enhanced potency and physical property enabled rapid progress from early leads to clinical compounds. An interdisciplinary design philosophy utilizing information from potency and pharmacokinetic/metabolism assays to simultaneously optimize key properties also contributed to the rapid progress observed in this series. The interdisciplinary nature of this effort cannot be emphasized enough, as all structural information, biological data, physical property data, and pharmacokinetic data combined to drive the next round of target design and synthesis. This series of compounds clearly demonstrates the multi-dimensional complexity of modern medicinal chemistry and drug design, and the critical importance of experienced teams of scientists with broad expertise working closely together to rapidly solve difficult drug development challenges. The entire program at Merck moved from screening lead, through multiple generations of design and synthesis of novel structures, to clinical development within a period of less than 2 years. This rapid success was driven largely by an interdisciplinary and highly cooperative team-based approach of optimizing multiple compound variables in a simultaneous manner, making optimal use of all available data, and applying that data directly to new compound design and synthesis.

11.6.2 Summary and Lessons Learned from the Process Development of MK-4965

A number of literations of the process development were carried out at various stages of the program depending on the API needs and timeline. Very early on when time pressure was high and the des-NH_2 compound **18** was available on large scale, we quickly developed a fit-for-purpose synthesis to install the amino group based on concurrent discovery of a general and efficient method for 2-amination of pyridines [41]. As the API needs became more significant, we continued to optimize the first-generation synthesis and address the key nonselective bromination issue by developing an expedient synthesis of 3-alkoxymethyl- and 3-aminomethyl-pyrazolo[3,4-b]pyridines [44]. In order to develop a manufacturing route, we avoided the oxidation process for the amination of the pyridine by installing the 2-amino group from the start via the selective *t*-butylamine addition to 2,6-difluoro-3-acylpyridines followed by efficient pyrazole ring formation [46]. Largely because of our development of these new methods, we were able to develop an efficient manufacturing route for the synthesis of the potent nonnucleoside RT inhibitor **19** in nine linear steps and 47% overall yield from 2,6-difluoropyridine **25**, which has been used successfully to prepare large quantities of **19**.

Process chemistry development plays a key role in drug development by providing large amounts of bulk drug in a timely manner. This is a complex and challenging process, and extensive creative thinking and problem solving skills are involved to generate a practical, efficient, and economical process for a drug candidate. This not only provides API to support further clinical studies, but also leads to the discovery of new synthetic methodologies impacting future science.

ACKNOWLEDGMENTS

The authors thank all the MK-4965 and HIV-associated team members at Merck as well as all collaborators.

REFERENCES

1. Tarby, C.M. Recent advances in the development of next generation non-nucleoside reverse transcriptase inhibitors. *Curr. Topics. Med. Chem.* **2004**, *4*, 1045–1057.
2. (a) Reviews of Efavirenz: Adkins, J.C. and Noble, S. *Efavirenz. Drugs.* **1998**, *56*(6),1055–1064; (b) Moyle, G.J. Efavirenz: shifting the HAART paradigm in adult HIV infection. *Expert Opin. Invest. Drugs.* **1999**, *8* (4),473–486.
3. Reviews of Nevirapine: (a) Mirochnick, M., Clarke, D.F., and Dorenbaum, A. Nevirapine. *Clin. Pharmacokinet.* **2000**, *39*, 281–293.
4. Reviews of Delavirdine: Scott, L.J. and Perry, C.M. Delavirdine: a review of its use in HIV infection. *Drugs.* **2000**, *60*(6),1411–1444.
5. Domaoal, R.A. and Demeter, L.M. Structure and biochemical effects of HIV mutants resistant to NNRTIs. *Int. J. Biochem. Cell Bio.* **2004**, *36*, 1735–1751.
6. Ren, J.S., Esnouf, R., Garman, E., Somers, D., Ross, C., Kirby, I., Keeling, J., Darby, G., Jones, Y., Stuart, D., and Stammers, D. High resolution structure of HIV-1 RT: insights from four RT-inhibitor complexes. *Nature Struct. Biol.* **1995**, *2*, 293–302.
7. Balzarini, J. and DeClerq, E. Analysis of inhibition of retroviral reverse transcriptase. *Meth. Enzymol.* **1996**, *275*, 472–502.
8. D'Aquila, R.T., Schapiro, J.M., Brun-Vezinet, F., Clotet, B., Conway, B., Demeter, L.M., Grant, R. M., Johnson, V.A., Kuritzkes, D.R., Loveday, C.,

SHAFER, R.W., and RICHMAN, D.D. Drug resistance mutations in HIV-1. *Top HIV Med.* **2003**, *11*(3),92–96.

9. REN, J.S., MILTON, J., WEAVER, K.L., SHORT, S.A., STUART, D.I., and STAMMERS, D.K. Structural basis for the resiliance of Efavirenz to mutations in HIV-1 RT. *Structure.* **2000**, *8*, 1089–1094.
10. ESNOUF, R., REN, J., ROSS, C., JONES, Y., STAMMERS, D., and STUART, D. Mechanism of inhibition of HIV-1 reverse transcriptase by non-nucleoside inhibitors. *Nature Struct. Biol.* **1995**, *2*, 303–308.
11. ADAMS, J., PATEL, N., MANKARYOUS, N., TADROS, M., and MILLER, C.D. Nonnucleoside reverse transcriptase inhibitor resistance and the role of second generation agents. *Ann. Pharmacother.* **2010**, *44*, 157–165.
12. DICKINSON, L., KHOO, S., and BACK, D. Pharmacokinetics and drug–drug interactions of antiretrovirals: an update. *Antiviral Res.* **2010**, *44*, 176–189.
13. HUGHES, C.A., ROBINSON, L., TSENG, A., and MACARTHUR, R.D. New antiretroviral drugs: a review of the efficacy, safety, pharmacokinetics, and resistance profile of tipranavir, darunavir, etravirine, rilpivirine, mavarivoc, and raltegravir. *Expert Opin. Pharmacother.* **2009**, *10*(15),2445–2466.
14. FRENKEL, Y.V., GALLICCHIO, E., DAS, K., LEVY, R.M., and ARNOLD, E. Molecular dynamics study of non-nucleoside reverse transcriptase inhibitor Rilpivirine (TMC278) aggregates: correlation between amphiphilic properties of the drug and oral bioavailability. *J. Med. Chem.* **2009**, *52*, 5986–5905.
15. FUJIWARA, T., SATO, A., EL-FARRASH, M., MIKI, S., ABE, K., ISAKA, I., KODAMA, M., WU, Y., CHEM, L.B., HARADA, H., SUGIMOTO, H., HATANAKA, M., and HINUMO, Y. S-1153 inhibits replication of known drug-resistat strains of HIV-1. *Antimicrob. Agents Chemother.* **1998**, *42* (6),1340–1345.
16. REN, J., NICHOLS, C., BIRD, L.E., FUJIWARA, T., SUGIMOTO, H., STUART, D.I., and STAMMERS, D.K. Binding of the second generation NNRTI S-1153 to HIV-1 RT involves extensive main chain hydrogen bonding. *J. Biol. Chem.* **2000**, *275*, 14316–14320.
17. GEWURZ, B.E., JACOBS, M., PROPER, J.A., DAHL, T.A., FUJIWARA, T., and BEZUBE, B.J. Capravirine, an NNRTI in patients infected with HIV-1: a phase 1 study. *Int. Conf. Retroviruses Opp. Infect.* **2000**, *7*, *Abst.* 669.
18. BU, H.Z., POOL, W.F., WU, E., RABER, S.R., AMANTES, M.A., and SHETTY, B.V. Metabolism and excretion of Capravirine, a new NNRTI, alone and in combination with Ritonavir in healthy volunteers. *Drug Metab. Dispos.* **2004**, *32*(7),689–698.
19. PESANO, R., PIRAINO, S., HAWLEY, P., HAMMOND, J., TRESSLER, R., RYAN, R., NICKENS, D., and RUIZ, R. 24 Week safety, tolerability, and efficacy of Capravirine as add-on therapy to Nelfinavir and 2 NRTIs in patients failing an NNRTI-based regimen. *Conf. Retroviruses Opp. Infect.* **2005**, *12*, *Abst.* 555.
20. WYATT, P.G., BETHELL, R.C., CAMMACK, N., CHARON, D., DODIC, N., DUMAITRE, B., EVANS, D.N., GREEN, D.V.S., HOPEWELL, P.L., HUMBER, D.C., LAMONT, R.B., ORR, D.C., PLESTED, S.J., RYAN, M.D., SOLLIS, S.L., STORER, R., and WEINGARTEN, G.C. Benzophenone derivatives: a novel series of potent and selective inhibitors of HIV-1 RT. *J. Med. Chem.* **1995**, *38*, 1657–1655.
21. CHAN, J.H., FREEMAN, G.A., TIDWELL, J.H., ROMINES, K.R., SCHALLER, L.T., COWAN, J.R., GONZALES, S.S., LOWELL, G.S., ANDREWS, III, C.W., REYNOLDS, D.J., ST. CLAIR, M., HAZEN, R.J., FERRIS, R.G., CREECH, K.L., ROBERTS, G.B., SHORT, S.A., WEAVER, K., KOSZALKA, G.W., and BOONE, L.W. Novel Benzophenones as NNRTIs of HIV-1 *J. Med. Chem.* **2004**, *47*, 1175–1182.
22. ROMINES, K.R., FREEMAN, G.A., SCHALLER, L.T., COWAN, J.R., GONZALES, S.S., TIDWELL, ANDREWS, III, C.W., STAMMERS, D.K., HAZEN, R.J., FERRIS, R.G., SHORT, S. A., CHAN, J.H., and BOONE, L.R. Structure–activity relationship studies of novel benzophenones leading to the discovery of a potent, next generation NNRTI. *J. Med. Chem.* **2006**, *49*, 727–739.
23. SCHALLER, L., BURNETTE, T., COWAN, J., FELDMAN, P., FREEMAN, G., MARR, H., QWENS, B., ROMINES, K., SHEPARD, J., BOONE, L., and CHAN, J.R. Prodrug strategies to deliver novel HIV-1 NNRTIs GW8248 and GW8635 ICAAC. **2003**, *43*, Abst. H-872.
24. TALLANT, M.D., EDELSTEIN, M.P., FERRIS, R.G., FREEMAN, G.A., CHONG, P.Y., ZHANG, H., MARR, H.B., TODD, D., LANG, D.G., and MCINTYRE, M.S. Lead optimization studies of GW8248X, a novel benzophenone NNRTI for the treatment of HIV-1. Abstracts of Papers, *236th ACS National Meeting* (Philadelphia, PA) **2008**, MEDI-236.
25. BECKER, S., LALEZARI, J., WALWORTH, C., KUMAR, P., CADE, J., NG-CASHIN, J., KIM, Y., SCOTT, J., ST. CLAIR, M., JONES, L., and SYMONDS, W. Antiviral activity and safety of GW695634, a novel next generation NNRTI in NNRTI-resistant HIV-1 infected patients. *AIDS Soc. Conf. HIV Path.* Treatment (Rio de Janero, Brazil). **2005**, *3*, Abst. WePe 6. 2 C03.
26. YOAKIM, C., BONNEAU, P.R., DEZIEL, R., DOYON, L., DUAN, J., GUSE, I., LANDRY, S., MALENFANT, E., NAUD, J., OGILVIE, W.W., O'MEARA, J.A., PLANTE, R., SIMONEAU, B., THAVONEKHAM, B., BOS, M., and CORDINGLEY, M.G. Novel nerivapine-like inhibitors with improved activity against NNRTI-resistant HIV: s-heteroaylthiomethyldipyridodiazepinone derivatives. *Bioorg. Med. Chem. Lett.* **2004**, *14*, 739–742.
27. BONNEAU, P.R., CYWIN, C.L., DEZIEL, R., DOYON, L., DUAN, J., GUSE, I., HACHE, B., HATTOX, S.E., LANDRY, S., MALENFANT, E., NAUD, J., OGILVIE, W.W., O'MEARA, J. A., PROUDFOOT, J.R., PLANTE, R., SIMONEAU, B., THAVONEKHAM, B., YAZDANIAN, M., YOAKIM, C., BOS, M., and CORDINGLEY, M.G. Towards a second generation NNRTI of HIV-1 with a broad spectrum of activity. *Abstracts of Papers, 226th ACS National Meeting* (New York, NY). **2003**, MEDI–326.
28. BONNEAU, P.R., DOYON, L., DUAN, J., SIMONEAU, B., YOAKIM, C., DEIZEL, R., OGILVIE, W.W., BOURGON, L., GARNEAU, M., LIARD, F., PLOUFFE, C., TREMBLAY, S., WARDROP, E.B., BOS, M., and CORDINGLEY, M.G. Nest

generation NNRTIs possessing broad spectrum activity. *11th CROI* (San Fransisco, CA). **2004**, Poster 530.

29. O'Meara, J.A., Yoakim, C., Bonneau, P.R., Bos, M., Cordingley, M.G., Deziel, R., Doyon, L., Duan, J., Garneau, M., Guse, I., Landry, S., Malenfant, E., Naud, J., Ogilvie, W.W., Thavonekham, B., and Simoneau, B. Novel 8-substituted dihydrodiazepinone inhibitors with a broad-spectrum of activity against HIV-1 strains resistant to NNRTIs. *J. Med. Chem.* **2005**, *48*, 5580–5588.
30. Bonneau, P., Robinson, P.A., Duan, J., Doyon, L., Simoneau, B., Yoakim, C., Garneau, M., Bos, M., Cordingley, M., Brenner, B., Spira, B., Wainberg, M., Huang, F., Drda, K., Ballow, C., Koenen-Bergmann, M., and Mayers, D.L. Antiviral characterization and human experience with BILR 355 BS, a novel next-generation NNRTI with a broad anti HIV-1 profile. *12th CROI* (Boston, MA). **2005**, Poster 558.
31. Coloumbe, R., Fink, D., Landry, S., Lessard, I., McCollum, R., Naud, J., O'Meara, J.A., Simoneau, B., Yoakim, C., and Bonneau, P. Crystallographic studies with BILR 355 BS, a novel NNRTI with a broad anti-HIV-1 profile. *Int. AIDS Soc. Conf. HIV Path.* (Rio de Janeiro, Brazil). **2005**, *3*, Abst. We PP 0105.
32. Tucker, T.J., Saggar, S.A., Sisko, J.T., Tynebor, R.M., Williams, T.M., Felock, P.J., Flynn, J.A., Lai, M., Liang, Y., McGaughey, M., Liu, M., Miller, M., Moyer, G., Munshi, V., Perlow-Poehnelt, R., Prasad, S., Sanchez, R., Torrent, M., Vacca, J.P., Wan, B., and Yan, Y. The design and synthesis of diaryl ether second generation HIV-1 NNTRIs with enhanced potency versus key clinical mutations. *Bioorg. Med. Chem. Lett.* **2008**, *18*, 2959–2966.
33. Tucker, T.J., Sisko, J.T., Tynebor, R.M., Williams, T. M., Felock, P.J., Flynn, J.A., Lai, M., Liang, Y., McGaughey, M., Liu, M., Miller, M., Moyer, G., Munshi, V., Perlow-Poehnelt, R., Prasad, S., Reid, J. C., Sanchez, R., Torrent, M., Vacca, J.P., Wan, B., and Yan, Y. Discovery of 3-{5-[(6-amino-1H-pyrazolo[3,4-b]pyridine-3-yl)methoxy]-2-chlorophenoxy}-5-chlorobenzonitrile (MK-4965): a potent, orally bioavailable HIV-1 NNRTI with improved potency against key mutant viruses. *J. Med. Chem.* **2008**, *51*, 6503–6511.
34. Tucker, T.J., Saggar, S., Sisko, J.T., Tynebor, R.M., Williams, T.M., Felock, P.J., Flynn, J.A., Lai, M., Liang, Y., McGaughey, M., Liu, M., Miller, M., Moyer, G., Munshi, V., Perlow-Poehnelt, R., Prasad, S., Reid, J.C., Sanchez, R., Torrent, M., Vacca, J.P., Wan, B., and Yan, Y. The discovery of MK-4965: a potent, orally bioavailable NNRTI with improved potenct versus key mutant viruses. Abstracts of Papers, *235th ACS National Meeting* (New Orleans, LA). **2008**, MEDI-174 and 175.
35. Tucker, T.J. The design and synthesis of novel second generation HIV-1 NNRTIs. *ACS Prospectives Series: Advances in Structure Based Drug Discovery* (San Francisco, CA). **2007**.
36. Tynebor, R.M., Tucker, T.J., Sisko, J.T., Anthony, N.J., DiStefano, D., Felock, P.J., Flynn, J.A., Gomez, R.P., Jolly, S.M., Lai, M., Liang, Y., Lim, J.J., McGaughey, G., Miller, M., Moyer, G., Munshi, V., Perlow-Poehnelt, R., Saggar, S., Sanchez, R.I., Su, D., Tinney, E., Torrent, M., Vacca, J.P., Williams, T., and Wan, B. Synthesis and SAR optimization of diaryl ether second generation NNRTIs. Abstracts of Papers, *2365th ACS National Meeting* (Philadelphia, PA). **2008**, MEDI-468.
37. Kuethe, J.T., Zhong, Y.-L., Alam, Mahbub, Alorati, Anthony D., Beutner, Gregory L., Cai, Dongwei, Fleitz, Fred J., Gibb, A.D., Kassim, A., Linn, K., Mancheno, D., Marcune, B., Pye, P.J., Scott, J.P., Tellers, D.M., Xiang, B., Yasuda, N., Yin, J., and Davies, I.W. Development of practical syntheses of potent non-nucleoside reverse transcriptase inhibitors. *Tetrahedron* **2009**, *65*, 5013–5023.
38. (a) For selected publications, please see: Kuramochi, T., Kakefuda, A., Yamada, H., Tsukamoto, I., Taguchi, T., and Sakamoto, S. Discovery of an *N*-(2-aminopyridin-4-ylmethyl)nicotinamide derivative: a potent and orally bioavailable NCX inhibitor. *Bioorg. Med. Chem.* **2005**, *13*, 4022–4036; (b) Ikemoto, T., Kawamoto, T., Wada, H., Ishida, T., Ito, T., Isogami, Y., Miyano, Y.o., Mizuno, Y., Tomimatsu, K., Hamamura, K., Takatani, M., and Wakimasu, M. Large-scale synthesis of new cyclazines, 5-thia-1, 8b-diazaacenaphthylene-3-carboxylic acid derivatives having the peripheral 12-electron ring system. *Tetrahedron* **2002**, *58*, 489–493; (c) Gudmundsson, K.S. and Johns, B.A. Synthesis of novel imidazo[1, 2-a]pyridines with potent activity against herpesviruses *Org. Lett.* **2003**, *5*, 1369–1372; (d) Bolm, C., Frison, J.-C., Paih, J.L., Moessner, C., and Raabe, G. Synthesis of C2-symmetric and unsymmetrically substituted 2,2′-dipyridylamines and crystal structure of a chiral 2, 2′-dipyridylamine copper (II) complex. *J. Organomet. Chem.* **2004**, *689*, 3767–3777; (e) Lang, F., Zewge, D., Houpis, I.N., and Volante, R.P. Amination of aryl halides using copper catalysis. *Tetrahedron Lett.* **2001**, *42*, 3251–3254; (f) Vedejs, E., Trapencieris, P., and Suna, E. Substituted isoquinolines by Noyori transfer hydrogenation: enantioselective synthesis of chiral diamines containing an aniline subunit. *J. Org. Chem.* **1999**, *64*, 6724–6729; (g) Huang, X. and Buchwald, S.L. New ammonia equivalents for the Pd-catalyzed amination of aryl halides. *Org. Lett.* **2001**, *3*, 3417–3419; (h) Mathes, B.M. and Filla, S.A. A general method for the preparation of 2,3,5-trisubstituted-furo[3, 2-b]pyridines. *Tetrahedron Lett.* **2003**, *44*, 725–728; (i) Imahori, T., Uchiyama, M., Sakamoto, T., and Kondo, Y. Regiocontrolled deprotonative-zincation of bromopyridines using aminozincates. *Chem. Commun.* **2001**, 2450–2451; (j) Alcázar, J., Alonso, J.M., Bartolomé, J.M., Iturino, L., and Matesanz, E. Synthesis of novel 3-substituted-2,3-

dihydro-1,4-dioxino[2, 3-b]pyridines as potential new scaffolds for drug discovery: selective introduction of substituents on the pyridine ring. *Tetrahedron Lett.* **2003**, *44*, 8983–8986; (k) Yamanaka, H., Araki, T., and Sakamoto, T. Site-selectivity in the reaction of 3-substituted pyridine 1-oxides with phosphoryl chloride. *Chem. Pharm. Bull.* **1988**, *36*, 2244–2247; (l) Klemm, L. H., Louris, J.N., Boisvert, W., Higgins, C., and Muchiri, D.R. Chemistry of thienopyridines. XXXIII. Synthetic routes to 5- and 7-substituted thieno[3,2-b]pyridines from the N-oxide *J. Heterocycl. Chem.* **1985**, *22*, 1249–1252; (m) Miura, Y., Takaku, S., Nawata, Y., and Hamana, M. Reactions of 3-substituted quinoline 1-oxides with acylating agents. *Heterocycles* **1991**, *32*, 1579–1586; (n) Bremner, D.H., Dunn, A.D., and Wilson, K.A. The synthesis of thienopyridines from ortho-halogenated pyridine derivatives. *Synthesis* **1992**, *6*, 528–530; (o) Ohta, A., Takahashi, N., and Shirokoma, Y. Syntheses of a naturally occurring hydroxamic acid and its analogues. *Heterocycles* **1990**, *30*, 875–884; (p) Itoh, T., Ono, K., Sugawara, T., and Mizuno, Y. Studies on the chemical synthesis of potential antimetabolites. 30. Regioselective introduction of a chlorine atom into the imidazo[4, 5-b]pyridine nucleus. *J. Heterocycl. Chem.* **1982**, *19, 513;* (q) Cuperly, D., Gros, P., and Fort, Y. First direct C-2-lithiation of 4-DMAP. Convenient access to reactive functional derivatives and ligands. *J. Org. Chem.* **2002**, *67*, 238–241; (r) Mathieu, J., Gros, P., and Fort, Y. Unprecedented C-6 functionalization of 3-picoline induced by a methyl to C-6 lithium shift. *Chem. Comm.* **2000**, 951–952; (s) Taylor, E.C. and Corvetti, A.J. Pyridine-1-oxides. i. Synthesis of some nicotinic acid derivatives. *J. Org. Chem.* **1954**, *19*, 1633–1640.

39. (a) Chichibabin, A.E. and Zeide, O.A. New reaction for compounds containing the pyridine nucleus. *J. Russ. Phys. Chem. Soc.* **1914**, *46*, 1216; (b) Leffler, M.T. Organic reactions. I: amination of heterocyclic bases by alkali amides. *Org. React.* **1942**, *1*, 91; (c) McGill, C.K. and Rappa, A. Advances in the chichibabin reaction. *Adv. Heterocycl. Chem.* **1988**, *44*, 1–79.

40. (a) Couturier, M. and Le, T. Safe and practical large-scale synthesis of 2-aminoquinoline-6-carboxylic acid benzyl ester. *Org. Proc. Res. Dev.* **2006**, *10, 534;* (b) Gerster, J.F., Lindstrom, K.J., Miller, R.L., Tomai, M. A., Birmachu, W., Bomersine, S.N., Gibson, S.J., Imbertson, L.M., Jacobson, J.R., Knafla, R.T., Maye, P.V., Nikolaides, N., Oneyemi, F.Y., Parkhurst, G.J., Pecore, S.E., Reiter, M.J., Scribner, L.S., Testerman, T.L., Thompson, N.J., Wagner, T.L., Weeks, C.E., Andre, J.-D., Lagain, D., Bastard, Y., and Lupu, M. Synthesis and structure–activity-relationships of 1H-imidazo[4, 5-c]quinolines that induce interferon production. *J. Med. Chem.* **2005**, *48*, 3481; (c) Storz, T., Marti, R., Meier, R., Nury, P., Roeder, M., and Zhang, K. First safe and practical synthesis of 2-amino-8-hydroxyquinoline. *Org. Proc. Res. Dev.* **2004**, *8*, 663; (d) Miura, Y., Takaku, S., Fujimura, Y., and Hamana, M. Synthesis of 2, 3-fused quinolines from 3-substituted quinoline 1-oxides. Part 1. *Heterocycles* **1992** *34*, 1055; (e) Glennon, R.A., Slusher, R.M., Lyon, R.A., Titeler, M., and McKenney, J.D. 5-HT1 and 5-HT2 binding characteristics of some quipazine analogues. *J. Med. Chem.* **1986**, *29*, 2375–2380.

41. Yin, J., Xiang, B., Huffman, M.A., Raab, C.E., and Davies, I.W. A general and efficient 2-amination of pyridines and quinolines. *J. Org. Chem.* **2007**, *72*, 4554–4557.

42. (a) Shi, C.-L., Shi, D.-Q., Kim, S.H., Huang, Z.-B., Ji, S.-J., and Ji, M. A novel and efficient one-pot synthesis of furo[3′,4′:5,6]pyrido[2, 3-c]pyrazole derivatives using organocatalysts. *Tetrahedron* **2008**, *64*, 2425–2432; (b) Stankovicová, H., Gáplovsky, A., Lácová, M., Chovancová, J., and Puchala, A. Transformation of 4-oxo-4H-(1)-benzopyran-3-carboxaldehydes into pyrazolo(3,4-b)pyridines. *J. Heterocyclic Chem.* **2006**, *43*, 843–848; (c) Ochiai, H., Ishida, A., Ohtani, T., Kusumi, K., Kishikawa, K., Yamamoto, S., Takeda, H., Obata, T., Nakai, H., and Toda, M. New orally active PDE4 inhibitors with therapeutic potential. *Bioorg. Med. Chem.* **2004**, *12*, 4089–4100; (d) de Mello, H., Echevarria, A.M., Canto-Cavalheiro, M., and Leon, L.L. Antileishmanial pyrazolopyridine derivatives: synthesis and structure–activity relationship analysis. *J. Med. Chem.* **2004**, *47*, 5427–5432; (e) Straub, A., Benet-Buckholz, J., Frode, R., Kern, A., Kohlsdorfer, C., Schmitt, P., Schwarz, T., Siefert, H.-M., and Stasch, J.-P. Metabolites of orally active NO-independent pyrazolopyridine stimulators of soluble guanylate cyclase. *Bioorg. Med. Chem.* **2002**, *10*, 1711–1717; (f) Bare, T.M., McLaren, C.D., Campbell, J.B., Firor, J.W., Resch, J.F., Walters, C.P., Salama, A.I., Meiners, B.A., and Patel, J.B. Synthesis and structure–activity relationships of a series of anxioselective pyrazolopyridine ester and amide anxiolytic agents. *J. Med. Chem.* **1989**, *32*, 2561–2573; (g) Lynch, B.M., Khan, M.A., Teo, H.C., and Pedrotti, F. Pyrazolo[3,4-b]pyridines: syntheses, reactions, and nuclear magnetic resonance spectra. *Can. J. Chem.* **1988**, *66*, 420–428;(h) Dorn, H. and Ozegowski, R. General syntheses and rational parameters for structural assignment of isomeric derivatives of [3,4]-fused pyrazoles. *J. Prakt. Chem.* **1979**, *321*, 881–98; (i) Chu, I. and Lynch, B.M. *J. Med. Chem.* **1975**, *18*, 161–165; (j) Sekikawa, I., Nishie, J., Tonooka, S., Tanaka, Y., and Kakimoto, S. Antituberculous compounds. XXVIII. Synthesis of pyrazolopyridines. *J. Heterocyclic Chem.* **1973**, *10*, 931–932; (k) Junek, H. and Aigner, H. Synthesen mit Nitrilen, XXXV. Reaktionen von Tetracyanäthylen mit Hete-rocyclen. *Chem. Ber.* **1973**, *106*, 914–921;(l) Imbach, J.L., Jacquier, R. and Vidal, J.L. Azoles. LXIX. Condensation of 3-amino-5-pyrazolone with several β-dicarbonyl compounds. *Bull. Chem. Soc. France* **1970**, 1929–1935 -5;(m) Junek, J. and Wrtilek, I. *Monatsh Chem.* **1969**, *100*, 1250–1255.

43. (a) Shi, C.-L., Shi, D.-Q., Kim, S.H., Huang, Z.-B., Ji, S.-J., and Ji, M. A novel and efficient one-pot synthesis of

furo[3′,4′:5,6]pyrido[2,3-c]pyrazole derivatives using organocatalysts. *Tetrahedron* **2008**, *64*, 2425–2432; (b) Sagitullina, G.P., Lisitskaya, L.A., Vorontsova, M.A., and Sagitullin, R.S. Facile synthesis of substituted 1H-pyrazolo[3,4-b]pyridines. *Mendeleev Commun.* **2007**, *17*, 192–193; (c) Revesz, L., Blum, E., Di Padova, F.E., Buhl, T., Feifel, R., Gram, H., Hiestand, P., Manning, U., Neumann, U., and Rucklin, G. Pyrazoloheteroaryls: novel p38α MAP kinase inhibiting scaffolds with oral activity. *Bioorg. Med. Chem. Lett.* **2006**, *16*, 262–266; (d) Shutske, G.M. and Roehr, J.E. Synthesis of some piperazinylpyrazolo[3,4-b]pyridines as selective serotonin re-uptake inhibitors. *J. Heterocyclic Chem.* **1997**, *34*, 789–795; (e) Henke, B.R., Aquino, C.J., Birkemo, L.S., Croom, D.K., Dougherty, R.W. Jr., Ervin, G.N., Grizzle, M.K., Hirst, G.C., James, M. K., Johnson, M.F., Queen, K.L., Sherrill, R.G., Sugg, E.E., Suh, E.M., Szewczyk, J.W., Unwalla, R.J., Yingling, J., and Willson, T.M. Optimization of 3-(1H-Indazol-3-ylmethyl)-1,5-benzodiazepines as potent, orally active CCK-A agonists. *J. Med. Chem.* **1997**, *40*, 2706–2725; (f) Bonnetaud, D., Queguiner, G., and Pastour, P. Synthesis of 3-formyl-2-hydroxypyridine and 2H-pyrano[2,3-b]pyridin-2-ones. *J. Heterocyclic Chem.* **1972**, *9*, 165–166.

44. Beutner, G.L., Kuethe, J.T., Kim. M., and Yasuda, N. Expedient synthesis of 3-alkoxymethyl- and 3-aminomethyl-pyrazolo[3,4-b]pyridines. *J. Org. Chem.* **2009**, *74*, 789–794.
45. Shutske, G.M. and Roehr, J.E. Synthesis of some piperazinylpyrazolo[3,4-b]pyridines as selective serotonin re-uptake inhibitors. *J. Heterocyclic Chem.* **1997**, *34*, 789–795.
46. Zhong, Y.-L., Lindale, M.G., and Yasuda, N. An efficient access to 3,6-disubstituted 1H-pyrazolo[3,4-b]pyridines via a one-pot double SnAr reaction and pyrazole formation. *Tetrahedron Lett.* **2009**, *50*, 2293–2297.
47. Previously unreported results from Merck Research Laboratories.
48. Kuethe, J.T., Tellers, D.M., Weissman, S.A., and Yasuda, N. Development of a sequential tetrahydropyran and tertiary butyl deprotection: high-throughput experimentation, mechanistic analysis, and DOE optimization. *Org. Process Res. Dev.* **2009**, *13*, 471–477.

CHAPTER 12

DISCOVERY OF BOCEPREVIR AND NARLAPREVIR: THE FIRST AND SECOND GENERATION OF HCV NS3 PROTEASE INHIBITORS

Kevin X. Chen and F. George Njoroge

12.1 INTRODUCTION

The hepatitis C virus (HCV) is a noncytopathic, hepatotropic member of the flavivirus family, that causes acute and chronic necroinflammatory liver diseases [1]. Levels of chronic HCV infection have reached pandemic proportions with approximately 170 million people infected worldwide and three to four million people newly infected each year [1,2]. In roughly 80% of cases, the virus leads to a chronic form of hepatitis, a condition that is incurable in many patients. Without therapeutic intervention, it can lead to morbidity or mortality in 10–20 years through either cirrhosis and hepatic failure or hepatocellular carcinoma [3–6]. It is anticipated that a significant percentage of those currently infected will develop cirrhosis and other associated hepatic sequelae. End-stage liver disease resulting from chronic HCV infection is the leading cause of liver transplantation in the western world [7].

The standard-of-care for HCV infection before the approval of protease drugs was a combination therapy of subcutaneous pegylated α-interferon (pegIFN) and the oral nucleoside drug ribavirin (RBV) for 24 to 48 weeks [8–10]. The primary goal of HCV treatment is to achieve a sustained viralogical response (SVR), which is defined clinically as an undetectable serum HCV-RNA level 24 weeks after cessation of therapy [7–9]. The combination therapy is relatively successful in patients infected with HCV genotypes 2 or 3, leading to an SVR in approximately 80 to 90% of patients treated [11]. In patients infected with HCV genotype 1, which is predominant in North America, Europe, and Japan, or genotype 4, however, only approximately 40–50% of patients achieve SVR [10]. The response rate can also be affected by host factors, such as age, race, gender, obesity, and degree of liver fibrosis [12–14]. Success of treatment has also been reported to be related to genetic polymorphisms near the IL28B gene on chromosome 19; patients with the CC genotype are more likely to achieve SVR than those with the TT genotype [15–17]. Some patients also experience significant side effects related to the pegylated interferon and ribavirin combination therapy treatment. The development of new antiviral drugs with higher treatment efficacy and more favorable side-effect profiles is thus of great clinical relevance and importance [8–10].

Case Studies in Modern Drug Discovery and Development, Edited by Xianhai Huang and Robert G. Aslanian.

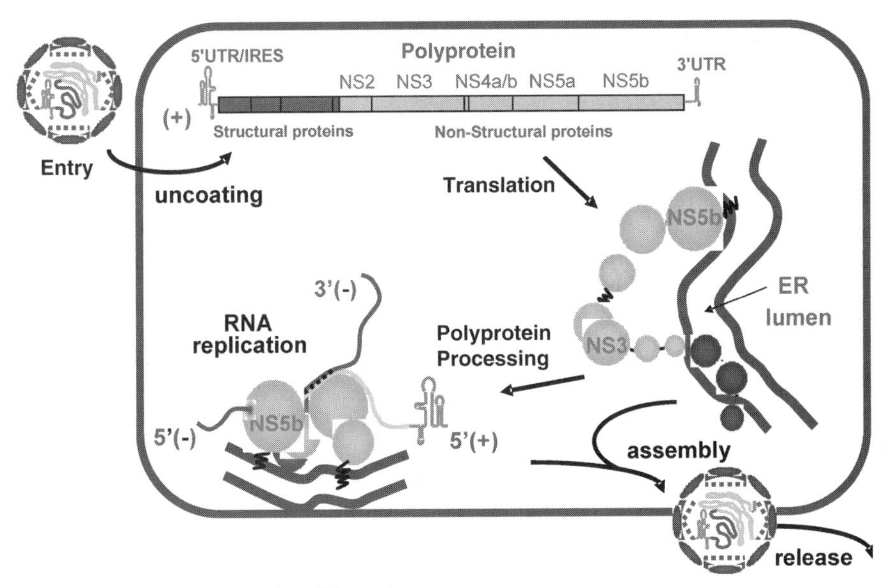

Figure 12.1 Hepatitis C virus life cycle.

HCV was identified in 1989 as a member of the Flaviviridae family [18]. The HCV genome is a 9.6 kb, uncapped, linear, single-stranded RNA (ssRNA) molecule with positive polarity that serves as a template for both translation and replication (Figures 12.1 and 12.2). Translation of the plus-strand RNA initiates at an internal ribosomal entry site (IRES) [19,20], resulting in the production of a single polyprotein precursor that is processed into structural (C, E1, E2, and p7) and nonstructural (NS2, NS3, NS4A, NS4B, NS5A, and NS5B) protein subunits by host and viral proteases [19–22]. The virally encoded protease responsible for processing the nonstructural portion of the polyprotein is located in the N-terminal third of the NS3 protein [19,20]. Besides autoproteolysis of the NS3–NS4A junction, the protease also cleaves the polyprotein at the NS4A–NS4B, NS4B–NS5A, and NS5A–NS5B junctions to release the downstream NS functional proteins (Figure 12.2). HCV replication proceeds via the synthesis of a complementary negative-strand RNA using the genome as a template and the subsequent synthesis of genomic positive-strand RNA from this negative-strand RNA template. The key enzyme, responsible for both of these

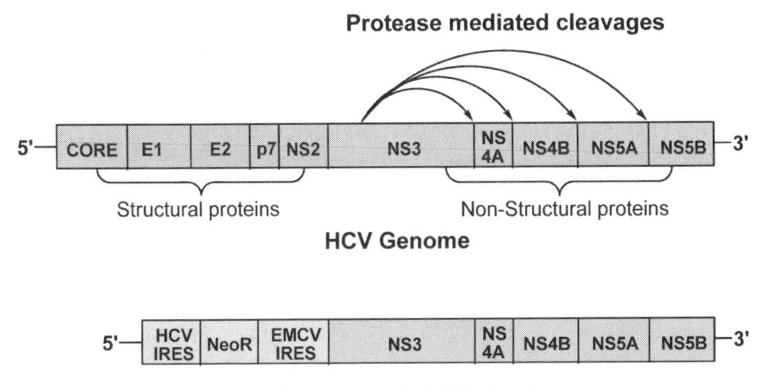

Figure 12.2 Schematic representation of the HCV genome, subgenomic HCV replicon, and NS3/NS4A protease mediated cleavage of four protein junctions (shown as arrows).

steps, is the NS5B RNA-dependent RNA polymerase (RdRp) [23,24]. The new RNAs are either translated to yield more polyprotein or, later in the infection cycle, encapsulated to generate progeny virions.

The essential roles played by HCV NS3 protease and NS5B polymerase in the virus replication life cycle have emerged as the most important targets for antiviral intervention drug development [25–27].

A large number of promising small-molecule inhibitors of these two enzymes are in clinical development. Many of them have demonstrated strong antiviral activity both *in vitro* and in patients. When they are combined with pegIFN and RBV, they are much more effective treatment for HCV infection than treatment with pegIFN and RBV alone [28,29]. Inhibitors toward other potential targets such as NS5A, IRES, and replicase are also under clinical or preclinical investigation [30,31]. Although efforts are ongoing to develop a vaccine, the unusually rapid genetic drift of HCV makes this a daunting task [31,32]. A major challenge for any successful direct acting anti-HCV therapy is the rapid emergence of the drug-resistant viruses under selective pressure. The fast turnover rate and the intrinsic low fidelity of the HCV replication machinery endow the virus with the ability to fully explore its genome space and quickly come up with mutations that render it resistant to antiviral drugs.

For more than a decade after the discovery and characterization of the virus, the development of HCV antiviral therapy has been severely hampered by the lack of an efficient cell-culture system and a small animal model for evaluating the clinical relevance of potential new drugs. However, this impediment has been largely overcome in the last 7–8 years by the development of subgenomic HCV RNA that replicate autonomously in transfected cells [33]. For example, the HCV-2a replicon JFH1 replicates efficiently when transfected into the human hepatoma cell line (Huh7) and supports the secretion of viral particles [34]. The high level of replication of this system opens new avenues for molecular studies of various aspects of the HCV life-cycle, including replication and viral entry, and also for the development of novel antiviral drugs. The chronically infected chimpanzee model [35] and the Severe Combined Immunodeficiency Disease (SCID) mouse with chimeric human liver model [36,37] also proved effective in limited preclinical evaluation of anti-HCV therapies, although both animal models suffer from limitations that make them less than ideal for expanded studies. HCV infects only humans and chimpanzees. The chronically infected chimpanzee model [35], the "gold standard" for HCV studies, is challenging and expensive because one out of three chimpanzees spontaneously resolves the HCV infection. In the immune deficient SCID mouse–human liver xenograft system, the liver of neonate SCID beige mice were colonized with infused human hepatocytes which rescued them from a fatal transgene. These human liver grafts were infected by several genotypes of HCV, and the HCV-infected mice are responsive to antiviral treatment. Thus, it appears that this human liver chimeric mouse model will be useful for studying HCV infection and may provide a valuable tool for antiviral drug testing [37]. Unfortunately, the animals are fragile and scale up of the colony has been slower than expected, thus limiting access to the system.

12.2 HCV NS3 PROTEASE INHIBITORS

The critical role played by NS3 protease in HCV viral replication makes it an attractive target for the creation of new HCV therapy [25,38,39]. Development of small-molecule inhibitors for this enzyme would potentially arrest the processing of the aforementioned polyprotein required for viral replication [40]. The X-ray crystal structures for

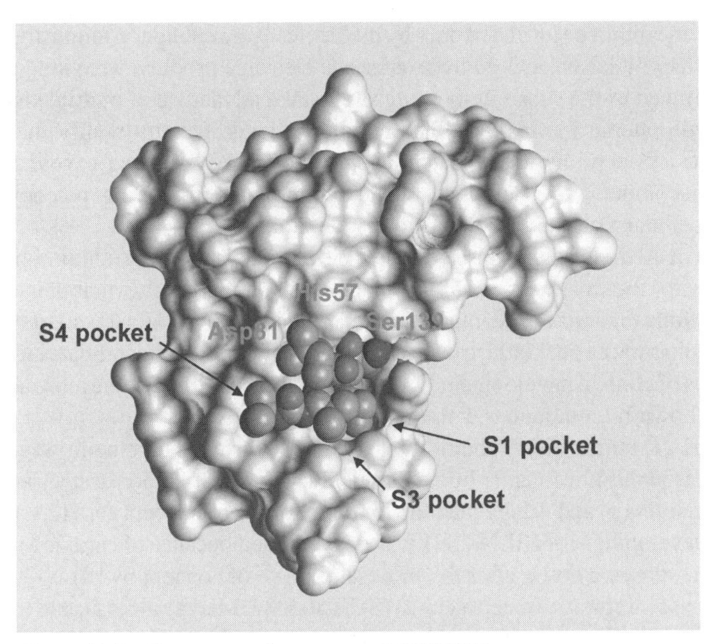

Figure 12.3 X-ray crystal structure of HCV NS3 protease.

either isolated domain or full-length protein of the HCV NS3 protease have been published [41,42]. The structural data provided detailed insights to facilitate potential rational design of inhibitors. The NS3 protease is, for the most part, a typical β-barrel serine protease, with a canonical Asp-His-Ser catalytic triad similar to the well-studied digestive enzymes, trypsin, and chymotrypsin (Figure 12.3). Histidine-57 and aspartic acid-81 of the catalytic triad are located in the N-terminal region, whereas serine-139 forms part of the C-terminal subdomain. The active site, located near the surface in a cleft between two β-barrel subdomains, is shallow, featureless, and highly solvent exposed. At other sites, cysteine is conserved in the P1 position of the natural substrate for the protease in all three trans-cleavage sites, and it is replaced by a threonine in the cis-cleavage event. The P1′ residue is a small hydrophobic amino acid, either a serine or an alanine. The P2, P3, and P4 sites are all amino acids with hydrophobic side chains, and P5 and P6 usually contain polar amino acids such as aspartic acid or glutamic acid. The NS3 protease uses an extended polydentate binding cleft, with several recognition subsites to ensure specificity. It forms a heterodimeric complex with the NS4A protein, an essential cofactor that activates the protease and assists in anchoring the heterodimer to the endoplasmic reticulum.

Although intensive research has focused on the development of HCV NS3 protease inhibitors as drug candidates, it has not been a smooth and productive journey for many years. At the beginning of these drug development efforts, there were no viable small-molecule leads from screening of millions of compound. Early inhibitors were derived from the product inhibition based on the substrate–enzyme active site interactions [43,44]. However, the HCV protease requires an extensive peptide substrate, with which it establishes multiple weak interactions distributed along an extended surface. The major concern was to develop orally bioavailable small-molecule drugs from such large substrates. The X-ray crystal structure of the enzyme revealed the fact that the substrate-binding sites of the protease were flat and shallow, lacking the deep binding pockets that had been exploited as anchor points to design potent and selective inhibitors for other protease targets. The fear was that the enzyme might be inhibited only by molecules large enough to mimic the natural substrate. Indeed, early leads, derived from substrate cleavage product, were long peptides which occupied much of the substrate-binding site to take advantage of multiple hydrogen bonding and hydrophobic interactions. The major challenge was to modify these large molecules to the less peptidic and lower molecular weight (MW) drug candidates with desirable pharmacokinetic (PK) profiles, while retaining or improving potency in the enzymatic and cellular assays.

As a result of all these challenges and difficulties, no HCV protease inhibitor has yet to reach the market for the treatment of HCV infection, in spite of the fact that the virus was discovered and fully characterized more than two decades ago. However, tremendous efforts from the pharmaceutical industry have resulted in a number of candidates which are at different stages of clinical development [25]. The structures of some of the more advanced candidates are shown in compounds **1** through **8**.

BILN-2061 (**1**, ciluprevir) (Scheme 12.1), from Boehringer Ingelheim was the first HCV NS3 protease inhibitor to enter human clinical trial [45]. It demonstrated rapid viral load reduction in humans and established the first-ever proof of concept for HCV protease inhibitors. The development of BILN-2061 was discontinued because of cardiac toxicity in monkeys at higher doses. Shortly after the successful proof of concept by BILN-2061, two other novel protease inhibitors, Boceprevir (**2**) (SCH 503034, Merck) [46,47], and telaprevir (**3**) (VX-950, Vertex) [48] were advanced into clinical studies in humans and demonstrated to be safe and efficacious. They have both completed phase III clinical trials and have been approved for marketing by FDA after expedited reviews. A number of other candidates are also at various stage of clinical or preclinical development. Among them, narlaprevir (**4**) (SCH 900518, Merck) [49], danoprevir (**5**) (ITMN-191, InterMune-Roche) [50], TMC435 (**6**) (Tibotec-Medivir) [51,52], Vaniprevir (**7**) (MK-7009, Merck) [53,54], and BI-201335 (**8**) (Boehringer Ingelheim) [55,56] have entered phase II and appear to be more advanced than others.

The NS3 protease inhibitors discovered to date can be divided into two classes based on the mechanism of action. One class consists of noncovalent inhibitors, such as BILN-2061 (**1**) and danoprevir (**5**). They are conventional reversible inhibitors.

The earliest conventional noncovalent protease inhibitors were peptide-based inhibitors derived from the enzyme cleavage product [57]. After extensive SAR development and optimization, compounds with much more complex P2 and P1 residues than the original natural amino acids emerged as potential drug candidate. BI-201335 from Boehringer Ingelheim (**8**) is the latest example of the linear elaborated potent peptide inhibitor. Since linear peptidic compounds were susceptible to hydrolysis by various peptidases, various depeptization strategies were investigated by different research groups in an attempt to achieve good PK properties. Macrocyclization was one such approach that has proven to be highly successful. The first small-molecule HCV clinical candidate, BILN-2061 (**1**), is a P1–P3 cyclized macrocyclic inhibitor. Danoprevir (**5**) and TMC435 (**6**) incorporated similar 15-membered P1–P3 macrocycle as that in compound **1**, while vaniprevir (**7**) had a unique 20-membered P2–P3 macrocycle.

One of the most successful strategies that was employed in the discovery of drug candidates for other serine, tyrosine, cysteine, or threonine protease targets [58–60] has been adapted to the development of HCV protease inhibitors. A covalent trap, or "warhead," such as an electrophilic aldehyde, ketone, α-ketoamide, α-ketoacid, boronic acid, or boronic ester group, was incorporated into a substrate-based inhibitor to react with the serine on the catalytic site of NS3 protease (Scheme 12.2) [58,60]. This represents the second class of NS3 inhibitors. Successful examples of α-ketoamides are boceprevir (**2**), telaprevir (**3**), and narlaprevir (**4**). It has been shown that the reaction of the active site serine

(Ser-139) with the α-ketoamide and subsequent trapping of the resulting transition-state analogues by the active site triad (Ser-139, His-57, and Asp-81) [48] provided effective inhibition through a stable, covalent, and reversible complex with the enzyme. The electrophilic "warhead" is essential for the protease inhibitory activity of these compounds. The time required for stable covalent adduct formation is in the order of minutes, which is much longer than that required in traditional noncovalent binding.

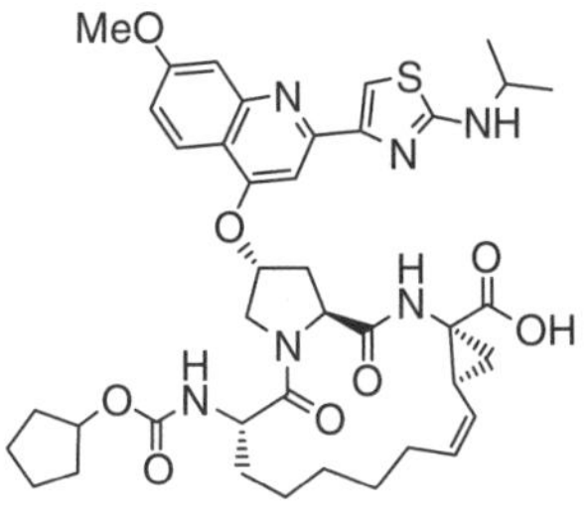

1
BILN-2061

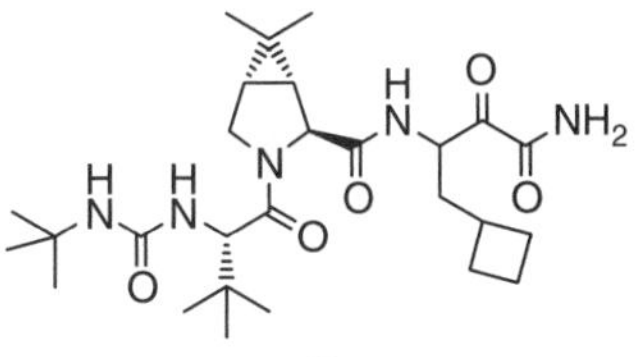

2
Boceprevir

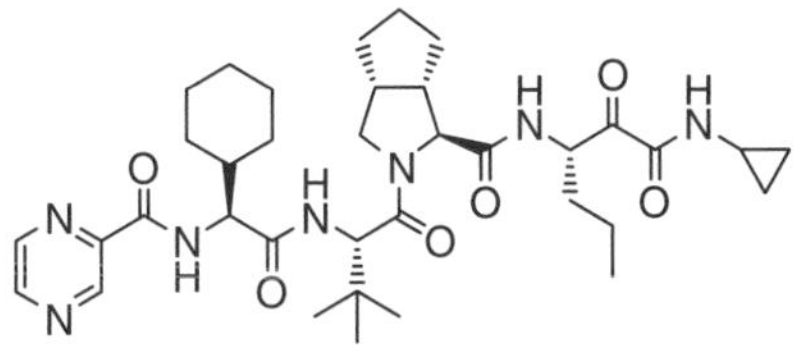

3
Telaprevir

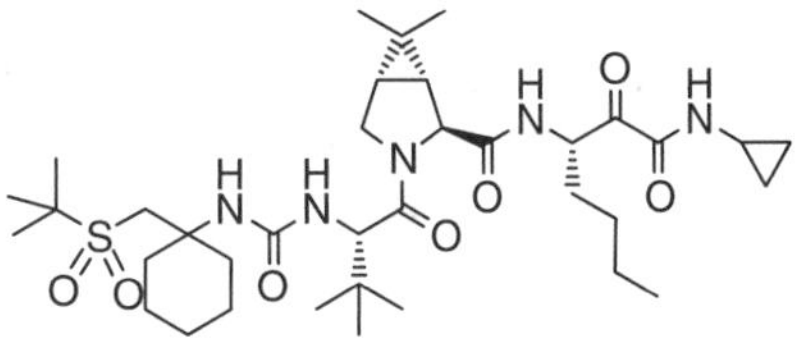

4
Narlaprevir

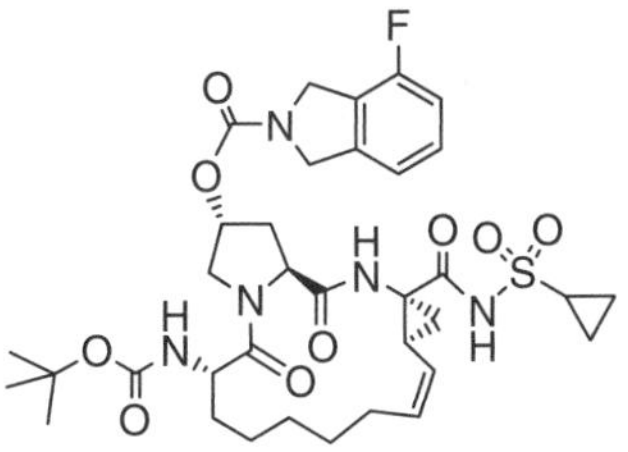

5
Danoprevir

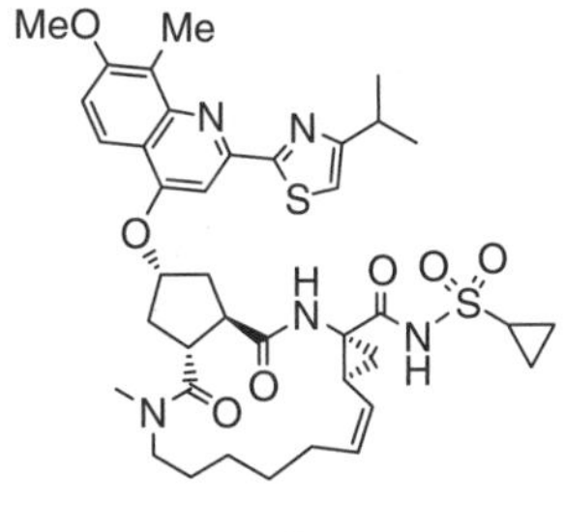

6
TMC435

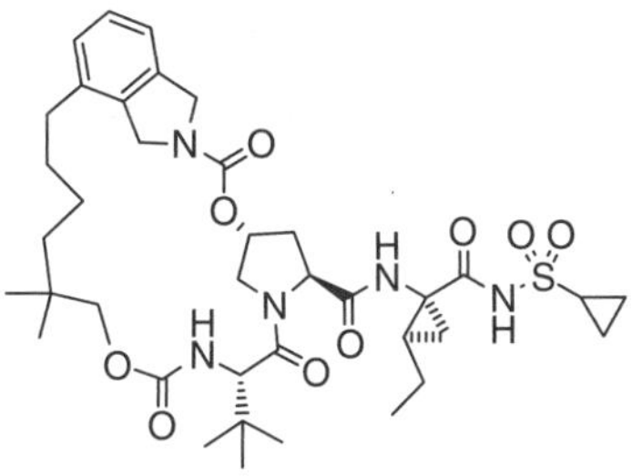

7
Vaniprevir

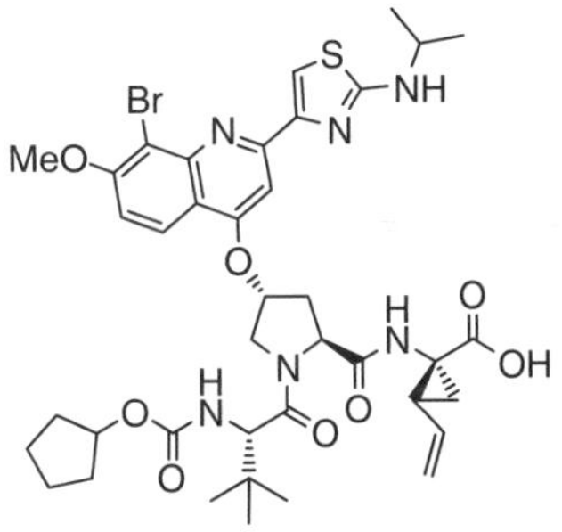

8
BI-201335

Scheme 12.1 Structures of boceprevir, telaprevir, and other advanced development candidates of HCV protease inhibitor.

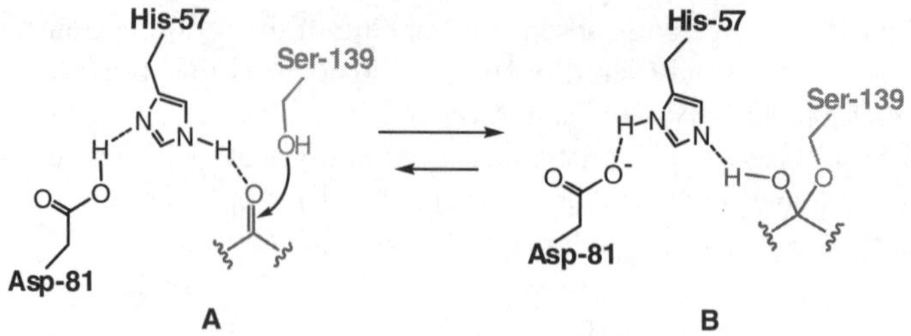

Scheme 12.2 Covalent bond formation between serine-139 hydroxyl and ketone carbonyl groups.

12.3 RESEARCH OPERATION PLAN AND BIOLOGICAL ASSAYS

12.3.1 Research Operation Plan

The development of HCV NS3 protease inhibitor started with the testing of a synthesized compound in a functional enzymatic assay. The compound was also simultaneously tested in a replicon cell-based assay. The activity of the compound against human neutrophil elastase (HNE) was also obtained as a measure of selectivity. Those inhibitors that met the potency criteria in both enzyme and cellular assays and selectivity requirement were submitted for rat PK study with oral dosing to assess the exposure (area-under-curve, AUC). If potency, selectivity, and rat oral PK AUC were all acceptable, the compound was then evaluated in rats, monkeys, and dogs with both oral and IV dosing to obtain bioavailability, clearance, and maximum concentration. Selected promising compounds were also examined in plasma protein binding, CACO-2 permeability, CYP P450 binding, hERG screening, hepatocyte clearance assays to have full profile of the molecules. The most advanced few compounds were finally tested in Kinase panel screenings, AMES tests, and small animal high-dosing tolerability studies to address potential toxicity issues. The compound with the best overall profile was selected as the development candidate for further preclinical and clinical evaluations.

12.3.2 Enzyme Assay

For noncovalent classical inhibitors, the binding constant K_i can be obtained through a conventional enzymatic assay using HCV NS3 protease. However, to accurately assess the potency of slow equilibrating (or “slow-binding”) covalently bonded inhibitors such as α-ketoamides, proteolytic reactions containing inhibitors are usually monitored until equilibrium is evident using progress curve analysis [61]. In this type of so-called continuous assay, the extent of hydrolysis of chromogenic 4-phenylazophenyl (PAP) ester from the peptide fragment Ac-DTEDVVP(Nva)-O-4-PAP was spectrophotometrically determined. To underscore the slow-binding nature of these molecules and distinguish them from simple, instantaneous competitive inhibitors, the equilibrium binding constant was usually designated as K_i^* [62], although for most purposes it could be considered equivalent to a traditional K_i.

12.3.3 Replicon Assay

Besides a functional biochemical assay, a cell-based assay is also essential for SAR studies in drug discovery. Almost a decade had past after the characterization of the hepatitis C virus before an HCV subgenomic replicon system was developed by Bartenschlager and colleagues in 1999 [33]. The replicon cell-based assay has since been used extensively to evaluate the functional potency and subsequent antiviral efficacy of HCV protease inhibitors. The HCV replicon is essentially a defective (i.e., noninfectious) viral genome in which the sequences encoding the structural proteins at the 5′ end of the RNA have been replaced by a selectable marker, the neomycin resistance gene (NeoR) (Figure 12.2). The NeoR marker allows selection of cells harboring functional replicons following transfection and antibiotic treatment. Replicon constructs, including those developed to evaluate potential antiviral agents, use a design where two independent IRES elements are present. The HCV IRES sequence drives expression of the neomycin resistance gene to allow selection of replicon bearing cells and a second IRES sequence from encephalomyocarditis virus (EMCV) initiates translation of the RNA segment encoding HCV nonstructural proteins from NS3 to NS5B. Even with full-length replicons expressing structural proteins, cells bearing HCV replicons do not generate progeny virions. This differs from a true HCV infection [15]. Until now the replicon system remains the only germane *in vitro* system for evaluating potential antiviral agents against the HCV nonstructural proteins. The EC_{50} and EC_{90} values for suppression of the bicistronic subgenomic replicon were obtained through a 72-h assay in HuH-7 cells. At 72 h, cells were lysed and the replicon RNA level determined using real-time polymerase chain reaction (PCR) analysis (Taqman™) that targeted the NS5B portion of the viral genome. Changes in replicon RNA level were compared to an internal control, cellular glyceraldehyde-3-phosphate dehydrogenase (GAPDH) messenger RNA levels, in a single-tube multiplex reaction. Dose response curves were generated and drug concentrations resulting in a twofold or a 10-fold reduction in replicon RNA were estimated using a grid search method to give EC_{50} and EC_{90} values.

12.3.4 Measure of Selectivity

One of the key elements contributing to the potency of an α-ketoamide is the electrophilic ketoamide functionality, which forms a reversible covalent bond with serine-139 (Ser-139) of the HCV protease. However, the ketoamide motif could also be susceptible to attack by a variety of other endogenous nucleophiles such as hydroxyl, amino, and thiol groups that are present in many biomolecules. To address the selectivity issue, inhibitory activity against HNE was measured as a gauge of selectivity (HNE/HCV) in the SAR development. The active site of HNE closely resembles in structure that of HCV NS3 protease, but with a much smaller S1 pocket [70]. Although the clinical relevance of this selectivity parameter has not been demonstrated, it helped to serve as a guide in designing selective inhibitors versus similar proteases, thereby, minimizing potential side effects that could surface in the clinic. A selectivity of greater than one thousand is desirable.

12.4 DISCOVERY OF BOCEPREVIR

12.4.1 Initial Lead Generation Through Structure-Based Drug Design

Our journey to the discovery of HCV NS3 protease inhibitors started with screening Schering-Plough and external compound libraries. Unfortunately, the screening effort of more than four million compounds did not generate any meaningful leads to initiate a drug discovery effort. We embarked on a structure-based drug design (SBDD) approach. Early research discovered that the protease is susceptible to marked inhibition by the cleavage products from the substrates. Learning from the strategy employed in developing other serine-protease inhibitors [58–60], we envisioned that trapping the catalytic site serine with an electrophile such as an aldehyde, ketone, or ketoamide would be a promising approach. However, when inhibitors with these traps were prepared and evaluated, most of them did not demonstrate any desired activity against the NS3 protease. After a considerable search, a few large peptidic molecules, mimicking the peptide substrate structures, but containing an α-ketoamide functionality, were found to be potent HCV protease inhibitors [46,63]. The discovery of the undecapeptide compound **9** (Scheme 12.3), which had a structure consisting of 11 amino acid residues spanning P6 to P5′, marked the first step in our long journey toward an HCV protease drug candidate. Compound **9** exhibited excellent potency in the enzyme assay ($K_i^* = 1.9$ nM) but was a mixture of two diastereomers at the epimerizable P1 α-center. Moreover, with a molecular weight of 1265 Da, it was not expected to display any desirable PK properties. Nonetheless, it served as a starting point for further SAR studies. With the aid of X-ray crystal structures, research focused on reducing the size of the molecule while improving its PK profile and maintaining good potency.

12.4.2 SAR Studies Focusing on Truncation, Depeptization, and Macrocyclization

12.4.2.1 Truncation Strategy To reduce the size of the molecule, a series of step-wise truncations at either or both the prime or nonprime side were performed [46,63,64]. Trimming the C-terminal (prime side) P_2'–P_5' tetrapeptide methionine–serine–tyrosine–serine from undecapeptide **9** yielded truncated compound **10** with a $K_i^* = 43$ nM (Scheme 12.3) [46]. The molecular weight of this heptapeptide was reduced to 796 from 1265, at a cost of only a 25-fold loss in potency. It seemed that those four amino acid residues provided some but not critical interactions. Next, a number of further modifications were investigated in a step-wise fashion to assess the importance of each segment: removal of the two polar glutamic acid residues and one valine residue on the nonprime side, introduction of phenylglycine dimethylamide on the prime side, changing the P3 amino acid to cyclohexylglycine and capping on P3 with isobutyl carbonyl (*i*-Boc) group. These changes eventually led to the pentapeptide **11** [64]. Unfortunately, this compound lost most of the activity with a K_i^* of 10 μM. Apparently, some important binding interactions contributed by the two aspartic acid residue in **10** were lost in compound **11**, even though phenylglycine was added as P2′ and P3 valine was extended to cyclohexylglycine. However, simply replacing P2 proline with a leucine resulted in pentapeptide **12** which had a very respectable K_i^* of 120 nM [64]. This evidence suggested the key role played by the P2 residue. The truncation exercise demonstrated that the large undecapeptide could be reduced to half its size to a pentapeptide while maintaining reasonable activity. Despite some good binding assay results, none of the compounds **9–12** had any appreciable activity in the replicon cell-based assay, probably due to the highly polar nature of the di-acid moiety in **9** and **10** and lack of good potency in **11** and **12**.

12.4.2.2 Depeptization Strategy Since large peptidic molecules are susceptible to hydrolysis *in vivo* by ubiquitous peptidases, it is difficult for them to process desirable pharmacokinetic properties. Thus, substantial effort was devoted to depeptize various amino acid residues of the lead compounds such as **9** so that the modified structures do not resemble natural amino acids and are therefore not recognized by peptidases *in vivo*. One way to depeptize a peptide is to employ modified α-amino acids or use non α-amino acid structure fragments, for example, isosteres, to replace α-amino acids and amide bonds, while maintaining hydrogen bonding and other key interactions with the enzyme backbone

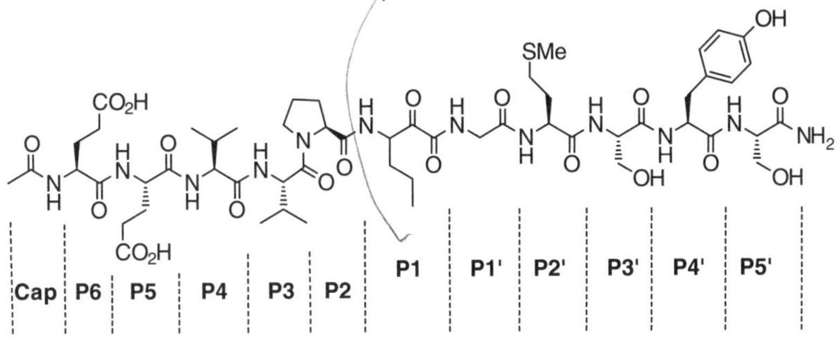

Cap P6 P5 P4 P3 P2 P1 P1' P2' P3' P4' P5'

9 Ki* = 1.9 nM

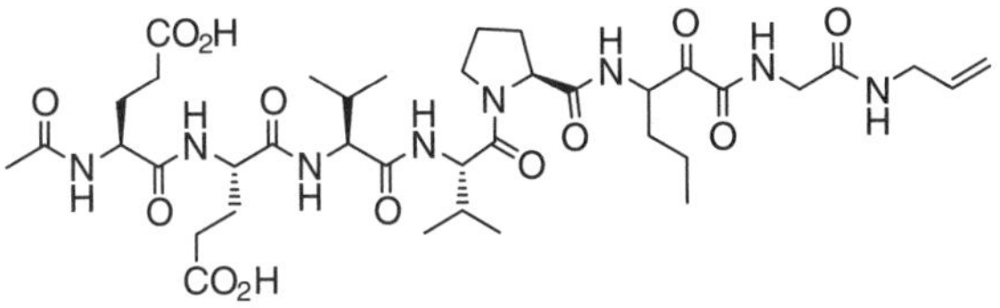

10 Ki* = 43 nM, EC_{90} > 5 μM

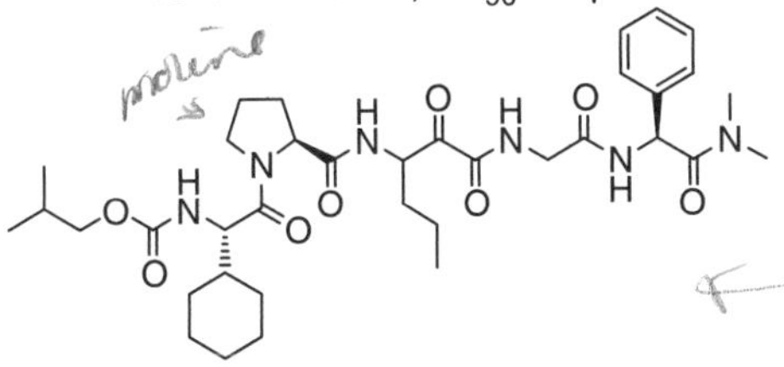

11 Ki* = 10000 nM, EC_{90} > 5 μM

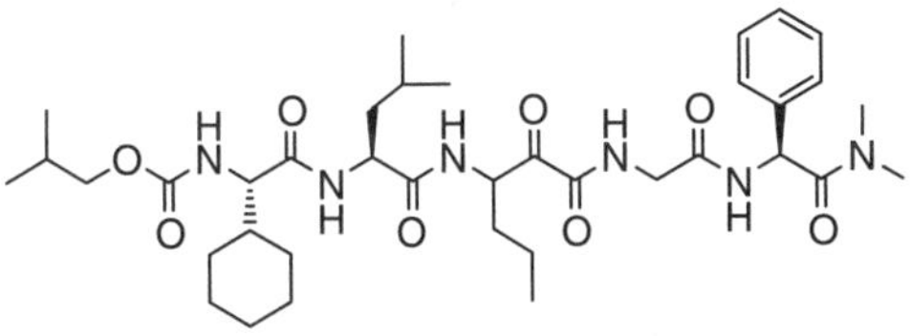

12 Ki* = 120 nM, EC_{90} > 5 μM

Scheme 12.3 Early lead structure and truncating excises.

or surface. The linear framework of the original peptide is also retained in this type of depeptization. The peptide inhibitor also incorporates some nonnatural amino acid, **13** was one of the more interesting compounds from our truncation studies (Scheme 12.4) [64]. It had a very good K_i^* of 15 nM in the enzyme assay, but didn't have any plasma levels in rats when dose orally. To improve the PK properties of this type of molecule, some depeptization studies were carried out. Compounds **14** and **15** are two examples of this effort. In the first analog, the positions of the nitrogen and α-carbon atoms of the P2 residue were switched, which resulted in a substituted urea connected to an α-amino ketone. Unfortunately, the final target (**14**) lost most potency ($K_i^* = 2100$ nM) compared to its peptide analog (**13**), presumably due to the fact that as a result of these modifications, the nature of the amide bond was changed (to a ketone) and one of the hydrogen bond forming N–Hs was lost. In the second compound (**15**), the α-carbon of the P2 residue was replaced with a nitrogen which resulted in a hydrazine urea motif between the P1 and P3 amino acids. Since all the amide bonds and hydrogen bond capabilities were preserved, the resulting inhibitor was still active ($K_i^* = 230$ nM), albeit with a 15-fold loss in potency. These two and a large number of other

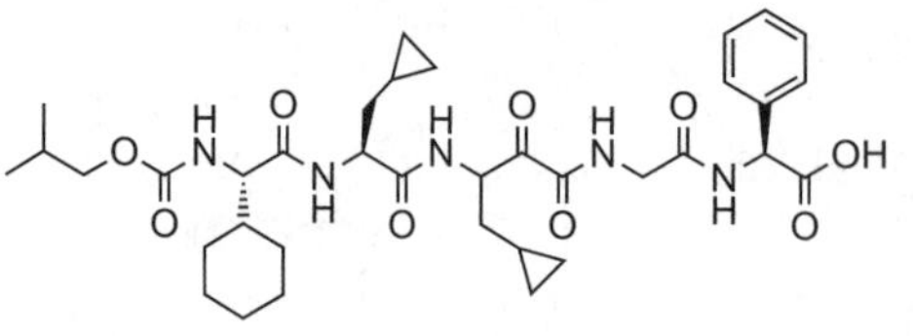

13 Ki* = 15 nM, EC_{90} = > 5 μM

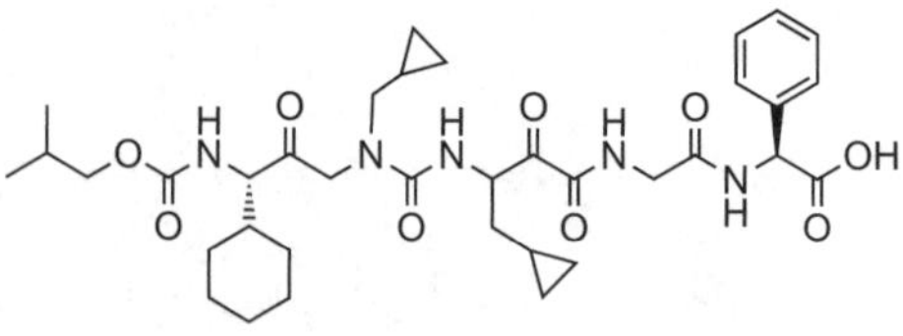

14 Ki* = 2100 nM, EC_{90} = > 5 μM

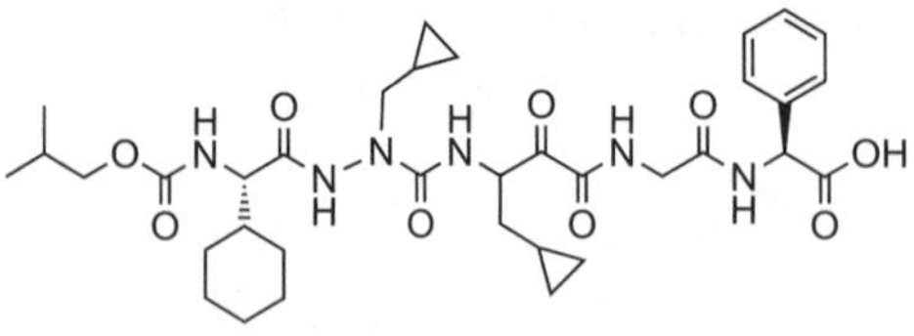

15 Ki* = 230 nM, EC_{90} = > 5 μM

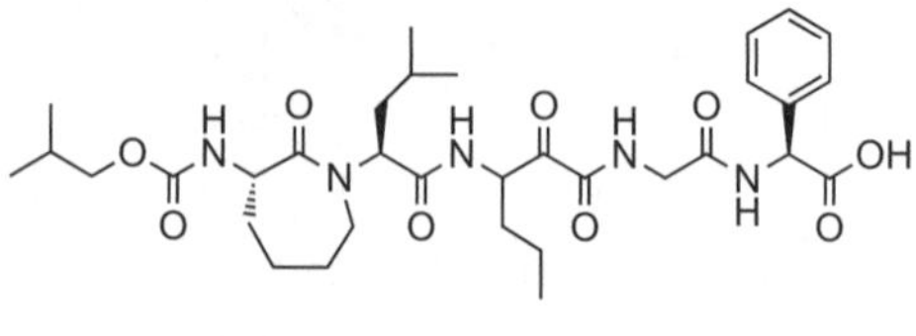

16 Ki* = 42000 nM, EC_{90} = > 5 μM

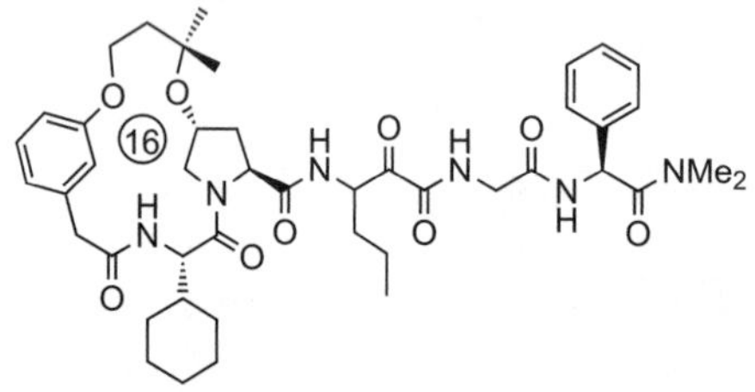

17 Ki* = 6 nM, EC_{90} = 0.9 μM

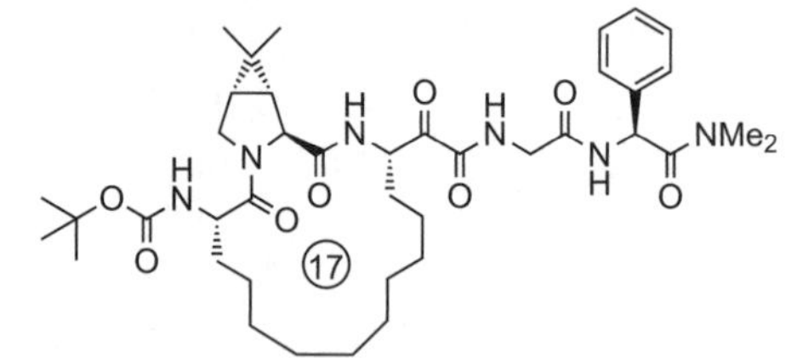

18 Ki* = 6 nM, EC_{90} = 0.6 μM

Scheme 12.4 Depeptization and macrocyclization strategy.

linear depeptized analogs did give rise to some inhibitors with reasonably good potency, but their PK profiles did not show marked improvement even at the cost of lowered potency.

12.4.2.3 Macrocyclization Strategy

Cyclization or macrocyclization between different amino acid residues or between an amino acid and an end-capping group is another common depeptization strategy. The resulting cyclic structures are difficult to be recognized by peptidases, thus potentially deterring hydrolysis and improving PK properties. The X-ray crystal structures of the inhibitors bound to NS3 protease were examined carefully to design structures that would have better fit against the enzyme surface and pockets.

P2–P3 Macrocycles Starting from reasonably potent pentapeptide inhibitors such as **12** (Scheme 12.3) or **13** (Scheme 12.4), the P3 amino acid side chain was cyclized to the P2–P3 amide nitrogen through a 7-membered ring to give structures of type **16** [47]. Unfortunately, this compound was almost inactive with a K_i^* of 42000 nM. Obviously, the cyclization changed the conformation of the peptide chain and disrupted some important interactions with the enzyme.

P2–P4 Macrocycles On the other hand, in the X-ray structures of pentapeptide inhibitors such as compound **11**, the proximity between the P2 proline and the *i*-butyl capping group raised the possibility of connecting them with a linker. Several series of P2–P4 macrocyclic inhibitors were investigated [25,47,65,66]. Macrocycles were prepared from P2 *m*-tyrosine through either a biphenyl ether linker or an alkyl phenyl ether linker cyclizing to P3 capping [66]. Some of the above mentioned inhibitors had moderate activities in the enzyme assay with K_i^* in the range of 100–900 nM. However, they were not potent enough to be explored further. In another series of P2–P4 macrocyclic inhibitors, 15- to 18-membered macrocycles were prepared from the P2 4-hydroxyl proline. One example is compound **17**, in which a *tert*-alkyl ether linkage connects the C4 hydroxyl of P2 proline to phenylacetamide moiety (P4) [67]. The X-ray structure demonstrated that the 16-membered macrocyclic ring formed a doughnut-shaped circle over the methyl group of protein backbone Ala156. This compound exhibited excellent potency ($K_i^* = 6$ nM) in the enzyme assay and also demonstrated moderate activity in the replicon assay ($EC_{90} = 0.90$ μM) which was lacking in many large peptide inhibitors so far. When evaluated for rat PK with oral dosing (10 mg kg^{-1}), **17** had a moderate AUC of 0.46 μM h, but a low bioavailability of only 2%.

P1–P3 Macrocycles The close proximity of the P1 and P3 side chains revealed by the X-ray structures of the early cleavage product derived peptide inhibitors bound to the protease had inspired the discovery of a number of P1–P3 macrocyclic inhibitors, including BILN-2061 (**1**). By cyclizing the P1 and P3 residues with a suitable linker, some of the resulting inhibitors demonstrated excellent potency in both enzyme and cell-based assays. Compound **18** was one of the early pentapeptide derivatives incorporating a 17-membered ring [68], and the more elaborated optimized dimethylcyclopropyl-proline P2 residue (see more details in P2 optimization section). As an added benefit of macrocyclization, the conformation of the macrocycle stabilized the α-center of the ketoamide, making it less likely to epimerize as evidenced by the resistance to racemize in the presence of a base. Thus, **18** was tested as a single diastereomer at P1 α-center, in contrast to the fact that other inhibitors were tested as a mixture of two P1 diastereomers. Compound **18** had an excellent potency in enzyme assay with a K_i^* of 6 nM. It also had good activity in cellular replicon assay with an EC_{90} of 0.6 μM. Despite excellent antiviral activities achieved by some macrocyclic inhibitors described earlier, they lacked the desired replicon potency and PK profile needed for further development.

12.4.3 Individual Amino Acid Residue Modifications

12.4.3.1 P2 Residue Optimization While the truncation and depeptization efforts were continued, modification and optimization of each individual amino acid residue were also carried out at the same time. Compound **19** was a dimethylamide analog of compound **13** (Table 12.1). Our structure–activity relationship studies had demonstrated that, in general, P2′ dimethylamide analogs were more potent in the replicon assay and gave better PK, presumably because they were less polar neutral molecules that possessed better cellular permeability. Compound **19** had no activity in cell-based replicon assay. However, when the P2 nitrogen was methylated [69], the resulting analog (**20**) demonstrated moderate activity in the replicon assay ($EC_{90} = 0.95$ μM), although the K_i^* was similar to that of **19**. This indicated that the proton on this amide bond was not involved in any important hydrogen bonding, and that the additional interaction provided by this methyl group was crucial for replicon activity. Analysis of the X-ray structure indicated that this methyl group was oriented to the same side of the P2 cyclopropyl methyl side chain. This fact prompted us to cyclize the methyl to the P2 side chain, which essentially led to the substituted proline for the P2 position. We learned earlier that the analog with a nonsubstituted proline as P2 had very weak activity (**11**, $K_i^* = 10000$ nM). By substituting proline with the 4,4-dimethyl groups and changing the P3 cyclohexylglycine to *tert*-butyl glycine, the resulting inhibitor **21** gave a good K_i^* of 36 nM. Not deterred by the fact that compound **21** did not have any cellular activity, prolines with larger substituents were investigated. The compound (**22**)

TABLE 12.1 P2 Residue Modifications

Compound	P2	R[1]	K_i^a (μM)	EC_{90} (μM)
19			50	>5.0
20			60	0.95
21		Me	36	>5.0
22		Me	19	2.0
23		Me	15	0.9
24*			5	0.1

[a]Compound **24** has a *t*-Boc P3 capping instead of *i*-Boc capping.

with a 4-*tert*-butyloxy proline P2 had an improved K_i^* of 19 nM. More importantly, it had some moderate replicon assay potency ($EC_{90} = 2\ \mu M$). Further elaboration of the substitution pattern led to the [3,3,1]-bicyclic P2 analog **23**, which not only exhibited better enzyme assay potency (K_i^* of 15 nM), but also gave improved cellular activity (EC_{90} of 0.9 μM). The bicyclic P2 was further optimized by reducing the ring size to a *gem*-dimethyl substituted cyclopropyl proline. With the concurrent evolution of moieties at other positions, for example, the *i*-Boc P3 capping group was changed to a *t*-Boc group, and P1 norvaline was changed back to cyclopropyl alanine, compound **24** (SCH 6) emerged as the final and best pentapeptide inhibitor [69]. It was dramatically more potent than its other linear pentapeptide analogs in both enzyme ($K_i^* = 5$ nM) and cellular assays ($EC_{90} = 0.1\ \mu M$).

The X-ray structure of **24** bound to the HCV protease demonstrated that the improvement in binding potency was probably a result of favorable interaction of the P2 *gem*-dimethylcyclopropylproline moiety with the methyl side chain of Ala-156 (Figure 12.4) [69]. The dimethylcyclopropyl group adopted a bent conformation, placing the two methyl groups in close proximity to Arg-155. However, compound **24** was still a large molecule with a MW of 725 [52], which may have been responsible for its poor PK profile in rats and monkeys. When dosed orally, it had an AUC of 0.35 μM h at 10 mg kg^{-1} with a bioavailability of 4% in rats, and an AUC of 0.03 μM h at 3 mg kg^{-1} with a bioavailability of 1% in monkeys. Clearly, to achieve desirable PK properties, further modifications such as reduction in molecular weight were needed. Nonetheless, **24** served as a lead compound for further SAR development. The most important achievement during this P2 optimization exercise was the discovery of the novel and unique new P2 moiety. The *gem*-dimethylcyclopropylproline was demonstrated to be a superior P2 residue, and it was used as the P2 of choice throughout further SAR investigations.

12.4.3.2 Tripeptides and Primary Amides

In a pentapeptide compound such as **25** (Table 12.2), which was a close analog of lead compound **24**, all remaining residues on the nonprime side were making important contributions to potency. Additional truncation efforts were then focused on the prime side. As the first step, the P2′ phenylglycine dimethylamide was converted to a benzyl group (**26**). Ki* changed from 10 nM for pentapeptide **25** to 56 nM for tetrapeptide **26**. Similarly, activity in the replicon assay

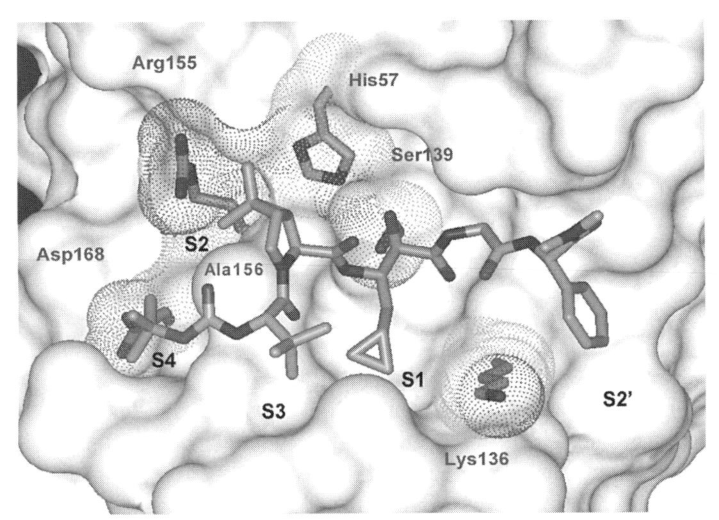

Figure 12.4 X-ray crystal structure of compound **24** (SCH-6) bound to HCV NS3 protease. (See color version of the figure in Color Plate section)

TABLE 12.2 Truncation from Pentapeptide to Tripeptide and Discovery of Primary Ketomide

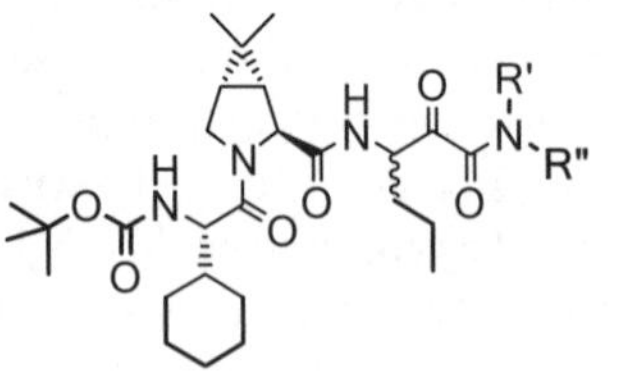

Compound	NR′R″	K_i^* (nM)	EC_{90} (μM)	Rat AUC (μM h)[a]
25[a]	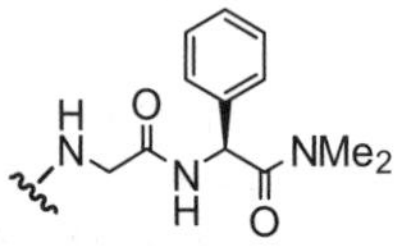 NH–CH2–C(O)–NH–CH(Ph)–C(O)NMe2	10	0.2	–
26	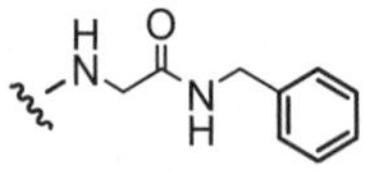 NH–CH2–C(O)–NH–CH2Ph	56	>1.0	–
27	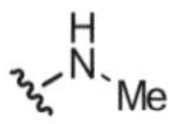 NHMe	1500	–	13
28	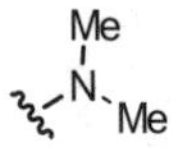 NMe2	>13000	–	–
29	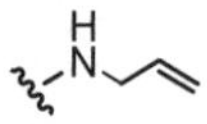 NH–CH2CH=CH2	280	>1.0	26
30	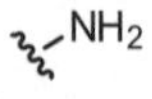 NH2	100	>1.0	2.5

[a]Compound 25 has an *i*-Boc P3 capping instead of a *t*-Boc capping.

[b]Rat PK AUC from 10 mpk oral dosing.

decreased from an EC_{90} of 0.2 μM to greater than 1 μM. At this stage, K_i^* was used as the sole tool to perform the truncation exercise and optimization process. Next, the P1′ glycine was replaced by alkyl groups with different characteristics such as short or long strait chains, saturated or unsaturated chains, aromatic substituted, small cyclic alkyls, etc. [46]. The secondary amides with a saturated alkyl group on the nitrogen, exemplified by compound **27** (K_i^* = 1500 nM), were significantly less potent than either tetrapeptide **26** or pentapeptide **25**. Not surprisingly, with two substituents on nitrogen, all tertiary ketoamides, such as compound **28** ($K_i^* > 13000$ nM), were basically inactive. However, when a small group with some sp^2-character, such as an allyl or cyclopropyl group, was put on the nitrogen, decent activity was observed. For example, allyl ketoamide analog **29** had a respectable K_i^* of 280 nM in the enzyme assay. Interestingly, it also had excellent PK in rats with a PO AUC of 26 μM h, far superior than that of most of its larger analogs. The most important finding in this round of truncation was the discovery of the primary amide. It was discovered that nonsubstituted primary ketoamides had better potency in the enzyme assay than most secondary and tertiary amides. At a MW of about 500, compound **30** demonstrated a good K_i^* of 100 nM, which was superior to all other substituted tripeptides such as **27**, **28,** and **29**. As expected, the rat oral exposure for the primary amide **30** was substantially lower than allyl amide **29** and methyl amide **27**, but at 2.5 μM h, it was very respectable. Although it did not possess any replicon potency at this stage, it definitely would serve as a good starting point for the search of the best tripeptide NS3 protease inhibitor. The selectivity HNE/HCV ratio for compound **30** was only 3, which meant that this number had to be improved significantly (see Section 12.3.4) in further SAR development.

12.4.3.3 P1 Side Chain Investigation Now that we had demonstrated the feasibility of a tripeptide as the lead structural type to optimize potency and PK properties, it was time to investigate the SAR at different parts of the molecule. The dimethylcyclopropylproline moiety had been established as the best P2 residue, it was incorporated in all inhibitors prepared in subsequent studies. From an analysis of the X-ray structure of the protease, the S1 pocket was small and had a hydrophobic surface. It was thus appropriate to put a series of small alkyl or cycloalkyl groups at this position (Table 12.3). With *tert*-Boc-capped cyclohexylglycine P3 and primary ketoamide, compounds **31** through **36** represent various P1 moieties that were examined. The α-carbon bearing the P1 side chain was adjacent to the electrophilic ketoamide moiety where Ser-139 of the enzyme attacks to form a covalent bond. The α-proton is fairly acidic, making this center readily epimerizable. If this α-center was made quaternary, then the potential for epimerization would be eliminated. Compound **31** incorporates a spirocyclopropyl P1 α-center. Unfortunately, it did not have any appreciable activity in the enzyme assay. The complete loss of potency could be a result of the difficulty for serine-139 to attack the sterically more hindered ketoamide functionality. The lack of activity of quaternary P1 analog prompted us to concentrate on monosubstituted P1 residues.

Since compound **30** had no cellular activity and poor selectivity, it was decided to try a few slightly larger alkyl or cycloalkyl groups such as isobutyl, cyclopropylmethyl, cyclobutylmethyl, cyclopentylmethyl, and trifluoropropyl groups. Apparently, the isobutyl group was not as good a fit as the *n*-propyl group because compound **32** ($K_i^* = 280$ nM) was almost threefold less active as compound **30**. However, when a cyclopropylmethyl P1 side chain was incorporated, a much improved inhibitor was obtained. Compound **33** had a very good K_i^* of 25 nM, and an even more impressive cellular potency (EC_{90}) of 0.4 μM. The selectivity (HNE/HCV) was also enhanced to 23. Equally impressive was the cyclobutylmethyl group in compound **34**, which had excellent K_i^* of 8 nM and EC_{90} of 0.7 μM. Although the replicon activity was slightly less than that of **33**, the selectivity margin was dramatically enhanced to 138. The 5-membered ring analog, **35**, however, lost potency in the enzyme and replicon assays gained in compounds **33** and **34**. It had a K_i^* of 150 nM and an EC_{90} of greater than 1 μM. However, it did give a high selectivity of 370. A trifluoropropyl group is slightly more hydrophobic than an *n*-propyl group and this effect was reflected in the improvement of potency of compound **36** compared to that of **30**: a twofold improvement of the K_i^* to 50 nM and improved replicon activity (EC_{90}) of 0.7 μM. The two compounds, however, had similar low selectivity (HNE/HCV = 2–3). The results from this

TABLE 12.3 P1 Side Chain SAR Investigation

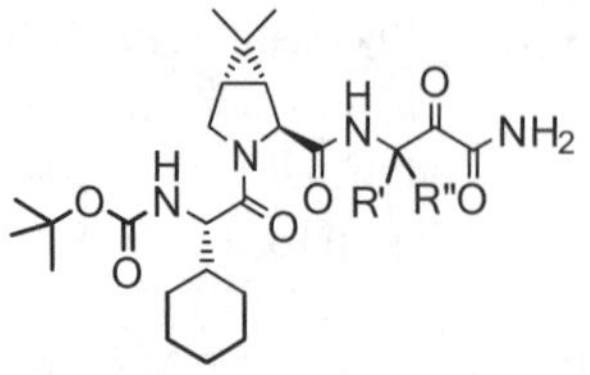

Compound	R′R″	K_i^* (nM)	EC_{90} (μM)	HNE/HCV
31		>13000	–	–
32	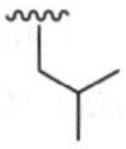	280	>1.0	–
33	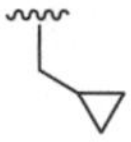	25	0.4	23
34	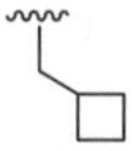	8	0.7	138
35	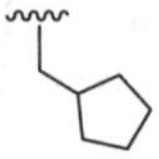	150	>1.0	370
36	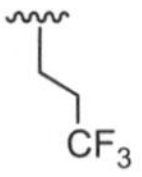 CF_3	50	0.7	2

series of P1 modifications clearly indicated that isobutyl and cyclopentylmethyl groups were too large to be accommodated in the S1 pocket, while the cyclopropylmethyl and cyclobutylmethyl groups were the best fit for the small space. It was also clear that larger P1 side chains provided higher selectivity against elastase. When both potency and selectivity were considered, cyclopropyl- and cyclobutyl-alanine appeared to be the best residues for the P1 position.

12.4.3.4 P3 Residue Modifications

P3 Side Chain Modifications The NS3 protease has a shallow and hydrophobic S3 pocket which is occupied by isoleucine in the natural substrate. The types of P3 residues that can be accommodated at this site are fairly limited. Our early studies revealed that polar

TABLE 12.4 P3 Residue Optimizations

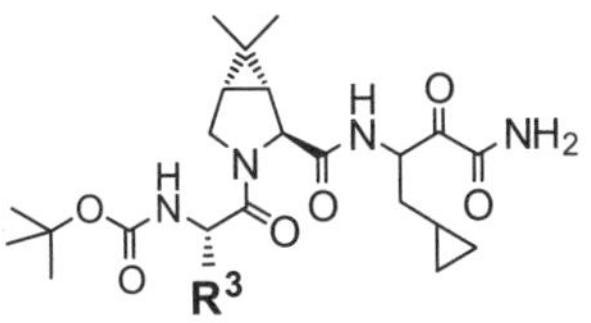

Compound	R^3	K_i^* (nM)	EC_{90} (μM)	HNE/HCV
37	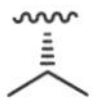	210	>1.0	19
38	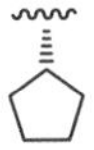	100	>1.0	11
39	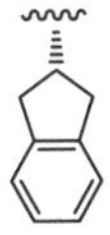	82	>1.0	50
40	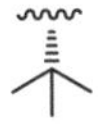	57	0.6	110

groups were not tolerated at all. Thus, only a small list of branched alkyl, and cycloalkyl P3 side chains were explored. Examples include compounds **37** to **40** (Table 12.4) [46,47]. Cyclopropylalanine was employed as the P1 residue.

Reducing the size of the cyclohexylglycine in **33** to valine at the P3 position resulted in inhibitor **37** with a K_i^* of 210 nM, an eightfold loss in activity, even though the selectivity (HNE/HCV) remained the same at about 19. If the isopropyl group in valine was too small to provide sufficient hydrophobic contact, the larger cyclopentane P3 side chain should have more contacts with the surface and thus better potency. Indeed, this analog (**38**) had a K_i^* of 100 nM, a twofold improvement over the valine derivative **37**, but still substantially less potent than cyclohexyl analog **33**. The selectivity of **38** against elastase was about half of that of **33**. Both compounds **37** and **38** did not show any activity in the replicon assay up to 1 μM. The loss of potency in compounds **37** and **38** compared to **33** could probably be attributed to less extensive van der Waals interactions between the P3 side chain and the enzyme surface. In an attempt to achieve more interactions, indanylglycine, which is larger and longer than cyclohexylglycine, was introduced as P3 residue in compound **39**. However, the K_i^* went up more than threefold to 82 nM. It also lost activity in the cellular assay (EC_{90} > 1 μM), although it did achieve higher selectivity. Presumably, the phenyl group of the indanylglycine moiety extended too far and caused some unfavorable interactions against the protein backbone. On the other hand, when the bulkier *tert*-butylglycine was incorporated as P3, the resulting inhibitor **40** was significantly better than the other three P3 alternatives. It had a K_i^* of 57 nM, which was only twofold less potent than **33**. But more importantly, it demonstrated good cellular activity with an EC_{90} of 0.60 μM, just slightly less than that of **33**. In addition, it had good selectivity of 110, much better than that for **33**. In summary, the P3 residue SAR study demonstrated that inhibitors with *tert*-butyl and cyclohexyl P3 side chains (**40** and **33**, respectively) were the most active in both enzyme and replicon assays, the former was more selective against elastase while the later was slightly more potent.

Optimization of P3-Capping Analysis of the X-ray structure of the NS3 protease surface revealed that P3 capping groups such as the *t*-Boc group were occupying the S4 pocket, and that there was more space and functionality in the pocket for the P3 cap to interact with. More binding could potentially be obtained with P3 cap incorporating different functionalities. To explore this possibility, a number of moieties were examined as potential P3 capping groups [46,47], and some representative examples are shown in Table 12.5 (compounds **41** to **46**). In this SAR investigation, *tert*-butylglycine was retained as the P3 moiety because of its ability to provide higher selectivity against elastase. Cyclopropylalanine was kept as the P1 residue.

In all the inhibitors discussed earlier, the capping groups were bonded to the P3 residue through a carbamate functionality such as the *i*-Boc or *t*-Boc P3 cappings. In this study, a number of alkyl groups other than *iso*- or *tert*-butyl groups were evaluated in carbamates. A cyclopropyl group is small and has some π-characteristics. Its carbamate-capped inhibitor **41** had a K_i^* of 300 nM, indicating that a small sp^2-character bearing moiety was not a good fit for the S4 pocket. The slightly larger isopropyl carbamate-capped derivative **42** faired somewhat better with a K_i^* of 150 nM, but it was still threefold less potent than the *tert*-butyl analog **40**, although the selectivity was maintained at the same level. The results from compounds **41** and **42** imply that smaller alkyl carbamates do not provide sufficient interaction with the protein to improve potency. Attention was then turned to carbamate analogs derived from larger alkyl groups. One example is compound **43**, which is capped by a 1-methylcyclohexyl carbamate. It turned out to be an excellent inhibitor with significant improvements on both potency and selectivity. The compound had a K_i^* of 13 nM, an impressive replicon EC_{90} of 0.23 μM and high selectivity of 390. It was very gratifying to observe that all three important parameters were improved three- to fourfold over those of reference compound **40**.

With the encouraging results from the carbamate investigation, it was natural to expand the scope of the SAR studies in this region. Cappings with other functionalities were tested. One example was to change the carbonyl group in the carbamate to a sulfonyl group. The resulting *tert*-butyl sulfonyl urea derivative **44** was prepared. Unfortunately, it lost most of the activity in the enzyme assay to a K_i^* of 1000 nM. Simple amide capping groups were also examined, and they were also ineffective. Parallel to the carbamate SAR development, a number of urea-capped inhibitors were also investigated. The two urea-capped compounds that corresponded to the two best carbamates (**40** and **43**) were prepared (compounds **45** and **46**). We were delighted to see that the *tert*-butyl urea analog **45** achieved significant improvement in all three measures compared to **40**: K_i^* (13 nM), EC_{90} (0.4 μM) and selectivity (HNE/HCV = 370). The 1-methylcyclohexyl urea-capped inhibitor **46**, as expected from the trend seen in carbamates, was indeed very active in the enzymatic assay with a K_i^* of 22 nM and had excellent potency in cell-based replicon assay with an EC_{90} of 0.27 μM, which was one of the best value that had ever been achieved in this assay. This compound also possessed excellent selectivity of 470 against elastase. Based on the results from these P3 capping studies, in general, the urea-capped inhibitors appeared to be more potent and selective than their corresponding carbamate analogs. Larger alkyl or cycloalkyl groups were better than smaller ones. But the compounds with larger

TABLE 12.5 P3 Capping SAR Development

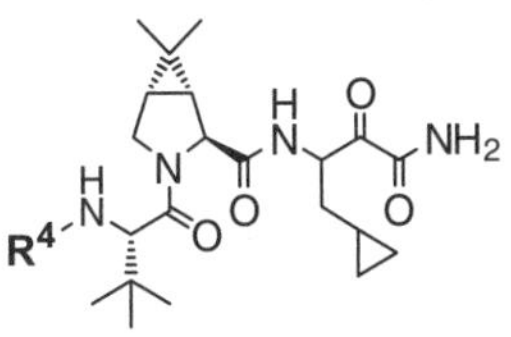

Compound	R^4	K_i^* (nM)	EC_{90} (μM)	HNE/HCV
41	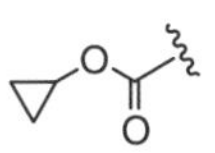	300	>1.0	–
42	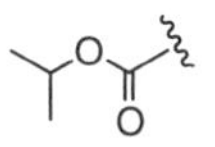	150	>1.0	100
43	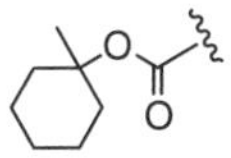	13	0.23	390
44	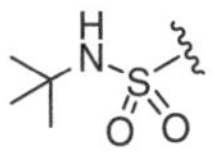	1000	>1.0	–
45	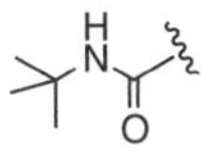	13	0.4	370
46	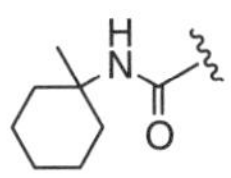	22	0.27	470

and more substituted capping groups such as 1-methylcyclohexyl carbamate or urea-capped analogs **43** and **46** usually gave poor results in rat PK studies. The *tert*-butyl urea or *tert*-butyl carbamate cappings were then the preferred cappings because of the balance of good potency, high selectivity, and reasonable PK profiles.

12.4.4 Correlations Between P1, P3, and P3 Capping: The Identification of Boceprevir

In the study of the effect of the modification of individual residues at various positions, we discovered that changes made at one position would affect the contribution from other

TABLE 12.6 Synergistic Effect Between P1, P3, and P3 Capping Groups and Discovery of Boceprevir

Compound	X	R^3	R^1	K_i^* (nM)	EC_{90} (μM)	HNE/HCV
47	O			76	0.8	680
48	NH			50	0.8	40
49	NH			50	0.5	90
2 Boceprevir	NH			14	0.35	2200

residues, that is, the individual modifications were not additive to each other. They might be synergistic in some cases, and antagonistic in other cases. Some interesting correlations between the potency and selectivity were observed. The synergistic effects between P1 and P3, P3 and P3 capping were among the most obvious [46,47]. For example, in a pair of compounds with a *t*-Boc capping and a cyclopropylalanine P1 (**33** and **40**), the analog bearing a cyclohexylglycine P3 had better enzyme activity (**33**, $K_i^* = 25$ nM) than the analog containing *tert*-butylglycine P3 (**40**, $K_i^* = 57$ nM). However, in a second pair of compounds with a *tert*-butyl urea capping and a cyclopropylalanine P1 (**48** and **45**) (Tables 12.5 and 12.6), the derivative with a cyclohexylglycine P3 (**48**, $K_i^* = 50$ nM) was found to be less potent than the *tert*-butylglycine P3 derivative (**45**, $K_i^* = 13$ nM). A similar trend was also observed in the two pairs with a cyclobutylalanine P1. Thus, comparing the pair with a *t*-Boc capping (**34** and **47**), the P3 cyclohexylglycine analog (**34**, $K_i^* = 8$ nM) was more potent than the P3 *tert*-butylglycine analog (**47**, $K_i^* = 76$ nM), while in the pair with a *tert*-butyl urea capping (**49** and **2**), the P3 cyclohexylglycine inhibitor (**49**, $K_i^* = 50$ nM) was less active than P3 *tert*-butylglycine derivative (**2**, $K_i^* = 14$ nM). The interesting phenomenon of the reversal of the activity from *t*-Boc to *tert*-butyl urea capping could not be explained by the X-ray structures of these compounds bound to the NS3 protease.

Another intriguing correlation was observed on the effect of pairing between P1 and P3 residues on the selectivity against human neutrophil elastase (HNE/HCV). A close examination of four pairs of inhibitors (**33**,**34**, **40**,**45**,**47**,**48**,**49**, and **2**) revealed that in a given pair of compounds with the same P3 and P3 capping, for example, **33** versus **34**, the analog with a cyclobutylalanine P1 (**34**, HNE/HCV = 138) was always more selective against elastase than the one with a cyclopropylalanine P1 (**33**, HNE/HCV = 23). The same was true in other three pairs, that is, **40** versus **47**,**48** versus **49**, and **45** versus **2**. On the other hand, in the pairs containing the same P1 residue and P3 capping, for example, **48** versuss **45**, inhibitors bearing a *tert*-butylglycine P3 (**45**, HNE/HCV = 370) were almost always more selective than their counterparts with a cyclohexylglycine P3 (**48**, HNE/HCV = 40). The same was also true in other three pairs, that is, **33** versus. **40**,**34** versus **47**, and **49** versus **2**.

Ultimately, it was gratifying that the combination of the *tert*-butyl urea capping, the *tert*-butylglycine P3, the cyclobutylalanine P1, and our unique and superior P2 residue gave rise to an inhibitor (**2**, boceprevir) that was selected for further preclinical and clinical development.

12.5 PROFILE OF BOCEPREVIR

12.5.1 *In Vitro* Characterization of Boceprevir

After thorough optimization at all positions of the molecule, the most potent and selective inhibitor **2** (SCH 503034, boceprevir) was selected as the clinical candidate based on its overall profile. In the HCV NS3 protease continuous assay, it had a potency of 14 nM (K_i^*) averaged over a large number of runs. In the 72-h subgenomic (genotype 1b) cell-based replicon assay in HuH-7 cells, the EC_{50} and EC_{90} values were determined to be 0.20 μM and 0.35 μM, respectively.

Since compound **2** contained an electrophilic α-ketoamide functionality which was susceptible to attack by a variety of activated nucleophiles present in many proteases and esterases, it was screened against various enzymes and proteins to examine its reactivity and selectivity toward other nucleophiles. It was found to be a very weak inhibitor ($K_i = 26$ μM) of human neutrophil elastase (a structurally closely related protease), representing a selectivity of 2200. No time dependence, suggestive of slow binding, was observed in the assay against elastase. The reactivity of **2** toward a panel of other serine proteases was measured and showed no cross-reactivity when tested up to 50 μM with trypsin, chymotrypsin, thrombin, or factor Xa. The cross-reactivity against a broad panel of other general enzymes was also evaluated. Only four enzymes were identified with weak cross-reactivity: human cathepsin B ($IC_{50} = 10.2 \pm 0.3$ μM, $n = 2$), cathepsin G ($IC_{50} = 2.2 \pm 1.1$ μM, $n = 2$), cathepsin L ($IC_{50} = 9.6 \pm 0.8$ μM, $n = 2$), and rat hepatic acyl CoA-cholesterol acyltransferase ($IC_{50} = 1.7 \pm 0.5$ μM, $n = 2$). However, in a separate cross-over study, compound **2** was shown to be inactive toward human adrenal acyl CoA-cholesterol acyltransferase with an $IC_{50} > 20$ μM. All of these studies indicated that (**2**) was highly selective toward the HCV serine protease. The α-ketoamide functionality was not reactive toward almost all other common known nucleophiles.

12.5.2 Pharmacokinetics of Boceprevir

Compound **2** was evaluated in several animal species (mouse, rat, dog, and monkey) to establish its pharmacokinetic profile (Table 12.7). With oral administration

TABLE 12.7 Pharmacokinetic Parameters of 2

Animal species	Mouse	Rat	Dog	Monkey
Dose (mg kg^{-1})	10	10	3	3
IV AUC (μM h)	2.7	5.9	5.8[a]	2.9
PO AUC (μM h)	0.93	1.5	3.1	0.12
Bioavailability (%)	34	26	30	4
C_{max} (μM)	2.3	0.66	2.3	0.09

[a]Dog PK IV dosing at 1.7 mg kg^{-1}.

(mean, $n = 3$) at specified doses (10 mg kg^{-1} in mouse and rats, and 3 mg kg^{-1} in dogs and monkeys), the observed AUCs were good in rats and dogs (1.5 and 3.1 μM h, respectively), moderate in mice (0.93 μM h) and poor in monkeys (0.12 μM h). The oral bioavailabilities were modest in mouse (34%), rats (26%), and dogs (30%) but low in monkeys (4%). The compound had no inhibition of CYPs 2D6, 2C9, 2C19 at greater 20 μM, either co- or preincubated. It had a weak inhibition of CYP3A4 with an IC50 of 8.5 μM when preincubated, which was considered not a concern at this range. Target organ analysis in rats 6 h after oral dosing revealed that **2** was highly concentrated in the liver, with a liver/plasma concentration ratio of 30.

12.5.3 The Interaction of Boceprevir with NS3 Protease

All the interactions between compound **2** and the NS3 protease were revealed in the X-ray structure of **2** bound to the enzyme (Figure 12.5). Clearly, the diastereomer with the (*S*)-configuration at the P1 α-center was the active inhibitor. The cyclobutylalanine P1 residue occupied most of the space available in the S1 pocket. This moiety made a large contribution to the excellent selectivity of **2** against human neutrophil elastase

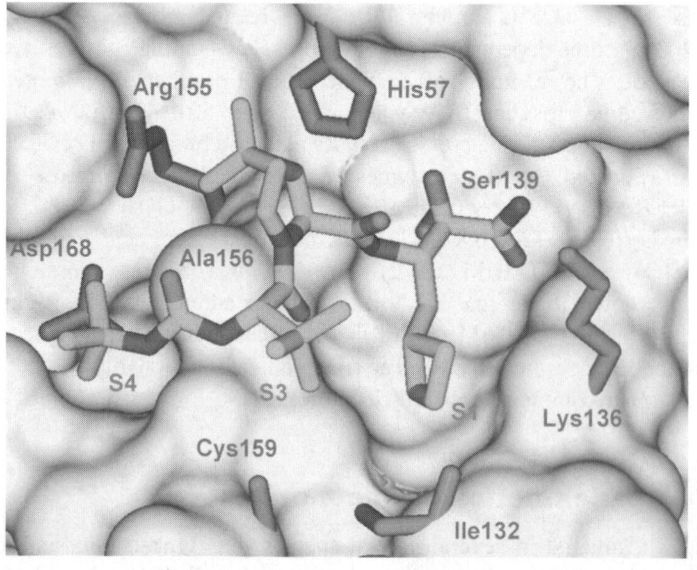

Figure 12.5 X-Ray structure of boceprevir bound to the NS3 protease.

(HNE/HCV = 2200), which has a much smaller S1 pocket [70]. A bent conformation was adopted by the P2 dimethylcyclopropylproline residue allowing maximum overlap of this moiety with Ala-156 of the protease, with the *exo*-methyl on the cyclopropane ring interacting favorably with the imidazole of the His-57 residue, and the *endo*-methyl making contact with both the Ala-156 and Arg-155 residues. At the P3 site, the *tert*-butyl side chain occupies the S3 pocket, having strong hydrophobic interaction with the surface. In the urea P3 capping group, the *tert*-butyl group extended into the S4 pocket and made good hydrophobic interactions with the underlying residue. As expected, the "war head" ketoamide formed a reversible covalent bond with active site Ser-139. It also formed a hydrogen bond with one of the backbone residues. In addition to hydrophobic van der Waals type interactions, compound **2** also formed several hydrogen bonds with the protein backbone. The functionalities involved in these hydrogen bonds were P1–NH, P3–carbonyl, and both urea NHs. It was evident that all these hydrophobic interactions and hydrogen bonds made important contributions toward the excellent potency and high selectivity of compound **2**.

12.6 CLINICAL DEVELOPMENT AND APPROVAL OF BOCEPREVIR

As a novel, potent, highly selective, orally bioavailable α-ketoamide HCV NS3 protease inhibitor, boceprevir was progressed through preclinical toxicology studies, and phase I first-in-human safety evaluations. It was safe and well tolerated. In the subsequent 14 days, phase Ib proof-of-concept trial, boceprevir (400 mg TID (three times daily)) in combination with PEG-Intron treatment in previously treated-but-failed genotype 1 patients delivered a mean 2.8 $\log_{10}$ viral load reduction [71,72]. In a phase II trial (SPRINT-1), patients treated with boceprevir (800 mg TID) for 48 weeks in combination with PEG-Intron and ribavirin regimens demonstrated SVR rates of 67 to 75% compared with SVR rates of 38% in the control arm [29].

Two phase III clinical trials, SPRINT-2 and RESPOND-2, have been completed recently in patients with difficult-to-treat genotype 1 HCV [73,74]. In SPRINT-2 trials of treatment naïve patients, up to 66% of patients achieved SVR with triple combination therapy while only 38% of patients achieved SVR with SOC. In the RESPOND-2 study of previously treated-but-failed patients, again up to 66% achieved SVR with triple combination therapy while only 21% of those on SOC achieved SVR. These results demonstrated the superior efficacy of boceprevir containing triple combination therapy compared to SOC for the treatment of chronic hepatitis C viral infections. A New Drug Application (NDA) has been filed with the Food and Drug Administration (FDA) and European Medicines Agency (EMA) to market boceprevir as a new drug in combination with PEG-interferon and RBV. FDA and EMA have accepted the NDA and promised an expedited review of the application. Boceprevir was approved by FDA on May 13, 2011. It is marketed as Victrelis by Merck.

12.7 SYNTHESIS OF BOCEPREVIR

Boceprevir was racemic at the α-center of the P1 residue. The two diastereomeric compounds could be separated by HPLC. However, when either pure isomer was treated with an organic or inorganic base (e.g., triethyl amine or lithium hydroxide) they underwent rapid isomerization. Fast equilibration was also observed under the conditions of biological assays. This obviated any need for separation of the two entities for pharmacological evaluations. The ratio of the two isomers varied significantly depending on the experimental conditions. As expected, the isomer with the natural (*S*)-configuration at the P1 α-center was the active isomer; fortunately, it was also the major isomer in most cases.

The synthetic route for the preparation of boceprevir by discovery medicinal chemists has been reported [46] and is presented here. The final routes for process and manufacturing of the drug substance will not be discussed since it has not been published, but some related chemistry can be found in a patent [75]. The discovery synthetic route to compound **2** is outlined in Scheme 12.5. The diphenylamine derivative of glycine ethyl ester (**50**) was alkylated with cyclobutylmethyl bromide (**51**) in the presence of potassium *t*-butoxide to give racemic α-substituted glycine derivative **52**. After hydrolysis of diphenylamine using 1 M hydrochloric acid, the resulting amine was protected with a Boc group to provide compound **53**. This ester was hydrolyzed to its corresponding carboxylic acid, which was then converted to a Weinreb amide (**54**) through coupling to *N*, *O*-dimethylhydroxyamine. Reduction of **54** gave rise to an aldehyde **55** [76], which, upon treatment with acetone cyanohydrin, afforded cyanohydrin **56** [77]. Intermediate **56** could be directly hydrolyzed to the corresponding α-hydroxy primary amide using basic aqueous hydrogen peroxide [78]. The product was treated with 4 M HCl to remove the Boc protecting group to yield α-hydroxy-β-aminoamide **57** as a hydrochloride salt. An alternative method to convert **56** to **57** through a four-step sequence could also be employed. Thus, **56** was hydrolyzed to the corresponding α-hydroxy methyl ester using methanolic HCl. The lost *N*-Boc protecting group was put back on the nitrogen and the methyl ester was hydrolyzed to the carboxylic acid, which was converted to a primary amide through a coupling with ammonium chloride. Finally, removal of the Boc group using 4 M HCl provided the desired P1 intermediate **57**.

The synthesis of the P2 moiety started with benzylidine protected bicyclic lactam **58**, which was derived from pyroglutamic acid [79]. Phenylselenation of compound **58** was followed by oxidation of resulting intermediate selenide with aqueous hydrogen peroxide and subsequent elimination to provide α,β-unsaturated lactam **59** [79]. Isopropylphosphonium ylide addition to the unsaturated lactam was followed subsequent cyclization afforded the isopropylidine lactam derivative **60**. The reduction of this product with lithium aluminum hydride (LAH) resulted in the 3,4-dimethylcyclopropyl-*N*-benzylprolinol [80], which was converted to the corresponding Boc-protected prolinol (**61**) via catalytic hydrogenation in the presence of Boc anhydride. Jones oxidation of the alcohol was followed by esterification of the resultant acid with trimethylsilyl (TMS) diazomethane and the removal of the Boc-protecting group to yield the desired advanced P2 intermediate **62** as a hydrochloride salt. Coupling of **62** with the P3 amino acid, *N*-Boc-*tert*-leucine, using BOP as the coupling agent provided a dipeptide which was treated with 4 M HCl to take off the Boc-protecting group to afford the dipeptide intermediate **63** as a hydrochloride salt. Reaction of the amine **63** with *tert*-butyl isocyanate delivered the *tert*-butyl urea P3-capped dipeptide that, upon hydrolysis of the methyl ester using lithium hydroxide, gave the advanced P2–P3 intermediate **64**. This carboxylic acid was then coupled to the P1 amine piece **57** under standard conditions of HOBt and EDC to yield the α-hydroxyamide tripeptide **65**. This primary amide was successfully oxidized to the corresponding α-ketoamide **2** under modified Moffat oxidation conditions using EDC, DMSO, and dichloroacetic acid [81]. Although this synthetic route designed by the discovery team was lengthy and had a low overall yield, it served the purpose of bringing up enough material for early testing.

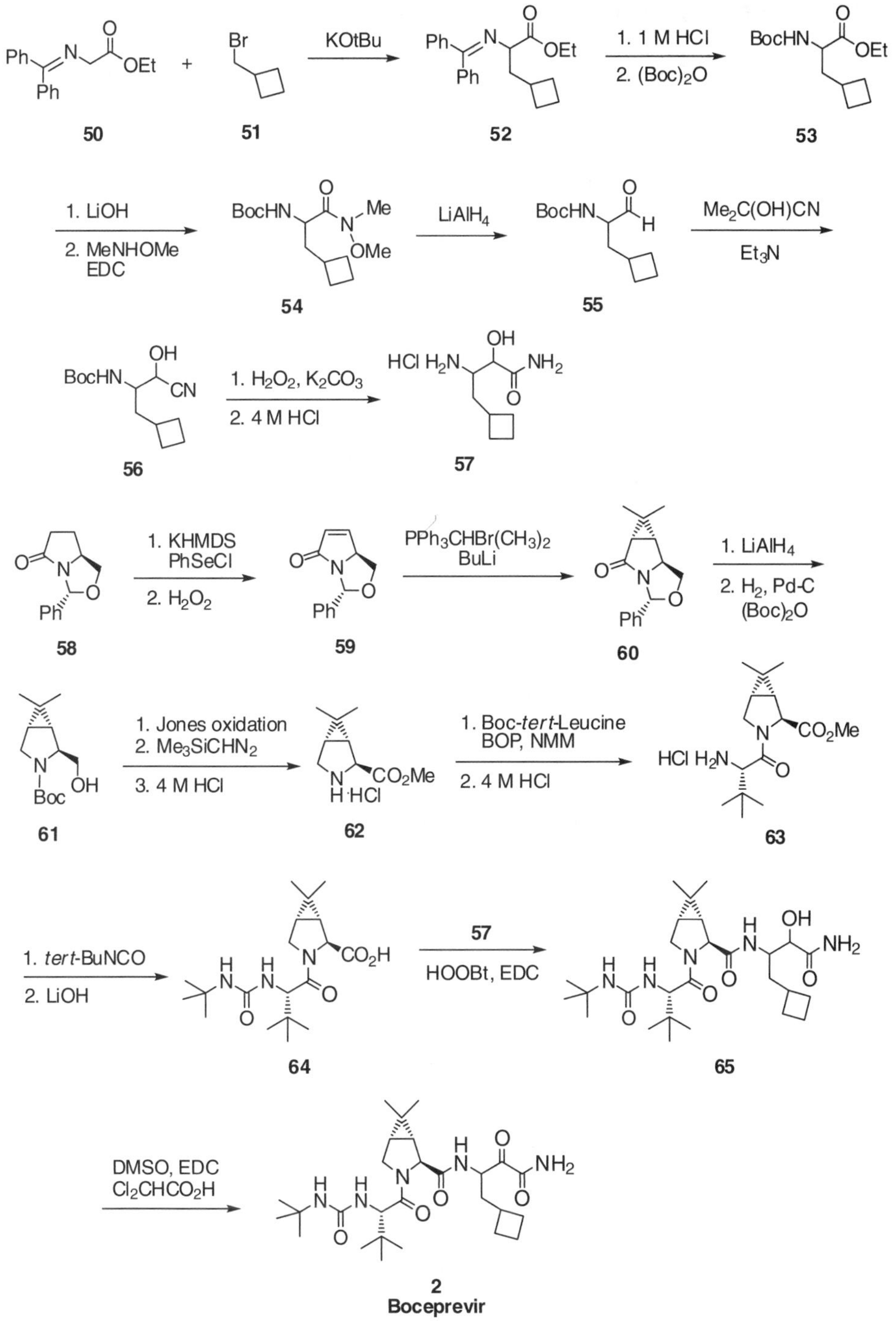

Scheme 12.5 Synthesis of boceprevir.

12.8 DISCOVERY OF NARLAPREVIR

12.8.1 Criteria for the Back-up Program of Boceprevir

With the recommendation of compound **2** (boceprevir) as the candidate for further preclinical and clinical development, search for a second-generation HCV NS3 protease inhibitor continued. The goal was to identify a candidate that had significantly improved (10-fold) *in vitro* potency, especially in the cell-based replicon assay, comparable PK profile in rats and dogs, and much better exposure in monkeys. Furthermore, to alleviate possible synthetic/purification issues that could arise during development, it was highly desirable to find a molecule that existed as a single isomer, unlike **2**, which was a mixture of two diastereomers at the P1 α-center.

12.8.2 SAR Studies

12.8.2.1 Extended P3 Cappings on Primary Ketoamides As discussed above, during earlier research that led to the discovery of boceprevir, extensive SAR development was conducted to optimize P′, P1, P2, P3, and the P3 capping moieties. Although incremental improvement was always possible through fine tuning at any of these sites, it was clear that major modifications at the P′, P1, P2, and P3 residues that could lead to significant enhancement in potency were probably difficult. Based on the X-ray crystal structure of **2** bound to the NS3 protease, there was plenty of room in the S4 and S5 pockets, and the extension of the P3 capping group into those areas seemed to be an attractive approach. Additional interactions with the enzyme surface or functional groups in those pockets could potentially improve potency. During the course of our original P3 capping SAR studies, the (*R*)-1-*tert*-butyl-ethylamine derived urea cap was found to be among the best. The X-ray structure indicated that the *tert*-butyl group extended into the S4 pocket, while the methyl group pointed toward the S5 pocket. This presented an opportunity for us to build additional moieties onto the methyl groups to improve binding affinity. Indeed, the capping groups derived from (*S*)-*tert*- leucinol or (*S*)-*tert*-leucine amine afforded inhibitors with significantly improved potency. Some examples representing a variety of structural types are shown in compounds **66** to **69** (Scheme 12.6). The P3 urea cap in **66** was an ethyl carbamate derived from (*S*)-*tert*-leucinol [82]. Together with the indanylglycine P3 and cyclobutylalanine P1, this compound had an enzyme assay K_i^* of 7 nM and cellular replicon assay EC_{90} of 0.1 μM, representing a 2- and 3.5-fold improvement, respectively, over boceprevir. The 4,4-dimethylglutaimide capping group, which was derived from (*S*)-*tert*-leucine amine, in compound **67** enhanced the potency in both enzyme and replicon assays even further to a K_i^* of 4 nM and an EC_{90} of 0.06 μM [83]. This was the first time ever the EC_{90} broke the 0.1 μM barrier. The thiophene sulfonamide cap from (*S*)-*tert*-leucine amine in compound **68**, combined with a P1–P3 16-membered macrocycle, also provided good enhancement in both K_i^* and EC_{90} (2 nM and 0.07 μM, respectively) [84], amounting to a more than fivefold improvement compared to boceprevir.

Previous P3 capping studies also demonstrated that 1-methylcyclohexyl carbamate or urea cappings delivered superior potency in replicon assay in inhibitors **43** and **46**. As in the case of *tert*-leucine amine derived analogs discussed earlier, the X-ray structure of these compounds revealed that the methyl group was pointing toward the direction of the S5 pocket while the cyclohexyl ring occupied the S4 pocket. Any substitution at the methyl group could extend into the S5 pocket. A number of alkyl and aryl substituents were introduced to the methyl group, with or without attachment of an additional functionality

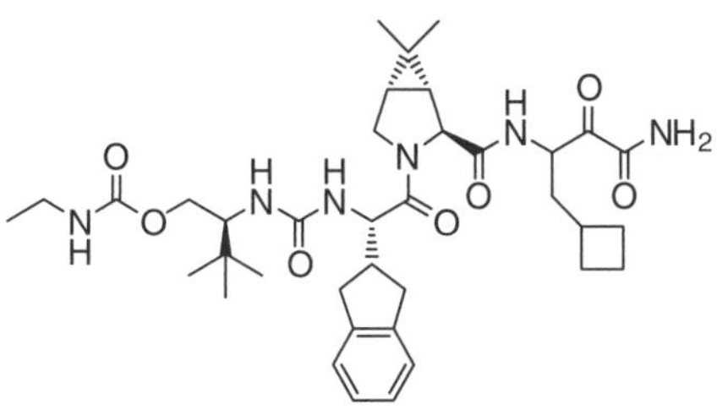

66 Ki* = 7 nM, EC_{90} = 0.1 μM

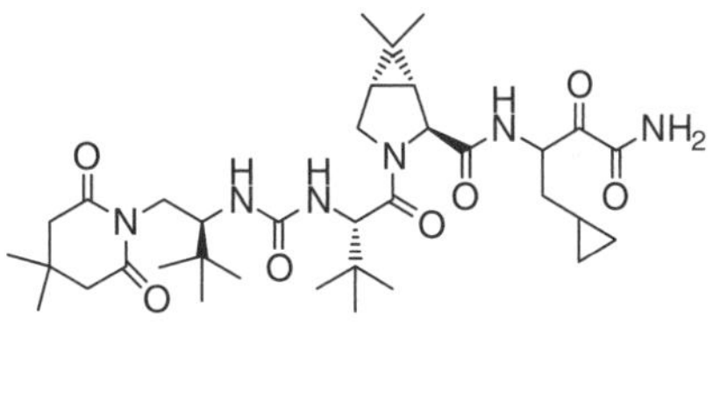

67 Ki* = 4 nM, EC_{90} = 0.06 μM

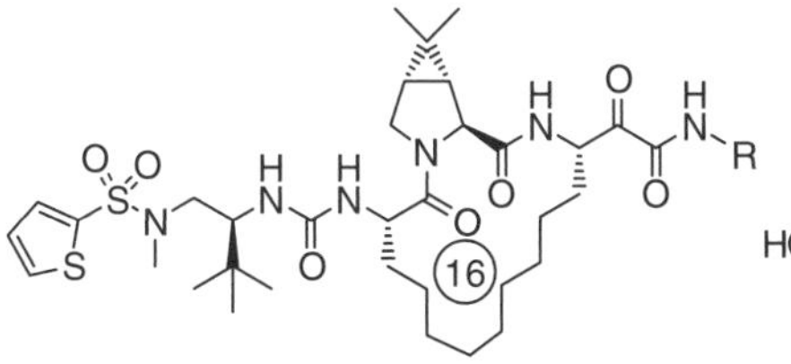

68 R = H, Ki* = 2 nM, EC_{90} = 0.07 μM
Rat PK AUC = 0.07 μM.h

69 R = allyl, Ki* = 2 nM, EC_{90} = 0.08 μM
Rat PK AUC = 1.3 μM.h

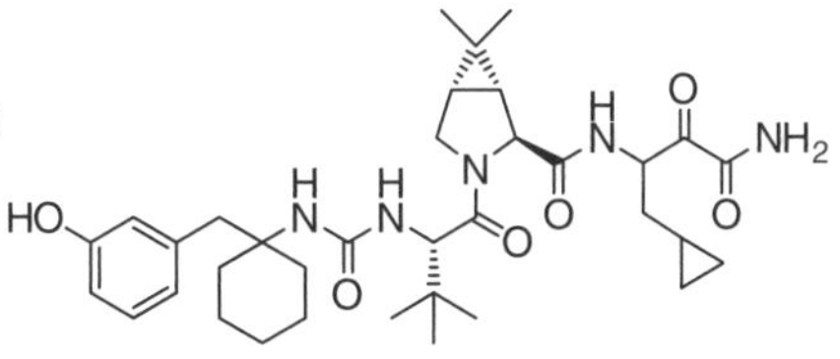

70 Ki* = 9 nM, EC_{90} = 0.07 μM

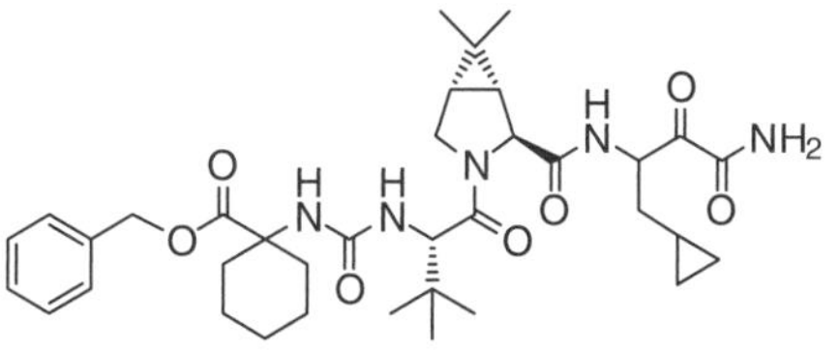

71 Ki* = 49 nM, EC_{90} = 0.02 μM

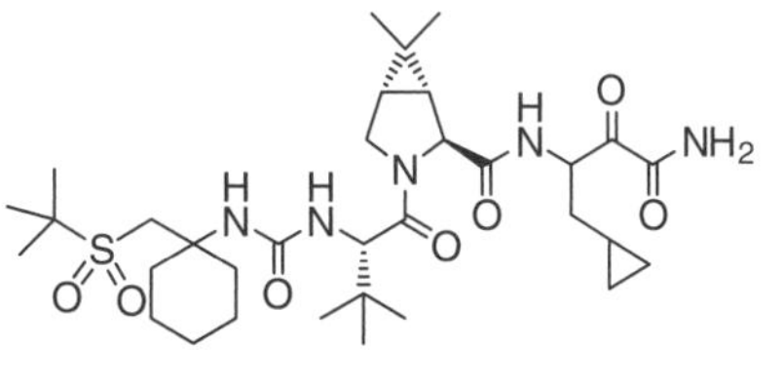

72 Ki* = 3 nM, EC_{90} = 0.08 μM
Rat PK AUC = 0.07 μM.h
Monkey PK AUC = 3.2 μM.h

Scheme 12.6 Primary ketoamide inhibitors with extended P3 cappings groups.

for potential hydrogen bonding [85,86]. Not surprisingly, most substituted compounds had better potency than their parent **46**. For example, the *m*-phenol substitution in analog **70** improved the enzyme potency ($K_i^* = 9$ nM) by more than twofold and the cellular activity by almost fourfold to an EC_{90} of 0.07 μM [85]. By incorporation of additional functionality, the ester analog **71** achieved even better replicon potency, $EC_{90} = 0.02$ μM, which was 13-fold more potent than **46** [86], although its K_i^* was somewhat worse. The *tert*-butyl sulfone substituted inhibitor **72** was also significantly more potent with a K_i^* of 3 nM and EC_{90} of 0.08 μM [85], representing sevenfold and threefold improvements, respectively.

12.8.2.2 Extended P3 Cappings, P′ and P1 Modifications on Secondary Ketoamides It was exciting that by introducing substitution, the resulting extended P3 cappings delivered inhibitors with badly needed potency improvements such as those from compounds **66** to **72**. However, these larger primary ketoamides rarely possessed desirable PK profiles in any animal species to be considered for further evaluation. For example, both compounds **68** and **72** had a negligible oral plasma exposure in rats (0.07 μM h). The ester-capped analog **71** also had no plasma levels in rat probably because the benzyl ester was readily hydrolyzed under physiological conditions. The liability of the primary amide was also confirmed by preclinical studies of boceprevir which determined that primary amide hydrolysis was one of the major metabolic pathways. Earlier results had indicated that secondary amides **27** and **29** had much better PK in rats (PO AUC = 13, and 26 μM h, respectively) compared to the primary amide analog **30** (2.5 μM h).

This phenomenon was also illustrated in the pair of compounds **68** and **69**. The allyl amide **69** had moderate oral exposure in the rat of 3.2 μM h while the corresponding primary amide **68** had no rat exposure. These facts prompted us to investigate the secondary ketoamide alternatives. Compound **29** demonstrated that ketoamides of smaller alkyl groups with sp^2-character, such as an allyl group, gave better potency than those of saturated alkyls. The advantage of the allyl group was even more evident in **69**, which possessed the same excellent activity as **68** in both enzyme and cellular assays. It is also well-known that the carbon atoms in a cyclopropyl ring have some sp^2-character. Thus, further SAR development would focus on the secondary α-ketoamides, mostly allyl and cyclopropyl amides.

Another interesting results from the extended P3 capping studies was that compound **72**, which was capped by a *tert*-butyl sulfone, gave respectable PK in monkeys (PO AUC = 3.2 μM h at 3 mpk), despite the fact that it had a poor oral exposure in rats (0.07 μM h). This unique phenomenon was also observed in many other sulfones which demonstrated good PK in monkeys even without appreciable rat exposure. This was very encouraging because none of any other capping groups had achieved good PK in monkeys. To overcome the lack of rat PK, we envisioned that the same secondary amide approach could be adapted.

Thus, a number of secondary ketoamides, particularly allyl and cyclopropyl amides, were prepared with various combinations of the best moieties at P1, P3, and P3 capping sites. To our delight, many of them had excellent potency, good PK, and high selectivity. Some representative examples are compounds **73–77** and **4** (Scheme 12.7). The *tert*-leucine amine derived bicyclic sultam (cyclic sulfonamide) capping group, in combination with *tert*-leucine P3, norleucine P1, and allyl ketoamide, resulted in compound **73** which had an excellent K_i^* of 5 nM and EC_{90} of 0.08 μM [87]. It also achieved extremely high selectivity of 6100× over HNE. Unfortunately, although its PK in rats was moderate with an oral AUC of 1.4 μM h, but in monkeys it was very poor. Similarly, the ethyl sulfonamide capping derived from *tert*-leucine amine, together with indanylglycine P3 and the same P1 and P′ moieties, afforded an inhibitor **74** [88], which also had excellent overall profile in potency (K_i^* = 6 nM, EC_{90} = 0.06 μM), selectivity (HNE/HCV = 1400) and moderate rat PK (oral AUC = 1.2 μM h), except that it still lacked the desired PK in monkeys (oral AUC = 0.69 μM h). The *tert*-leucine amine glutaimide derived capping in compound **75** improved potency to a K_i^* of 4 nM and replicon potency EC_{90} of 0.03 μM which were among the best activities ever achieved in our ketoamide inhibitors [83]. Its selectivity was the highest (HNE/HCV = 7100). This compound also demonstrated moderate oral PK in rats and dogs with a PO AUC of 0.9 μM h and 1.2 μM h, respectively. The only shortcoming for inhibitor **75** was the low PK in monkeys (PO AUC = 0.1 μM h at 3 mpk). When the two diastereomers at the P1 residue were separated by HPLC, the active (*S*)-isomer of **75** had lower PK values in dogs than the parent **75** as a diastereomeric mixture.

While exploring SAR relationships using the allyl group as the P′ substituent to improve potency and PK profile of the inhibitors, we were cognizant of the fact that a terminal double bond may potentially be a toxicological liability. In order to assess this potential liability, one allyl ketoamide analog (structure not shown) was subjected to a rat *in vivo* study. Results indicated that trace amount of hydroxy-glutathione (GSH) adduct were formed [49]. This observation raised the possibility of *in vivo* formation of a reactive epoxide from the terminal olefin, which would be highly undesirable and would have potential drug safety concerns. Thus, we focused more on P′ cyclopropyl ketoamide analogs to develop a likely candidate for further evaluation. Toward this end, the unique combination of a cyclopropyl ketone capping derived from cyclohexyl glycine, the *tert*-leucine P3, a new butynyl glycine P1 and cyclopropyl ketoamide in compound **76** also provided a very good

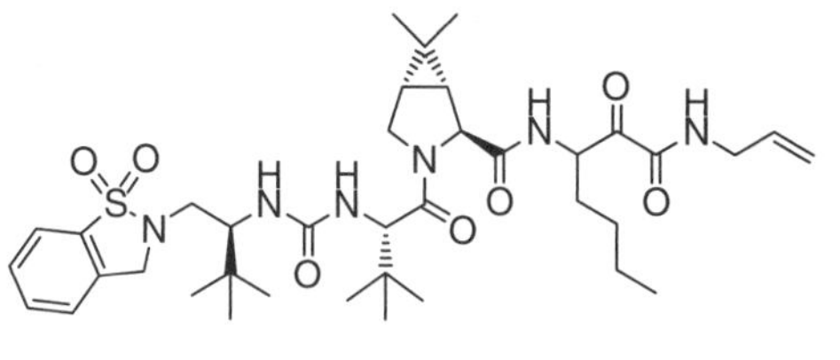

73 Ki* = 5 nM, EC_{90} = 0.08 μM
HNE/HCV = 6100
Rat PK AUC = 1.4 μM.h
Monkey PK AUC = 0.03 μM.h

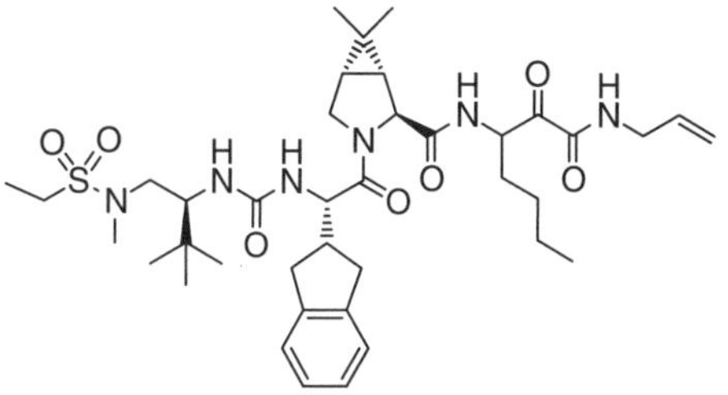

74 Ki* = 6 nM, EC_{90} = 0.06 μM
HNE/HCV = 1400
Rat PK AUC = 1.2 μM.h
Monkey PK AUC = 0.69 μM.h

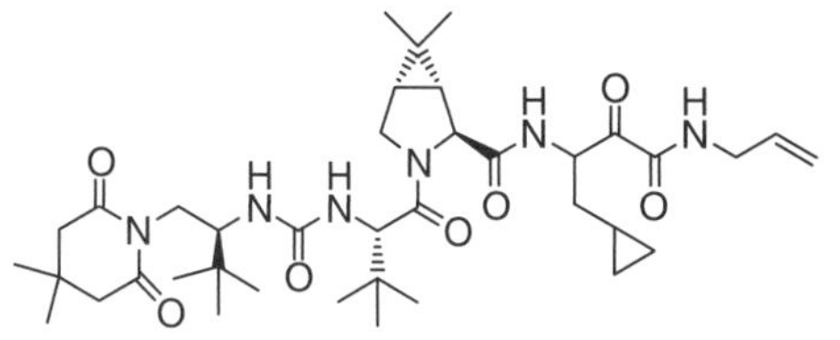

75 Ki* = 4 nM, EC_{90} = 0.03 μM
HNE/HCV = 7100
Rat PK AUC = 0.9 μM.h
Monkey PK AUC = 0.1 μM.h
Dog PK AUC = 1.2 μM.h

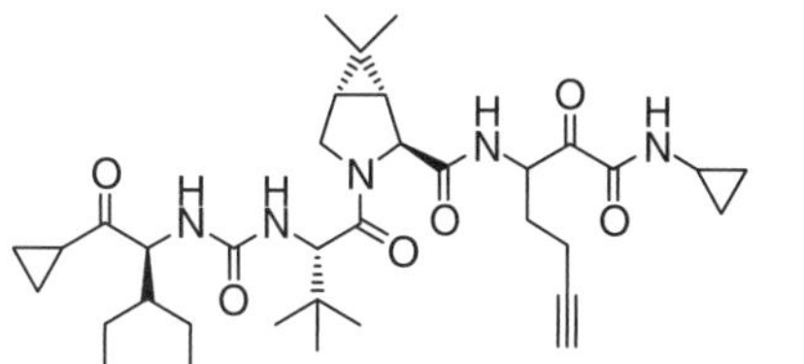

76 Ki* = 4 nM, EC_{90} = 0.055 μM
HNE/HCV < 100
Rat PK AUC = 11 μM.h

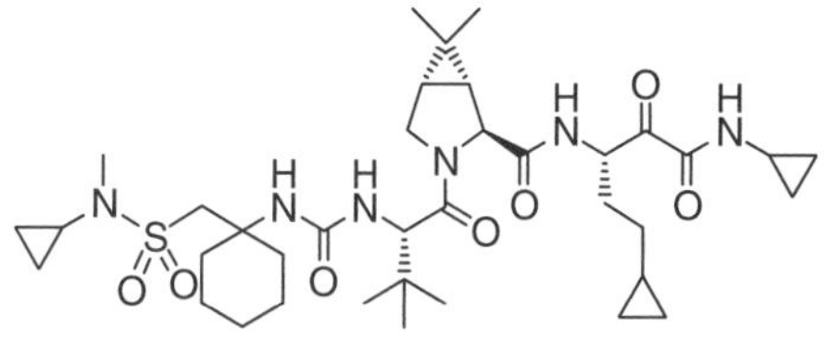

77 Ki* = 6 nM, EC_{90} = 0.075 μM
HNE/HCV = 2500
Rat PK AUC = 0.9 μM.h
Monkey PK AUC = 5.4 μM.h
Dog PK AUC = 4 μM.h

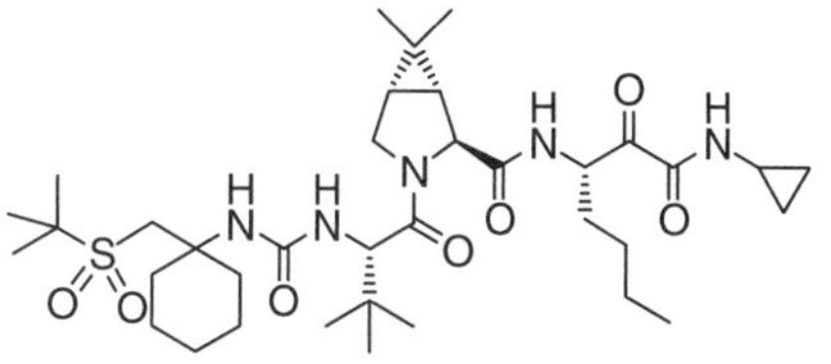

Narlaprevir
4 Ki* = 6 nM, EC_{90} = 0.04 μM
HNE/HCV = 600
Rat PK AUC = 6.5 μM.h
Monkey PK AUC = 1.1 μM.h
Dog PK AUC = 0.9 μM.h

Scheme 12.7 Secondary ketoamide with extended P3 cappings. Discovery of narlaprevir.

inhibitor with an excellent K_i^* of 4 nM and EC_{90} of 0.055 μM [86]. This inhibitor had excellent rat PK with an oral dosing AUC of 11 μM h. The drawback for this compound was its low selectivity (HNE/HCV < 100). Although inhibitors described above were mostly diastereomeric mixtures at P1, similar to **2**, our ultimate goal was to identify and develop an appropriate candidate as a single isomer. Hence we synthesized and evaluated many good compounds as single isomers with an *S*-stereocenter at the P1 position. Compound 77 was an excellent example: an *N*-methyl-*N*-cyclopropylamine sulfonamide substituted 1-methyl-cyclohexyl urea capping, the usual *tert*-leucine P2, the unique cyclopropylethyl glycine P1, and cyclopropyl ketoamide [89]. Besides very good potency in both enzyme and replicon assays (K_i^* of 6 nM, EC_{90} of 0.075 μM), this analog demonstrated unusually high oral exposures in monkeys and dogs with PO AUCs of 5.4 and 4 μM h, respectively. Its PK in rats was moderate (PO AUC = 0.9 μM h). It also had very high selectivity of 2500. Although **77** was an excellent compound in many aspects, its EC_{90} and rat PK were slightly less than desired.

TABLE 12.8 Pharmacokinetic Parameters of Compound 4

Animal species	Rat	Monkey	Dog
Dose (IV/PO, $mg\,kg^{-1}$)	4/10	1/3	1/3
IV AUC (μM h)	5.7	0.8	1.0
PO AUC (μM h)	6.5	1.1	0.9
Bioavailability (%)	46	46	29
C_{max} (μM)	1.3	–	0.8
$T_{1/2}$ (h)	4.8	–	2

Finally, we prepared the compound with a *tert*-butyl sulfone capping, a *tert*-leucine P3, a norleucine P1, and a cyclopropyl ketoamide line up of residues which resulted in inhibitor **4** (narlaprevir) [49].

12.8.3 Profile of Narlaprevir

12.8.3.1 *In vitro and Pharmacokinetic Profile of Narlaprevir* Compound **4** (narlaprevir) was very active in both enzyme and replicon assays achieving a K_i^* of 6 nM and EC_{90} of 0.04 μM. Its selectivity against elastase was adequate with a HNE/HCV = 600. The most important attribute about this molecule was that it exhibited moderate to good exposure in all three animal PK studies (Table 12.8). In rats at 10 mpk oral dosing, it achieved a very good AUC of 6.5 μM h with reasonable bioavailability (46%) and moderate half life of 4.8 h. The PO AUC (1.1 μM h at 3 mpk) and bioavailability (46%) in monkeys were also quite respectable. In dogs, PO AUC (0.9 μM h at 3 mpk) and bioavailability (29%) were moderate. The excellent potency coupled with good PK exhibited by compound **4** represented the best overall profile among the second-generation inhibitors with extended capping moieties (also named as P4 in some publications). Thus, compound **4** was selected for further preclinical evaluation. Resistance studies indicated that **4** was cross-resistant to mutations raised against boceprevir in both enzymatic and replicon assays. However, inhibitor **4** retained more activity against many of these mutants due to its higher intrinsic potency compared to **2** [90]. Compound **4** displayed no significant issues in the *in vitro* CYP or hERG assays. No glutathione or acyl glucuronide conjugates were observed with **4** in rats, dogs, and monkeys, thus indicating no reactive metabolite concerns. Crystalline material was also obtained for inhibitor **4** which resulted in improved physicochemical properties. With the results from these preclinical studies, and the fact that all the goals for a second-generation candidate (~10-fold more potent, improved monkey and rat PK, single isomer, crystalline) were achieved, this compound (**4**, narlaprevir) was selected as a development candidate.

12.8.3.2 *The Interaction of Narlaprevir with NS3 Protease* The X-ray crystal structure of **4** bound to the NS3 protease was solved (Figure 12.6). Similar to boceprevir, the α-ketoamide reacted with Ser-139 hydroxyl to form a reversible covalent bond, the P1, P2, and P3 side chains bound to the enzyme through hydrophobic interactions and the peptide chain formed a series of hydrogen bonding with the protein backbone [46]. The P3 capping cyclohexyl moiety was extending further into the enzyme S4 pocket than the *tert*-butyl group in **2** for additional hydrophobic contacts. More importantly, one of the newly introduced P4 sulfone oxygen atoms was in close proximity for hydrogen bonding interaction with the N–H of Cys-159. Presumably, these two additional favorable interactions with the enzyme resulted in improved potency.

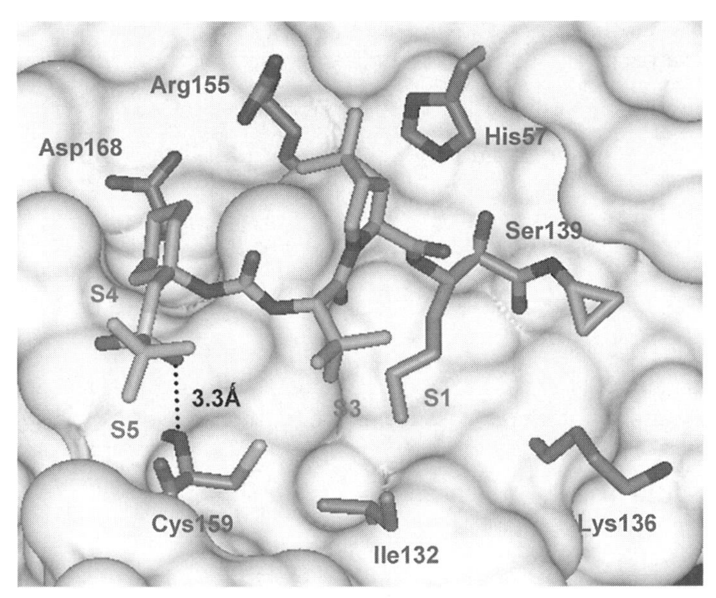

Figure 12.6 Compound **4** (narlaprevir) bound to HCV NS3 protease

12.8.4 Clinical Development Aspects of Narlaprevir

With improved potency, pharmacokinetic profile and physicochemical characteristics, compound **4** was evaluated in animal toxicological studies and was found to be safe [90,91]. It was then advanced to human clinical trials. It was found to be generally safe and well-tolerated in phase I safety studies [91]. In a phase Ib clinical trials, with 400 mg BID dosing, the sustained virological response rates were up to 81% in the treatment-naïve patients [92]. In a phase II trial with 200 mg QD dosing, when co-dosed with a P450 CYP3A4 inhibitor ritonavir, narlaprevir-based triple combination therapy achieved early virological response (EVR) (undetectable HCV-RNA levels at week 12) in 84–87% of patients [93]. These results demonstrated the potential that narlaprevir could be developed as a once-daily therapy. Further development of this compound will not be discussed here since it is out of the scope of the chapter.

12.8.5 Synthesis of Narlaprevir

Similar to the synthesis of boceprevir shown in Scheme 12.1, the P2–P3 dipeptide and the α-hydroxy-β-aminopropanamide P1–P′ advanced intermediate were prepared before the assembly of the final target molecule. Synthesis of narlaprevir is outlined in Scheme 12.8 [49]. The P2–P3 intermediate **63** was the same as that in boceprevir preparation. The P1–P′ moiety was synthesized in a five-step sequence starting from L-norleucine. Thus, reduction of L-norleucine **78** followed by amino protection provided Boc-protected amino alcohol **79** which was oxidized under mild conditions employing bleach/TEMPO to afford aldehyde **80**. Passerini reaction of **80** with cyclopropylisonitrile **81** in the presence of acetic acid provided the intermediate acetate **82**. Sequential deprotection of the acetate and the Boc-protecting group unraveled the required P1–P′ intermediate **83** in approximately 60% overall yield after five steps. To prepare the sulfone capping group, ester **84** was alkylated with benzyloxymethyl chloride to give **85**. Removal of the benzyl protecting group and subsequent conversion to the alcohol provided mesylate **86**. Displacement of the mesylate group with sodium *tert*-butylthiolate and hydrolysis of the ester

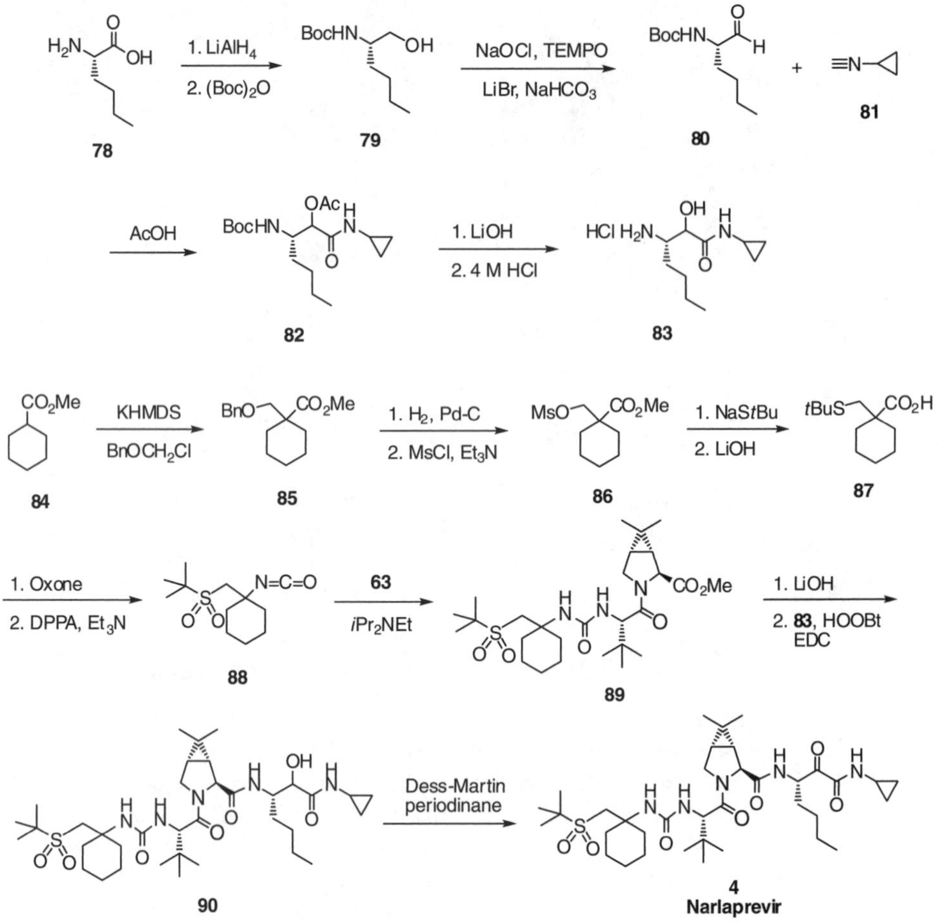

Scheme 12.8 Synthesis of narlaprevir.

resulted in thioether **87**. Oxidation of the thioether to a sulfone and Curtius rearrangement of acid afforded the isocyanate capping intermediate **88**. The reaction between the isocyanate and the previously described dipeptide intermediate **63** gave rise to the left-hand fragment (**89**) of the target molecule. Hydrolysis of the ester to its corresponding acid, and subsequent coupling with P1–P′ intermediate **83** provided an α-hydroxyamide **90**. Finally, oxidation with Dess–Martin periodinane afforded the target compound **4**.

While the above synthetic sequence described in Scheme 12.2 was useful for SAR studies, a better route that was amenable for scale-up was highly desirable. Thus, the synthetic route was redesigned and several major improvements were made (Scheme 12.9) [49]. Lewis acid mediated alkylation of silylenol ether of **84** with chloromethyl-*tert*-butylthioether provided **91** in one step. Hydrolysis of the methyl ester, followed by oxidation with Oxone, afforded sulfone acid **92** in 62% yield (three steps). Curtius rearrangement of the acid afforded isocyanate **88** as described above. Reaction of **88** with *L-tert*-leucine in a biphasic medium provided a urea-capped P3 acid, which could be crystallized from ethyl acetate. The coupling of this acid with P2 intermediate dimethylcyclopropylproline methyl ester **62** gave the capping-P3–P2 dipeptide **89**. Hydrolysis of the methyl ester afforded the corresponding advanced intermediate acid in 86% yield (four steps), which could, again, be crystallized. The coupling between this acid and the P1–P′

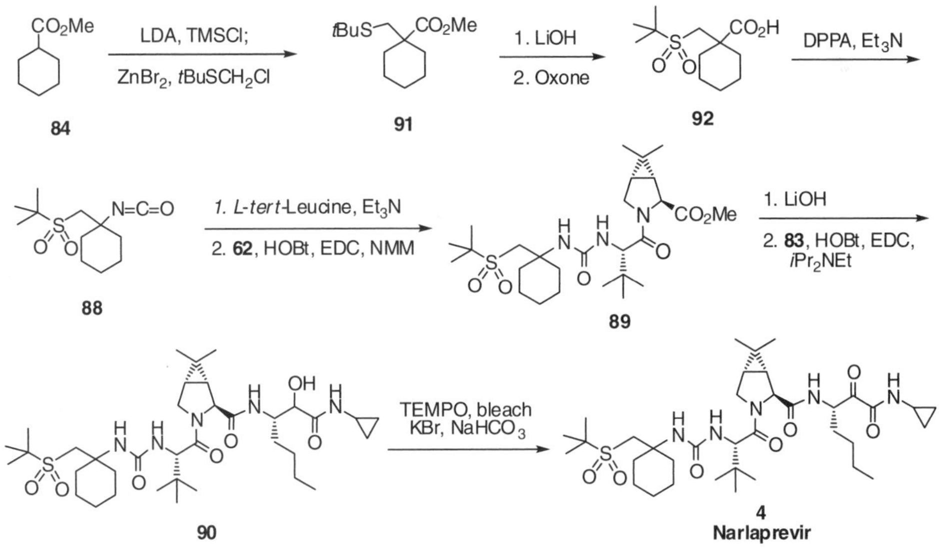

Scheme 12.9 Improved synthesis of narlaprevir.

intermediate **83** provided **90**. After a brief investigation, we identified the best oxidation conditions for the conversion of **90** to **4** was to use bleach/TEMPO combination in a buffer. The product was crystallized from acetone–water solvent mixture to provide **4** in high yield. It is noteworthy that the entire sequence for the synthesis of **4** in Scheme 12.3 was carried out without any chromatography purification, and the integrity of the P1 stereocenter was maintained. The improved synthetic route was used to bring up more than one kilogram each of the advanced intermediates **83** and **89**.

12.9 SUMMARY

The standard-of-care for HCV infection has been improved during last decade following the advancement of pegylated α-interferon and ribavirin combination therapy; however, the overall SVR rate for this combination therapy is only ~40 to 50% [1,10]. Recent emergence of directly acting antiviral (DAA) agents gives new hope for a cure for patients with chronic HCV infection. The HCV NS3 protease is considered to be among the most important drug targets and its relevance was demonstrated by the first clinical proof-of-concept of ciluprevir. However, it has been a long journey to pursue a potent and orally bioavailable HCV NS3 protease inhibitor as a drug candidate for the treatment of hepatitis C virus infection. The shallow and flat active site and nearby pockets of the protease presented significant challenges for the discovery of active inhibitors. With no viable leads from large scale screening efforts, a structure-based drug design approach guided by an X-ray crystal structure of the enzyme was pursued. The endeavor started with large peptide inhibitors mimicking protease cleavage products, stepwise truncations and systematic optimizations on each prime and nonprime amino acid residue gave rise to potent pentapeptides, and eventually to small tripeptide inhibitors. The combination of optimized moieties at each position led to the discovery of boceprevir (**2**). It has a K_i^* of 14 nM in enzyme assay and an EC_{90} of 0.35 μM in cell-based replicon assay. Boceprevir demonstrated good oral bioavailability in rats and dogs, and was found to be highly concentrated in the liver. It has completed phase I to III clinical trials, where it is shown to be safe and well-tolerated, and efficacious as a component of a triple combination therapy together with pegIFN and ribavirin for the treatment of hepatitis C viral infections. It was accepted by FDA for an expedited review and has been approved for marketing as Victrelis.

The discovery effort continued to seek a second-generation NS3 protease candidate. The criteria for the new clinical candidate were a 10-fold improvement in cellular assay potency, better monkey PK and single isomer at the P1 α-center. The strategy of extending the P3 capping group further into the S4 pocket and establishing additional interactions in the S5 pocket was adapted. After extensive efforts, a number of extended novel P3 capping chemo types such as sulfonamide, sultam, carbamate, ketone, and imide were discovered to be highly potent inhibitors. But they did not possess adequate monkey PK. The sulfone capping, however, exhibited respectable monkey PK in many compounds. Further optimization of the sulfone group and other moieties delivered the final candidate compound **4** (narlaprevir). Narlaprevir had a K_i^* of 6 nM in enzyme assay and an EC_{90} of 0.04 μM. It demonstrated good oral bioavailability in rats, dogs, and monkeys. It was found to be safe in animal toxicology studies, and was advanced to phase I clinical trials where it was shown to be safe and well-tolerated. Results from phase II clinical trials indicated that narlaprevir was highly efficacious for the treatment of HCV infection.

Extensive research in the pharmaceutical industry has resulted in a number of other novel drug candidates which have entered clinical evaluation to establish their effectiveness for HCV patients. The success of any of these agents will be largely dependent on its ability to inhibit all viral variants and prevent the emergence of escape mutants, because HCV has a high rate of turnover and high replication activity [94]. A large number of viral variants are produced continuously [95]. The fact that HCV has at least six different genotypes and more than 100 subtypes complicates treatment even further [96]. The current consensus is that combinations of several antiviral agents attacking different targets in the viral life cycle and perhaps, the hosts themselves will almost certainly be required to eliminate the infection and prevent the emergence of drug-resistant viral mutants. Ultimately, an all oral combination of two or more direct acting antiviral agents would be highly desirable. On the other hand, recent reports suggest that a polymorphism upstream of IL-28B is associated with a twofold difference in SVR rates for pegIFN and RBV combination therapy [97,98]. Some IL-28B gene variant is associated with increased SVR and is a potential effective bio-marker of treatment outcome [98]. This raises the hope that genetically guided therapy will lead to better HCV treatment selection and higher SVR rates in different groups of patients.

REFERENCES

1. Lauer, G. M. and Walker, B. D. Hepatitis C virus infection. *N. Engl. J. Med.* **2001**, *345*, 41–52.
2. Pawlotsky, J. M. Treating hepatitis C in "difficult-to-treat" patients. *N. Engl. J. Med.* **2004**, *351*, 422–423.
3. Alter, H. J. HCV natural history: the retrospective and prospective in perspective. *J. Hepatol.* **2005**, *43*, 550–552.
4. Shepard, C. W., Finelli, L., and Alter, M. J. Global epidemiology of hepatitis C virus infection. *Lancet. Infect. Dis.* **2005**, *5*, 558–567.
5. Wasley, A. and Alter, M. J. Epidemiology of hepatitis C: geographic differences and temporal trends. *Semin. Liver Dis.* **2000**, *20*, 1–16.
6. Alter, H. J. and Seeff, L. B. Recovery, persistence, and sequelae in hepatitis C virus infection: a perspective on long-term outcome. *Semin. Liver Dis.* **2000**, *20*, 17–35.
7. Brown, R. S. Jr. and Gaglio, P. J. Scope of worldwide hepatitis C problem. *Liver Transplant.* **2003**, *9*, S10–S13.
8. Feld, J. J. and Hoofnagle, J. H. Mechanism of action of interferon and ribavirin in treatment of hepatitis C. *Nature (London)* **2005**, *436*, 967–972.
9. Neumann, A. U., Lam, N. P., Dahari, H., Gretch, D. R., Wiley, T. E., Layden, T. J., and Perelson, A. S. Hepatitis C viral dynamics *in vivo* and the antiviral efficacy of

interferon-α therapy. *Science (Washington D.C.)* **1998**, *282*, 103–107.
10. Fried, M. W., Shiffman, M. L., Reddy, D. K. R., Smith, C., Marinos, G., Gonçales, F. L., Häussinger, D., Diago, M., Carosi, G., Dhumeaux, D., Craxi, A., Lin, A., Hoffman, J., and Yu, J. PEGinterferon-α-2a plus ribavirin for chronic hepatitis C virus infection. *N. Engl. J. Med.* **2002**, *347*, 975–982.
11. Shiffman, M. L., Suter, F., Bacon, B. R., Nelson, D., Harley, H., Sola, R., Shafran, S. D., Barange, K., Lin, A., Soman, A., and Zeuzem, S. Peginterferon alfa-2a and ribavirin for 16 or 24 weeks in HCV genotype 2 or 3. *N. Engl. J. Med.* **2007**, *357*, 124–134.
12. Chung, R. T., Andersen, J., Volberding, P., Robbins, G. K., Liu, T., Sherman, K. E., Peters, M. G., Koziel, M. J., Bhan, A. K., Alston, B., and Colquhoun, D. Peginterferon alfa-2a plus ribavirin versus interferon alfa-2a plus ribavirin for chronic hepatitis C in HIV-coinfected persons. *N. Engl. J. Med.* **2004**, *351*, 451–459.
13. Muir, A. and Rockey, D. C. Treatment of acute hepatitis c with interferon alfa-2b. *N. Engl. J. Med.* **2002**, *346*, 1091–1092.
14. Davis, G. L., Esteban-Mur, R., Rustgi, V., Hoefs, J., Gordon, S. C., Trepo, C., Shiffman, M. L., Zeuzem, S., Craxi, A., Ling, M. H., and Albrecht, J. Interferon alfa-2b alone or in combination with ribavirin for the treatment of relapse of chronic hepatitis c. International hepatitis interventional therapy group. *N. Engl. J. Med.* **1998**, *339*, 1493–1499.
15. Honda, M., Sakai, A., Yamashita, T., Nakamoto, Y., Mizukoshi, E., Sakai, Y., Nakamura, M., Shirasaki, T., Horimoto, K., Tanaka, Y., and Tokunaga, K. Hepatic isg expression is associated with genetic variation in interleukin 28B and the outcome of ifn therapy for chronic hepatitis C. *Gastroenterology* **2010**, *139*, 499–509.
16. Tanaka, Y., Nishida, N., Sugiyama, M., Kurosaki, M., Matsuura, K., Sakamoto, N., Nakagawa, M., Korenaga, M., Hino, K., Hige, S., and Ito, Y. Genome-wide association of IL28B with response to pegylated interferon-alpha and ribavirin therapy for chronic hepatitis C. *Nat. Genet.* **2009**, *41*, 1105–1109.
17. Ge, D., Fellay, J., Thompson, A. J., Simon, J. S., Shianna, K. V., Urban, T. J., Heinzen, E. L., Qiu, P., Bertelsen, A. H., Muir, A. J., and Sulkowski, M. Genetic variation in IL28B predicts hepatitis C treatment-induced viral clearance. *Nature* **2009**, *461*, 399–401.
18. Choo, Q. L., Kuo, G., Weiner, A. J., Overby, L. R., Bradley, D. W., and Houghton, M. Isolation of a cDNA clone derived from a blood-borne non-A, non-B viral hepatitis genome. *Science (Washington D. C.)* **1989**, *244*, 359–362.
19. Lindenbach, B. D. and Rice, C. M. Unravelling hepatitis C virus replication from genome to function. *Nature (London)* **2005**, *436*, 933–938.
20. Kolykhalov, A. A., Mihalik, K., Feinstone, S. M., and Rice, C. M. Hepatitis C virus-encoded enzymatic activities and conserved RNA elements in the 3′ nontranslated region are essential for virus replication *in vivo*. *J.Virol.* **2000**, *74*, 2046–2051.
21. Tellinghuisen, T. L. and Rice, C. M. Interaction between hepatitis C virus proteins and host cell factors. *Curr. Opin. Microbiol.* **2002**, *5*, 419–427.
22. Gale, M., Jr. and Foy, E. M. Evasion of intracellular host defence by hepatitis C virus. *Nature* **2005**, *436*, 939–945.
23. Behrens, S. E., Tomei, L., and De Francesco, R. Identification and properties of the RNA-dependent RNA polymerase of hepatitis C virus. *EMBO J.* **1996**, *15*, 12–22.
24. Lohmann, V., Korner, F., Herian, U., and Bartenschlager, R. Biochemical properties of hepatitis C virus ns5b RNAdependent RNA polymerase and identification of amino acid sequence motifs essential for enzymatic activity. *J. Virol.* **1997**, *71*, 8416–8428.
25. Chen, K. X. and Njoroge, F. G. A review of HCV protease inhibitors. *Curr. Opin. Invest. Drugs.* **2009**, *10*, 821–837.
26. Watkins, W. J., Ray, A. S., and Chong, L. S. HCV NS5B polymerase inhibitors. *Curr. Opin. Drug Dis. Dev.* **2010**, *13*, 441–465.
27. Legrand-Abravanel, F., Nicot, F., and Izopet, J. New NS5B polymerase inhibitors for hepatitis C. *Expert Opin. Investig. Drugs* **2010**, *19*, 963–975.
28. Hezode, C., Forestier, N., Dusheiko, G., Ferenci, P., Pol, S., Goeser, T., Bronowicki, J. P., Bourliere, M., Gharakhanian, S., Bengtsson, L., and McNair, L. Telaprevir and peginterferon with or without ribavirin for chronic HCV infection. *N. Engl. J. Med.* **2009**, *360*, 1839–1850.
29. Kwo, P. Y., Lawitz, E. J., McCone, J., Schiff, E. R., Vierling, J. M., Pound, D., Davis, M. N., Galati, J. S., Gordon, S. C., Ravendhran, N., Rossaro, L., Anderson, F. H., Jacobson, I. M., Rubin, R., Koury, K., Pedicone, L. D., Brass, C. A., Chaudhri, E., and Albrecht, J. K. Efficacy of boceprevir, an NS3 protease inhibitor, in combination with peginterferon alfa-2b and ribavirin in treatment-naive patients with genotype 1 hepatitis C infection (SPRINT-1): an open-label, randomised, multicentre phase 2 trial. *Lancet* **2010**, *376*, 705–716.
30. Gao, M., Nettles, R. E., Belema, M., Snyder, L. B., Nguyen, V. N., Fridell, R. A., Serrano-Wu, M. H., Langley, D. R., Sun, J. -H., O'BoyleII, D. R., Lemm, J. A., Wang, C., Knipe, J. O., Chien, C., Colonno, R. J., Grasela, D. M., Meanwell, N. A., and Hamann, L. G. Chemical genetics strategy identifies an HCV NS5A inhibitor with a potent clinical effect. *Nature* **2010**, *465*, 96–100.
31. Manns, M. P., Foster, G. R., Rockstroh, J. K., Zeuzem, S., Zoulim, F., and Houghton, M. The way forward in HCV treatment – finding the right path. *Nat. Rev. Drug Discov.* **2007**, *6*, 991–1000.
32. Houghton, M. and Abrignani, S. Prospects for a vaccine against the hepatitis C virus. *Nature (London)* **2005**, *436*, 961–966.

33. Lohmann, V., Korner, F., Koch, J., Herian, U., Theilmann, L., and Bartenschlager, R. Replication of subgenomic hepatitis C virus RNAs in a hepatoma cell line. *Science* **1999**, *285*, 110–113.
34. Wakita, T., Pietschmann, T., Kato, T., Date, T., Miyamoto, M., Zhao, Z., Murthy, K., Habermann, A., Krausslich, H. G., Mizokami, M., and Bartenschlager, R. Production of infectious hepatitis C virus in tissue culture from a cloned viral genome. *Nat. Med.* **2005**, *11*, 791–796.
35. Walker, C. M. Comparative features of hepatitis C virus infection in humans and chimpanzees. *Springer Semin. Immunopathol.* **1997**, *19*, 85–98.
36. Mercer, D. F., Schiller, D. E., Elliott, J. F., Douglas, D. N., Hao, C., Rinfret, A., Addison, W. R., Fischer, K. P., Churchill, T. A., Lakey, J. R. T., Tyrrell, D. L. J., and Kneteman, N. Hepatitis C virus replication in mice with chimeric human livers. *Nat. Med.* **2001**, *7*, 927–933.
37. Bissig, K. D., Wieland, S. F., Tran, P., Isogawa, M., Le, T. T., Chisari, F. V., and Verma, I. M. Human liver chimeric mice provide a model for hepatitis B and C virus infection and treatment. *J. Clin. Invest.* **2010**, *120*, 924–930.
38. White, P. W., Llinas-Brunet, M., and Bos, M. Blunting the Swiss army knife of hepatitis C virus: inhibitors of NS3/4A protease. in *Progress in Medicinal Chemistry* (eds. F. D. King and G. Lawton), Vol. 44, Elsevier, New York, **2006**, pp. 65–107.
39. De Francesco, R. and Migliaccio, G. Challenges and successes in developing new therapies for hepatitis C. *Nature (London)* **2005**, *436*, 953–960.
40. Malcolm, B. A., Liu, R., Lahser, F., Agrawal, S., Belanger, B., Butkiewicz, N., Chase, R., Gheyas, F., Hart, A., Hesk, D., Ingravallo, P., Jiang, C., Kong, R., Lu, J., Pichardo, J., Prongay, A., Skelton, A., Tong, X., Venkatraman, S., Xia, E., Girijavallabhan, V., and Njoroge, F. G. SCH 503034, a mechanism-based inhibitor of hepatitis C virus NS3 protease, suppresses polyprotein maturation and enhances the antiviral activity of alpha interferon in replicon cells. *Antimicrob. Agents Chemother.* **2006**, *50*, 1013–1020.
41. Yan, Y., Li, Y., Munshi, S., Sardana, V., Cole, J. L., Sardana, M., Steinkuehler, C., Tomei, L., De Francesco, R., Kuo, L. C., and Chen, Z. Complex of NS3 protease and NS4A peptide of BK strain hepatitis C virus: a 2.2 Å resolution structure in a hexagonal crystal form. *Protein Sci.* **1998**, *7*, 837–847.
42. Love, R. A., Parge, H. E., Wichersham, J. A., Hostomsky, Z., Habuka, N., Moomaw, E. W., Adachi, T., and Hostomska, Z. The crystal structure of hepatitis C virus NS3 proteinase reveals a trypsin-like fold and a structural zinc binding site. *Cell* **1996**, *87*, 331–342.
43. Llinas-Brunet, M., Bailey, M. D., Fazal, G., Goulet, S., Halmos, T., LePlante, S., Maurice, R., Poirier, M., Poupart, M. -A., Thibeault, D., Wernic, D., and Lamarre, D. Peptide-based inhibitors of the hepatitis C virus serine protease. *Bioorg. Med. Chem. Lett.* **1998**, *8*, 1713–1718.
44. Steinkühler, C., Biasiol, G., Brunetti, M., Urbani, A., Koch, U., Cortese, R., Pessi, A., and De Francesco, R. Product inhibition of the hepatitis C virus NS3 protease. *Biochemistry* **1998**, *37*, 8899–8905.
45. Lamarre, D., Anderson, P. C., Bailey, M., Beaulieu, P., Bolger, G., Bonneau, P., Bös, M., Cameron, D. R., Cartier, M., Cordingley, M. G., Faucher, A -M., Goudreau, N., Kawai, S. H., Kukolj, G., Lagacé, L., LaPlante, S. R., Narjes, H., Poupart, M. -A., Rancourt, J., Sentjens, R. E., George, T. S., Simoneau, B., Steinmann, G., Thibeault, D., Tsantrizos, Y. S., Weldon, S. M., Yong, C. -L., and Llinàs-Brunet, M. An NS3 protease inhibitor with antiviral effects in humans infected with hepatitis C virus. *Nature (London)* **2003**, *426*, 186–189.
46. Venkatraman, S., Bogen, S. L., Arasappan, A., Bennett, F., Chen, K., Jao, J., Liu, Y. -T., Lovey, R., Hendrata, S., Huang, Y., Pan, W., Parekh, T., Pinto, P., Popov, V., Pike, R., Ruan, S., Santhanam, B., Vibulbhan, B., Wu, W., Yang, W., Kong, J., Liang, X., Wong, J., Liu, R., Butkiewicz, N., Chase, R., Hart, A., Agrawal, S., Ingravallo, P., Pichardo, J., Kong, R., Baroudy, B., Malcolm, B., Guo, Z., Prongay, A., Madison, V., Broske, L., Cui, X., Cheng, K. -C., Hsieh, Y., Brisson, J. -M., Prelusky, D., Korfmacher, W., White, R., Bogdanowich-Knipp, S., Pavlovsky, A., Bradley, P., Saksena, A. K., Ganguly, A., Piwinski, J., Girijavallabhan, V., and Njoroge, F. G. Discovery of (1*R*,5*S*)-*N*-[3-amino-1-(cyclobutylmethyl)-2,3-dioxopropyl]-3-[2(S)-[[[(1,1-dimethylethyl)amino] carbonyl]amino]-3,3-dimethyl-1-oxobutyl]-6,6-dimethyl-3-azabicyclo[3.1.0]hexan-(*S*)-carboxamide (SCH 503034), a selective, potent, orally bioavailable hepatitis C virus NS3 protease inhibitor: a potential therapeutic agent for the treatment of hepatitis C infection. *J. Med. Chem.* **2006**, *49*, 6074–6086.
47. Chen, K. X. and Njoroge, F. G. The journey to the discovery of boceprevir: an NS3-NS4 HCV protease inhibitor for the treatment of chronic hepatitis C. in *Progress in Medicinal Chemistry* (eds. G. Lawton and D. R. Witty), Vol. 49, Elsevier, New York, **2010**, pp. 1–36.
48. Perni, R. B., Almquist, S. J., Byrn, R. A., Chandorkar, G., Chaturvedi, P. R., Courtney, L. F., Decker, C. J., Dinehart, K., Gates, C. A., Harbeson, S. L., Heiser, A., Kalkeri, G., Kolaczkowski, E., Lin, K., Luong, Y. -P., Rao, B. G., Taylor, W. P., Thomson, J. A., Tung, R. D., Wei, Y., Kwong, A. D., and Lin, C. Preclinical profile of VX-950, a potent, selective, and orally, bioavailable inhibitor of hepatitis C virus NS3-4A serine protease. *Antimicrob. Agents Chemother.* **2006**, *50*, 899–909.
49. Arasappan, A., Bennett, F., Bogen, S. L., Venkatraman, S., Blackman, M., Chen, K. X., Hendrata, S., Huang, Y., Huelgas, R. M., Nair, L., Padilla, A. I., Pan, W., Pike, R., Pinto, P., Ruan, S., Sannigrahi, M., Velazquez, F., Vibulbhan, B., Wu, W., Yang, W., Saksena, A. K., Girijavallabhan, V., Shih, N. -Y., Kong, J., Meng, T., Jin, Y., Wong, J., McNamara, P., Prongay, A., Madison, V., Piwinski, J., Cheng, K. -C.,

Morrison, R., Malcolm, B., Tong, X., Ralston, R., and Njoroge, F. G. Discovery of narlaprevir (SCH 900518): a potent, second generation HCV NS3 serine protease inhibitor. *ACS Med. Chem. Lett.* **2010**, *1*, 64–69.

50. Seiwert, S. D., Andrews, S. W., Jiang, Y., Serebryany, V., Tan, H., Kossen, K., Rajagopalan, P. T., Misialek, S., Stevens, S. K., Stoycheva, A., Hong, J., Lim, S. R., Qin, X., Rieger, R., Condroski, K. R., Zhang, H., Do, M. G., Lemieux, C., Hingorani, G. P., Hartley, D. P., Josey, J. A., Pan, L., Beigelman, L., and Blatt, L. M. Preclinical characteristics of the hepatitis C virus NS3/4A protease inhibitor ITMN-191 (R7227). *Antimicrob. Agents Chemother.* **2008**, *52*, 4432–4441.
51. Raboisson, P., de Kock, H., Rosenquist, A., Nilsson, M., Salvador-Oden, L., Lin, T. I., Roue, N., Ivanov, V., Wähling, H., Wickström, K., and Hamelink, E. Structure–activity relationship study on a novel series of cyclopentane-containing macrocyclic inhibitors of the hepatitis C virus NS3/4A protease leading to the discovery of TMC435350. *Bioorg. Med. Chem. Lett.* **2008**, *18*, 4853–4858.
52. Lin, T. I., Lenz, O., Fanning, G., Verbinnen, T., Delouvroy, F., Scholliers, A., Vermeiren, K., Rosenquist, A., Edlund, M., Samuelsson, B., and Vrang, L. *In vitro* activity and preclinical profile of TMC435350, a potent hepatitis C virus protease inhibitor. *Antimicrob. Agents Chemother.* **2009**, *53*, 1377–1385.
53. McCauley, J. A., McIntyre, C. J., Rudd, M. T., Nguyen, K. T., Romano, J. J., Butcher, J. W., Gilbert, K. F., Bush, K. J., Holloway, M. K., Swestock, J., Wan, B. -L., Carroll, S. S., DiMuzio, J. M., Graham, D. J., Ludmerer, S. W., Mao, S. -S., Stahlhut, M. W., Fandozzi, C. M., Trainor, N., Olsen, D. B., Vacca, J. P. and Liverton, N. J. Discovery of vaniprevir (MK-7009), a macrocyclic hepatitis C virus NS3/4a protease inhibitor. *J. Med. Chem.* **2010**, *53*, 2443–2463.
54. Liverton, N. J., Carroll, S. S., Di Muzio, JRRCR.R. Fandozzi, C., Graham, D. J., Hazuda, D., Holloway, M. K., Ludmerer, S. W., McCauley, J. A., McIntyre, C. J., Olsen, D. B., Rudd, M. T., Stahlhut, M., and Vacca, J. P. MK-7009, a potent and selective inhibitor of hepatitis C virus NS3/4A protease. *Antimicrob. Agents Chemother.* **2010**, *54*, 305–311.
55. Llinas-Brunet, M., Bailey, M. D., Goudreau, N., Bhardwaj, P. K., Bordeleau, J., Bos, M., Bousquet, Y., Cordingley, M. G., Duan, J., Forgione, P., Garneau, M., Ghiro, E., Gorys, V., Goulet, S., Halmos, T., Kawai, S. H., Naud, J., Poupart, M. -A., and White, P. W. Discovery of a potent and selective noncovalent linear inhibitor of the hepatitis C virus NS3 protease (BI 201335). *J. Med. Chem.* **2010**, *53*, 6466–6476.
56. White, P. W., Llinas-Brunet, M., Amad, M., Bethell, R. C., Bolger, G., Cordingley, M. G., Duan, J., Garneau, M., Lagace, L., Thibeault, D., and Kukolj, G. Preclinical characterization of BI 201335, a C-terminal carboxylic acid inhibitor of the hepatitis C virus NS3-NS4A protease. *Antimicrob. Agents Chemother.* **2010**, *54*, 4611–4618.
57. Ingallinella, P., Altamura, S., Bianchi, E., Taliani, M., Ingenito, R., Cortese, R., De Francesco, R., Steinkühler, C., and Pessi, A. Potent peptide inhibitors of human hepatitis C virus NS3 protease are obtained by optimizing the cleavage products. *Biochemistry* **1998**, *37*, 8906–8914.
58. Sanderson, P. E. J. and Naylor-Olsen, A. M. Thrombin inhibitor design. *Curr. Med. Chem.* **1998**, *5*, 289–304.
59. Turk, B. Targeting proteases: successes, failures and future prospects. *Nat. Rev. Drug Discov.* **2006**, *5*, 785–799.
60. Powers, J. C., Asgian, J. L., Ekici, D., and James, K. E. Irreversible inhibitors of serine, cysteine, and threonine proteases. *Chem. Rev.* **2002**, *102*, 4639–4750.
61. Zhang, R., Beyer, B. M., Durkin, J., Ingram, R., Njoroge, F. G., Windsor, W. T., and Malcolm, B. A. A continuous spectrophotometric assay for the hepatitis C virus serine protease. *Anal. Biochem.* **1999**, *270*, 268–275. The substrate Ac-DTEDVVP(Nva)-O-PAP was used in the study.
62. Morrison, J. and Walsh, C.T. The behavior and significance of slow-binding enzyme inhibitors. in *Advanced Enzymolology* (ed. Meister, A.), Vol. 61, John Wiley & Sons, Inc., New Jersey, **1988**, pp. 201–301. For definition of K_i^* and discussions.
63. Njoroge, F. G., Chen, K. X., Shih, N. -Y., and Piwinski, J. J. Challenges in modern drug discovery: a case study of boceprevir, an HCV protease inhibitor for the treatment of hepatitis C virus infection. *Acc. Chem. Res.* **2008**, *41*, 50–59.
64. Bogen, S. L., Ruan, R., Saksena, A. K., Njoroge, F. G., Girijavallabhan, V., Agrawal, S., Liu, R., Pichardo, J., Baroudy, B., and Prongay, A. Depeptidization efforts on P3 - P2′ α-ketoamide inhibitors of HCV NS3-4A serine protease: Effect on HCV replicon activity. *Bioorg. Med. Chem. Lett.* **2006**, *16*, 1621–1627.
65. Chen, K. X., Njoroge, F. G., Vibulbhan, B., Prongay, A., Pichardo, J., Madison, V., Buevich, A., and Chan, T. -M. Proline-based macrocyclic inhibitors of the hepatitis C virus: stereoselective synthesis and biological activity. *Angew. Chem. Int. Ed.* **2005**, *44*, 7024–7028.
66. Chen, K. X., Njoroge, F. G., Pichardo, J., Prongay, A., Butkiewicz, N., Yao, N., Madison, V., and Girijavallabhan, V. Design, synthesis and biological activity of m-tyrosine-based 16- and 17-membered macrocyclic inhibitors of hepatitis C virus NS3 serine protease. *J. Med. Chem.* **2005**, *48*, 6229–6235.
67. Chen, K. X., Njoroge, F. G., Arasappan, A., Venkatraman, S., Vibulbhan, B., Yang, W., Parekh, T. N., Pichardo, J., Prongay, A., Cheng, K. -C., Butkiewicz, N., Yao, N., Madison, V., and Girijavallabhan, V. Novel potent hepatitis C virus NS3 serine protease inhibitors derived from proline-based macrocycles. *J. Med. Chem.* **2006**, *49*, 995–1005.
68. Venkatraman, S., Velazquez, F., Wu, W., Blackman, M., Chen, K. X., Bogen, S., Nair, L., Tong, X., Chase, R., Hart, A., Agrawal, S., Pichardo, J., Prongay, A., Cheng, K. -C., Girijavallabhan, V., Piwinski, J., Shih,

N. -Y., and Njoroge, F. G. Discovery and structure–activity relationship of P1-P3 ketoamide derived macrocyclic inhibitors of hepatitis C virus NS3 protease. *J. Med. Chem.* **2009**, *52*, 336–346.

69. Bogen, S. L., Arasappan, A., Bennett, F., Chen, K., Jao, E., Liu, Y. -T., Lovey, R. G., Venkatraman, S., Pan, W., Parekh, T., Pike, R. E., Ruan, S., Liu, R., Baroudy, B., Agrawal, S., Ingravallo, P., Pichardo, J., Prongay, A., Brisson, J. -M., Hsieh, T. Y., Cheng, K. -C., Kemp, S. J., Levy, O. E., Lim-Wilby, M., Tamura, S. Y., Saksena, A. K. Girijavallabhan, V., and Njoroge, F. G. Discovery of SCH 446211 (SCH6): a new ketoamide inhibitor of the HCV NS3 serine protease and HCV subgenomic RNA replication NS3 serine. *J. Med. Chem.* **2006**, *49*, 2750–2757.
70. Sinha, S., Watorek, W., Karr, S., Giles, J., Bode, W., and Travis, J. Primary structure of human neutrophil elastase. *Proc. Natl. Acad. Sci. U.S.A.* **1987**, *84*, 2228–2232.
71. Mederacke, I., Wedemeyer, H., and Manns, M. P. Boceprevir, an NS3 serine protease inhibitor of hepatitis C virus, for the treatment of HCV infection. *Curr. Opin. Investig. Drugs* **2009**, *10*, 181–189.
72. Sarrazin, C., Rouzier, R., Wagner, F., Forestier, N., Larrey, D., Gupta, S., Hussain, M., Shah, A., Cutler, D., Zhang, J., and Zeuzem, S. SCH 503034, a novel hepatitis C virus protease inhibitor, plus pegylated interferon alpha-2b for genotype 1 nonresponders. *Gastroenterology* **2007**, *132*, 1270–1278.
73. Bacon, B. R., Gordon, S. C., and Lawitz, E. HCV RESPOND-2 final results: high sustained virologic response among genotype 1 previous non-responders and relapsers to peginterferon/ribavirin when re-treated with boceprevir plus pegIntron (peginterferon alfa-2b)/ Ribavirin. *61st Annual Meeting of the American Association for the Study of Liver Diseases*, Boston, October 29–November 2, 2010. Abstract 216.
74. Poordad, F., McCone, J., and Bacon, B. R. Boceprevir (BOC) combined with peginterferon alfa-2b/ribavirin (P/R) for treatment-naive patients with hepatitis C virus (HCV) genotype (G) 1: SPRINT-2 final results. *61st Annual Meeting of the American Association for the Study of Liver Diseases*, Boston, October 29–November 2, 2010. Abstract LB-4.
75. Sudhakar, A., Dahanukar, V., Zavialov, I., Orr, C., Nguyen, H. N., Weber, J., Jeon, I., Chen, M., Green, M. D., Wong, G. S., Park, J., and Iwama, T. Process and intermediates for the preparation of (1*R*,2*S*,5*S*)-*N*-[3-amino-1-(cyclobutylmethyl)-2,3-dioxopropyl]-3-[(2*S*)-2-[[[[1,1-dimethylethyl]amino]carbonyl]amino]-3,3-dimethyl-1-oxobutyl]-6,6-dimethyl-3-azabicyclo [3. 1. 0]hexane-2-carboxamide. *PCT Int. Appl.* **2004**. *WO 2004113294*.
76. Nahm, S. and Weinreb, S. M. *N*-Methoxy-*N*-methylamides as effective acylating agents. *Tetrahedron Lett.* **1981**, *22*, 3815–3818.
77. Van der Veken, P., Senten, K., Kertèsz, I., Haemers, A., and Augustyns, K. β-Fluorinated proline derivatives: potential transition state inhibitors for proline selective serine dipeptidases. *Tetrahedron Lett.* **2003**, *44*, 969–972.
78. Seebach, D., Imwinkelried, R., and Stucky, G. Preparation of optically active alcohols from 1,3-dioxan-4-ones. A practical version of the asymmetric synthesis with nucleophilic substitution at acetal centers. *Angew. Chem., Int. Ed. Engl.* **1986**, *25*, 178–180.
79. Zhang, R., Mamai, A., and Madalengoitia, J. S. Cyclopropanation reactions of pyroglutamic acid-derived synthons with alkylidene transfer reagents. *J. Org. Chem.* **1999**, *64*, 547–555.
80. Ahmad, S., Doweyko, L. M., Dugar, S., Grazier, N., Ngu, K., Wu, S. C., Yost, K. J., Chen, B. -C., Gougoutas, J. Z., DiMarco, J. D., Lan, S. -J., Gavin, B. J., Chen, A. Y., Dorso, C. R., Serafino, R., Kirby, M., and Atwal, K. S. Arylcyclopropanecarboxyl guanidines as novel, potent, and selective inhibitors of the sodium hydrogen exchanger isoform-1. *J. Med. Chem.* **2001**, *44*, 3302–3310.
81. Norbeck, D. W. and Kramer, J. B. Synthesis of (−)-oxetanocin. *J. Am. Chem. Soc.* **1988**, *110*, 7217–7218.
82. Arasappan, A., Padilla, A. I., Jao, E., Bennett, F., Bogen, S. L., Chen, K. X., Pike, R. E., Sannigrahi, M., Soares, J., Venkatraman, S., Vibulbhan, B., Saksena, A. K., Girijavallabhan, V., Tong, X., Cheng, K. -C., and Njoroge, F. G. Toward second generation hepatitis C virus NS3 serine protease inhibitors: discovery of novel P4 modified analogues with improved potency and pharmacokinetic profile. *J. Med. Chem.* **2009**, *52*, 2806–2817.
83. Chen, K. X., Nair, L., Vibulbhan, B., Yang, W., Arasappan, A., Bogen, S. L., Venkatraman, S., Bennett, F., Pan, W., Blackman, M. L., Padilla, A. I., Prongay, A., Cheng, K. -C., Tong, X., Shih, N. -Y., and Njoroge, F. G. Second-generation highly potent and selective inhibitors of the hepatitis C virus NS3 serine protease. *J. Med. Chem.* **2009**, *52*, 1370–1379.
84. Venkatraman, S., Velazquez, F., Wu, W., Blackman, M., Chen, K. X., Bogen, S. L., Nair, L., Tong, X., Chase, R., Hart, A., Agrawal, S., Pichardo, J., Prongay, A., Cheng, K. -C., Girijavallabhan, V., Piwinski, J., Shih, N. -Y., and Njoroge, F. G. Discovery and structure–activity relationship of P1-P3 ketoamide derived macrocyclic inhibitors of hepatitis C virus NS3 protease. *J. Med. Chem.* **2009**, *52*, 336–346.
85. Bennett, F., Huang, Y., Hendrata, S., Lovey, R., Bogen, S. L., Pan, W., Guo, Z., Prongay, A., Chen, K. X., Arasappan, A., Venkatraman, S., Velazquez, F., Nair, L., Sannigrahi, M., Tong, X., Pichardo, J., Cheng, K. -C., Girijavallabhan, V. M., Saksena, A. K., and Njoroge, F. G. The introduction of P4 substituted 1-methylcyclohexyl groups into Boceprevir: a change in direction in the search for a second generation HCV NS3 protease inhibitor. *Bioorg. Med. Chem. Lett.* **2010**, *20*, 2617–2621.

86. Bogen, S. L., Pan, W., Ruan, S., Nair, L. G., Arasappan, A., Bennett, F., Chen, K. X., Jao, E., Venkatraman, S., Vibulbhan, B., Liu, R., Cheng, K. -C., Guo, Z., Tong, X., Saksena, A. K., Girijavallabhan, V., and Njoroge, F. G. Toward the back-up of boceprevir (SCH 503034): discovery of new extended P4-capped ketoamide inhibitors of hepatitis C virus NS3 serine protease with improved potency and pharmacokinetic profiles. *J. Med. Chem.* **2009**, *52*, 3679–3688.
87. Chen, K. X., Vibulbhan, B., Yang, W., Nair, L. G., Tong, X., Cheng, K. -C., and Njoroge, F. G. Novel potent inhibitors of hepatitis C virus (HCV) NS3 protease with cyclic sulfonyl P3 cappings. *Bioorg. Med. Chem. Lett.* **2009**, *19*, 1105–1109.
88. Venkatraman, S., Blackman, M., Wu, W., Nair, L., Arasappan, A., Padilla, A., Bogen, S. L., Bennett, F., Chen, K. X., Pichardo, J., Tong, X., Prongay, A., Cheng, K. -C., Girijavallabhan, V., and Njoroge, F. G. Discovery of novel P3 sulfonamide-capped inhibitors of HCV NS3 protease. Inhibitors with improved cellular potencies. *Bioorg. Med. Chem.* **2009**, *17*, 4486–4495.
89. Bogen, S. L., Arasappan, A., Velazquez, F., Blackman, M., Huelgas, R., Pan, W., Siegel, E., Nair, L. G., Venkatraman, S., Guo, Z., Doll, R., Shih, N. -Y., and Njoroge, F. G. Discovery of potent sulfonamide P4-capped ketoamide second generation inhibitors of hepatitis C virus NS3 serine protease with favorable pharmacokinetic profiles in preclinical species. *Bioorg. Med. Chem.* **2010**, *18*, 1854–1865.
90. Tong, X., Arasappan, A., Bennett, F., Chase, R., Feld, B., Guo, Z., Hart, A., Madison, V., Malcolm, B., Pichardo, J., Prongay, A., Ralston, R., Skelton, A., Xia, E., Zhang, R., and Njoroge, F. G. Preclinical characterization of the antiviral activity of SCH 900518 (Narlaprevir), a novel mechanism-based inhibitor of hepatitis C virus NS3 protease. *Antimicrob. Agents Chemother.* **2010**, *54*, 2365–2370.
91. Reesink, H. W., Bergmann, J. F., de Bruijne, J., Weegink, C. J., van Lier, J. J., van Vliet, A., Keung, A., Li, J., O'Mara, E., Treitel, M. A., Hughes, E. A., Janssen, H. L. A., and de Knegt, R. J. Safety and antiviral activity of SCH 900518 administered as monotherapy and in combination with peginterferon alfa-2b to naive and treatment-experienced HCV-1 infected patients. *J. Hepatol.* **2009**, *50 (Suppl 1)*, S35–S36.
92. de Bruijne, J., Bergmann, J. F., Reesink, H. W., Weegink, C. J., Molenkamp, R., Schinkel, J., Tong, X., Li, J., Treitel, M. A., Hughes, E. A., van Lier, J. J., van Vliet, A., Janssen, H. L. A., and de Knegt, R. J. Antiviral activity of narlaprevir combined with ritonavir and pegylated interferon in chronic hepatitis C patients. *Hepatology* **2010**, *52*, 1590–1599.
93. Vierling, J.Once daily narlaprevir (SCH 900518) in combination with PEGINTRON (peginterferon alfa-2b)/ribavirin for treatment-naïve subjects with genotype-1 CHC: interim results from NEXT-1, a Phase 2a study. *American Association for the Study of Liver Diseases 2009*, Boston, Abstract LB4.
94. Wieland, S.F. and Chisari, F.V. Stealth and cunning: hepatitis B and hepatitis C viruses. *J. Virol.* **2005**, *79*, 9369–9380.
95. Bartenschlager, R. and Lohmann, V. Replication of hepatitis C virus. *J. Gen. Virol.* **2000**, *81*, 1631–1648.
96. Simmonds, P., Bukh, J., Combet, C., Deleage, G., Enomoto, N., Feinstone, S., Halfon, P., Inchauspe, G., Kuiken, C., Maertens, G., and Mizokami, M. Consensus proposals for a unified system of nomenclature of hepatitis C virus genotypes. *Hepatology* **2005**, *42*, 962–973.
97. McCarthy, J. J., Li, J. H., Thompson, A., Suchindran, S., Lao, X. Q., Patel, K., Tillmann, H. L., Muir, A. J., and McHutchison, J. G. Replicated association between an IL28B gene variant and a sustained response to pegylated interferon and ribavirin. *Gastroenterology* **2010**, *138*, 2307–2314.
98. Thompson, A. J., Muir, A. J., Sulkowski, M. S., Ge, D., Fellay, J., Shianna, K. V., Urban, T., Afdhal, N. H., Jacobson, I. M., Esteban, R., and Poordad, F. Interleukin-28B polymorphism improves viral kinetics and is the strongest pretreatment predictor of sustained virologic response in genotype 1 hepatitis C virus. *Gastroenterology* **2010**, *139*, 120–129. e118.

CHAPTER **13**

THE DISCOVERY OF SAMSCA® (TOLVAPTAN): THE FIRST ORAL NONPEPTIDE VASOPRESSIN RECEPTOR ANTAGONIST

Kazumi Kondo and Yoshitaka Yamamura

13.1 BACKGROUND INFORMATION ABOUT THE DISEASE

Otsuka's mission to develop a drug for the treatment of volume overload in congestive heart failure (CHF) was initiated in 1983. Before the drug discovery program started, in 1982, Prof. Dr. Masayoshi Orita[1] in Osaka University advised that the water diuretics, aquaretics, could be a promising medication for treating CHF.

Several classes of compounds are currently prescribed for treating CHF, including cardiac glycosides,[2]angiotensin-converting enzyme inhibitors (ACE inhibitors), and diuretics.[3] Diuretics can reduce the accumulation of fluid in the legs, abdomen, and lungs, lower blood pressure, and improve the signs and symptoms related to volume overload in CHF. Diuretics are effective for treating CHF; however, these drugs also lead to the excretion of salts and water, and chronic treatment with diuretics causes hyponatremia [1].

Water diuretics (aquaretics) are expected to induce excretion of water without loss of salts. The neurohypophysial nonapeptide hormone arginine vasopressin (AVP, Figure 13.1) is well known for its pressor response and antidiuretic activities in mammals [2]. AVP exerts vasoconstriction by interacting with the vascular V_{1a} receptors and causes antidiuresis by interacting with the renal V_2 receptors. These mechanisms help to maintain normal plasma osmolality, blood volume, and blood pressure. AVP antagonists are expected to be novel therapeutic agents for the treatment of diseases characterized by the excessive renal reabsorption of free water. Therefore, AVP V_2 receptor antagonists are expected to be water diuretics. Both chronic treatment of CHF and treatment of hyponatremia will become possible using water diuretics.

Since vasopressin was first prepared by total synthesis, numerous analogs of AVP have been synthesized and evaluated to identify the structural features responsible for their respective biological features [3]. At the beginning of Otsuka's research in this area, many attempts to develop a V_2 antagonist for treating diseases characterized by

[1] Current address: Osaka Jikei Gakuen, Osaka Jikei Gakuen Godo Bldg 9th Floor, 1-2-8 Miyahara, Yodogawa-ku, Osaka city, 532-0003 Osaka, Japan.

[2] http://en.wikipedia.org/wiki/Cardiac_glycoside

[3] http://www.heartsite.com/html/chf_5.html

Case Studies in Modern Drug Discovery and Development, Edited by Xianhai Huang and Robert G. Aslanian.

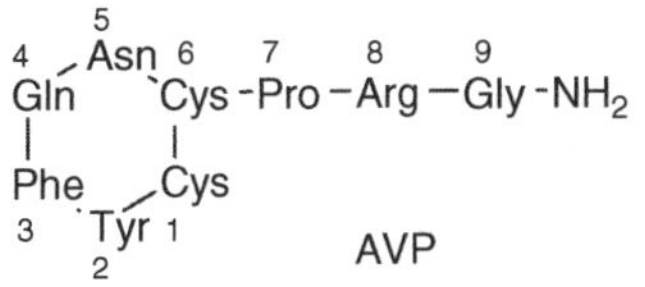

Figure 13.1 Neurohypophysial nonapeptide hormone arginine vasopressin (AVP).

excess renal reabsorption of free water have been reported, because V_2 antagonists may correct the fluid retention and hyponatremia observed in congestive heart failure, liver cirrhosis [6m], and nephrotic syndrome [6n]. However, marked species differences and inconsistencies have been revealed between the *in vivo* and *in vitro* assay systems as reported in the case of SK&F-101926 and SK&F-105494 (Figure 13.2) [4]. These compounds showed antagonist activity in an *in vitro* study and in animal models, including the rhesus monkey, but showed a full antidiuretic response in humans. It was assumed that such species differences originated from the structural resemblance of the peptide derivatives to AVP itself. Therefore, the effort on AVP receptor antagonists was focused on the discovery of nonpeptide compounds. Another drawback of peptide antagonists is poor bioavailability by oral administration. Chronic treatment by oral administration is generally preferred, and patients with conditions such as CHF and hyponatremia are also amenable to this route of treatment. Before 1983, no nonpeptide compounds had been reported to show an affinity for any vasopressin receptors.

13.2 BIOLOGICAL RATIONAL

Figure 13.3 shows the coupling mechanisms of vasopressin receptors. AVP receptors are members of the superfamily of G-protein coupled receptors with seven trans-membrane domains. AVP binding to the V_2 receptors activates the Gs, followed by an increase in the intracellular cAMP synthesis. Finally, the synthesis of aquaporin-2 water channel proteins and their shuttling to the apical surface of the collecting ducts allow free water to be reabsorbed. On the other hand, AVP binding to the V_{1a} or V_{1b} receptors activates the Gq, which leads to an increase in the intracellular levels of diacylglycerol (DAG) and inositol (1,4,5)-triphosphate (IP3). IP3 stimulates calcium release from the endoplasmic reticulum, and the emptying of calcium stores activates calcium influx. The increase in intracellular calcium concentration activates the cascade of calcium-mediated effects, which lead to the activation of PKC (protein kinase C).

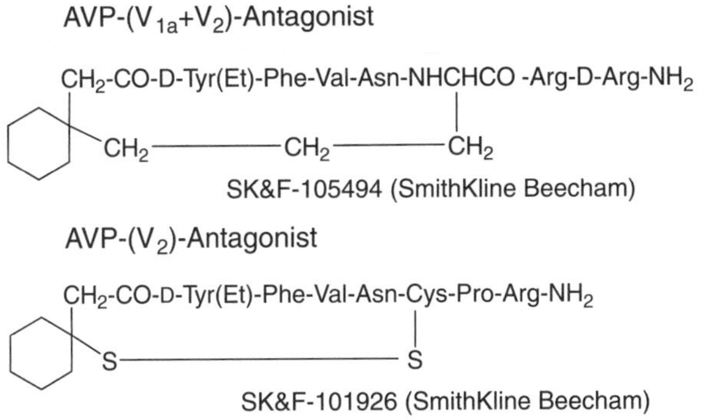

Figure 13.2 SK&F-101926 and SK&F-105494.

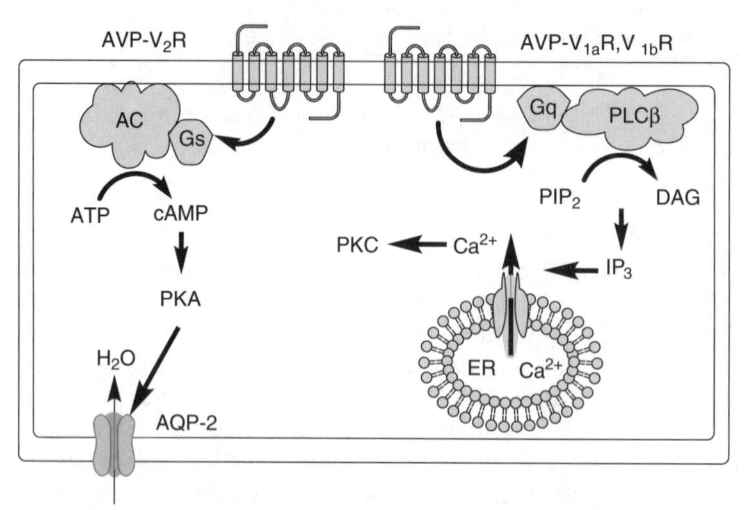

Abbreviations: AC, adenylyl cyclase; AQP-2, aquaporin, AVP-regulated water channel; AVP, arginine vasopressin; DAG, diacylglycerol; ER, endoplasmic reticulum; IP3, inositol (1,4,5)-trisphosphate; PIP2, phosphatidylinositol (4,5)-bisphosphate; PKA, protein kinase A; PKC, protein kinase C; PLC β, phospholipase Cβ.

Figure 13.3 Coupling mechanisms of vasopressin receptors.

13.3 LEAD GENERATION STRATEGIES: THE DISCOVERY OF MOZAVAPTAN

No reports about nonpeptide vasopressin receptor antagonists or agonists were found in patents or in the literature; therefore, in-house compound library screening was initiated. The competition binding experiments were performed using ^{3}H-AVP as a natural ligand with rat V_{1a} and rat V_2 receptors [5]. No receptor cloning was reported when the binding experiment was initiated; therefore, experiments in a HTS manner could not be performed.

After about 20,000 compounds from the in-house library were screened, several compounds were found that showed potent inhibition of binding at the 3×10^{-4} M concentration (Figure 13.4). Interestingly, some of these compounds contained a

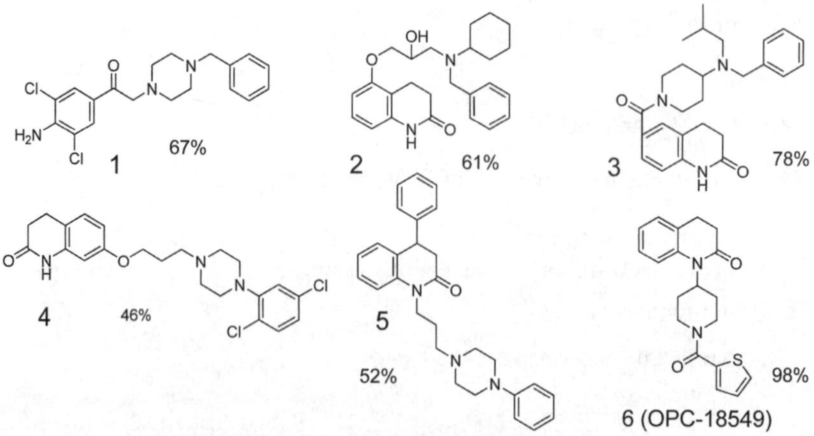

1 67%
2 61%
3 78%
4 46%
5 52%
6 (OPC-18549) 98%

Figure 13.4 In-house library screening leads.

TABLE 13.1 Initial Modifications Based on Compound 6

1-(1-R-piperidin-4-yl)-3,4-dihydroquinolin-2(1H)-one (N–R)

No.	R	Receptor affinity IC_{50} (μM)[a]	
		V_{1a}	V_2
6	CO–(2-thienyl)	2.5	>100
7	CO–(2-furyl)	11	>100
8	CO–(4-pyridyl)	37	>100
9	CO–(2-pyrazinyl)	26	>100
10	CO–phenyl	1.9	>50
11	CH_2–phenyl	>100	>100
12	$COCH_2$–phenyl	12	>100

[a]Compounds were tested for their ability to displace [^{3}H]AVP from its specific binding sites in rat liver (V_{1a}) and kidney (V_2 receptor) plasma membrane preparations.

3,4-dihydroquinolin-2-one, dihydrocarbostyril as a scaffold. Among them, compound **6**, **OPC-18549**, showed IC_{50} values for the rat V_{1a} and V_2 receptors of 2.5 μM and >100 μM, respectively. Because compound **6** has a simple structure with V_{1a}-selective inhibition, the optimization of this molecule as the lead structure to identify compounds with high affinity of V_2 receptor was initialized to enhance its activity and oral bioavailability.

The initial modifications of compound **6** were focused on the terminal thiophenecarboxamide substituent. Replacement of this thiophene ring with another heteroaromatic ring did not lead to any increase in activity, as shown by the selected analogs **7–12** in Table 13.1. Among these compounds, the simple phenyl derivative **10** showed modest improvement for the V_{1a} receptor over lead compound **6**. The insertion of a methylene group between the carbonyl and phenyl ring as in **12** reduced the affinity. Conversion of the amido bond into the aminomethylene group as in compound **11** eliminated the binding affinity.

The substituent effects on the phenyl-ring are shown in Table 13.2. Substitution on the para-position almost always led to a greater binding affinity for the V_{1a} receptor compared to the ortho- or meta-positions. More interestingly, para-substitution with

TABLE 13.2 SAR Studies Based on Compound 10

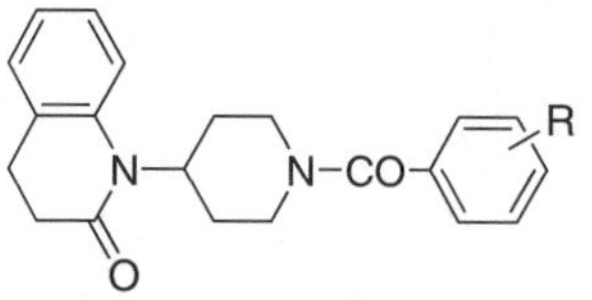

No.	R	Receptor affinity IC_{50} (μM)		Antipressor activity
		V_{1a}	V_2	% Inhibition[a]
13	2-Cl	9.9	>100	
14	3-Cl	4.4	>100	
15	4-Cl	1.2	78	
16	2-Me	8.4	>100	
17	3-Me	1.3	>100	
18	4-Me	0.5	>100	23 ± 8.9 (100)
19	2-NO_2	8.4	>100	
20	3-NO_2	3.1	>100	
21	4-NO_2	2.0	>100	
22	2-OMe	0.65	36	
23	3-OMe	2.6	>100	
24	4-OMe	0.49	>100	
25	4-OEt	0.21	>100	75 ± 3.4 (30)
26	4-O-nPr	0.32	>100	65 ± 6.1 (30)
27	4-O-nBu	0.42	>100	
28	4-O-nHex	1.5	54	
29	4-Et	0.5	80	
30	4-nPr	0.33	>100	86 ± 6.0 (100)
31	4-nBu	0.35	83	

[a]The inhibition was expressed as percentage change in diastolic blood pressure increased by AVP (30 mU/kg, iv) before and after test compounds po administration. Except where indicated, a number of determination was four. Dosage in parentheses (mg/kg).

methyl or methoxy (**18**,**24**) provided a substantial increase in the affinity for the V_{1a} receptor compared to nonsubstituted compound **10**. More analogs of the alkoxy- and alkyl-substituted compounds were synthesized and evaluated (compounds **25**–**31**). The 4-ethoxy (**25**) and 4-*n*-propyl (**30**) derivatives showed the most potent affinity for the V_{1a} receptor among the alkoxy and alkyl derivatives, respectively. It seems that the chain length at the para-position does not affect the V_{1a} receptor affinity. It is noteworthy that a relatively long substituent, such as *n*-hexyloxy (**28**), at the para-position did not lower the affinity to V_{1a} receptor compared to the nonsubstituted analog (compound **10**).

The antivasopressor activity was then examined by oral administration to conscious rats, as illustrated by the selected analogs in Table 13.2. These compounds were found to be orally effective V_{1a} antagonists, although the antagonist potency was not satisfactory. Encouraged by these results, effort was continued to modify this new lead compound (**25**). In order to improve oral activity, it was hypothesized that this compound had sufficient lipophilicity but poor water solubility, suggesting the introduction of a hydrophilic group at the terminal would enhance its oral activity.

TABLE 13.3 SAR Studies Based on Compound 10 with Hydrophilic Substituents

N–⟨piperidine⟩N–CO–⟨phenyl⟩–$O(CH_2)_n$-X

No.	n	X	Receptor affinity IC_{50} (μM) V_{1a}	V_2	Antipressor activity % Inhibition[a]	ID_{50} (mg/kg)
32	2	NH_2	2.0	>100		
33	3	NH_2	0.75	>100		
34	4	NH_2	0.33	>100	31 ± 14 (10)	
35	5	NH_2	0.28	>100	NE (10)	
36	6	NH_2	0.10	>100		
37	8	NH_2	0.068	44	NE (10)	
38	3	NHCHO	0.24	>100	50 ± 13 (10)	
39	4	NHCHO	0.25	>100		
40	2	NHAc	0.42	>100	80 ± 4.7 (10)	3.4
41	3	NHAc	0.44	>100	93 ± 4.0 (10)	2.0
42	4	NHAc	0.21	>100	78 ± 9.3 (10)	2.5
43	5	NHAc	0.16	>100	81 ± 6.3 (10)	2.3
44	6	NHAc	0.12	>100	72 ± 12 (10)	5.0
45	8	NHAc	0.30	>100	NE (10)	
46	3	NHCOEt	0.78	>100		
47	3	$NHCO_2Me$	0.36	>100	73 ± 9.2 (10)	4.0
48	3	N(Me)Ac	0.54	>100		

[a]The inhibition was expressed as percentage change in diastolic blood pressure increased by AVP (30 mU/kg, iv) before and after test compounds po administration. Except where indicated, a number of determination was four. Dosage in parentheses (mg/kg). ID50 represents the 50% inhibition dose for AVP (30 miliunits/kg, iv) induced vasoconstriction when test compounds are orally administrated.

The results of the hydrophilic substituent series are shown in Table 13.3. The effects of such hydrophilic substituents differ entirely from the unsubstituted series **24–28** presented in Table 13.2. In the simple amino series **32–37**, it seems that the longer chain showed more potent V_{1a} binding affinity, and compound **37** showed the highest binding affinity (IC_{50} = 0.068 μM). However, both in the formyl amino series **38–39** and the acetyl amino series **40–45**, the potency of binding affinity was not as greatly changed as in the simple amino series. The optimal length of the alkoxy chain with regard to binding affinity is six carbons when the terminal hydrophilic substituent is acetamide.

The comparison of binding affinities between a series of compounds (**33–36** and **41–44**), whose chain length (n) is 3–6 atoms, indicates that the basicity of the terminal amino group is not critical. *N*-Methylation of the amide nitrogen (**48**) had virtually no effect on V_{1a} binding compared to **41** or **46**, which suggests that the terminal amide bond does not act as a hydrogen bond donor with the receptor. Furthermore, none of the compounds in Tables 13.1, 13.2, or 13.3 exhibited apparent V_2 receptor binding affinity.

The data in Table 13.3 shows, however, that the relative orders of potency of the various analogs in the *in vitro* assay do not always translate well into *in vivo* antagonistic activity. For example, the potent *in vitro* compounds (**34,35,37**) did not show potent

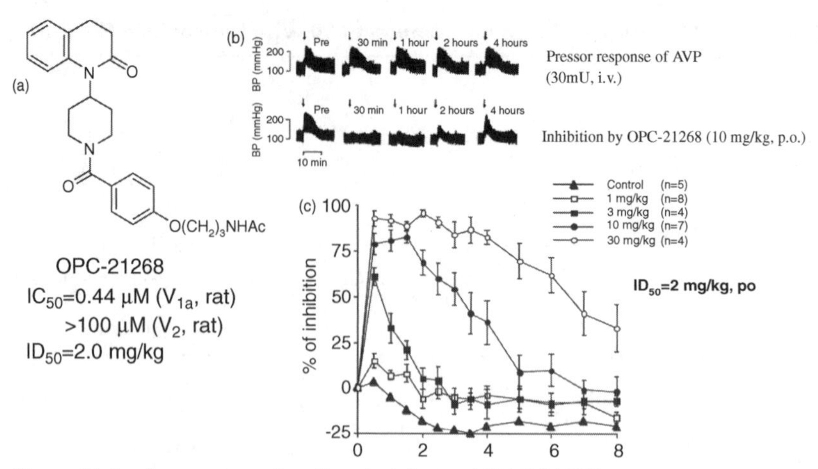

Figure 13.5 Antagonism of orally administrated **OPC-21268** on pressor responses to AVP in conscious rats.

activity *in vivo*. The enhancement of antivasopressor activity by oral administration was achieved by adding an acetyl group to the amine on the terminal of the alkoxy chain, such as in **40–44**. Of note, compound **40** (**OPC-21268**), which did not show potent binding affinity, showed the most potent oral activity. Replacement of the amide linkage of **40** with urethane, as in **47**, was slightly detrimental to the *in vivo* activity. Conversion of the acetyl group of **40** into a formyl or propyl (such as in **38** and **46**) lowered the oral activity [6].

Figure 13.5a shows the chemical structure of **OPC-21268** (compound **40**). The oral efficacy of **OPC-21268** was examined in conscious rats (male Sprague–Dawley rats, 300–400 g, Charles River Labs). Exogeneously administrated AVP (30 mU kg^{-1} i.v.) induced an increase in blood pressure in conscious rats (Figure 13.5b). After oral administration of **OPC-21268** (10 mg kg^{-1}), the vasoconstriction induced by exogenous AVP was inhibited in a time-dependent manner (Figure 13.5c). The inhibitory effect of **OPC-21268** was dose-dependent, and the effect lasted for more than 8 h at 30 mg kg^{-1}. The 50% inhibition dose (ID_{50}) for AVP-induced vasoconstriction was estimated as 2 mg kg^{-1} [7].

Although none of the 2-quinolone derivatives exhibited any apparent V_2 receptor binding affinity, further investigations were conducted to find a V_2 antagonist. Some compounds shown in Table 13.2 did exhibit moderate affinity to the V_2 receptor (**15**, **22**, etc.). Encouraged by these results, a series of more rigid analogs were synthesized by replacing the piperidyl moiety of compound **15** with a phenyl ring. In the study of the V_{1a} antagonist series, it was found out that the two amide moieties in compound **15** were essential for the affinity of the AVP receptors. Furthermore, the team was interested in reversing the amide linkage in the 3,4-dihydro-2(1H)-quinolinone core of compound **15** and achieving a normal peptide bond arrangement (from CON-spacer-NCO (**15**) to NCO-spacer-NCO (**49**)). The resultant structure is shown as **49** in Figure 13.6.

Replacement of the piperidine ring of compound **15** by a phenyl ring resulted in a benzamide **49**, which greatly enhanced V_2 binding affinity (Table 13.4). The success of compound **49** encouraged effort to search for a V_2 receptor antagonist. The longer alkoxy chain was introduced on the terminal phenyl ring as seen with compounds **50–52**, because 4-OEt was the optimal substituent for binding in the V_{1a} antagonist series. However, the introduction of a longer alkoxy chain, as in compounds **51** and **52**, drastically lowered not

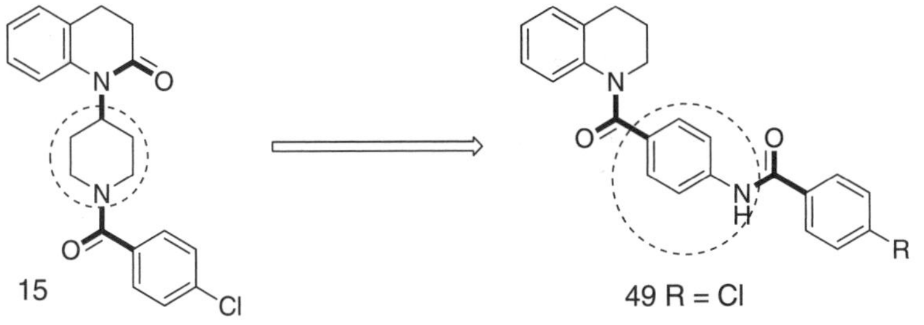

Figure 13.6 Core modification of compound **15**.

only the V_2 binding affinity, but also the V_{1a} binding affinity. The binding mode of compound **49** with the AVP receptor seems to be different from that of the 2(1*H*)-quinolinones in the V_{1a} antagonist series.

Comparison of **55**, **66**, and **67** showed that the substituted position of the benzamide must be para to the tetrahydroquinolinylcarbonyl group for the greatest binding affinity to both V_{1a} and V_2 receptors, while ortho (**67**) followed by meta-substitution (**66**) decreases the

TABLE 13.4 SAR Studies Based on Compound 15

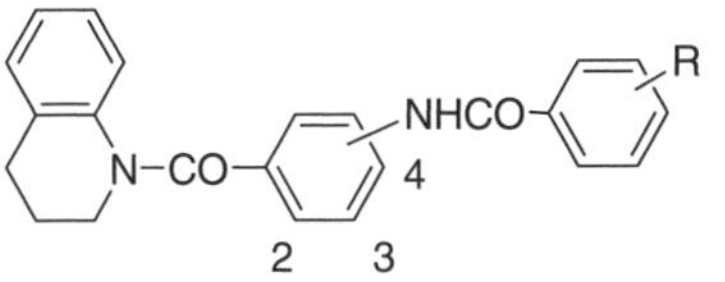

			Receptor affinity IC_{50} (μM)	
No.	Position	R	V_{1a}	V_2
49	4	4-Cl	5.1	1.9
50	4	4-OMe	2.2	1.8
51	4	4-OEt	14	>100
52	4	4-OnBu	>100	>100
53	4	4-Me	10	1.4
54	4	4-NO_2	>100	6.5
55	4	H	1.6	0.98
56	4	2-Cl	1.6	0.42
57	4	2-OMe	1.9	2.1
58	4	2-Me	1.4	0.20
59	4	3-Cl	6.4	0.20
60	4	3-OMe	2.8	0.40
61	4	3-Me	3.1	0.68
62	4	3,4-Me_2	>100	1.2
63	4	2,4-Me_2	3.3	0.21
64	4	2,4-Cl_2	>100	0.25
65	4	3,5-Cl_2	9.4	0.082
66	3	H	>100	40
67	2	H	88	22

affinity. The substitution on the terminal phenyl ring showed that the ortho- and meta-positions were always superior to the para position for V_2 affinity (**49**, **50**, **53**–**61**), except for the 2-OMe group (**57**). Thus, compounds **49**, **50**, **53**, and **54** have lower V_2 binding affinities than the unsubstituted benzamide **55** due to increased steric interactions between this region of the terminal aromatic ring and the receptor site. Substituents on the meta- and ortho-positions (**56**, **58**–**61**) showed a slight enhancement of V_2 binding affinity. The most potent compound in the series was the 3,5-dichloro substituted compound (**65**), a significant 22-fold improvement over the 4-Cl lead **49**. Surprisingly, the 2,4-di-substitution on the phenyl ring led to a retention of V_2 binding (**63**, **64** vs. **53**, **58** and **49**, **56**). It is unclear why **63** and **64** do not show lower binding affinity than the ortho-monosubstitution (**56**, **58**). The presence of the ortho-substituent on the phenyl ring might force a conformational change, consequently reducing the interactions between the para-substituent and the receptor site.

More modifications on the benzamide are shown in Table 13.5. The alkyl group (**68**–**70**) produced a substantial decrease in V_2 affinity. Insertion of a methylene spacer between the carbonyl and phenyl ring proved compatible with V_2 affinity (**71** vs. **55**); however, the insertion of a longer chain, as in **72**, reduced the affinity. Other replacements of the phenyl ring, such as with pyridyl (**73**), furyl (**74**), or thienyl (**75**) groups, provided less effective compounds.

TABLE 13.5 Further Modifications of the Benzamide Side Chain

N-CO—(phenylene)—NHCO—R

No.	R	Receptor affinity IC_{50} (μM)	
		V_{1a}	V_2
68	Me	74	>100
69	n-Pr	4.3	7.1
70	i-Pr	2.4	8.1
71	CH_2Ph	3.2	1.0
72	CH_2CH_2Ph	2.3	6.1
73	3-pyridyl (N)	11	7.6
74	2-furyl (O)	4.0	6.4
75	3-thienyl (S)	1.7	1.7

Based on these studies, the 2-methylbenzamide **58** was selected for further investigation. Replacements of the tetrahydroquinoline ring of the new lead **58** with other benzoheterocycles are shown in Table 13.6. In the six-membered ring series, the insertion of a hetero atom onto the tetrahydroquinoline ring decreases the V_2 binding affinity, as seen with compounds **76** and **77**. However, the enlargement of six-membered rings to seven-membered rings showed a striking effect on V_2 binding affinity (**76** vs. **81**, **77** vs. **83**, and **58** vs. **78**). Remarkably, compounds **78** and **79** bound to the V_2 receptor with an affinity approximately one order of magnitude higher than **58** and **56**, respectively. Moreover, **78** and **79** showed more potent binding affinity for the V_{1a} receptor by two orders of magnitude over **58** and **56**, respectively. The increased steric bulkiness and/or lipophilicity of the seven-membered ring compared to that of between 2- and 3-position on six-membered ring might be responsible for the enhanced binding affinity. Interestingly, compound **83** showed selectivity on the binding affinity for the V_2 receptor. The eight-membered ring substituted analog, benzazocine **85**, 5-*N*-methyl-1,5-benzodiazepine **83**, and benzazepine **78**, all have very similar binding affinity for the V_2 receptor.

Compounds **86–88** in Table 13.7 were prepared to evaluate the roles of the amide linkage of the benzamide substructure in compound **80**. Replacement with the urethane **86**, sulfonamide **87**, or urea **88** caused a substantial decrease in V_2 receptor affinity when compared with **80**.

The potent V_2 binders **78**, **79**, and **85** in Table 13.6 failed to demonstrate oral diuretic activity. However, the 1,4-benzodiazepine derivative **84**, which showed lower V_2 affinity than those, did provide some diuretic activity, with a 5- to 6-fold increase in urine volume being observed for 4 h at 100 mg kg^{-1} after oral administration in normally hydrated conscious rats ($n=3$) compared to the control rats ($n=6$). This may have been due to the better oral bioavailability of the 1,4-benzodiazepine than the other heterocycles. In an attempt to produce an analog having greater potency, bioavailability, and V_2 selectivity on binding affinity, the effect of introducing a basic amino group was investigated, such as a dimethylamine, on the benzazepine ring of compounds **78** and **79**, which showed potent binding affinity to both V_{1a} and V_2 receptors. To make the synthesis easier, an amino group was introduced at the 5-position on the benzazepine ring.

The 5-dimethylamino substituted analogs **89–93** led to the retention of potent binding affinity for the V_2 receptor but a reduction of the binding affinity for the V_{1a} receptor (Table 13.8). The effect of the substituents on the terminal phenyl ring followed the same trends as those observed earlier. Thus, the replacement with 2-Me (**90**) and 3-Me (**91**) increased the V_2 binding affinity over the nonsubstituted congener (**89**), while the para-substituent (**92**) was slightly detrimental to V_2 binding. A comparison of the V_2 binding affinity of compounds (**90**, **94–100**, **102**) indicates that this series of V_2 receptor antagonists, with the exception of the cyclic analog **103**, are relatively insensitive to an alkyl substituent on the amino group at the 5-position of the benzazepine ring. The replacement with acetamide in **105** and urea in **106** led to poor affinity for the V_2 receptor when compared with the amine **102** or monoalkylamino series **94–96**. The basicity of an amino group at the 5-position is not essential for potent affinity for the V_2 receptor, because the hydroxyl compound **104** showed potent affinity for the V_2 receptor.

The introduction of a 3,5-dichloro substituent on the terminal phenyl ring, which showed the highest binding affinity for the V_2 receptor in the tetrahydroquinoline series, resulted in about the same potency as 2,4-dichloro or 2-chloro (**108** vs. **109** and **93**) with regard to the binding affinity for the V_2 receptor.

N-Methylation of the amide nitrogen, as in compound **107**, drastically lowered the V_2 binding affinity by two orders of magnitude when compared with compound **90**. It seems

TABLE 13.6 Replacements of the Tetrahydroquinoline Ring of Compound 58

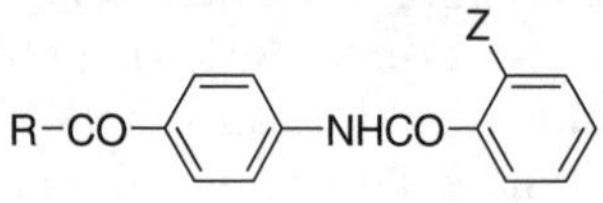

R–CO–(C6H4)–NHCO–(C6H4)–Z

No.	R	Z	Receptor affinity IC_{50} (μM)	
			V_{1a}	V_2
76	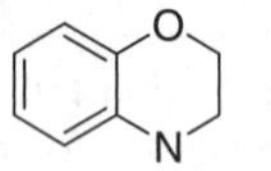	Me	7.7	4.1
77	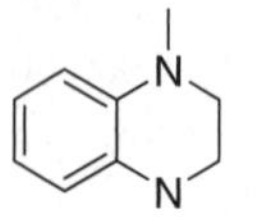	Me	5.1	0.40
78	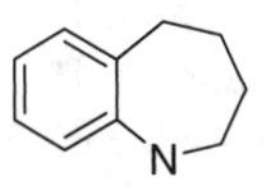	Me	0.056	0.018
79	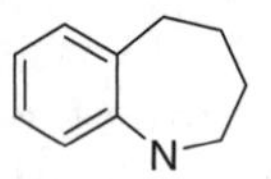	Cl	0.045	0.029
80	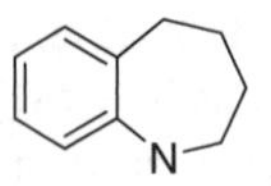	H	0.095	0.070
81	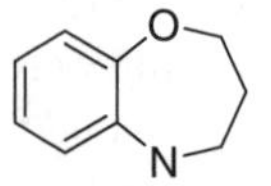	Me	1.2	0.11
82	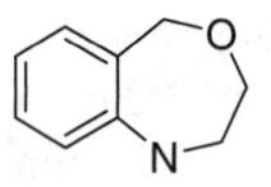	Me	0.63	0.30
83	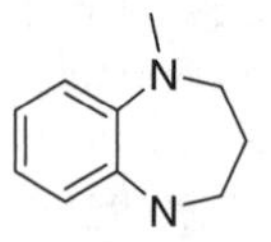	Me	0.38	0.014
84	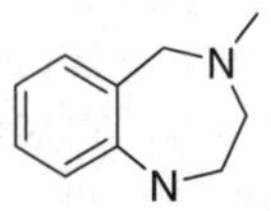	Me	1.8	0.17
85	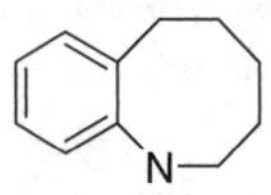	Me	0.41	0.028

TABLE 13.7 Modification of the Amide Linkage

N−CO−(C6H4)−NH-A−(C6H5)

		Receptor affinity IC_{50} (μM)	
No.	-A-	V_{1a}	V_2
86	-COO-	7.8	0.79
87	$-SO_2-$	2.5	1.6
88	-CONH-	0.76	0.18

that either the tertiary amide was arranged into an unfavorable conformation for binding or it is necessary to have a hydrogen-bonding interaction between the amide moiety and the receptor.

More importantly, some of the analogs showed oral efficacy. In the 5-dimethylamino series **89–93**, the 2-Me (**90**) demonstrated potent oral efficacy in rats, whereas H (**89**) and 3-Me (**91**) showed no activity. In a simple 5-alkylamino series (**90, 93–97**), the relative orders of binding affinity for the V_2 receptor translated well into *in vivo* diuretic activity. However, additional substitutents on the alkyl group, as seen with compounds **98–100**, are detrimental to oral efficacy.

Compounds **110–113** were prepared for comparison with 2-Me (**90**). The replacement of the methyl with OMe (**110**) or NO_2 (**111**) lowered the V_2 binding affinity, as was seen previously in the tetrahydroquinoline series. The amine **112** and the acetamide **113** showed much less activity than **90**. Lipophilic groups at this position seemed to show better binding affinity for the V_2 receptor [8].

The results of *in vitro* and *in vivo* evaluations with **90** (mozavaptan) are presented in detail in separate reports [9]. These studies indicated that the compound is an effective, orally bioavailable vasopressin V_2 receptor antagonist. In alcohol-anesthetized rats, **90** effectively blocked AVP-induced antidiuretic action with no agonistic properties. In normal conscious rats, it increased urine flow and decreased urine osmolality following oral administration (1–30 mg kg^{-1}). Thus, **90** (mozavaptan, **OPC-31260**) is a selective V_2 receptor antagonist, which acts as an aquaretic agent. Physuline® (mozavaptan hydrochloride) is commercially available in Japan (since October 2006) as a drug to treat paraneoplastic SIADH (the syndrome of inappropriate antidiuretic hormone).

13.4 LEAD OPTIMIZATION: FROM MOZAVAPTAN TO TOLVAPTAN

Although the amino group at the 5-position seemed essential for oral bioavailability as described in the discovery of mozavaptan, further modification of the amino moiety to enhance binding affinity failed. Further studies were focused on the effects of other additional substituents on the benzazepine scaffold.

As shown in Table 13.9, the substitution of a Cl moiety at the 6 and 9 positions (**114**, **117**) lowered the affinity for the V_2 receptor by 16- and 11.6-fold compared to compound **90**

TABLE 13.8 The Effect of Basic Amino Groups

No.	X	R	Y	IC_{50} (nM)		*in vivo*
				V_{1a}	V_2	UV (ml)
89	NMe_2	H	H	3.0	0.027	(>30)
90	NMe_2	H	2-Me	1.4	0.012	12.3 ± 2.3 ($ED_3 = 3.8$)
91	NMe_2	H	3-Me	2.4	0.014	(>30)
92	NMe_2	H	4-Me	26	0.044	
93	NMe_2	H	2-Cl	3.0	0.027	7.0 ± 0.5 (4.2)
94	NHMe	H	2-Me	0.72	0.024	8.3 ± 2.5 (4.6)
95	NHEt	H	2-Me	1.6	0.029	5.4 ± 0.6 (8.0)
96	NHnPr	H	2-Me	0.89	0.050	5.6 ± 1.0 (6.6)
97	N(Me)nPr	H	2-Me	1.2	0.022	8.3 ± 1.8 (4.9)
98	$N(Me)CH_2CO_2Et$	H	2-Me	0.98	0.029	(>30)
99	$N(Me)CH_2CN$	H	2-Me	3.2	0.025	(>30)
100	$N(Me)CH_2CONH_2$	H	2-Me	0.29	0.013	6.2 ± 0.6 (6.4)
101	=N-OAc	H	2-Me	2.3	0.058	(>30)
102	NH_2	H	2-Me	0.39	0.032	
103	piperidyl	H	2-Cl	2.8	0.14	
104	OH	H	2-Me	0.14	0.029	3.6 ± 0.8
105	NHAc	H	2-Me	3.2	0.15	(>30)
106	NHCONHMe	H	2-Me	2.8	0.096	
107	NMe_2	Me	2-Me	19	1.0	
108	NMe_2	H	3,5-Cl_2	2.6	0.020	
109	NMe_2	H	2,4-Cl_2	1.3	0.013	
110	NMe_2	H	2-OMe	1.0	0.077	
111	NMe_2	H	2-NO_2	2.6	0.071	
112	NMe_2	H	2-NH_2	1.9	0.19	
113	NMe_2	H	2-NHAc	16	0.64	

[a]UV values mean 2 hr urine volume (mL) when the test compounds were administrated orally at a dose of 10 mg/kg and are expressed as a mean ± SEM (n = 4). The mean value of 2 hr urine volume of control rats was 1.1 ± 0.2 mL (n = 4). Values in parentheses indicate ED_3 value. ED_3 represents the dose (mg/kg) required for a 3 fold increase in the 2 hr urine volume over the control rats. Values such as >30 designate that at this dose (mg/kg) a 3 fold increase in the 2 hr urine volume was not observed when compared with that of the control rats.

(mozavaptan), respectively. The substitution at the 8-position (**116**) lowered the affinity by about fivefold. Interestingly, the binding affinity for the V_{1a} receptor was enhanced (7.4-fold) by the Cl-substitution at the 7-position (**115**) compared to compound **90**. The diuretic activity after oral administration was enhanced by introducing a Cl atom at the 7-position compared to compound **90**, as shown by the ED_3 values.

Several derivatives were synthesized focusing on the effects of substituents at the 5-position of the benzazepine ring (Table 13.10). It was clearly demonstrated that steric size

TABLE 13.9 Substitution Effects of Compound 90

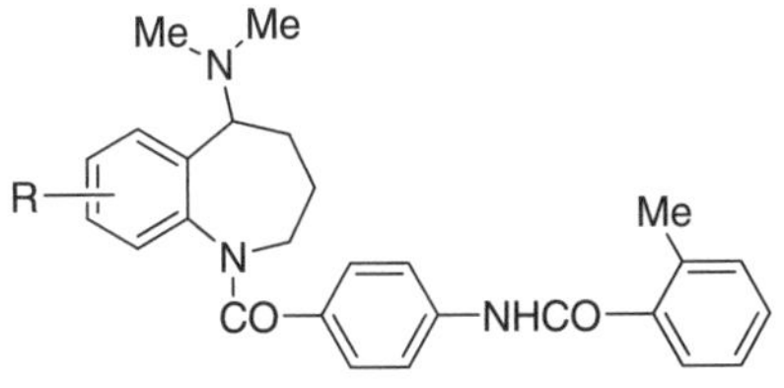

		Receptor affinity IC_{50} (μM)		*In vivo*	
No.	R	V_{1a}	V_2	UV (mL)	ED_3
114	6-Cl	1.7	0.19	1.6	
115	7-Cl	0.19	0.025	14.6	1.5
116	8-Cl	1.2	0.063	3.4	
117	9-Cl	0.54	0.14	2.4	
90	H	1.4	0.012	12.3	3.8

was important for the V_2-affinity in the case of the amine derivatives. The monomethylamino derivative **118** was 3.6-fold more potent than dimethylamino derivative **115** with regard to the V_2 receptor affinity. A longer chain (**119**) lowered the affinity compared with **118**. Di-substitution (**120**) eliminated the binding affinity for the V_2 receptor. The steric effects of the hydroxyl or alkoxy derivatives seemed to be smaller (**121, 122, 123**) compared to the amino series (**118, 119**). It was not clear why there are differences in the binding affinity between the alkoxy and amino derivatives. The oral activity of **118** and **119** was similar to **114**. The OH group was chosen as the substituent at the 5-position for further

TABLE 13.10 The Effects of Substituents at the 5-Position of the Benzazepine Ring

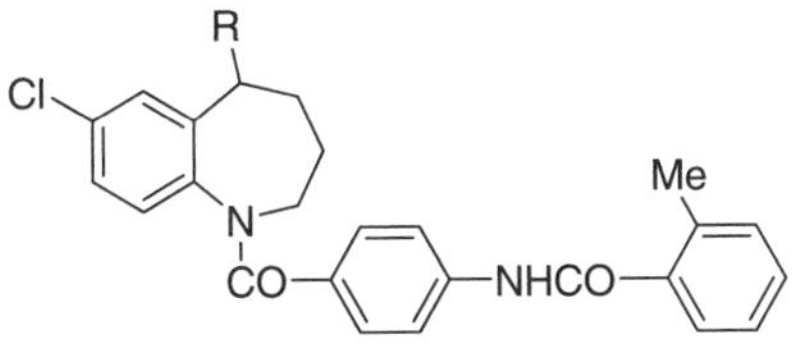

		Receptor affinity IC_{50} (μM)		*In vivo*	
No.	R	V_{1a}	V_2	UV (mL)	ED_3
118	NHMe	0.064	0.007	15.5	1.4
119	NH-Allyl	0.045	0.018	15.4	3.3
120	N(Me)-Allyl	0.35	0.097		
121	OH	0.017	0.003	7.2	
122	OMe	0.034	0.005	6.3	
123	O-Allyl	0.053	0.009	7.6	

TABLE 13.11 Final Modification Leading to the Discovery of Tolvaptan

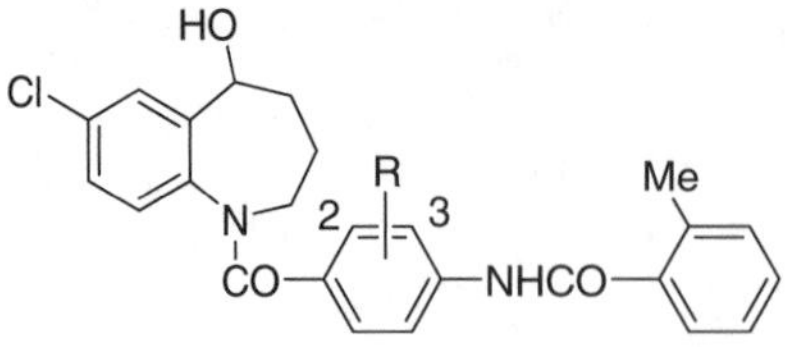

		Receptor affinity IC_{50} (μM)		*In vivo*	
No.	R	V_{1a}	V_2	UV (mL)	ED_3
124	2-Cl	0.29	0.008	16.8	1.6
125	3-Cl	0.031	0.028	3.0	
126	2-Me	0.58	0.003	17.3	0.54
127	2-OMe	0.039	0.013	15.2	1.4
128	3-OMe	0.007	0.005	3.5	

optimization because the OH derivative **121** showed the highest affinity for the V_2 receptor, although the oral activity and selectivity for the V_{1a} receptors did not improve compared to mozavaptan.

The final optimization was carried out on the rest of the structure (Table 13.11). The binding affinity for the V_2 receptors was slightly diminished by the 3-Cl (**125**) and 2-OMe (**127**) substituents compared to **121**. Interestingly, the binding affinity for the V_{1a} receptor and the oral activity (shown as urine volume) dramatically changed due to one substituent on the aminobenzoyl moiety (*R*-). The 2-Cl (**124**) and 2-Me (**126**) substitutions lowered the affinity for the V_{1a} receptor, but 3-OMe (**128**) enhanced this affinity. As previously reported on the V_{1a} selective nonpeptide antagonists, the binding affinity for the V_{1a} receptor was enhanced by one substituent due to its hydrogen bonding ability. Therefore, the enhancement by the 3-OMe group might be explained in the same manner. The substitution at the 2-position enhanced the oral activity (**124**, **126**, **127**).

Based on the better selectivity for the V_2 receptor compared to the V_{1a} receptor ($V_{1a}/V_2 = 193$, based on IC_{50}, Table 13.11) and its potent oral activity ($ED_3 = 0.54\ mg\ kg^{-1}$), compound **126** (tolvaptan, OPC-41061) was selected for advanced *in vivo* studies and for clinical trials [10].

Compound **126** (tolvaptan) also showed a very high affinity for human receptors (V_{1a}: $K_i = 12.3 \pm 0.8$ nM, V_2: $K_i = 0.43 \pm 0.06$ nM) as characterized in HeLa cells expressing cloned human AVP receptors.

13.5 PHARMACOLOGICAL PROFILES OF TOLVAPTAN

13.5.1 Antagonistic Affinities of Tolvaptan for AVP Receptors

As shown in Table 13.12, HeLa cells transfected with each subtype of human AVP receptor constantly expressed a sufficient number of receptors for the [^{3}H]-AVP binding assay through repeated passaging. In V_2-HeLa cells, the expressed V_2 receptors were functional and stimulated adenylate cyclase after stimulation by AVP (Figure 13.7). AVP, even at the

TABLE 13.12 Characterization of Human AVP Receptor Expressed on Cultured HeLa Cells for [^{3}H]-AVP Binding[a]

	V_2	V_{1a}	V_{1b}
Kd (nM)	1.09 ± 0.05	2.29 ± 0.11	1.68 ± 0.06
B_{max} (fmol/mg protein)	1021 ± 98	519 ± 45	69 ± 5.7

[a]Values are expressed as the mean ± S.E.M. of at least four separate determinations performed in duplicate.

minimum concentration of 10^{-12} M, increased the production of cAMP ($281 \pm 98\%$ from the basal value), with the maximum increase achieved at 10^{-8} M.

Tolvaptan and mozavaptan displaced [^{3}H]-AVP binding to human V_2 receptors expressed on HeLa cells in a concentration-dependent manner, and the inhibition curve paralleled the curve for AVP (Figure 13.8). The K_i value for tolvaptan was 1.8 times higher than that for AVP and 22 times higher than that for mozavaptan, indicating that tolvaptan had the most potent affinity for human V_2-receptors. Both compounds also inhibited [^{3}H]-AVP binding to V_{1a} receptors, but not to human V_{1b} receptors (Table 13.13). In comparison with

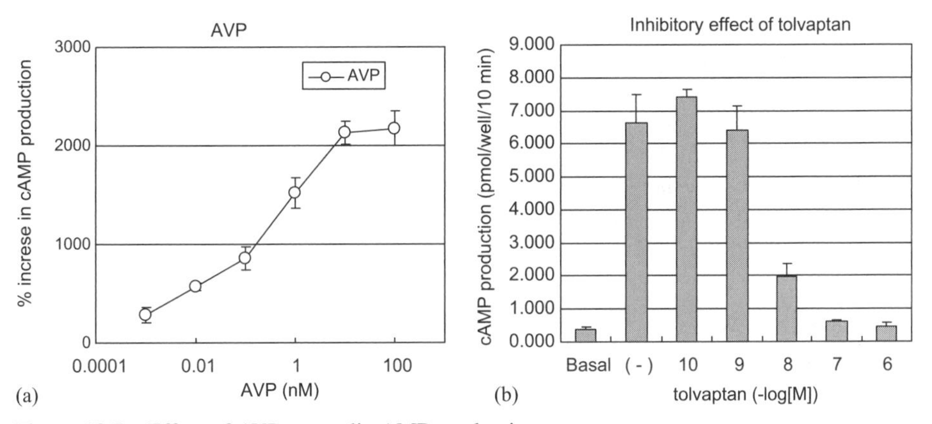

Figure 13.7 Effect of AVP on cyclic AMP production.

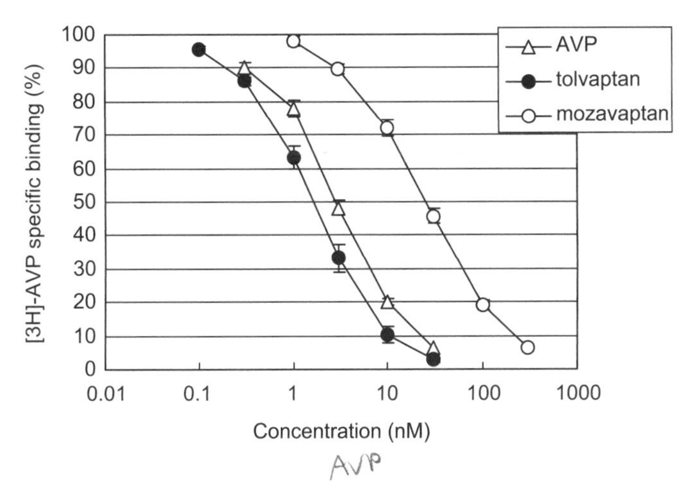

Figure 13.8 Effect of tolvaptan and mozavaptan on [3H]-AVP binding to V_2-HeLa cells.

TABLE 13.13 Antagonistic Potency of Tolvaptan and Mozavaptan for Human and Rat AVP Receptors[a]

	Ki (nM)				
	Human			Rat	
	V_2	V_{1a}	V_{1b}	V_2	V_{1a}
AVP	0.78 ± 0.08	0.84 ± 0.08	0.59 ± 0.05	0.95 ± 0.31	1.45 ± 0.26
Tolvaptan	0.43 ± 0.06	12.3 ± 0.8	$> 100{,}000$	1.33 ± 0.30	325 ± 41
Mozavaptan	9.42 ± 0.90	150 ± 15	$> 100{,}000$	6.36 ± 1.56	524 ± 119

[a]Values are expressed as the mean ± S.E.M. of at least four separate determinations performed in duplicate.

the affinity for rat AVP receptors, tolvaptan showed 3 times more potent antagonism of V_2 receptors and 26 times more potent antagonism of V_{1a} receptors in humans than in rats, indicating that tolvaptan is a more potent antagonist of human AVP receptors than rat AVP receptors. However, mozavaptan showed almost the same affinity for both human and rat V_2 receptors. Tolvaptan was also 29 times more selective for human V_2 receptors than for human V_{1a} receptors and 244 times more selective for rat V_2 receptors than for rat V_{1a} receptors (Table 13.13).

Furthermore, to confirm the antagonistic activity, the effect of tolvaptan on the adenylate cyclase activity induced by AVP in V_2-HeLa cells (Figure 13.7) was examined. At the submaximal concentration of 10^{-9} M, AVP increased cAMP generation by 1520% from the control. Tolvaptan dose-dependently inhibited the increase in cAMP production induced by 1 nM of AVP. However, tolvaptan alone did not increase cAMP production at up to 10^{-6} M (data not shown). These data clearly show that tolvaptan possesses a more potent affinity for human V_2 receptors than native AVP, and that tolvaptan can clearly antagonize V_2 receptors with no intrinsic agonistic activity.

13.5.2 Aquaretic Effect Following a Single Dose in Conscious Rats

A single oral dose of tolvaptan increased urine volume and decreased urine osmolality in a dose-dependent manner at doses of 0.3–10 mg kg^{-1} in normally hydrated conscious rats (Figure 13.9). The maximum urine output for 2-h postdosing was 18.0 ± 2.6 mL, which was 12 times higher than the control, and urine osmolality reached a minimum of

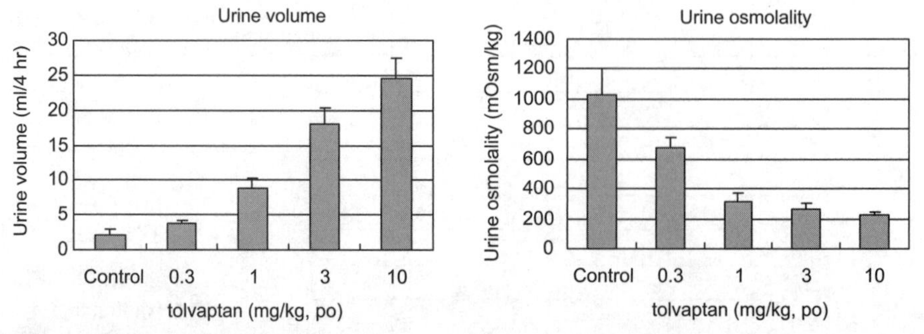

Figure 13.9 Aquaretic effect of a single oral administration of Tolvaptan in normally hydrated conscious rats.

TABLE 13.14 Effect of Single Oral Administration of Tolvaptan on Serum Parameters at 4-h Postdosing in Normally Hydrated Male SD Rats[a]

Dose (mg/kg)	Osmolality (mOsm/kg)	Na (meq/L)	BUN (mg/dL)	Creatinine (mg/dL)	AVP (pg/mL)
Control	293 ± 2	145 ± 0	17.1 ± 0.7	0.58 ± 0.01	<0.2
1 mg/kg	294 ± 1	147 ± 1	14.7 ± 0.6	0.60 ± 0.02	0.4 ± 0.1
3 mg/kg	294 ± 2	148 ± 1	12.0 ± 0.4	0.58 ± 0.01	1.2 ± 0.2
10 mg/kg	301 ± 3	152 ± 1	12.6 ± 0.5	0.71 ± 0.02	4.4 ± 0.9

[a]Values are expressed as the mean ± S.E.M.

$175 \pm 15\,\mathrm{mOsm\,kg^{-1}}$ (vs. $714 \pm 136\,\mathrm{mOsm\,kg^{-1}}$ for the control). No significant increase in urine output was seen after 4-h postdosing (data not shown). Urinary Na excretion during the 4-h postdosing increased dose-dependently. However, the magnitude of the increase was considerably smaller than that by natriuretic agents such as furosemide (data shown previously) [9a].

At 4-h postdosing, the serum osmolality and Na and creatinine concentrations were significantly elevated, presumably by the decreased body fluid resulting from the aquaresis induced by tolvaptan (Table 13.14). The serum AVP concentration also increased dose-dependently following the elevation of serum osmolality. In spite of the hemoconcentrated status at 4-h postdosing, blood urea nitrogen (BUN) was dose-dependently decreased, presumably by tolvaptan-mediated inhibition of urea reabsorption at the terminal of the inner medullary collecting duct, and thus leading to an increase in the urinary urea excretion.

13.6 DRUG DEVELOPMENT

13.6.1 Synthetic Route of Discovery and Commercial Synthesis [10a]

The synthesis of tolvaptan is shown in Scheme 13.1. Commercially available 5-chloro-2-nitrobenzoic acid (**129**) was converted to methyl ester (**130**) using dimethyl sulfate and K_2CO_3 in acetone. The nitro group of (**130**) was reduced with tin(II) chloride in ethanol to afford the aniline (**131**). Tosylation of **131** with *p*-toluenesulfonyl chloride in pyridine provided tosylamide (**132**). Compound **132** was reacted with ethyl 4-bromobutyrate (**133**) to give **134**. The Dieckmann condensation of **134** (heating with potassium *t*-butoxide in toluene) provided the benzazepine (**135**). Compound **135** was decarboxylated by heating with concentrated hydrochloric acid in acetic acid to give **136**. The key intermediate (**137**) was obtained by deprotection of the tosylate (**136**) by heating in polyphosphoric acid. Compound **137** was reacted with 4-nitro-2-methylbenzoyl chloride (**138**) to give the amide (**139**). The nitro group of **139** was reduced by reacting with $SnCl_2{\cdot}2H_2O$ in a mixture of concentrated hydrochloric acid and EtOH. The amino intermediate (**140**) was condensed with 2-methylbenzoyl chloride (**141**) to give the amide (**142**). The subsequent reduction of the 5-keto moiety of **142** with sodium borohydride led to compound **126** (tolvaptan). The commercial synthesis (racemic at the hydroxyl group) is performed using a modified scheme for reagents and conditions to provide the scale-up.

13.6.2 Nonclinical Toxicology

The nonclinical safety profile of tolvaptan was evaluated in a series of safety pharmacology and toxicology studies using mice, rats, dogs, rabbits, guinea pigs, and *in vitro* systems.

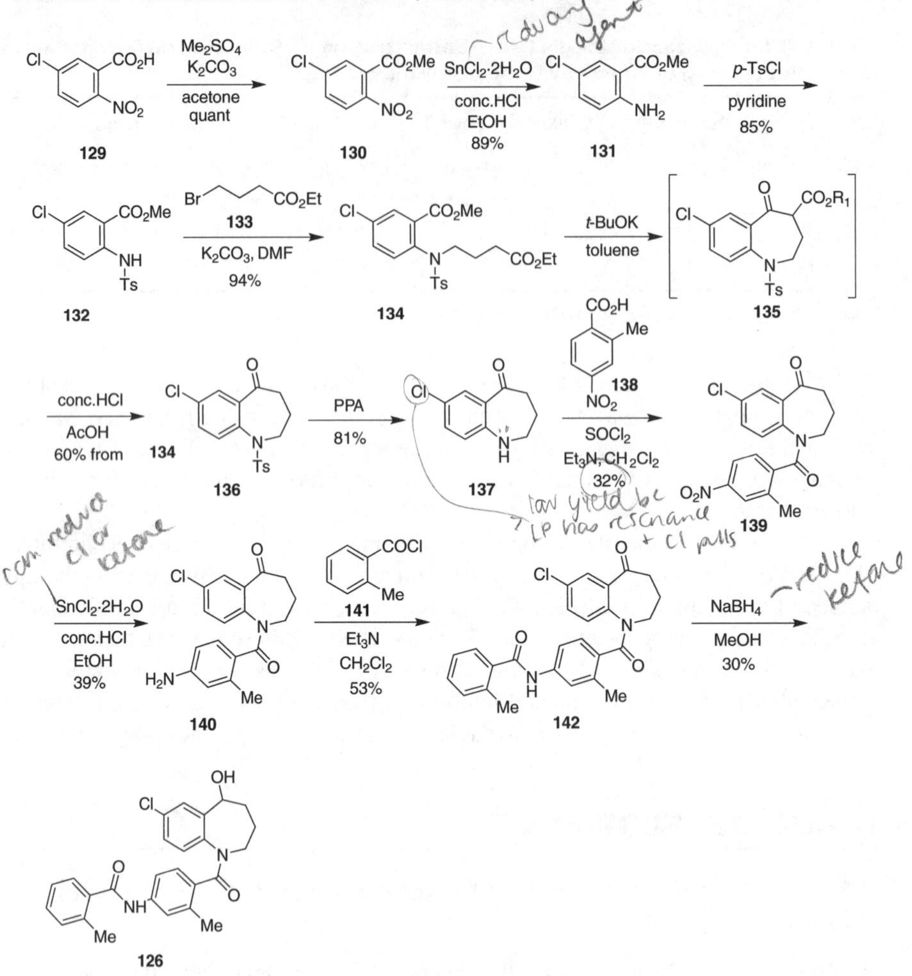

Scheme 13.1 The synthesis of tolvaptan.

In safety pharmacological studies, tolvaptan has demonstrated no adverse effects on the central nervous system, somatic nervous system, autonomic nervous system, smooth muscle, respiratory and cardiovascular system, or digestive systems.

In general toxicity studies, a single oral dose of tolvaptan was not lethal at doses up to 2000 mg kg^{-1} in rats and dogs. Tolvaptan did not cause any target organ toxicity in rats for 26 weeks or in dogs for 52 weeks at oral doses up to 1000 mg kg^{-1} day^{-1}, though the toxicities attributable to the exaggerated pharmacological action of tolvaptan were noted at 1000 mg kg^{-1} day^{-1} in female rats and male and female dogs.

In reproductive and developmental toxicity studies in rats orally administered with tolvaptan, fertility was not adversely affected in both male and female animals, and, when administered to pregnant animals, viability or growth was suppressed at the maternal toxic dose of 1000 mg kg^{-1} day^{-1}. In rabbits, tolvaptan showed teratogenicity at the oral dose of 1000 mg kg^{-1} day^{-1}, at which dose evident maternal toxicity, including abortion, occurred.

Tolvaptan showed weak phototoxicity in an *in vitro* study but no phototoxicity was observed in an *in vivo* study using guinea pigs and rabbits.

Tolvaptan had no potential of genotoxicity, carcinogenicity, antigenicity, or immunotoxicity.

13.6.3 Clinical Studies[4]

In healthy subjects, the pharmacokinetics of tolvaptan after single doses of up to 480 mg and multiple doses up to 300 mg once daily have been examined [11]. The area under the curve (AUC) increases proportionally with dose. After the administration of doses $\geq$ 60 mg, however, the C_{max} increases less than proportionally with dose. As the plasma tolvaptan concentration increased, the duration that the urine excretion rate above baseline rate also increased. The most frequent adverse events-excess thirst, frequent urination, and dry mouth appeared to be related to the pharmacological action of tolvaptan. No dose-limiting toxicities were observed.

The pharmacokinetic properties of stereospecific tolvaptan were assessed using a steady-state ratio of the *S*-(−) to the *R*-(+) enantiomer of about 3. Peak concentrations of tolvaptan are observed between 2- and 4-h postdose. Food does not impact the bioavailability of tolvaptan. Tolvaptan is highly plasma protein bound (99%) and distributed into an apparent volume of distribution of about 3 L kg^{-1}. Tolvaptan is eliminated entirely by nonrenal routes and mainly, if not exclusively, metabolized by CYP 3A4. No clinically significant drug interactions were found when tolvaptan was administered with furosemide, hydrochlorothiazide, amiodarone, warfarin, or lovastatin. Tolvaptan does not appear to be an inhibitor of either CYP3A4 or CYP2C9 isozymes. Tolvaptan metabolism is significantly decreased by CYP3A4 inhibitors. The coadministration of ketoconazole significantly inhibited the metabolism of tolvaptan. Tolvaptan bioavailability was increased when administered with grapefruit juice. Tolvaptan concentrations were reduced by 85% when administered with rifampin. Steady-state digoxin concentrations (as determined by the area under the concentration-time curve during a dosing interval [τ] at steady state [AUCτ]) were increased by approximately 20%; *in vitro* studies indicate that tolvaptan is capable of binding to *p*-glycoprotein.

After oral dosing, clearance is about 4 mL min^{-1} kg^{-1}, and the terminal phase half-life is about 12 h. The accumulation factor of tolvaptan with the once-daily regimen is 1.3, and the trough concentrations amount to $\leq$ 16% of the peak concentrations, suggesting a dominant half-life somewhat shorter than 12 h.

In a large phase three trial in subjects hospitalized with worsening heart failure and symptoms of fluid overload, [12] tolvaptan, in addition to continued conventional therapy including diuretics, had the following effects: increased weight reduction, improvement in both the patient-assessed dyspnea and pedal edema in the first 7 days, normalized the serum sodium concentrations in subjects with hyponatremia (maintained for more than 6 months), and maintained renal function in comparison to placebo. No differences between tolvaptan (30 mg) and placebo were observed in mortality or heart failure-related morbidity in these subjects.

In subjects with cardiac edema that had not resolved with furosemide treatment, tolvaptan (15, 30, and 45 mg) significantly reduced body weight and dose-dependently increased urine volume [13]. Congestive symptoms such as lower limb edema and jugular venous distension also improved with tolvaptan compared to placebo. In subjects with lower limb edema or ascites secondary to hepatic disease, whose condition had not improved with furosemide treatment, tolvaptan dose-dependently improved hepatic edema and reduced the abdominal circumference [14].

Moreover, in subjects with hyponatremia (serum sodium < 135 mEq L^{-1}), tolvaptan increased the serum sodium concentrations in the overall population as well as in subjects with mild and severe hyponatremia (serum sodium concentrations $\geq$ 130 mEq L^{-1} and < 130 mEq L^{-1}, respectively) [15]. Improvements in serum sodium concentrations were

[4] http://www.samsca.com/clinical-studies.aspx

statistically significant for tolvaptan compared with placebo. These improvements were observed in the tolvaptan group within 8 h after initiating treatment and persisted throughout the treatment duration, reaching normalization (defined as serum sodium concentrations > 135 mEq L^{-1}) in many cases. A decline in serum sodium concentrations compared to that of serum sodium concentrations in placebo-treated subjects was observed within 7 days after discontinuation of tolvaptan. Importantly, the increases in serum sodium concentrations in the tolvaptan group were steady, with few adverse effects from over- or too-rapid serum sodium correction. These changes were attributed to removal of excess free water and led to significant changes in the mental component summary composite score of the SF-12 quality of life measure. Changes were seen in the mental components of an exploratory patient-reported health outcomes instrument as well.

13.7 SUMMARY FOCUSING ON LESSONS LEARNED

On 21st May, 2009, the US Food and Drug Administration (FDA) approved Samsca® (tolvaptan) as the only oral selective vasopressin antagonist for the treatment of hypervolemic and euvolemic hyponatremia, including patients with heart failure, cirrhosis, and the syndrome of inappropriate antidiuretic hormone (SIADH) [16]. In August, 2009, the European Commission approved the Marketing Authorization Application for the oral once-daily medication Samsca® for the treatment of hyponatraemia secondary to syndrome of inappropriate antidiuretic hormone secretion (SIADH) in adults. On 27th October, 2010, samsca® has been approved for use in Japan for the treatment of volume overload in heart failure when adequate response is not obtained with other diuretics (e.g., loop diuretics).

The in-house drug discovery efforts to find an aquaretic in progress since 1983 finally led to a vasopressin V_2 receptor selective antagonist, Samsca®. It is very rewarding to have been part of this adventure in uncovering the mysteries of a drug having a novel mechanism of action.

Vincent H. Gattone II, Vincente E. Torres and colleagues reported the "Inhibition of renal cystic disease development and progression by a vasopressin V_2 receptor antagonist" in Nature Medicine in 2003 [17]. The polycystic kidney diseases (PKDs) are hereditary disorders causing significant renal failure and death in children and adults. There is no therapeutic drug available that slows or prevents cyst formation and kidney enlargement in humans [18].

A number of reports have shown that cAMP play a major role in cyst fluid accumulation and cystgenesis, [19] and one of the agonists, AVP, has emerged as a potent modulator of cystogenesis in recent years. Gattone, Torres and colleagues demonstrated the inhibition of cystogenesis by blocking cAMP pathway with a V_2 receptor antagonist.

Encouraged by these results, a clinical trial in humans with autosomal dominant polycystic kidney disease (ADPKD) using tolvaptan was performed. A phase III multicenter, double-blind, placebo-controlled, parallel-arm, 3-year trial to determine the long-term safety and efficacy of oral tolvaptan tablets in adult subjects with ADPKD has been initiated [20].

The biological effects of AVP are mediated through three receptor subtypes (Figure 13.3.) [21]. Some actions of the receptor subtypes have only been studied *in vitro*, and their significance *in vivo* and in disease states is still unknown. V_2-receptor-mediated antagonism in disease states has been evaluated in clinical studies. Many questions remain to be answered and need to be the focus of further research [22]. In addition, V_{1a}- or V_{1b}-mediated antagonism in disease states has not been sufficiently evaluated. The stimulation with AVP through the V_{1a} or V_{1b} receptor is likely to be observed at a much higher concentration of AVP than that through the V_2 receptor. Thus, it will be challenging to determine the roles of V_{1a} and V_{1b} receptors in disease states. Under such a situation, the drug discovery efforts do not come to an end and projects will continue to understand the physiological roles of AVP receptors and to find better compounds that will be beneficial for patients.

ACKNOWLEDGMENTS

The authors greatly appreciate Mr. Akihiko Otsuka and Dr. Youichi Yabuuchi for their continuous encouragement.

REFERENCES

1. Oren, R. M. Hyponatremia in congestive heart failure. *Am. J. Cardiol.* **2005**, *95*, 2B–7B.
2. (a) Altura, B. M. and Altura, B. T. Vascular smooth muscle and neurohypophysical hormones. *Fed. Proc.* **1977**, *36*, 1853–1860; (b) Howl, J., Ismail, T., Strain, A. J., Kirk, C. J., Anderson, D., and Wheatley, M. Characterization of human liver vasopressin receptor. *Biochem. J.* **1991**, *276*, 189–195; (c) Jard, S., Lombard, C., Marie, J., and Devilliers, G. Vasopressin receptors from cultured mesangial cells resemble V_{1a} type. *Am. J. Physiol.*, **1987**, *253*, F41–F49; (d) Penit, J., Faure, M., and Jard, S. Vasopressin and angiotensin II receptors in rat aortic smooth muscle cells in culture. *Am. J. Physiol.* **1983**, *244*, E72–E82; (e) Thibonnier, M. and Roberts, J. M. Characterization of human platelet vasopressin receptors. *J. Clin. Invest.* **1985**, *76*, 1857–1964; (f) Dorsa, D. M., Majumdar, L. A., Petracca, F. M., Baskin, D. G., and Cornett, L. E. Characterization and localization of ^{3}H-arginine^8-vasopressin binding to rat kidney and brain tissue, *Peptides* **1983**, *4*, 699–706; (g) Birnbaumer, M. Vasopressin receptors. *Trends Endocrinol. Metab.* **2000**, *11*, 406–410.
3. (a) Manning, M., and Sawyer, W. H. Discovery, development, and some uses of vasopressin and oxytocin antagonists. *J. Lab. Clin. Med.* **1989**, *114*, 617–632; (b) László, F. A., László, F., Jr., and Wied, D. D. Parmacology and clinical perspectives of vasopressin antagonists. *Pharmacol. Rev.* **1991**, *43*, 73–108; (c) Kruszynski, M., Lammek, B., and Manning, M. [1-β-Mercapto-β,β-cyclopentamethylene-propionic acid), 2-(*O*-methyl)tyrosine] argine-vasopressin and [1-β-mercapto-β,β-cyclopentamethylenepropionic acid)] argine-vasopressine, two highly potent antagonists of the vasopressor response to arginine-vasopressin. *J. Med. Chem.* **1980**, *23*, 364–368; (d) Manning, M., Lammek, B., Bankowski, K., Seto, J., and Sawyer, W. H. Synthesis and some pharmacological properties of 18 potent *O*-alkyltyrosine-substituted antagonists of the vasopressor responses to arginine-vasopressin. *J. Med. Chem.* **1985**, *28*, 1485–1491; (e) Manning, M., Olma, A., Klis, W., Kolodziejczyk, A., Nawrocka, E., Misicka, A., Seto, J., and Sawyer, W. H. Carboxy terminus of vasopressin required for activity but not binding. *Nature*, **1984**, *308*, 652–653; (f) Huffman, W. F., Ali, F. E., Bryan, W. M., Callahan, J. F., Moore, M. L., Silvestri, J. S., Yim, N. C. F., Kinter, L. B., McDonald, J. E., Ashton-Shue, D., Stassen, F. L., Heckman, G. D., Schmidt, D. B., and Sulat, L. Novel vasopressin analogues that help define a minimum effective antagonist pharmacophore. *J. Med. Chem.* **1985**, *28*, 1759–1760; (g) Ali, F. E., Bryan, W., Chang, H.-L., Huffman, W. F., Moore, M. L., Heckman, G., Kinter, L. B., McDonald, J., Schmidt, D., Shue, D., and Stassen, F. L. Potent vasopressin antagonists lacking the proline residue at position 7. *J. Med. Chem.* **1986**, *29*, 984–988; (h) Moore, M. L., Albrightson, C., Brickson, B., Bryan, H. G., Caldwell, N., Callahan, J. F., Foster, J., Kinter, L. B., Newlander, K. A., Schmidt, D. B., Sorenson, E., Stassen, F. L., Yim, N. C. F., and Huffman, W. F. Dicarbavasopressin antagonist analogs exhibit reduced in vivo agonist activity. *J. Med. Chem.* **1988**, *31*, 1487–1489; (i) Manning, M., Misicka, A., Olma, A., Klis, W. A., Bankowski, K., Nawrocka, E., Kruszynski, M., Kolodziejczk, A., Cheng, L.-L., Seto, J., Wo, N. C., and Sawyer, W. H. C-Terminal deletions in antagonistic analogs of vasopressin that improve their specificities for antidiuretic V_2 and vasopressor V_1 receptors. *J. Med. Chem.* **1987**, *30*, 2245–2252; (j) Lammek, B., Rekowski, P., Kupryszewski, G., Melin, P., and Ragnarsson, U. Synthesis of arginine-vasopressins, modified in positions 1 and 2, as antagonists of the vasopressor response to the parent hormone. *J. Med. Chem.* **1988**, *31*, 603–606; (k) Manning, M., Stoev, S., Kolodziejczyk, A., Klis, W. A., Kruszynski, M., Misicka, A., and Olma, A. Design of potent and selective linear antagonists of vasopressor (V_1-receptor) responses to vasopressin. *J. Med. Chem.* **1990**, *33*, 3079–3086; (l) Manning, M., Przybylski, J., Grzonka, Z., Nawrocka, E., Lammek, B., Misicka, A., Cheng, L.-L., Chan, W. Y., Wo, N. C., and Sawyer, W. H. Potent V_2/V_{1a} vasopressin antagonists with C-terminal ethylenediamine-linked retro-amino acids. *J. Med. Chem.* **1992**, *35*, 3895–3904; (m)

CASTELLO, L., PIRISI, M., SAINAGHI, P. P., and BARTOLI, E. Hyponatremia in liver cirrhosis: pathophysiological principles of management, *Dig. Liver Dis.* **2005**, *37*, 73–81; (n) HURLEY, J. K. Symptomatic hyponatremia in nephrotic syndrome. *Am. J. Dis. Child.* **1980**, *134*, 204–206.

4. (a) BROOKS, D. P., KOSTER, P. F., ALBRIGHTSON-WINSLOW, C. R., STASSEN, F. L., HUFFMAN, W, F., and KINTER, L. B. SK&F 105494 is a potent antidiuretic hormone antagonist in the rhesus Monkey (Macaca mulata). *J. Pharmacol. Exp. Ther.* **1988**, *245*, 211–215; (b) CALDWELL, N., BRICKSON, B., KINTER, L. B., BROOKS, D. P., HUFFMAN. W. F., STASSEN, F. L., and ALBRIGHTSON-WINSLOW, C. SK&F 105494: a potent antidiuretic hormone antagonist devoid of partial agonist activity in dogs. *J. Pharmacol. Exp. Ther.* **1988**, *247*, 897–901; (c) BROOKS, D. P., KOSTER, P. F., ALBRIGHTSON, C. R., HUFFMAN, W. F., MOORE, M. L., STASSEN, F. L., SCHMIDT, D. B., and KINTER, L. B. Vasopressin receptor antagonism in rhesus monkey and man: stereochemical requirements. *Euro. J. Pharmacol.* **1989**, *160*, 159–162; (d) RUFFOLO, R. R., JR, BROOKS, D. P., HUFFMAN, W. F., and POSTE, G. From Vasopressin antagonist to agonist: a saga of surprise! *Drug News Perspect.* **1991**, *4*, 217–222.
5. (a) NAKAMURA, T., TOMOMURA, A., NODA, C., SHIMOJI, M., and ICHIHARA, A. Acquisition of a β-adrenergic response by adult rat hepatocytes during primary culture. *J. Biol. Chem.* **1983**, *258*, 9283–9289; (b) NAKAHARA, T., TERADA, S., PINCUS, J., FLOURET, G., and HECHTER, O. Neurohypophyseal hormone-responsive renal adenylate cyclase. *J. Biol. Chem.* **1978**, *253*, 3211–3218.
6. (a) OGAWA, H., YAMAMURA, Y., MIYAMOTO, H., KONDO, K., YAMASHITA, H., NAKAYA, K., CHIHARA, T., MORI, T., TOMINAGA, M., and YABUUCHI, Y. Orally active, nonpeptide vasopressin V1 antagonists. A novel series of 1-(1-substituted 4-piperidyl)-3,4-dihydro-2(1H)-quinolinone. *J. Med. Chem.* **1993**, *36*, 2011–2017; (b) KONDO, K., OGAWA, H., NAKAYA, K., TOMINAGA, M., and YABUUCHI, Y. Structure-activity relationships of non-peptide vasopressin V_{1a} antagonists: 1-(1-multi-substituted benzoyl 4-piperidyl)-3,4-dihydro-2(1H)-quinolinones. *Chem. Pharm. Bull.* **1996**, *44*, 725–33.
7. YAMAMURA, Y., OGAWA, H., CHIHARA, T., KONDO, K., ONOGAWA, T., NAKAMURA, S., MORI, T., TOMINAGA, M., and YABUUCHI, Y. OPC-21268, an orally effective, nonpeptide vasopressin V1 receptor antagonist. *Science*, **1991**, *252*, 572–574.
8. OGAWA, H., YAMASHITA, H., KONDO, K., YAMAMURA, Y., MIYAMOTO, H., KAN, K., KITANO, K., TANAKA, M., NAKAYA, K., NAKAMURA, S., MORI, T., TOMINAGA, M., and YABUUCHI, Y. Orally active, nonpeptide vasopressin V_2 receptor antagonists: a novel series of 1-[4-(benzoylamino)benzoyl]-2,3,4,5-tetrahydro-1H-benzazepines and related compounds. *J. Med. Chem.* **1996**, *39*, 3547–3555.
9. (a) YAMAMURA, Y., OGAWA, H., YAMASHITA, H., CHIHARA, T., MIYAMOTO, H., NAKAMURA, S., ONOGAWA, T., YAMASHITA, T., HOSOKAWA, T., MORI, T., TOMINAGA, M., and YABUUCHI, Y. Characterization of a novel aquaretic agent, OPC-31260, as an orally effective, nonpeptide vasopressin V_2 receptor antagonist. *Br. J. Pharmacol.* **1992**, *105*, 787–791; (b) OHNISHI, A., ORITA, Y., OKAHARA, R., FUJIHARA, H., INOUE, T., YAMAMURA, Y., YABUUCHI, Y. and TANAKA, T. Potent aquaretic agent. *J. Clin. Invest.* **1993**, *92*, 2653–2659; (c) OHNISHI, A., ORITA, Y., TAKAGI, N., FUJITA, T., TOYOKI, T., IHARA, Y., YAMAMURA, Y., INOUE, T., TANAKA, T. Aquaretic effect of a potent, orally active, nonpeptide V_2 antagonist in men, *J. Pharmacol. Exp. Ther.* **1995**, *272*, 546–551.
10. (a) KONDO, K., OGAWA, H., YAMASHITA, H., MIYAMOTO, H., TANAKA, M., NAKAYA, K., KITANO, K., YAMAMURA, Y., NAKAMURA, S., ONOGAWA, T., MORI, T., and TOMINAGA, M. 7-Chloro-5-hydroxy-1-[2-methyl-4-(2-methylbenzoyl-amino)benzoyl]-2,3,4,5-tetrahydro-1H-1-benzazepine (OPC-41061): a potent, orally active nonpeptide arginine vasopressin V_2 receptor antagonist. *Bioorg. Med. Chem.* **1999**, *7*, 1743–1754. (b) YAMAMURA, Y., NAKAMURA, S., ITO, S., HIRANO, T., ONOGAWA, T., YAMASHITA, T., YAMADA, Y., TSUJIMAE, K., AOYAMA, M., KOTOSAI, K., OGAWA, H., YAMASHITA, H., KONDO, K., TOMINAGA, M., TSUJIMOTO, G., and MORI, T. OPC-41061, a potent human vasopressin V_2-receptor antagonist: pharmacological profile and aquaretic effect by single and multiple oral dosing in rats. *J. Pharmacol. Exp. Ther.* **1998**, *287*, 860–867.
11. SHOAF, S. E., WANG, Z., BRICMONT, P., and MALLIKAARJUN, S. Pharmacokinetics, Pharmacodynamics, and safety of Tolvaptan, a nonpeptide AVP antagonist, during ascending single-dose studies in healthy subjects. *J. Clin. Pharmacol.* **2007**, *47*, 1498–1507.
12. (a) GHEORGHIADE, M., KONSTAM, M. A., BURNETT, J. C., JR., GRINFELD. L., MAGGIONI, A. P., SWEDBERG, K., UDELSON, J. E., ZANNAD, F., COOK, T., OUYANG, J., ZIMMER, C., and ORLANDI, C. Short-term clinical effects of tolvaptan, an oral vasopressin antagonist, in patients hospitalized for heart failure: the EVEREST Clinical Status Trials. *JAMA* **2007**, *297*, 1332–1343; (b) KONSTAM, M. A., GHEORGHIADE, M., BURNETT, J. C., JR., GRINFELD, L., MAGGIONI, A. P., SWEDBERG, K., UDELSON, J. E., ZANNAD, F., COOK, T., OUYANG, J., ZIMMER, C., and ORLANDI, C. Effects of oral tolvaptan in patients hospitalized for worsening heart failure: the EVEREST outcome trial. *JAMA* **2007**, *297*, 1319–1331.
13. YAMAMURA, Y. unpublished result.
14. OKITA, K., SAKAIDA, I., OKADA, M., KANEKO, A., CHAYAMA, K., KATO, M., SATA, M., YOSHIHARA, N., ONO, N., and MURAWAKI, Y. A multicenter, open-label, dose-ranging study to exploratively evaluate the efficacy, safety, and dose-response of tolvaptan in patients with decompensated liver cirrhosis. *J Gastroenterol.* **2010**, *45*, 979–987.
15. SCHRIER, R. W., GROSS, P., GHEORGHIADE, M., BERL, T., VERBALIS, J. G., CZERWIEC, F. S., and ORLANDI, C. Tolvaptan, a selective oral vasopressin V_2-receptor

antagonist, for hyponatremia. *N. Engl. J. Med.* **2006**, *355*, 2099–2112.

16. GHALI, J. K., HAMAD, B., YASOTHAN, U., and KIRKPATRICK. P. Tolvaptan. *Nature Rev. Drug Discov.* **2009**, *8*, 611–612.
17. (a) GATTONEII, V. H., WANG, X., HARRIS, P. C., and TORRES, V. E. Inhibition of renal cystic disease development and progressionby a vasopressin V_2 receptor antagonist. *Nature Med.* **2003**, *9*, 1323–1326; (b) TORRES, V. E., WANG, X., QIAN, Q., SOMLO, S., HARRIS, P. C., and GATTONEII, V. H. Effective treatment of an orthologous model of autosomal dominant polycystic kidney disease. *Nature Med.* **2004**, *10*, 363–364; (c) WANG, X., GATTONE, V., HARRIS, P. C., and TORRES, V. E. Effectiveness of vasopressin V_2 receptor antagonists OPC-31260 and OPC-41061 on polycystic kidney disease development in the PCK rat. *J. Am. Soc. Nephrol.* **2005**, *16*, 846–851.
18. BELIBI, F. A. and EDELSTEIN, C. L. Novel targets for the treatment of autosomal dominant polycystic kidney disease. *Expert Opin. Investig. Drugs.* **2010**, *19*, 315–328.
19. (a) IBRAGHIMOV-BESKROVNAYA, O. and BUKAN, N. Polycystic kidney diseases: From molecular discoveries to targeted therapeutic strategies. *Cell. Mol. Life Sci.*, **2008**, *65*, 605–619; (b) GALLAGHER, A. R., GERMINO, G. G., and SOMLO, S. Molecular advances in autosomal dominant polycystic kidney disease. *Adv. Chronic Kidney Dis.* **2010**, *17*, 118–130.
20. (a) IGARASHI, P. and SOMLO, S. Genetics and pathogenesis of polycystic kidney disease. *J Am. Soc. Nephrol.* **2002**, *13*, 2384–2393; (b) BENNETT, W. M. V_2 receptor antagonists in cystic kidney diseases: an exciting step towards a practical treatment. *J. Am. Soc. Nephrol.* **2005**, *16*, 838–839; (c) TORRES V. E. Role of vasopressin antagonists. *Clin. J. Am. Soc. Nephrol.* **2008**, *3*, 1212–1218; (d) TORRES, V. E. Treatment strategies and clinical trial design in ADPKD. *Adv. Clin. Kidn. Dis.* **2010**, *17*, 190–204; (e) NEMEROVSKI, C. and HUTCHINSON, D. J. Treatment of hypervolemic or euvolemic hyponatremia associated with heart failure, cirrhosis, or the syndrome of inappropriate antiuretic hormone with tolvaptan: a clinical review. *Clin. Ther.* **2010**, *32*, 1015–1032.
21. BIRNBAUMER, M. Vasopressin Receptors. *Trends Endocrinol. Metab.* **2000**, *11*, 406–410.
22. COSTELLO-BOERRIGTER, L. C., BOERRIGTER, G., and BURNET, J. C., JR., Pharmacology of vasopressin antagonists. *Heart Fail. Rev.* **2009**, *14*, 75–82.

CHAPTER 14

SILODOSIN (URIEF®, RAPAFLO®, THRUPAS®, UROREC®, SILODIX™): A SELECTIVE α_{1A} ADRENOCEPTOR ANTAGONIST FOR THE TREATMENT OF BENIGN PROSTATIC HYPERPLASIA

Masaki Yoshida, Imao Mikoshiba, Katsuyoshi Akiyama, and Junzo Kudoh

14.1 BACKGROUND INFORMATION

14.1.1 Benign Prostatic Hyperplasia

Benign prostatic hyperplasia (BPH) is a common progressive disease among men, with an incidence that is age dependent. Histologic BPH, which typically develops after the age of 40 years, ranges in prevalence from >50% at 60 years to as high as 90% by 85 years [1–3]. BPH contributes to, but is not the single cause of, bothersome lower urinary tract symptoms (LUTS) that may affect quality of life (QoL). The prevalence of troublesome symptoms increases with age, with symptoms typically occurring in men aged ≥50 years [3].

Histologically, BPH is characterized by a progressive increase in the number of epithelial and stromal cells that develops initially in the periurethral area of the prostate gland [1,4,5]. This cellular proliferative process increases prostatic smooth muscle tone, resulting in urethral constriction [6]. Benign prostatic enlargement (BPE) may also result from the proliferation of epithelial and stromal cells and may further contribute to constriction of the urethra, leading to bladder outlet obstruction (BOO). BPE and BOO do not occur in all men with histopathologic BPH/LUTS, and the presence of BPE does not necessarily mean that BOO will develop [5].

Approximately 50% of patients with histologic BPH report moderate to severe LUTS [2], consisting of storage and voiding symptoms [2,3]. Commonly reported storage-related symptoms include urinary frequency, urgency, and nocturia. Voiding symptoms, typically attributable to urethral obstruction, consist of decreased and intermittent force of the urinary stream and the sensation of incomplete bladder emptying [1]. Although bothersome LUTS may affect quality of life by altering normal daily activities and sleep patterns, mortality associated with BPH is rare [1,7]. Although uncommon, serious complications of BPH may occur, including acute urinary retention, renal insufficiency, urinary tract infection, hematuria, bladder stones, and renal failure [6,8].

Case Studies in Modern Drug Discovery and Development, Edited by Xianhai Huang and Robert G. Aslanian.

These complications may be triggered or worsened by inadequate management of BPH. The incidence of acute urinary retention in untreated patients ranges from 0.3% to 3.5% per year; the risk of developing other long-term complications is unclear [8].

The management of patients with BPH includes nonpharmacologic, pharmacologic, and procedural/surgical options, with the choice of therapy typically depending on the presence and severity of symptoms [1,9]. Watchful waiting is the preferred management strategy for patients with mild LUTS and those who do not perceive their symptoms to be particularly bothersome. Pharmacologic treatments include α_1-adrenergic receptor (AR) antagonists (or blockers) and 5α-reductase inhibitors, which are recommended for use alone or in combination in patients with bothersome moderate to severe LUTS.

Treatment with 5α-reductase inhibitors is reserved for those with demonstrated prostatic enlargement [1,9]. Minimally invasive procedures such as transurethral needle ablation of the prostate, an outpatient procedure, are alternative options for men with mild to moderate [9] or severe symptoms [1]. Patients presenting with severe symptoms of BPH may undergo surgical procedures such as transurethral resection of the prostate or transurethral incision of the prostate.

14.1.2 α_1-Adrenergic Receptors

Adrenergic receptors (ARs) were originally divided into α-AR and β-AR categories [8], but application of molecular biologic methods has confirmed nine total AR subtypes: α_{1A} (formerly named α_{1C}), α_{1B}, α_{1D}, α_{2A}, α_{2B}, α_{2C}, β_1, β_2, and β_3 [10,11]. α_1-ARs generally mediate their actions through members of the Gq/11 family of G proteins that stimulate inositol phosphate (membrane phospholipid) hydrolysis, with each subtype demonstrating different efficacy of coupling to phosphoinositide hydrolysis: $\alpha_{1A}>\alpha_{1B}>\alpha_{1D}$ [12]. In addition, α_1-AR subtypes can be pharmacologically distinguished on the basis of differential binding to α_1-antagonists (blockers) [13], as well as differential inactivation by the alkylating agent chloroethylclonidine [12,14].

All 3 α_1-AR subtypes exist in a wide range of human tissues [15]. The α_{1A}-AR subtype shows the highest levels of expression in human liver, followed by slightly lower levels in heart, cerebellum, and cerebral cortex; the α_{1B}-AR subtype has highest expression in human spleen, kidney, and fetal brain; α_{1D}-AR has the highest levels in the cerebral cortex and human aorta [15].

In terms of male LUTS, α_1-AR expression in prostate, urethra, spinal cord, and bladder is important. Molecular and contraction studies in human prostate tissue demonstrate the α_{1A}-AR subtype predominates (70%–100%) in prostate stroma [16,17]. Because baseline tone is present in prostate smooth muscle (due to its rich sympathetic innervation), blockade of prostate α_{1A}-ARs results in relaxation of prostate smooth muscle. Hence, α_1-AR blockade is capable of modifying the dynamic (prostate smooth muscle contraction) component in BPH. Another tissue important in LUTS is the urethra. To date, most studies show that all regions of human urethra (including bladder neck and intraprostatic urethra) contain only α_{1A}-ARs. Because of reflex arcs, spinal cord α_1-AR expression may be important in LUTS [18].

Normal detrusor (bladder smooth muscle tissue) obtained from surgical patients expresses predominantly α_{1D}-ARs, although other subtypes are present to a lesser extent [19]. Studies demonstrating increased α_{1D}-AR expression and function in models of bladder hypertrophy provide a mechanistic explanation for increased irritability symptoms associated with LUTS [20,21].

α_1-AR antagonists mediate vasodilation in vasculature; therefore, one of the side effects of treating LUTS with α_1-AR antagonists is hypotension. α_{1A}-ARs predominate in human splanchnic (mesenteric, splenic, hepatic, and distal omental) resistance arteries [22]. Interestingly, α_1-AR expression increases 2-fold in representative (mammary) arteries with aging, with the ratio of α_{1B}:α_{1A} increasing, whereas no alteration occurs in veins [22]. Studies of pharmacy databases in Europe suggest that the administration of α_1-AR blockers increases the incidence of hip fractures (chosen as a surrogate for clinically important orthostatic hypotension); [23] further analysis with regard to the precise α_1-AR antagonists prescribed suggests that avoidance of α_{1B}-AR blockade may result in fewer overall hip fractures [3].

14.2 THE DISCOVERY OF SILODOSIN

14.2.1 Medicinal Chemistry

Therapy with α_1-AR antagonists generally leads to rapid improvement in LUTS; thus, these agents are commonly used as first-line treatments for LUTS associated with BPH [3,6]. A number of α_1-AR antagonists (alfuzosin, doxazosin, tamsulosin, and terazosin) have been approved for the treatment of BPH in the United States; of these, tamsulosin is selective for the α_{1A}-AR. In patients with BPH-related LUTS, α_1-AR antagonists relax prostate smooth muscle and decrease urethral resistance, thereby relieving LUTS [9] and BOO [10]. According to the American Urological Association (AUA) Practice Guidelines Committee [1], these agents have comparable clinical effectiveness, although differences in their pharmacologic profiles imply differences in their adverse-effect profiles. The greatest safety concern associated with the use of these agents is the occurrence of vasodilatory symptoms resulting from inhibition of α_1-ARs in the systemic vasculature; this effect is minimized by use of agents that selectively antagonize the α_{1A}-AR [7].

Previous α_1-AR antagonists have vasodilatory symptoms including postural hypotension and dizziness, and have to be carefully employed for patients, especially aging, suffering from dysuria. Thus, for the treatment of BPH, it has long been desired to develop a therapeutic agent having a selective suppressive action on urethral contractions with less hypotension including postural hypotension: this effect may be minimized by use of agents that selectively antagonize the α_{1A}-AR [7].

At the start of the 1990s, Kissei Pharmaceutical Co., Ltd. began development of α_1-AR antagonists highly selective to the LUT without affecting blood pressure [24,25]. Since conventional drugs for the treatment of dysuria, such as prazosin, were non selective α_1-AR antagonists, and were associated with undesired side effects such as postural hypotension, their efforts were focused on the improvement of the selectivity of urethral contraction over hypotension including postural hypotension [26,27], and led to the discovery of a series of novel indoline derivatives. Focusing on α_1-AR antagonists with the conventional quinazoline and phenylpiperazine motifs with low selectivity to α_{1A}-AR, amide group and trifluoroethoxy group were introduced into their indoline structure to optimize the structure to increase the α_{1A}-AR blocking action and organ selectivity. Compounds were then assessed for their pharmacokinetics, to develop a drug product characterized by high intestinal absorption, long-lasting action, and less CNS penetration after oral administration. The eventual product was silodosin (Figure 14.1B), which showed high selectivity to the LUT, suggesting a higher efficacy and less effect on the circulatory system (blood pressure, etc.). Regarding the action of silodosin at the molecular level, in contrast to the quinazoline based α_1-AR antagonists, which all are strong inverse agonists, silodosin is a neutral antagonist [28,29] and this difference may have consequences for some of its *in vivo* effects [30].

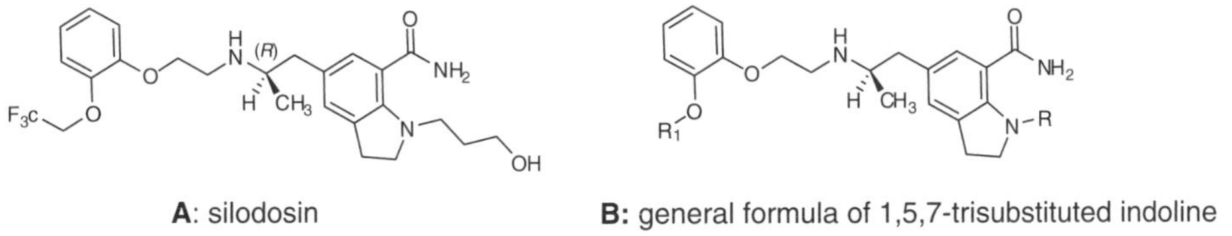

A: silodosin

B: general formula of 1,5,7-trisubstituted indoline

Figure 14.1 Chemical structures of silodosin (A) and general formula of 1, 5, 7-trisubstituted indoline (B).

The initial medicinal chemistry effort focused on modifications of the R and R1 group in the initially identified indoline scaffold (Figure 14.1B) since low doses of these compounds specifically suppress urethral contractions induced by agents such as phenylephrine without affecting blood pressure. Thus they may not induce hypotension including postural hypotension. SAR efforts have generated alkyl substituted (R and R1) compounds with desirable properties. In an experiment using anesthetized rats, these compounds suppressed urethral contraction by 50% at a dose of about 0.5 to 60 μg/kg induced by an intravenous administration of phenylephrine (30 $\mu g\,kg^{-1}$), and showed a little blood pressure lowering activity at a higher dose. Some of them lowered blood pressure 10% at an intravenous dose of 10 to 100 $\mu g\,kg^{-1}$. Among the compounds tested, compound KMD-3213 (silodosin, Figure 14.1A) produced 50% suppressive activity at about 1.3 $\mu g\,kg^{-1}$ and showed a 10% decrease in blood pressure at an intravenous dose of about 26 $\mu g\,kg^{-1}$. Due to these favorable properties, KMD-3213 (silodosin) was selected as a development candidate for treatment of BPH.

14.2.2 The Synthesis of Silodosin (Discovery Route) [26,27]

The preparation of Silodosin was straight forward and the chemistry is summarized here. Silodosin is prepared from optically active indoline derivative **1** in 6 steps (Figure 14.2). The phenethylamino group in **1** was protected by Boc group to give carbamate **2**, and the acetyl group of **2** was removed under basic condition to yield compound **3** which was converted to primary amide **4** with hydrogen peroxide in the presence of NaOH. The introduction of the *tert*-butylyldimethlsilyloxypropyl group into the N1 position of the indoline skeleton of **4** was achieved by alkylation to give *N*-alkylindoline **5**. The TBS group of **5** was deprotected with tetrabutylammonium fluoride, and the Boc group was removed under acidic condition to give silodosin.

The optically active indoline **1** (*R*-enantiomer) was prepared by the condensation of 2-aminopropylindoline **7** with phenoxyethylbromide **8** followed by optical resolution with (+)-mandelic acid (Figure 14.3) and recrystallization.

The phenoxyethylbromide **8** was synthesized in four steps from guaiacol (**10**) as follows (Figure 14.4). The alkylation of **10** with 2,2,2-trifluoroethyl iodide under basic condition gave corresponding ether **11**. Demethylation of **11** in the presence of BBr_3 provided phenol **12** which was alkylated with 1,2-dibromoethane using NaOH to yield **8**.

The synthetic route of 2-aminopropylindoline **7** is shown in Figure 14.5. 1-Acetyl-5-propionylindoline **13** was treated with pyrrolidone hydrotribromide (PTBr) and sulfuric acid to yield α-bromoketone 14. The reduction of α-bromoketone **14** with triethylsilane

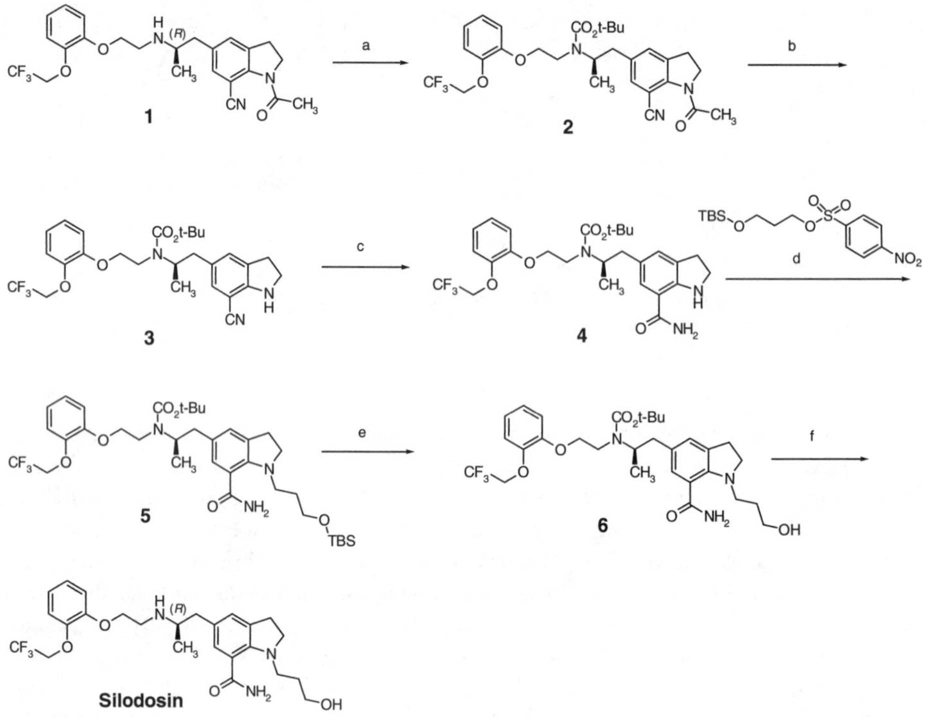

Figure 14.2 Synthesis of silodosin from compound **1**. Reagents: (a) Boc_2O; (b) NaOH; (c) H_2O_2, NaOH; (d) K_2CO_3; (e) TBAF; (f) TFA.

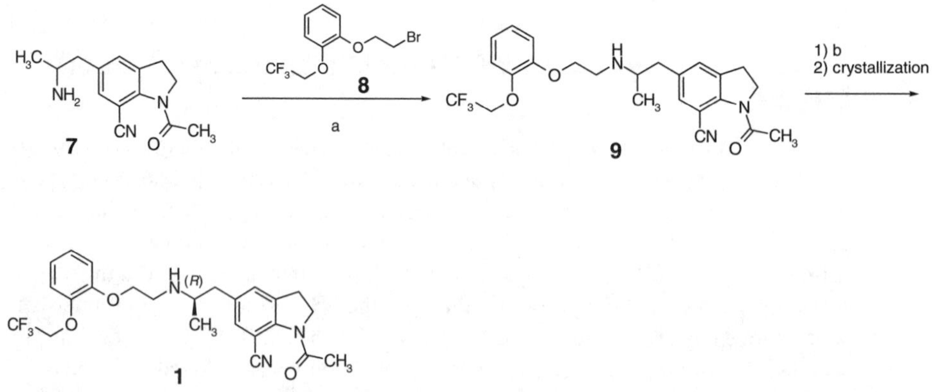

Figure 14.3 Preparation of optically active indoline **1**. Reagents: (a) $NaHCO_3$; (b) (+)-mandelic acid.

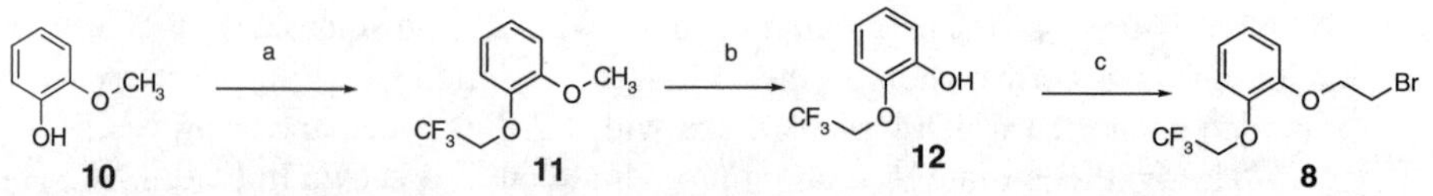

Figure 14.4 Synthesis of phenoxyethylbromide **8**. Reagents: (a) CF_3CH_2I, K_2CO_3; (b) BBr_3; (c) $BrCH_2CH_2Br$, NaOH.

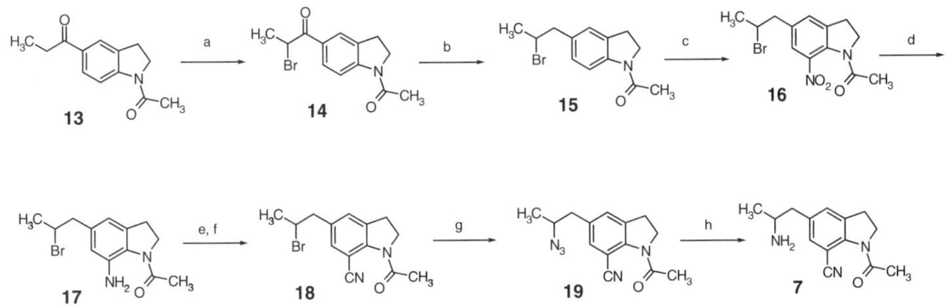

Figure 14.5 Synthesis of 2-aminopropylindoline **7**. Reagents: (a) PTBr, H_2SO_4; (b) Et_3SiH/TFA; (c) $HNO_3/AcOH$; (d) H_2, PtO_2; (e) $NaNO_2$, HCl; (f) CuCN; (g) NaN_3; (h) H_2, Pd-$BaSO_4$.

in trifluoroacetic acid gave 2-bromopropylindoline **15**. Nitration of C7 position of indoline skeleton with HNO_3 provided 7-nitroindoline 16 which was hydrogenated in the presence of platinum dioxide to obtain the aniline **17**. Aniline **17** was treated with sodium nitrite in hydrochloric acid solution followed by the reaction with copper cyanide to give nitrile **18**. Upon reaction with sodium azide, compound **18** was converted to alkylazide **19**, which was hydrogenated in the presence of 5% Pd/$BaSO_4$ to yield the corresponding alkylamine (**7**).

14.2.3 Receptor Binding Studies

Receptor-binding studies (saturation and replacement experiments) were performed using membrane fractions prepared from mouse-derived LM (tk-) cells expressing human α_{1A}-, α_{1B}-, or α_{1D}-AR, and ^{3}H-prazosin hydrochloride, to study the affinities of various drugs (Figure 14.6) for human α_1-AR subtypes. As indicated in Table 14.1 [31], the affinity of silodosin for α_{1A}-AR was 162 times higher than for the α_{1B}-AR and 55 times higher than for the α_{1D}-AR (calculated as the ratio of 162/2.95), having the highest selectivity for α_{1A}-AR among the tested α_1-AR antagonists.

It has long been suggested that a fourth subtype of α_1 adrenoceptors may exist, the α_{1L} receptor [33]. Prazosin showed low affinity for this subtype. α_{1L} receptor is a phenotype at

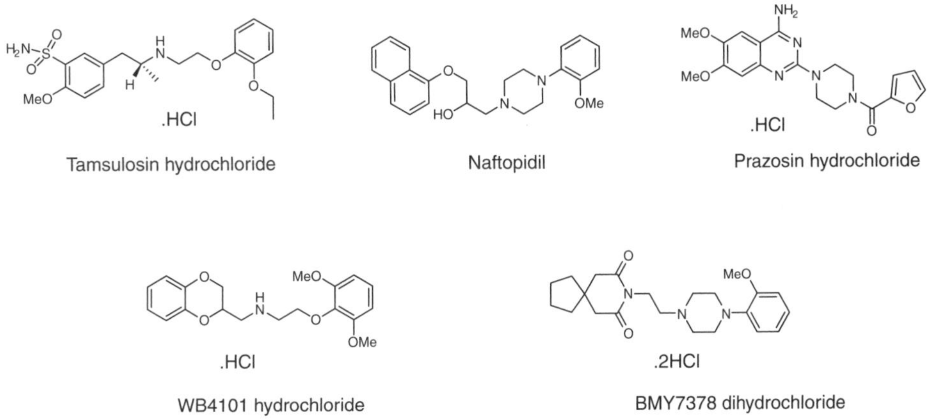

Figure 14.6 Chemical structures of tamsulosin hydrochloride, naftopidil, prazosin hydrochloride, WB4101 hydrochloride, BMY7378 dihydrochloride.

TABLE 14.1 Affinity and Selectivity for Human α_1-AR Subtype of Silodosin and other α_1-AR Antagonists

	K_i value[a] (nmol L^{-1})			α_1-AR subtype selectivity[b]	
Compound	α_{1A}-AR	α_{1B}-AR	α_{1D}-AR	α_{1A}/α_{1B} ratio	α_{1D}/α_{1B} ratio
Silodosin	0.039 ± 0.006	6.5 ± 0.6	2.2 ± 0.1	162	2.95
Tamsulosin hydrochloride	0.012 ± 0.002	0.12 ± 0.00	0.030 ± 0.005	9.55	3.80
Naftopidil	23 ± 7	7.8 ± 0.0	4.4 ± 0.4	0.372	1.78
Prazosin hydrochloride	0.12 ± 0.01	0.028 ± 0.002	0.078 ± 0.007	0.204	0.316
WB4101 hydrochloride	0.17 ± 0.01	1.1 ± 0.1	0.22 ± 0.04	6.03	5.01
BMY7378 dihydrochloride	75 ± 21	28 ± 7	0.43 ± 0.06	0.389	64.6

The K_i value in the table presents the mean ± SE of three experiments. [This table was cited from reference No. 31 with permission.]

[b]The subtype selectivity (α_{1A}/α_{1B} and α_{1D}/α_{1B} ratios) was calculated from the ratio after converting the concentration, specifically, using 10 M [$M = pK_i$ (α_{1A} or α_{1D}) $- pK_i$ (α_{1B})].

protein level (functional contribution) of α_{1A}-AR in the native tissue especially in human prostate. While it is clear that this is the functional state of the α_{1A}-AR, it is nevertheless of relevance because some drugs exhibit similar potency for the α_{1A} and α_{1L} state (e.g., tamsulosin), whereas others have much lower affinity for the α_{1L} state (e.g., all quinazolines). It has been reported that silodosin has high affinity for α_{1L}, as well as α_{1A}-AR [34,35]. It has been reported that the prostatic contraction was mediated mainly via α_{1L} (but not α_{1A}) adrenoceptor in human, so that the effective inhibition of prostatic contraction was made by suppressing α_{1L} as well as α_{1A}-mediated response.

As many studies have demonstrated that prostate, urethra, and bladder neck tissues have abundant α_{1A}-AR [36–38], it is suggested that silodosin selectively binds to α_{1A}-AR present in these tissues to suppress sympathetic stimulation, which results in relaxation of smooth muscle and to facilitate smooth urination, leading to improvement in both voiding and storage symptoms associated with BPH.

To investigate the interaction in the bindings of silodosin to α_1-AR subtypes and understand the improved selectivity of silodosin, molecular modeling was performed on Octane 2 workstation (Silicon Graphics) using Discover/Insight II software (Molecular Simulations Inc., San Diego, CA) [39] and binding profiles were compared with those of tamsulosin and prazosin. Through molecular modeling, possible binding sites for these drugs were suggested to lie between transmembrane domains (TM) 3, 4, 5, and 6 of the α_1-AR subtypes. Figure 14.7 depicts the lateral view of the binding site between amino acid of seven TM of α_1-ARs and the functional groups of silodosin.

Ethylamine nitrogen, amide nitrogen, and indoline nitrogen of silodosin possibly form hydrogen bonds with Asp106 (TM3), Gln167 (TM4), and Ser188 (TM5) of α_{1A}-AR, Asp125 (TM3), and Ser207 (TM5) of α_{1B}-AR and Asp176 (TM3) and Ser258 (TM5) of α_{1D}-AR. Glu186 (α_{1B}) being negatively charged would form a salt bridge with positively charged Lys185 (α_{1B}) in extracellular loops (EL) 2 and Glu237 (α_{1D}) with Lys236 (α_{1D}) in TM4. The bonding energy of the amide group in silodosin is not sufficient to break the salt bridges in α_{1B} and α_{1D}. Thus, Glu186 and Glu237 in α_{1B} and α_{1D}-ARs, respectively, may not contribute to the interaction with silodosin. On the other hand, Arg166 (α_{1A}) at the same position of lysine in α_{1B} may not interact with the neutral residue Gln167 (α_{1A}). Therefore,

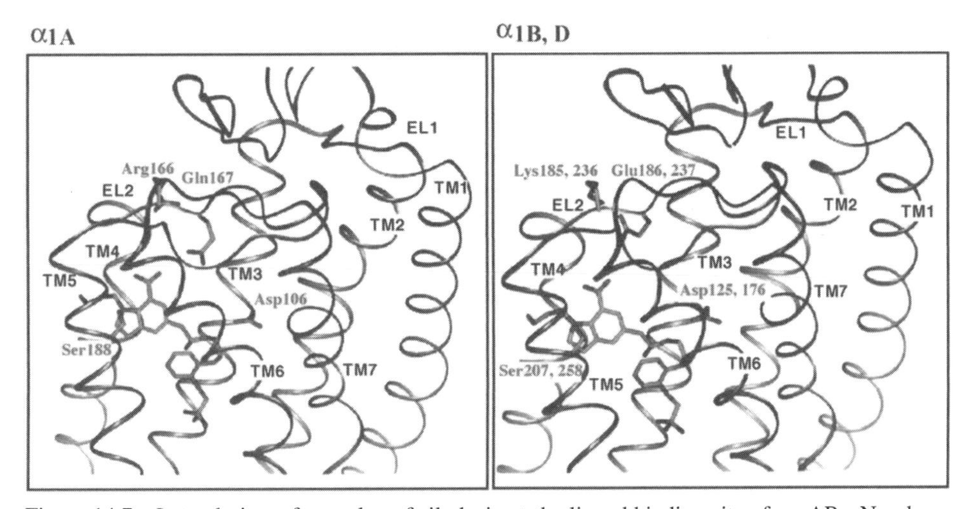

Figure 14.7 Lateral view of complex of silodosin at the ligand binding site of α_1-ARs. Numbers with TM and EL denote those of transmembrane helices and extracellular loops. [This figure was cited from reference No. 39 with permission.]

Gln167 may be able to orient to the ligand-binding site for binding with the amide group of silodosin. Figure 14.8A schematically shows the binding sites with silodosin in α_{1A}-ARs.

In the case of tamsulosin (Figure 14.8B), ethylamine nitrogen, sulfonamide nitrogen, and methoxy oxygen of the benzene ring may interact with Asp106 (TM3) and Ser188 (TM5) of α_{1A}-AR, Asp125 (TM3), and Ser207 (TM5) of α_{1B}-AR and Asp176 (TM3), Glu237 (TM4) and Ser258 (TM5) of α_{1D}-AR. Sulfonamide nitrogen of tamsulosin would interact with Glu237 in TM4 of α_{1D}-AR. This is probably due to the more acidic nature of sulfonamide and the longer bond lengths of the C–S and S–N bonds, which would enable the sulfonamide to bind with Glu237 of α_{1D}-AR.

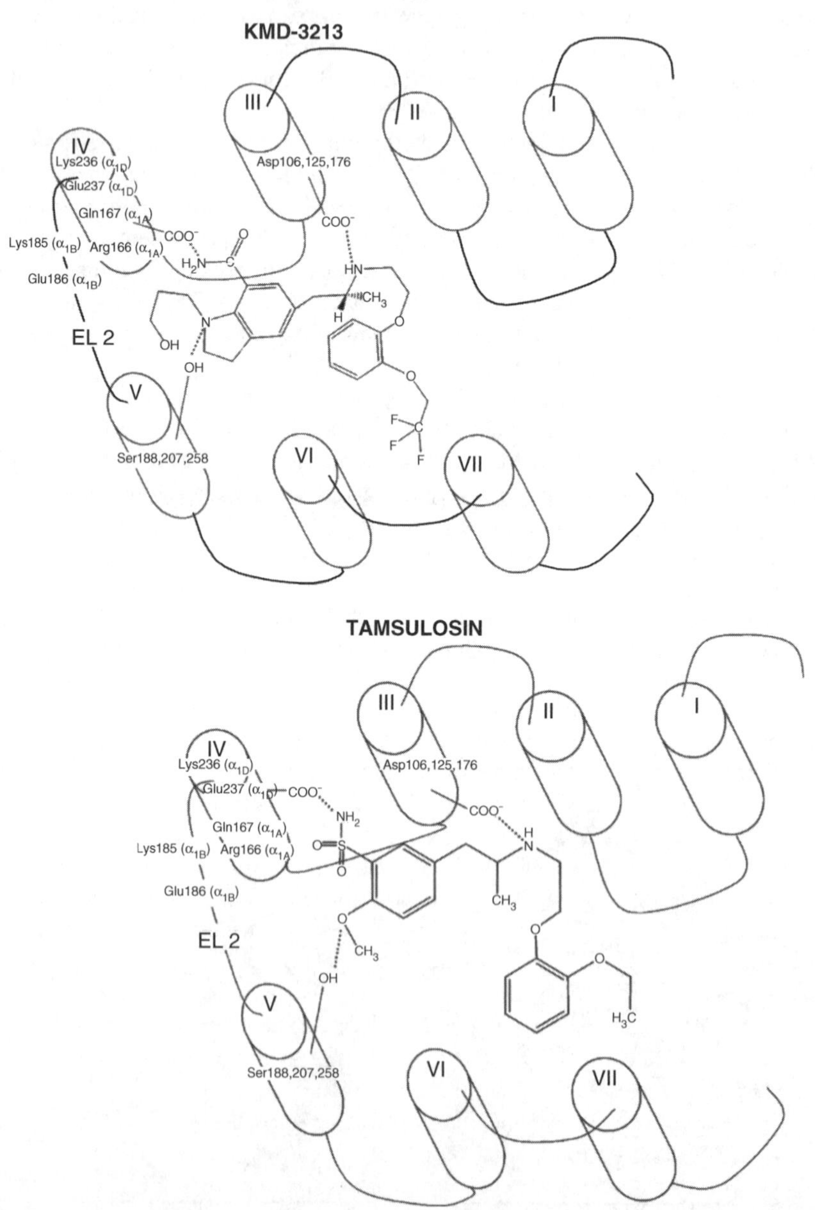

Figure 14.8 Bindings of silodosin (A) and tamsulosin (B) with α_1-ARs. Interaction between the functional groups and amino acids is shown in dotted lines indicating electrostatic interactions. [This figure was cited from reference No. 39 with permission.]

Thus, Glu237 of TM4 in α_{1D}-AR and Gln167 of TM4 in α_{1A}-AR clearly justify the selective binding profile of tamsulosin and silodosin for α_{1D}- and α_{1A}-AR, respectively.

For reference, the number of binding sites of prazosin in all the subtypes is the same. Prazosin interacts with amino acids in the same positions and in the identical helices of all the α_1-AR subtypes. This may account for the nonselectivity of prazosin to all the α_1-AR subtypes.

Silodosin's affinity for β_2-AR (pK_i value: 8.25) was almost equal to that for α_{1D}-AR subtype (pK_i value: 8.66) and α_{1B}-AR subtype (pK_i: 8.19), but showed affinity only at higher concentrations for α_2- and β_1-AR, muscarinic receptor, serotonin (5-HT1) receptor and dopamine (D1, D2 long, D3, and D4.2) receptors [36]. The affinities of silodosin for other receptor subtypes were lower than that for α_{1A}-AR. A uterus specimen isolated from a pregnant rat was used to determine the functional effect on β_2-AR. Silodosin showed antagonism of the β_2-AR at concentrations of 3×10^{-6} mol L^{-1} and higher. The affinity of KMD-3213G (a glucuronide conjugate of silodosin, see Figure 14.10), which is one of the major metabolites of silodosin in humans, for the dopamine D3 receptor was almost equal to that of silodosin, although its affinities for α_2-, β_1- and β_2-ARs, muscarinic receptor, serotonin (5-HT1) receptor and dopamine (D1, D2 long, D3, and D4.2) receptors were lower than the corresponding affinities of silodosin [39]. Another major metabolite in humans is KMD-3293 in which the primary hydroxyl group was oxidized to the carboxylic acid, showed a lower affinity for all tested receptors than did silodosin [39].

14.3 PHARMACOLOGY OF SILODOSIN

14.3.1 Action Against Noradrenalin-Induced Contraction of Lower Urinary Tract Tissue

The study was designed to determine the native tissue selectivity and α_1-adrenoceptor subtype selectivity of silodosin by conduction functional studies on contraction of isolated muscular preparations from rabbit and rat.

Tissue samples of α_{1A}-AR-rich prostate, urethra, and bladder trigone isolated from male Japanese white rabbits, α_{1B}-AR-rich spleen isolated from male SD rats, and α_{1D}-AR-rich thoracic aorta isolated from male SD rats were suspended in an organ bath filled with 10-mL Krebs solution aerated with 95% O_2 and 5% CO_2 at 37°C, to study the suppression of noradrenalin (NA)-induced contraction by silodosin, using tamsulosin hydrochloride, naftopidil, and prazosin hydrochloride for comparison. The results showed that all of the tested α_1-AR antagonists shifted the NA dose–response curves of the rabbit prostate, rat spleen, and rat thoracic aorta to the right in a concentration-dependent manner [31,32].

The antagonistic action of silodosin against NA-induced contraction of each isolated tissue was compared with those of α_1-AR antagonists by the pA_2 (negative logarithmic value of molar concentration of antagonistic blockers necessary to parallel shift 2 times the independent stimulant concentration-reaction curve to the higher concentration side) or the pK_b value (negative logarithmic value of dissociation constant for binding of antagonistic blockers to receptors) (Table 14.2) [31].

The tissue selectivity was calculated from the data of Table 14.2. Silodosin was about 280 times more selective for prostate tissue versus spleen and about 50 times more selective versus thoracic aorta which shows that silodosin is significantly more selective for prostate tissue compared to other α_1-AR antagonists. Furthermore, the selectivity for the urethra and bladder trigone was found to be comparable to the prostate. The selectivity of tamsulosin hydrochloride of the prostate was about 20 times higher that for the selectivity to spleen, but

TABLE 14.2 pA_2 or pK_b Values of Silodosin, Tamsulosin Hydrochloride, Naftopidil and Prazosin Hydrochloride for Noradrenaline-Induced Contraction in the Isolated Rabbit Prostate, Isolated Rabbit Urethra, Isolated Rabbit Trigone of Bladder, Isolated Rat Spleen and Isolated Rat Thoracic Aorta[a]

	pA_2 or pK_b values				
	α_{1A}-AR			α_{1B}-AR	α_{1D}-AR
Compound	Prostate[b]	Urethra[b]	Bladder trigone[b]	Spleen[c]	Thoracic aorta[c]
Silodosin	9.60 ± 0.05^c	8.71 ± 0.09 (0.98 ± 0.32)	9.35 ± 0.15^d	7.15 ± 0.05 ($0.67 \pm 0.09^*$)	7.88 ± 0.05 (1.00 ± 0.18)
Tamsulosin hydrochloride	9.93 ± 0.07^c	9.00 ± 0.06 (1.16 ± 0.27)	9.48 ± 0.14^d	8.64 ± 0.06 ($0.61 \pm 0.18^*$)	9.82 ± 0.06 (0.91 ± 0.20)
Naftopidil	6.69 ± 0.05^c (1.13 ± 0.21)	6.48 ± 0.11 (0.93 ± 0.39)	6.80 ± 0.07 (0.91 ± 0.25)	6.30 ± 0.07 (0.69 ± 0.23)	7.48 ± 0.06 (1.14 ± 0.23)
Prazosin hydrochloride	7.91 ± 0.02 (1.08 ± 0.09)	7.96 ± 0.04 ($0.85 \pm 0.13^*$)	8.10 ± 0.05 (0.97 ± 0.18)	9.34 ± 0.13 ($0.56 \pm 0.26^*$)	9.17 ± 0.06 (1.11 ± 0.23)

[a]Each value in the table presents mean $\pm$ SE of 4 to 5 animals. Each value in parenthesis presents the slop of the Schild plot. [This table was cited from reference No. 31 with permission.]

[b]Rabbits.

[c]Rats.

[d]pK_b value.

*Significantly different from the unity at $P < 0.05$ by paired-t test.

comparable to the thoracic aorta. On the other hand, naftopidil and prazosin hydrochloride were more selective for spleen and thoracic aorta, 0.4 and 5 times for naftopidil and 25 and 20 times for prazosin hydrochloride, respectively, showing the selectivity to the prostate to be lower.

These results demonstrate that silodosin has a higher selectivity to the LUT, especially the prostate, as compared to other tested α_1-AR antagonists.

14.3.2 Actions Against Phenylephrine-Induced Increase in Intraurethral Pressure and Blood Pressure

It is so essential to experiment in *in vivo* uroselectivity (ratio of reactivities for LUT against blood pressure) of bland-new compound, that this study was conducted to confirm the effectiveness of silodosin using rats and dogs.

Intravenous dosing of the α_1-AR agonist phenylephrine (PE) through the femoral vein increases intraurethral pressure (IUP) in urethane-anesthetized male Sprague–Dawley (SD) rats. This effect should be blocked by an α_1-AR antagonist. A comparison of silodosin, tamsulosin hydrochloride, naftopidil, and prazosin hydrochloride is given in Table 14.3. The results showed that each of α_1-AR antagonists dose dependently suppressed the PE-induced increase in IUP, lowering the MBP [40,41]. Silodosin potently suppressed the PE-induced increase in IUP, but tamsulosin hydrochloride equally suppressed the PE-induced increase in IUP but also decreased the mean blood pressure (MBP) at a similar dose. Naftopidil and prazosin hydrochloride showed a greater ability to decrease the MBP in contrast to silodosin. Heart rate (HR) was decreased about 10% by naftopidil at doses of 1000 and 3000 $\mu g\ kg^{-1}$. No other antagonists had this effect. The efficacy to suppress the PE-induced IUP increase defined by the ID_{50} value (the dose to suppress IUP increase by 50%) decreased in order of tamsulosin hydrochloride, silodosin, prazosin hydrochloride, naftopidil, and the efficacy to decrease the MBP defined by the ED_{15} value (the dose to decrease the MBP by 15%) decreased in order of prazosin hydrochloride, tamsulosin hydrochloride, silodosin, naftopidil, showing that silodosin (ED_{15}/ID_{50}) has the highest selectivity for the LUT at 11.7, followed by tamsulosin hydrochloride, prazosin hydrochloride, and naftopidil in this order (Table 14.3) [40].

In a study designed to gauge the time cause of α_1-AR antagonists given intraduodenally on IUP and MBP, silodosin (3–300 $\mu g\ kg^{-1}$), tamsulosin hydrochloride (3–100 $\mu g\ kg^{-1}$), or naftopidil (300–10,000 $\mu g\ kg^{-1}$) were dosed intraduodenally to fasted anesthetized male SD rats, followed by intravenous PE administration 5, 30 min and 1, 2, 3, and 4 h

TABLE 14.3 ID_{50} Value, ED_{15} Value, and Uroselectivity of Silodosin, Tamsulosin Hydrochloride, Naftopidil and Prazosin Hydrochloride after Intravenous Administration in the Anesthetized Rat[a]

	IUP	MBP	Uroselectivity
Drug	ID_{50} ($\mu g\ kg^{-1}$)	ED_{15} ($\mu g\ kg^{-1}$)	(ED_{15}/ID_{50})
Silodosin	0.932	10.9	11.7
Tamsulosin hydrochloride	0.400	0.895	2.24
Naftopidil	361	48.1	0.133
Prazosin hydrochloride	4.04	0.792	0.196

[a]The ID_{50} or ED_{15} value is the average value from five animals. [This table was cited from reference No. 40 with permission.]

Abbreviations: IUP, intraurethral pressure; MBP, mean blood pressure.

TABLE 14.4 ID_{50} Value, ED_{15} Value, and Uroselectivity of Silodosin, Tamsulosin hydrochloride, Naftopidil after Intraduodenal Administration in the Anesthetized Rat[a]

	IUP	MBP	Uroselectivity
Drug	ID_{50} ($\mu g\ kg^{-1}$)	ED_{15} ($\mu g\ kg^{-1}$)	ED_{15}/ID_{50}
Silodosin	10.6	276	26.0
Tamsulosin hydrochloride	5.45	20.8	3.82
Naftopidil	1200	1666	1.39

[a]The ID_{50} or ED_{15} value is the average value from 5 to 6 animals. [This table was cited from reference No. 40 with permission.]

Abbreviations: IUP, intraurethral pressure; MBP, mean blood pressure.

after administration and compare with the baseline. In a separate experiment, silodosin (100–3000 $\mu g\ kg^{-1}$), tamsulosin hydrochloride (10–300 $\mu g\ kg^{-1}$), and naftopidil (300–30,000 $\mu g\ kg^{-1}$) were administered intraduodenally to a separate set of animals to observe the MBP and HR until 4 h after administration. Each drug was found to dose dependently suppress the PE-induced IUP increase and lower the MBP, starting immediately after administration [41,42]. The values of various drugs to suppress 50% of the PE-induced IUP increase and to lower the MBP by 15% are shown in Table 14.4.

In brief, the above study results demonstrate that silodosin has a greater impact on LUT symptom, with a decreased ability to cause a decrease in blood pressure, suggesting that silodosin can be a useful candidate for a therapeutic drug of micturition disorder associated with BPH.

14.3.3 Actions Against Intraurethral Pressure Increased by Stimulating Hypogastric Nerve and Blood Pressure in Dogs with Benign Prostatic Hyperplasia

Male dogs are reported to have age-specific prostatic hyperplasia. However, it develops into prostatic cancer at a lower frequency than in humans. Nevertheless, this animal species is considered to be an important model to study prostatic hyperplasia and cancer [42]. Dogs with excessive hyperplastic prostate are known to show clinical symptoms like dysuria as humans do, with morphologic similarity such as gonadal hyperplasia and interstitial hyperplasia due probably to mechanical and functional obstruction being reported. Therefore, dogs with prostatic hyperplasia are considered to be a useful animal model to study the pharmacologic efficacy of a drug for micturition disorder associated with BPH in humans [42].

The hypogastric nerve is a sympathetic nerve mediating prostatic contraction. In male beagles diagnosed by veterinary palpation as having prostatic hyperplasia, electrical stimulation of this nerve induces increases in IUP. This effect can be blocked by administration of α_1-AR antagonists. After blood pressure, HR, and transient increase in IUP induced by electrical stimulation to hypogastric nerve were stabilized, silodosin, tamsulosin hydrochloride, or naftopidil was intravenously administered at intervals of 30 min starting with a low dose and titrating upward. The study results showed that all these drugs dose dependently suppressed the increase in IUP and lowered the MBP. The ID_{50} to increase the IUP, the ED_{15} to lower MBP and the selectivity for the LUT (ED_{15}/ID_{50}) are shown in Table 14.5. The results demonstrate that silodosin has less of an effect on blood pressure and may be a useful drug to improve micturition associated with BPH.

TABLE 14.5 ID_{50} Value, ED_{15} Value, and Uroselectivity of Silodosin, Tamsulosin Hydrochloride, and Naftopidil after Intravenous Administration in the Anesthetized BPH Dog[a]

	IUP	MBP	Uroselectivity
Drug	ID_{50} ($\mu g\ kg^{-1}$)	ED_{15} ($\mu g\ kg^{-1}$)	ED_{15}/ID_{50}
Silodosin	1.97	35.9	19.8
Tamsulosin hydrochloride	0.855	0.736	0.939
Naftopidil	35.3	156	4.94

[a]The ID_{50} or ED_{15} value is the average value from 4 animals. [This table was cited from reference No. 42 with permission.]

Abbreviations: IUP, intraurethral pressure; MBP, mean blood pressure.

14.3.4 Safety Pharmacology

The safety profile of silodosin was systematically investigated [43]. Orally administered silodosin showed no effects on the central nervous system of rats at doses up to 2 mg kg^{-1}. After administration of silodosin at 20 mg kg^{-1}, trembling, increased somnolence and decreased body temperatures were observed. The glucuronide metabolite of silodosin, KMD-3213G (or KMD127K) did not show any CNS effects in rats after intravenous injections up to the highest dose of 3 mg kg^{-1}. In terms of cardiovascular effects, orally administered silodosin in conscious dogs decreased blood pressure at doses as low as 0.2 mg kg^{-1}. No effect on heart rate and electrocardiograph (ECG) was observed at doses up to 20 mg kg^{-1}. Silodosin inhibited hERGtail current with the IC_{50} value of 8.91×10^{-6} mol L^{-1}. It prolonged APD90 in the papillary muscle isolated from guinea pig by 6.4% at 1×10^{-6} mol L^{-1} and by 17.1 % at 1×10^{-5} mol L^{-1}. KMD-3213G did not show any effect on the cardiovascular systems in dogs after intravenous injections up to the highest dose of 3 mg g^{-1}. It also did not show any effect on HERO tail current and myocardial action potential waveform in the papillary muscle isolated from guinea pigs at concentrations up to 1×10^{-5} mol L^{-1}. For pulmonary effects, orally-administered silodosin increased the respiratory rates in conscious dogs at a dose as low as 2 mg kg^{-1}, though it did not show any effect on blood gas parameters even at the highest dose of 20 mg kg^{-1}. KMD-3213G did not show any effect on the respiratory system in dogs after intravenous injections up to the highest dose of 3 mg kg^{-1}. The results of these studies have supported the further development of KMD-3213 (silodosin).

14.4 METABOLISM OF SILODOSIN [43]

The evaluation of the metabolism is one of the essential processes in the drug development. Thus, absorption, distribution, metabolism, and excretion studies of silodosin were performed in mice, rats, and dogs (ICR mice, Sprague–Dawley (SD) rats and Beagle dogs), using nonlabeled and ^{14}C-labeled silodosin (Figure 14.9). An *in vitro* metabolism study in monkeys used hepatocytes from Cynomolgus monkeys.

Concentrations of silodosin and its metabolites in plasma and tissues were determined by high performance liquid chromatography (HPLC) fluorescent or liquid chromatography tandem mass spectrometry (LC/MS/MS) after extraction from measured samples. The analytical method was validated for intraassay and interassay reproducibility and if necessary, specificity, dilution effects, freeze/thaw stability and storage stability. Radioactivity in samples was determined using a liquid scintillation counter for studies using

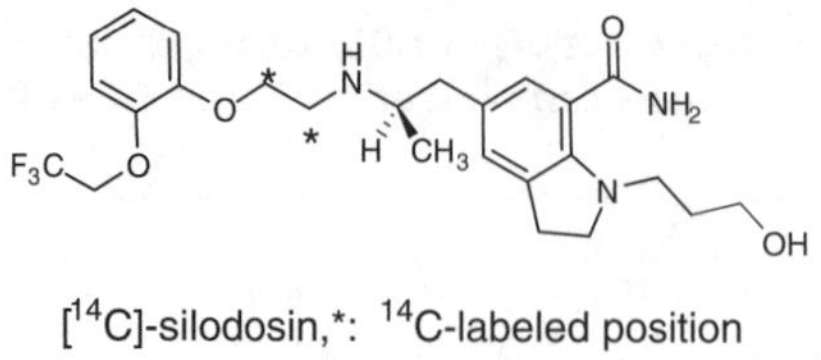

[^{14}C]-silodosin,*: ^{14}C-labeled position

Figure 14.9 ^{14}C-labeled silodosin.

^{14}C-KMD-3213. In the metabolite identification study using ^{14}C-silodosin, the amount of each metabolite of silodosin was determined using HPLC with a radioactivity detector, and metabolites were measured by liquid chromatography/mass spectrometry (LC/MS).

In vitro metabolism studies using rat, dog, and human hepatocytes showed that a glucuronide conjugate of silodosin (KMD-3213G) and a metabolite in which the primary hydroxyl group was oxidized (KMD-3293) were mainly synthesized in hepatocytes and are the major metabolites in humans (Figure 14.10). KMD-3293 was also synthesized in rat and dog hepatocytes, but KMD-3213G was not seen in rat and dog hepatocytes. The major human glucuronidated metabolite KMD-3213 (silodosin) was minimally produced in monkey hepatocytes.

In order to study the ability of silodosin in inducing or inhibiting the cytochrome P450 (CYP450) enzymes responsible for drug metabolism, rats were orally-administered silodosin at dose of 1, 10, and 30 mg kg^{-1} once daily for 7 days. The livers were removed and microsomes were prepared from the isolated liver. Enzyme activity was determined using the liver microsomes. Cytochrome P450 was increased in the rats receiving repeat oral administration of 10 and 30 mg kg^{-1} daily compared to the negative control group.

The activity of aniline 4-hydroxylase, a kind of drug-metabolizing enzyme decreased only in those rats given 10 mg kg^{-1} daily compared to rats in the negative control group with 0.83 times the activity of the negative control. The uridine diphosphate glucuronyl transferase (UDP-GT) activity significantly decreased in rats receiving 1 mg kg^{-1} daily compared to rats in the negative control group with a 0.78-fold difference. There were no difference in the amount of liver microsome protein, the amount of cytochrome *b*5, aminopyrine *N*-dimethyl enzyme activity, 7-ethoxy cumarine *O*-deethylase enzyme activity, or glutathione *S*-transferase activity between silodosin-treated rats and control rats.

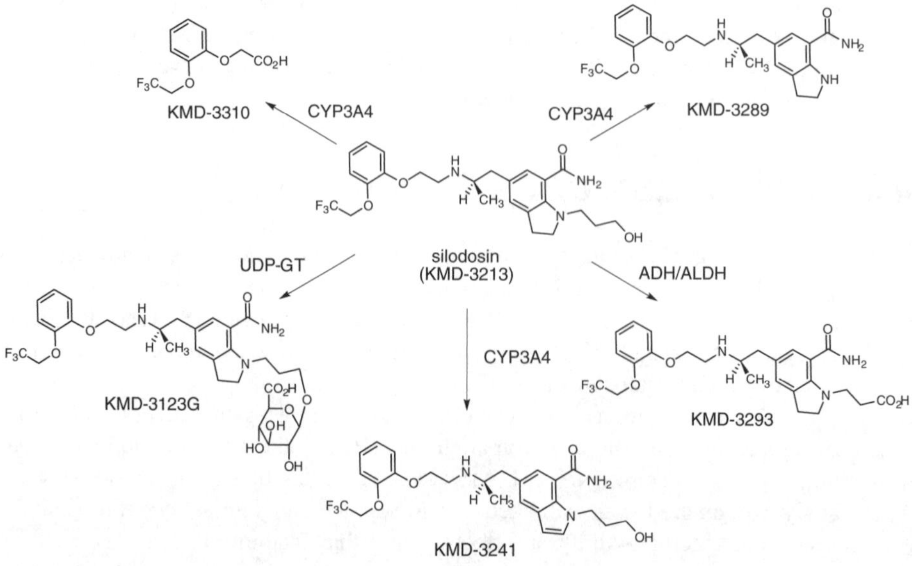

Figure 14.10 Metabolic pathway of silodosin.

From these results, rats receiving a dose that is 100-fold higher than the pharmacologic dose (0.1 mg kg^{-1}) had a statistically greater increase in the amount of cytochrome P450 compared to the control group, that was 20% greater than control.

To further understand the metabolism of KMD-3213 (silodosin), studies were carried out to determine the enzymes responsible for the generation of these metabolites. In an attempt to identify the enzymes responsible for the metabolism of KMD-3213 (silodosin) to its main metabolite KMD-3293, the rate of KMD-3293 formation was measured using human liver microsomal or S9 fractions in the presence of NADPH, NADP, or NAD. S9 fraction is supernatant of liver homogenate centrifuged at 9000 *g*, that contains many kind of liver metabolizing enzymes. An insignificant amount of KMD-3293 was formed using microsomes in the absence or presence of NADPH or S9 in the absence of NAD or NADP. In S9 the rates of formation in the presence of NAD and NADP were 2.5 and 0.2 nmol 30 min^{-1} 2 mg^{-1} protein, respectively. Based on the above data, it was proposed that alcohol dehydrogenase and aldehyde dehydrogenase are involved in the metabolism of KMD-3213 (silodosin) to KMD-3293.

The enzyme responsible for production of metabolite KMD-3310 from KMD-3213 (silodosin) was also identified. The rate of KMD-3310 formation was measured using human liver microsomes, S9 fractions, or cytosol in the presence or absence of ß-NADPH or ß-NADH. It was concluded that CYP3A4 is involved in the metabolism of KMD-3213 (silodosin) to KMD-3310.

An *in vitro* study to determine the UGT isoforms responsible for the metabolism of KMD-3213 (silodosin) was carried out using ^{14}C-KMD-3213 and microsomes expressing human UGT. The K_m and V_{max} values were also determined. The glucuronidated metabolite MD127 (KMD-3213G) was formed in the presence of human UGT2B7 microsomes (but not in 1A3, 1A6, 1A9, 1A10, 2B7, or 2B15). The mean percent formation of KMD-3213G was 1.69%, 5.02%, and 8.49% after incubation for 10, 30, and 60 min, respectively. The K_m and V_{max} for glucuronidation of ^{14}C-KMD-3213 by human UGT2B7 were 401.0 μmol L^{-1} and 670.7 pmol min^{-1} mg^{-1} protein.

Radiolabeled KMD-3213 (silodosin) was used to determine the metabolic profile of the compound *in vivo*. The percentages of unchanged drug and metabolites in the plasma, liver, kidneys, prostate, bile, urine, and feces were measured by RI-HPLC. KMD-3250 was primarily detected in the liver, feces, and bile, and KMD-3310 in the kidneys, prostate, plasma, and urine of male SD rats. The percentages of unchanged drug at 0.5 and 4 h after administration were 4.8% and 11.9%, in the plasma, 1.4% and 4.0%, in the liver, 3.8% and 12.7%, in the kidneys, and 26.7% and 32.3% in the prostate, respectively.

The percentages of unchanged drug in the urine, feces, and bile by 24 h after administration were 12.8%, 12.7%, and 2.3%, respectively. In addition, the metabolic profile in the plasma, liver, kidneys, and prostate was specific to each organ, showing no marked change over time.

The effects of KMD-3213 (silodosin) on drug-metabolizing enzymes in hepatic microsomes after repeated oral administration to rats at doses of 1, 10, or 30 mg kg^{-1} once daily for 7 days were investigated. All of the indexes (body weight, liver weight, microsomal protein content, cytochrome content, metabolic enzyme activities) tested in this study except rat body weight increased significantly in the positive control group, that is, phenobarbital group (80 mg g^{-1}, intraperitoneally). Cytochrome P450 contents significantly increased in the 10 and 30 mg kg^{-1} KMD-3213 (silodosin) groups and increases were by 1.2- and 1.23-fold of those in negative control group, respectively.

Aniline 4-hydroxylase activity and UDPG transferase activity decreased significantly in the 10 or 1 mg kg^{-1} groups, respectively, however, those decreases were 0.83 or 0.78 to those in negative control group, respectively, and not dose dependent. There were no effects on microsomal protein content, aminopyrine *N*-demethylase activity, 7-ethoxycoumarin *O*-deethylase activity, and glutathione *S*-transferase activity. These results indicated that the effects of KMD-3213 (silodosin) on drug-metabolizing enzymes in rat liver are slight.

These results indicated that the effect of KMD-3213 (silodosin) on drug-metabolizing enzymes in rat liver are slight, so that there seemed to have little risk of drug–drug interaction with KMD-3213 (silodosin). This information is very important for clinical use of silodosin.

14.5 PHARMACOKINETICS OF SILODOSIN [43]

14.5.1 Absorption

The purpose of this study was to estimate absorption of KMD-3213 (silodosin) in alimentary tract of male rats.

Absorption of KMD-3213 (silodosin) was evaluated in fasting rats given a single oral dose of 0.3, 1, and 3 mg kg^{-1} silodosin. The t_{max} in plasma was 0.10 to 0.15 h. The C_{max} and AUC increased with increasing dose from 0.3 to 1 mg kg^{-1}, but was not dose proportional at higher levels. The dose independency at the higher dose is a usual phenomenon. In nonfasting rats given a single intravenous injection of 0.03, 0.1, 0.3, and 1 mg kg^{-1} silodosin, the AUC increased with increasing dose over a range of 0.03 to 0.3 mg kg^{-1}. The $t_{1/2}$ of silodosin in rats after a single oral administration or intravenous injection was 1.5 to 2.0 h and 2.4 to 3.2 h, respectively. The bioavailability (BA) of silodosin in rats receiving a single oral dose of 0.3 and 1 mg kg^{-1} was about 9%. The CL_{tot} of silodosin after a single intravenous administration of silodosin to rats was 55 to 72 mL min^{-1} kg^{-1}. Liver blood flow rate is an average of 60 mL min^{-1} kg^{-1}. Thus, CL_{tot} value of silodosin was in equivalent in liver blood flow rate. This means silodosin shows the liver blood flow rate-controlling metabolism.

The bioavailability of KMD-3213 (silodosin) in dog was favorable. In fasting dogs receiving a single oral dose of 0.5 mg g^{-1} silodosin, the plasma concentration reached the C_{max} within 1 h and the $t_{1/2}$ was 2 h. The BA in dogs after a single oral dose was about 25% and CL_{tot} was 22.3 mL^{-1} min^{-1} g^{-1}.

The metabolism of KMD-3213 (silodosin) was farther studied in mice (Slc:ICR) and dogs (male Beagle). After a single oral dose of silodosin in male and female mice at doses of 20, 100, and 500 mg kg^{-1} for males and 60, 150, and 400 mg kg^{-1} for females, the T_{max} of silodosin in plasma occurred within 2.0 h in both sexes. The $AUC_{0\text{-}24}$ and C_{max} of silodosin and its metabolites increased with increasing doses. The percentage of the $AUC_{0\text{-}24}$ of silodosin relative to the total $AUC_{0\text{-}24}$ was 50% or more. After a single oral dose of silodosin in male and female dogs at doses of 100 and 200 mg kg^{-1}, the plasma concentration of silodosin reached C_{max} within 2.0 h. However, the $AUC_{0\text{-}24}$ of silodosin did not show a dose proportional increase. The percentage of the $AUC_{0\text{-}24}$ of silodosin was not less than 50% of the total $AUC_{0\text{-}24}$ of determined substances.

The site of absorption of ^{14}C-KMD-3213 in male rats (SD) was studied. Plasma radioactivity was measured after injections of ^{14}C-KMD-3213 (1 mg kg^{-1}) into ligated, isolated gut loops of the stomach and intestinal tract (duodenum, jejunum and ileum) in rats. The radioactivities of the residual and the tissues in gut loop were measured. The maximum radioactivity in plasma after the administration to ligated stomach, duodenum, jejunum and ileum were 11.6 ± 6.8 (4 h after administration), 251.0 ± 119.6 (1 h after administration), 275.3 ± 65.0 (2 h after administration), and 202.6 ± 68.7 ng equivalent. of KMD-3213 mL^{-1} (1 h after administration), respectively. Therefore, plasma radioactivity was similar after injection into the ligated duodenum, jejunum, and ileum. In contrast, plasma radioactivity after administration to ligated stomach was significantly lower than the others. The dose recovery at 4 h after administration to ligated stomach, duodenum, jejunum, and ileum were 91.0 ± 7.4, 16.8 ± 4.9, 31.1 ± 14.7, and $24.5 \pm 11.6\%$, respectively. These results indicate that KMD-3213 (silodosin) is widely absorbed throughout the intestine of rat, but poorly absorbed from the stomach.

In repeated doses, the AUC and C_{max} increased in a dose-dependent manner for both silodosin and its metabolites in mice, rats and dogs.

These studies using experimental animals made it possible to predict of the absorption of KMD-3213 (silodosin) administered orally in human.

14.5.2 Organ Distribution [43]

The quantitative tissue distribution of radioactivity was investigated in male rats in order to examine tissue affinity, accumulation and elimination, etc., of KMD-3213 (silodosin).

In fasting rats receiving a single oral dose of 1 mg kg^{-1} ^{14}C-KMD-3213, radioactivity was rapidly distributed into the organs and tissues.

High concentrations of radioactivity were detected in the liver, kidneys, and bladder 30 min after oral administration in addition to the intestinal tract. High concentrations of radioactivity were also detected in the liver and kidneys, and comparatively high concentrations were in the pituitary, the pancreas, and the bladder, 4 h after administration. At 24 h postdose, the highest concentration of radioactivity was detected in the liver and the second highest concentration was in the pituitary. Radioactivity decreased with time in most of the organs and tissues. Higher concentrations of radioactivity remained in the liver and the kidneys than in the other organs and tissues 168 h after administration. Radioactivity disappeared more rapidly from plasma compared to other organs and tissues, and at 168 h after administration, was below the level of detection. In the prostate, concentrations of radioactivity equaled the concentrations in plasma, and persisted with radioactivity being detected even 168 h after administration. In addition, the elimination half-lives of radioactivity in the testis, brown fat, white fat, skin, and heart were longer than those in other organs and tissues. Throughout all the time points, radioactivity in the cerebrum and the cerebellum were lower than those in plasma indicating that the distribution of silodosin to the central nervous system was low.

In nonfasting rats given repeat oral administrations of ^{14}C-KMD-3213 at 1 mg kg^{-1} once daily for 21 days, high concentrations of radioactivity were distributed to the liver, followed by the kidneys, pituitary, and skin.

Distribution in blood cells test, the blood cell association of silodosin was about 30% to 60% of the administered dose in rat and dog blood, whereas it was not greater than 5% in humans.

In order to further understand the extent of liver and kidney accumulation and pharmacokinetics of KMD-3213 (silodosin) and metabolites KMD-3241 and KM-3289, a 4-week oral capsule study in dogs at a dose of 25 mg kg^{-1} day^{-1} was conducted. Blood samples were taken on days 1, 14, 21, and 28 following daily oral administration of KMD-3213 (silodosin). Plasma concentrations of KMD-3213 (silodosin), and the metabolites KMD-3241 and KMD-3289 (Figure 14.10), were measured by a validated high-performance liquid chromatographic (HPLC) method up to 24 h postdose. Samples of liver and kidney tissue were taken from animals on days 1, 14, 21, and 28 after the 24 h blood samples had been taken. The concentrations of KMD-3213 (silodosin), KMD-3241, and KMD-3289 were also measured by validated HPLC methods. The terminal half-lives of KMD-3213 (silodosin), KMD-3241 and KMD-3289 on days 1, 14, 21, and 28 were similar, and in the range 1.3 to 4.9 h. There was little or no evidence of accumulation of KMD-3213 (silodosin) or KMD-3241 in liver and kidney tissue (accumulation ratios <2), however, KMD-3289 concentrations in liver and kidney were higher after repeated oral doses of KMD-3213 (silodosin) than after a single dose, and were similar on days 21 and 28 indicating that steady-state had been attained by day 21.

The qualitative tissue distribution of radioactivity in male and pregnant female rats after a single oral administration was performed by whole blood autoradiography. This study was conducted to confirm whole body distribution and placenta permeability of silodosin. Following a single oral administration of ^{14}C-KMD-3213 at a dose of 1 mg kg^{-1} 24 h after a single oral dose of ^{14}C-KMD-3213 to male rats (versus at 0.5, 4, or 24 h postdose), the highest concentration of radioactivity was found in the gastrointestinal tract contents and urinary bladder, while medium levels were generally associated with the liver, pituitary, preputial gland, prostate, and urethra. The lowest levels of radioactivity were detected in many other tissues, including the adrenal gland, blood, exorbital and intraorbital lacrimal glands, harderian gland, kidney, lung, myocardium, pancreas, salivary gland, spleen, thyroid, and uveal tract, but not in the brain, eye, or spinal cord.

At 48 and 72 h postadministration, concentrations of radioactivity in all tissues had declined considerably, such that none contained relatively high levels, and only the gastrointestinal tract, liver, pituitary, and preputial gland contained medium levels at the former time and only liver at the latter time. The only other tissue associated with radioactivity (at low levels) at both of these times was the kidney.

During the 24 h after single oral doses of ^{14}C-KMD-3213 to pregnant female rats (viz at 0.5, 4, or 24 h postdose), the highest concentrations of radioactivity were present in the gastrointestinal tract contents and urinary bladder (as was also the case for male rats).

In pregnant female rats, however, medium levels were generally associated with a larger number of tissues, namely, the exorbital and intraorbital lacrimal glands, fat, kidney, harderian gland, liver, pituitary, preputial gland, salivary gland, uterus wall, and uveal tract. The lowest levels of radioactivity were detected in the adrenal glands, bone marrow, lung, myocardium, ovary, pancreas, placenta, and spleen, but none was detected in the brain, eye, spinal cord, or fetuses. By 48 h after dosing, concentrations of radioactivity in all tissues had declined considerably, such that none contained relatively high levels. Medium levels were present in the gastrointestinal tract, kidney, liver, preputial gland, and uterus wall, and low levels were detected in the exorbital and intraorbital lacrimal glands, fat, harderian gland, pituitary, placenta, salivary gland, small intestine contents, and uveal tract.

In summary, radioactivity was rapidly and widely distributed throughout the animal body, although highest tissue concentrations were largely confined to the gastrointestinal tract and urinary bladder, that is, the principal excretory organs. Medium levels of radioactivity were generally present in liver and certain glandular tissues, but only low levels were found in the brain and spinal cord of both sexes and in the fetuses of pregnant females, thereby demonstrating that the drug did not readily penetrate the blood–brain barrier or undergo appreciable transplacental transfer in rats.

14.5.3 Excretion

The excretion of silodosin[43] was studied using labeled KMD-3213 (silodosin). In fasting rats given a single oral dose of ^{14}C-KMD-3213 at 1 mg kg^{-1}, urine, feces, and expired air accounted for 15.3%, 81.7%, and 0.5%, respectively, of the total administered radioactivity 168 h after administration. In fasting dogs administered a single oral administration of

^{14}C-KMD-3213 at 0.5 mg g^{-1}, radioactivity excreted in urine and feces, and recovered from the cage wash, was 24.62%, 61.8%, and 3.73%, respectively, of the administered radioactivity, and 89.53% in total.

In nonfasting rats receiving repeat oral doses of ^{14}C-KMD-3213 at 1 mg g^{-1} once daily for 21 days, urinary and fecal excretion fractions were 9.9% and 87.4%, respectively, of the administered radioactivity and 97.3% in total. In addition, the urinary excretion fraction was constant 12 days after administration.

These results indicated that excretion dynamics of repeated oral administration of silodosin was not different from that of single oral administration.

14.6 TOXICOLOGY OF SILODOSIN [43]

Since evaluation of toxicology of silodosin is one of the essential parts of development processes, toxicokinetic studies were also conducted in conjunction with pivotal toxicology studies and indicated that silodosin and its metabolites were adequately included in those studies, except for the glucuronidated metabolite which circulates at approximately four times the plasma levels of silodosin in humans.

In a 26-week study in rats, at 15 mg kg^{-1} day^{-1} (approximately equal to the expected clinical exposure via AUC), pharmacologic signs included ptosis, lacrimation, and salivation. Slight to moderate fatty degeneration of hepatocytes (males) and slight swelling of centrilobular hepatocytes (males) were also observed. Increased lipid droplets were observed in the liver by electron microscopy in males. At 60 mg kg^{-1} day^{-1} (about 5–7 times the expected clinical exposure), discoloration of the liver was observed. Histopathology included slight to moderate fatty degeneration of hepatocytes (males), slight swelling of centrilobular hepatocytes (males), slight eosinophilic changes of centrilobular hepatocytes (males), slight dilatation of the adrenal cortex (males), hypertrophy of the vaginal mucous epithelium, and slight mammary gland hyperplasia (females). Increased lipid droplets were observed in the liver by electron microscopy in males. At 300 mg kg^{-1} day^{-1} (estimated 20 times the expected clinical exposure), clinical signs also included deep respiration and decrease in locomotor activity. Increased relative liver and relative adrenal weights and decreased uterine weight were observed.

Slight fatty degeneration of hepatocytes was observed in females and moderate to severe fatty degeneration was observed in males. Histopathology included slight swelling of centrilobular hepatocytes (males and females), slight eosinophilic changes of centrilobular hepatocytes (males and females), slight dilatation of the adrenal cortex (males), hypertrophy of the vaginal mucous epithelium, and slight to moderate mammary gland hyperplasia (females) with increased secretory activity. Increased cytochrome p450 content was observed in the liver at this dose and was higher in males than in females (p450s were not measured at 60 mg kg^{-1} day^{-1}). Proliferation of the smooth-surfaced endoplasmic reticulum was observed by electron microscopy in the liver but not the kidney. Increased lipid droplets were observed in the liver by electron microscopy in males and females. In an additional 26-week study in rats, at 0, 1, and 5 mg kg^{-1} day^{-1}, slight fatty degeneration of hepatocytes was observed. No other effects were observed in this study.

In a 52-week oral dose study in dogs, 20 mg kg^{-1} day^{-1} (about 12–19 times the expected clinical exposure via AUC) was a No Observed Adverse Effect Level (NoAEL). Although pharmacologic signs were observed at this dose (and at 5 mg kg^{-1} day^{-1}), their severity was decreased by week 3. Brown discoloration was observed in liver and kidney at all treated doses, and liver tissue stained slightly positive for neutral lipids. At 80 mg kg^{-1} day^{-1}

(about 51–118 times), pharmacologic signs were observed for the duration of the study (52 weeks), for several hours following administration. Decreased body weights/body weight gain and decreased hemoglobin were observed. Liver tissue stained positive (slight to moderate) for neutral lipids. No indication of tissue damage was observed, but an apparent increase in alkaline phosphatase was observed (without statistical significance).

In dogs and rats, liver hypertrophy is commonly seen due to a proliferation of cytochrome p450s and is usually not considered relevant to clinical use if no signal is observed in the clinic. Accumulation of lipid and discoloration of the liver was not accompanied by toxicity in dogs, but slight fatty degeneration of hepatocytes was observed in rats at all doses tested, including the control. No clearly drug-related hepatic effects were observed in clinical studies, but clinical monitoring of liver effects will continue into phase IV of development.

In a 13-week oral dose study in dogs, a NoAEL for delayed maturation of testes and epididymis and the absence of sperm was $10\,mg\,kg^{-1}\,day^{-1}$. At $50\,mg\,kg^{-1}\,day^{-1}$, these effects were observed in the 13-week study; however, they were not apparent at termination of the $80\,mg\,kg^{-1}\,day^{-1}$ group in the 52-week study. It may be speculated that differences between these studies reflect the different maturation levels of the dogs at the time of termination.

In a 2-week intravenous toxicity study of the major human glucuronidated metabolite, KMD127 (KMD-3213 glucuronide, KMD-3213G), it was found to be similar both in pharmacology and toxicology to the parent drug, silodosin. Pharmacology studies showed this metabolite to be slightly less active than the parent drug, and distribution studies in rats showed it to be distributed to tissue, including the prostate.

Neither silodosin nor its glucuronidated metabolite increased the number of revertant colonies at any dose tested, and both were judged to be not mutagenic in bacterial mutation assays.

Increases in mutant frequency were not observed at any dose of silodosin tested, and it was concluded that it was not genotoxic under the conditions tested in a mammalian cell mutation assay.

In Chinese hamster lung fibroblast cells, no increase in chromosomal aberrations were observed at any dose of silodosin tested by the 24- or 48-h direct method or by the 6-h treatment activation method in the presence of S9. However, in the 6-h treatment in the absence of S9, chromosomal aberrations were observed and confirmed in an additional assay. Although mitotic index was not measured in this study, an additional study was also performed, in which decreased mitotic index (toxicity) was found to be associated with chromosomal aberrations under similar conditions at similar concentrations. Chromosomal aberrations in cell culture at high, cyotoxic doses, are not expected to be relevant to clinical use.

The glucuronide metabolite of silodosin was found to be not mutagenic under the conditions of a chromosomal aberration assay in cultured Chinese hamster cells.

No increase in micronuclei was observed in mice at doses up to $1000\,mg\,kg^{-1}$ silodosin, and it was judged to be not genotoxic under the conditions of this assay.

In a rat liver DNA repair (UDS) test, silodosin did not cause any significant increases in either the gross nuclear grain count or the net nuclear grain count (i.e., the gross nuclear grain count minus the cytoplasmic grain count) at any dose level at either sampling time, and was therefore judged to be not genotoxic under the conditions of this assay.

In a carcinogenicity study by dietary administration of silodosin to CD-l mice for 104 weeks at doses up to $100\,mg\,kg^{-1}\,day^{-1}$ (about 19 times the exposure of the maximum recommended human dose or MHRE via AUC) in males and $400\,mg\,kg^{-1}\,day^{-1}$ in females (about 68 times the MRHE via AUC), there were no significant tumor findings in male mice. Female mice treated for 2 years with doses of $150\,mg\,kg^{-1}\,day^{-1}$ (about 29 times the MRHE via AUC) or greater had statistically significant increases in the incidence of mammary gland adenoacanthoma and adenocarcinomas, associated with hyperprolactinemia. Mice do not produce glucuronidated silodosin, which is present in human serum at approximate four times the level of circulating silodosin. In an additional carcinogenicity study by dietary administration to male CD-l mice for 104 weeks (replacement study for male mice killed in excessive numbers through fighting during the previous 2-year assay), the study was negative for drug-related neoplasms.

In a 2-year oral carcinogenicity study in rats administered doses up to 150 mg kg^{-1} day^{-1} (about 8 times the exposure of the maximum recommended human dose or MHRE via AUC of silodosin), an increase in thyroid follicular cell tumor incidence was seen in male rats, along with increased metabolism of and decreased circulating levels of thyroxine (T4). Although the incidence of follicular cell adenomas in female rats was increased, the incidence in dosed groups was not statistically significant. There was increased incidence and severity, although minimal to slight of thyroid follicular cell hypertrophy in the female rats, as well as in the male rats.

An embryo/fetal study in rabbits showed decreased maternal body weight at the high dose of 200 mg kg^{-1} day^{-1} (approximately 13–25 times the maximum recommended human exposure of parent drug via AUC). No evidence of teratogenicity was observed at this dose. Variations of lung location were observed at 20, 60, and 200 mg kg^{-1} day^{-1} and one fetus in each treated group ($<1\%$, not statistically significant) had a ventricular septal defect.

Embryo/fetal studies in rats showed no maternal or fetal effects at a high dose of 1000 mg kg^{-1} day^{-1}. In a combined male/female rat fertility study, at 60 mg kg^{-1} day^{-1} and above, prolongation or disappearance of the estrous cycle was observed in females. Decreased copulation index was observed at 200 mg kg^{-1} day^{-1} and above and decreased fertility index was observed at 20 mg kg^{-1} day^{-1} and above (all treated doses).

In a male rat fertility study, sperm viability and count were significantly lower in the 600 mg kg^{-1} day^{-1} (about 65 times the exposure of the maximum recommended human dose via AUC) group after one month. Histopathologic examination of infertile males revealed changes in the testes and epididymis in the 200 (about 30 times) and 600 mg kg^{-1} groups which were considered to be due to treatment with KMD-3213 (silodosin). The copulation and fertility indices indicated no significant differences between the treated groups and the control group. However, the fertility index was somewhat lower in the 600 mg kg^{-1} group. Implantation index observed at cesarean section was significantly lower in the 600 mg kg^{-1} group. The noobserved adverse effect level (NOAEL) of KMD-3213 (silodosin) for general toxicity was 200 mg kg^{-1} in male rats. The NOAEL of KMD-3213 (silodosin) for male reproductive function was 60 mg kg^{-1} and that for early embryonic development was 200 mg kg^{-1}. These effects are at relatively high multiples of the expected clinical exposures.

Treatment of male rats with silodosin for 15 days resulted in decreased fertility and implantation index at the high dose of 20 mg kg^{-1} day^{-1} (about twice the exposure of the maximum recommended human dose via AUC). Effects on fertility and implantation indices recovered after a 2 weeks recovery period. No effect was observed at 6 mg kg^{-1} day^{-1}. The high dose effects appear to be in an exposure range which may be relevant to clinical use, similar to effects reported for other drugs in this class.

In a female rat fertility study, no effect on fertility parameters was observed at the high dose of 20 mg kg^{-1} day^{-1} (about 1 to 4 times the exposure of the maximum recommended human dose via AUC). This dose did result in estrus cycle changes. No effect on the estrus cycle was observed at 6 mg kg^{-1} day^{-1}. Silodosin is not approved for use in women.

No effects on physical or behavioral development of offspring were observed when rats were treated during pregnancy and lactation at up to 300 mg kg^{-1} day^{-1}.

In an evaluation of silodosin *in vitro* for phototoxicity in Balb/c 3T3 fibroblasts using a neutral red assay, a small increase in phototoxicity over control (classified as a "probable" level of phototoxicity) was observed in the presence of silodosin. However, in a single dose oral phototoxicity study in hairless mice, only mild erythema was observed after 4 h simulated sunlight exposure at high silodosin exposure levels.

These toxicity studies revealed that KMD-3213 (silodosin) was expected to have little incidence of adverse events for clinical use.

14.7 CLINICAL TRIALS

Clinical trials are consisted of three phases. Phase I study is to evaluate the pharmacokinetics, pharamacodynamics, and safety of the drug in healthy adult human volunteers. Phase II studies are "proof of concept" and "dose-finding" studies, in which the drug is prescribed multiple dosages for the target populations. In case of silodosin, the target populations are patients with BPH. This study clarifies the optimal dosage of the drugs. In phase III study, the drug is evaluated for the efficacy and safety for the target populations, as compared to placebo and/or active comparator. Although silodosin is now approved in many countries, initial clinical trials were conducted in Japan. Those results are presented here. Although silodosin is now approved in many countries, initial clinical trials were conducted in Japan. Those results are presented here.

14.7.1 Phase I Studies

In the single rising dose studies, silodosin was administered orally to fasting healthy male adult subjects (aged 20–29 years; six subjects per group) at doses of 0.5, 1, 1.5, 2, 2.5, 4, 8, and 12 mg [44]. The plasma concentration of silodosin dose dependently increased, with the C_{max} and $AUC_{0-\infty}$ linearly increasing in parallel. In addition, the T_{max} was 0.9 to 2.3 h, with a $t_{1/2}$ of 3.0 to 6.5 h. The cumulative urinary excretion rate of silodosin up to 48 h after administration of either the conjugate or nonconjugate form was low, with no substantial difference among the doses.

In healthy male human volunteers given a single oral dose of 8 mg of ^{14}C-KMD-3213, KMD-3213G, and KMD-3293 were mainly detected in plasma, along with silodosin.

The effects of food were studied to determine the optimum use of the drug. A single 4 mg dose of silodosin was orally administered to 11 healthy male adult volunteers (aged 20–28 years) 30 min after breakfast or fasted (for more than 12 h before administration) using the open-label crossover method [44]. The T_{max} was shortened from 2.1 to 1.4 h after having a meal, and the $t_{1/2}$ was reduced from 6.0 to 4.7 h. On the other hand, the C_{max} was increased from 23.0 to 28.0 ng mL^{-1}, reaching 1.3-fold high geometric mean least square, but the 1.1-fold high geometric mean least square of AUC_{0-48}, suggesting that the AUC is less likely to be affected.

In a multiple fixed dose study of the drug, silodosin, 4 mg, was orally administered to 5 healthy male adult volunteers (aged 20–25 years) twice daily for 7 days (once daily 30 min after breakfast on days 1 and 7 and twice daily 30 min after breakfast and dinner on day 2 through 6) [40]. The plasma concentration of silodosin reached a steady state on day 3 of administration, where the cumulative rate from the initial administration (C_{max} at the steady state/C_{max} at the first administration after correction for accumulation) was 1.1, suggesting that accumulation will not be an issue chemically. On the other hand, the $t_{1/2}$ of silodosin after repeated administration was prolonged to about 10 h on day 7 from 6.9 h on day 1. Silodosin and its metabolites did not accumulate in urine until 192 h after administration, with the urinary accumulation rate on day 2 or 3 or later after administration being kept almost constant.

A study comparing the pharmacokinetics of silodosin in elderly subjects and young subjects was conducted. Silodosin, 4 mg, was orally administered once to 12 healthy male elderly subjects (aged 65–75 years) and nonelderly subjects (aged 21–31 years) 30 min after breakfast [44]. The $t_{1/2}$ in elderly subjects was slightly prolonged as compared to the nonelderly subjects, although no other pharmacokinetic parameters showed notable differences. The cumulative urinary excretion rate of silodosin showed no significant difference between the elderly and nonelderly subjects. The cumulative urinary excretion rate of primary metabolites (silodosin-glucuronic acid conjugate and KMD-3293) was slightly lower in the elderly subjects than in the nonelderly subjects, though notable difference was not obvious. In addition, the cumulative urinary excretion rate of KMD-3241, KMD-3295, and KMD-3289 was lower in the elderly subjects than in the nonelderly subjects, but excretion of these metabolites was far less as compared to silodosin and primary metabolites, suggesting that the effect of aging on urinary excretion of silodosin is small.

In a study to determine the effect of impaired renal function on the pharmacokinetics, silodosin, 4 mg, was orally administered to six fasted patients with impaired renal function [creatinine clearance (CCr) 27 to 49 mL min^{-1} (mean 39.2 mL min^{-1}), aged 53–72 years] and seven subjects with normal renal function [Ccr: 125–176 mL min^{-1} (mean 138.7 mL min^{-1}), aged 21–46 years] [44]. The plasma concentration of total drugs (protein-bound and nonbound drugs) was higher in the patients with impaired renal function than in the subjects with normal renal function, and the geometric mean least square of C_{max} and $AUC_{0–48}$ of silodosin was 3.1 and 3.2 times high in the patients with lowered renal function as compared to the subjects with normal renal function. In patients with impaired renal function, the plasma concentration of α_1-acid glycoprotein was higher as compared to the subjects with normal renal function, where the C_{max} and $AUC_{0–48}$ of plasma total drugs are highly positively correlated with the plasma concentration of α_1-acid glycoprotein. This suggests that silodosin was bound to α_1-acid glycoprotein in plasma, and the total drug concentration was increased as the plasma concentration of α_1-acid glycoprotein was increased. On the other hand, the plasma concentration of free, unbound silodosin and nonbound drugs in plasma that is likely to be involved in the efficacy and adverse drug reactions seemed to result in the geometric mean least square of C_{max} and $AUC_{0\text{-}\infty}$ that were 1.5 and 2.0 times higher, respectively, in the patients with lowered renal function as compared to the subjects with normal renal function, suggesting that they were less increased than the total drugs.

During the clinical trials, human metabolites of silodosin were monitored [44]. In the mass-balance study of healthy human volunteer, the $AUC_{0–12h}$ values of silodosin, KMD-3213G, and KMD-3293 after oral administration of ^{14}C-silodosin were 24.0%, 21.9%, and 34.9%, respectively, of total serum radioactivity ($AUC_{0–12h}$). The amounts of other metabolites were less than 5% in these studies. KMD-3293, KMD-3310, and KMD-3213G were identified in the urine within 48 h after administration of ^{14}C-silodosin. On the other hand, KMD-3293, KMD-3241, KMD-3295, and KMD-3289 (structures shown in Figure 14.10) were identified in the feces. As previously discussed, the estimated metabolic enzymes involved in the metabolisms of silodosin to KMD-3213G and KMD-3293 were UDP-GT (UGT2B7 as an isoform) and alcohol dehydrogenase/aldehyde dehydrogenase (ADH/ALDH). CYP3A4 was involved in the conversion of silodosin to other oxidative metabolites.

14.7.2 Phase III Randomized, Placebo-Controlled, Double-Blind Study [45]

Phase II study revealed that the clinically optimal dosage of silodosin was 4 mg twice daily. Then, Phase III randomized, double-blind, placebo controlled study was conducted at 88 centers in Japan.

The men included were $\geq$50 years old, outpatients, and had LUTS associated with BPH, the latter diagnosed based on a DRE or ultrasonographic findings. Inclusion criteria were a total IPSS of ≥8, an associated quality-of-life (QoL) score of ≥3, prostate volume (measured by transabdominal ultrasonography or TRUS) of ≥20 mL, a maximum urinary flow rate (Q_{max}) of <15 mL s^{-1} with a voided volume of ≥100 mL and a residual urine volume of < 100 mL. Patients were excluded if they had received antiandrogen therapy for 1 year before the study or had a prostatectomy, intrapelvic radiation therapy or prostatic hyperthermia (transurethral microwave hyperthermia or transurethral needle ablation). Patients who had prostate cancer or suspected prostate cancer, neurogenic bladder, bladder neck constriction, urethral stricture, bladder calculus, severe bladder diverticulum, active urinary tract infection requiring medical treatment, renal impairment (serum creatinine ≥2.0 mg dL^{-1}) and other complications considered likely to affect micturition, were excluded, as were those with severe hepatic and cardiovascular disease and a history of orthostatic hypotension.

After completing a 7-day "washout" and 7-day a single-blind placebo run-in period, patients were randomized to receive oral silodosin 4 mg twice daily, tamsulosin 0.2 mg day^{-1}, or placebo twice daily for 12 weeks. This study was performed as a double dummy design. Drugs were prescribed as follows: silodosin group (silodosin 4 mg twice a day, tamsulosin placebo twice a day); tamsulosin group (tamsulosin 0.2 mg once a day in the morning, tamsulosin placebo once a day, silodosin placebo twice a day), placebo group (silodosin placebo twice a day, tamsulosin placebo twice a day).

At the end of the washout period and at 1, 2, 4, 8, and 12 weeks during the treatment period subjective symptoms (IPSS and QOL scores) and medication compliance were recorded, and uroflowmetry and physical examinations (blood pressure and HR) conducted. Clinical laboratory tests were conducted at the start of the observation period and at 4 and 12 weeks of treatment. All adverse events were recorded and assessed for severity and causal relationship with taking the investigational product.

The primary endpoint of evaluation for efficacy was the change in the total IPSS from baseline; secondary endpoints were change in Q_{max}, and evaluation of subjective symptoms, for example, the IPSS voiding and storage scores and QOL score.

The results of primary endpoints are summarized here. In all, 457 patients were enrolled and randomized to receive silodosin (176), tamsulosin (192), or placebo (89). One patient in the silodosin group was excluded from the full analysis set due to protocol violation. There were no significant differences among the three groups in baseline characteristics, except for the QoL score. Therefore, an adjusted analysis by baseline QoL score was used for the primary endpoint.

The results of the primary outcome measure are shown in Figure 14.11: the change in total IPSS from baseline was -8.3 ± 6.4, -6.8 ± 5.7, and -5.3 ± 6.7 in the silodosin, tamsulosin, and placebo groups, respectively. As shown in Table 14.6, there were significantly greater decreases with silodosin than placebo from 1 week after starting treatment. In the early-stage comparison, silodosin elicited a significantly larger decrease in IPSS than did tamsulosin at 2 weeks. The mean (95% CI) intergroup differences in the total IPSS between silodosin and placebo, and between silodosin and tamsulosin, were −3.0 (−4.6, −1.3) and −1.4 (−2.7, −0.2), respectively, thus confirming that silodosin was better than placebo and not inferior to tamsulosin (both $P < 0.001$).

The results of the secondary outcome measures are also shown in Table 14.6. Silodosin was significantly better than placebo in QoL score ($P < 0.002$). Silodosin also showed significant improvements in voiding symptoms (symptoms attributable to urethral obstruction such as slow stream, straining, intermittency, and feeling of incomplete voiding) and storage symptoms (daytime frequency, urinary urgency, and nocturia) over placebo. In addition to significant effects in patients with moderate symptoms (IPSS 8–19), silodosin also showed significant improvements in total IPSS over placebo in patients with severe

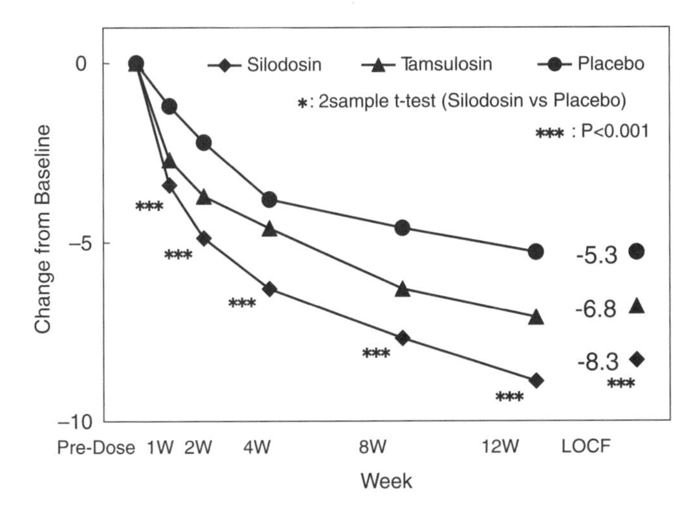

Figure 14.11 Time course of change in IPSS total score in Phase III randomized, placebo-controlled, double-blind study. [This figure was cited from reference No. 45 with permission.]

symptoms (IPSS ≥ 20). It is known that maximum flow rate (Q_{max}) depends on the voided volume at measurement. Therefore, the change in Q_{max} was compared among the three treatment groups in the overall subgroup of patients with a change in voided volume of <50% before and after treatment. In this *post hoc* investigation, the change in Q_{max} from baseline in the silodosin group was significantly ($P = 0.005$) better than placebo.

For adverse events, the incidence rates of adverse events were 88.6%, 82.3%, and 71.6% in the silodosin, tamsulosin, and placebo groups, respectively. Inter group comparisons showed that adverse events were significantly ($P < 0.001$) more frequent in the silodosin than in the placebo group. Adverse events are summarized in Table 14.7. The incidence rates of drug-related adverse events were 69.7%, 47.4%, and 36.4% in the three groups, respectively, showing a significantly ($P < 0.001$) higher frequency of adverse events in the silodosin than in the placebo and tamsulosin groups. Adverse events resulting in withdrawal occurred in 18 (10.2%), 11 (5.7%), and 4 (4.5%) patients in the silodosin, tamsulosin and placebo groups, respectively. All of these adverse events resolved after discontinuing treatment. The most common adverse event in the silodosin group was abnormal ejaculation. However, only five men (2.9%) discontinued treatment due to abnormal ejaculation. There were no clinically significant differences of systolic/diastolic blood pressure or HR between the silodosin and tamsulosin groups. In addition, incidence of side effects relating to hypotension (such as dizziness) by silodosin was similar to tamsulosin and placebo.

14.7.3 Long-Term Administration Study [46]

The efficacy and safety of long-term administration of silodosin in patients with LUTS associated with BPH were investigated in a 52-week open-label oral administration study in 361 outpatients aged 50 years or older (mean age of 67.3 ± 6.7 years: safety was assessed in an initial 364 patients from whom 3 patients were later excluded) with a total IPSS score of 8 or higher, QOL score of 3 or higher, prostate volume of 20 mL or more, voiding volume of 100 mL or more, and Q_{max} of 15 mL s^{-1} or less at this time point. Silodosin, 4 mg, (reduced to 2 mg when an adverse event occurred) was administered twice daily after breakfast and dinner. This study was not an open-label extension of the pivotal phase III study, but a stand-alone open label study.

The study results[1] showed that the total IPSS score was 18.4 ± 6.3 at baseline, 13.1 ± 6.3 at week 4, 10.6 ± 6.0 at week 12, 9.4 ± 6.1 at week 28, and 8.2 ± 5.7 at week 52,

TABLE 14.6 Change in Efficacy Measures from Baseline[a]

Variable	Silodosin	Tamsulosin	Placebo	P^c	P^d
N	175	192	89		
Total IPSS at LOCF[b]	−8.3 ± 6.4	−6.8 ± 5.7	−5.3 ± 6.7	<0.001[&]	
Total IPSS at week 1	−3.4 ± 4.2	−2.7 ± 4.1	−1.2 ± 3.4	<0.001	0.110
Total IPSS at week 2	−4.9 ± 4.9	−3.7 ± 4.4	−2.2 ± 4.1	<0.001	0.011
IPSS voiding symptoms	−5.8 ± 4.6	−4.8 ± 4.1	−3.8 ± 4.8	<0.001	0.023
IPSS storage symptoms	−2.5 ± 2.9	−2.1 ± 2.6	−1.5 ± 2.6	<0.006	0.106
Patients with ≥25% improvement in IPSS	133/174 (76.4%)	126/192 (65.6%)	45/89 (50.6%)	<0.001	0.028
IPSS in severe (IPSS ≥ 20) patients	−12.4 ± 7.3	−10.1 ± 6.1	−8.7 ± 8.4	0.044	0.063
IPSS in moderate (8–19) patients	−6.3 ± 4.9	−5.3 ± 4.9	−3.8 ± 5.3	0.001	0.105
QoL score	−1.7 ± 1.4	−1.4 ± 1.3	−1.1 ± 1.2	0.002	0.052
Q_{max}[e]	1.70 ± 3.31	2.60 ± 3.98	0.26 ± 2.21	0.005	0.063

[a]Data given as mean ± SD or *n*/*N* (%). [This table was cited from reference No. 45 with permission.]

[b]LOCF, last observation carried forward.

[c]Silodosin versus placebo.

[d]Silodosin versus tamsulosin.

[e]Values from subgroup analysis of patients with a change of voided volume from baseline of <50%.

TABLE 14.7 Lists of Adverse Events (cited from ref. No. 45 with permission)

	Clinical symptoms, *n* (%)		
	Silodosin (175)	Tamsulosin (192)	Placebo (89)
Abnormal ejaculation	39 (22.3)	3 (1.6)	0
Upper respiratory tract infection	33 (18.9)	53 (27.6)	17 (19.1)
Thirst	18 (10.3)	7 (3.6)	4 (4.5)
Loose stool	16 (9.1)	7 (3.6)	5 (5.6)
Diarrhea	12 (6.9)	13 (6.8)	5 (5.6)
Urinary incontinence	11 (6.3)	11 (5.7)	0
Dizziness	9 (5.1)	14 (7.3)	4 (4.5)
	Laboratory test values, *n/N* (%)		
	Silodosin	Tamsulosin	Placebo
Elevated triglyceride	44/175 (25.1)	42/192 (21.9)	18/88 (20.5)
Elevated C-reactive protein	22/175 (12.6)	32/192 (16.7)	13/88 (14.8)
Elevated γ-GTP	13/175 (7.4)	7/192 (3.6)	6/88 (6.8)
Urinary sediment abnormality	12/173 (6.9)	13/192 (6.8)	7/87 (8.0)
Elevated total cholesterol	9/175 (5.1)	6/192 (3.1)	2/88 (2.3)
Glycosuria	9/175 (5.1)	16/192 (8.3)	6/88 (6.8)

demonstrating a benefit for 52 weeks beginning at week 4. Of IPSS subscores, the score for voiding symptoms was 10.9 ± 4.5 at baseline, 7.5 ± 4.5 at week 4, and 4.4 ± 3.9 at week 52, and for storage symptoms, 7.5 ± 3.2 at baseline, 5.6 ± 2.9 at week 4, and 3.8 ± 2.4 at week 52, demonstrating sustained improvement from as early as week 4 ($P = 0.000$). Additionally, the IPSS subscores for residual sensation, intermittency of urination, urinary stream, straining urination, pollakisuria, urinary urgency, and nocturia similarly lasted for 52 weeks from as early as week 4 ($P = 0.000$).

The improvement in the total I-PSS score by severity showed that 214 moderate cases (60.5%) and 140 severe cases (39.5%) at baseline were changed to 165 mild cases (46.6%), 156 moderate cases (44.1%), and 33 severe cases (9.3%) at completion of administration (or study discontinuation). The final disposition of patients in whom symptoms were moderate at baseline was in 112 mild patients (52.3%), 98 moderate patients (45.8%), and 4 severe patients (1.9%) at completion of administration (or study discontinuation), and in patients in whom the symptom severity was severe, 53 patients (37.9%) were mild, 58 patients (41.4%) were moderate, and 29 patients (20.7%) were severe at completion of administration.

In patients in whom the dose was not reduced or reduced to 2 mg b.i.d, the variation of total IPPS scores from baseline at week 4, 12, 28, and 52 was -5.3 ± 5.2, -8.0 ± 6.1, -9.2 ± 6.8, and -10.2 ± 6.8 in the patients whose dose was not reduced, and -5.3 ± 5.1, -5.8 ± 4.6, -7.3 ± 6.1, and -8.9 ± 6.7 in the dose-reduced patients, respectively, showing improvement at all assessment time points in both of the patients population ($P = 0.000$). The score change in the patient group whose dose was reduced to 4 mg day^{-1} was slightly inferior to the patient group in which the dose of 8 mg day^{-1} was not reduced, although the improved efficacy lasted for 52 weeks from as early as week 4 ($P = 0.000$).

The QOL score of all patients administrated silodosin was 4.8 ± 0.9 at baseline, and 3.7 ± 1.3 at week 4, 3.3 ± 1.3 at week 12, 3.0 ± 1.4 at week 28, and 2.7 ± 1.3 at week 52, also showing that the improvement of QOL lasted for 52 weeks from as early as week 4 ($P = 0.000$).

The Q_{max} was $9.51 \pm 3.09\,mL\,s^{-1}$ at baseline, $11.35 \pm 4.68\,mL\,s^{-1}$ at week 4, $10.57 \pm 4.68\,mL\,s^{-1}$ at week 12, $11.07 \pm 4.69\,mL\,s^{-1}$ at week 28, and $12.36 \pm 5.74\,mL\,s^{-1}$ at week 52, also showing that the improving efficacy lasted for 52 weeks from as early as week 4. In addition, the residual urine volume was 44.5 ± 61.1 mL at baseline and 30.2 ± 39.2 mL at week 52, showing improvement ($P = 0.000$).

The overall efficacy (excluding "Unevaluable" cases) defined as "Effective" or better was 40.0% (92/230 patients) at week 52 and as "Slightly effective" or better was 82.2% (189/230 patients).

The percent of adverse drug reactions was 65.4% (238/364 patients). Adverse drug reactions whose incidence was 5% or higher included ejaculation disorder (25.0%: 91/364 patients), diarrhea (7.4%: 27/364 patients), thirst (7.1%: 26/364 patients), dizziness on standing up (6.6%: 24/364 patients), nasal congestion (5.8%: 21/364 patients), and light-headed feeling (5.2%: 19/364 patients). On the other hand, the incidence of abnormal clinical laboratory test values was 31.1% (112/360 patients), and the abnormality whose incidence was 5% or higher was increased TG (9.2%: 33/359 patients).

The cumulative incidences of adverse drug reactions extrapolated by the Kaplan--Meier method were 61.0% and 67.7% at week 28 and 52, respectively, indicating that more adverse drug reactions developed earlier, although delayed type adverse drug reactions to be noted were not observed.

The percent of patients who discontinued treatment because of adverse drug reactions and abnormal clinical laboratory values was 12.1% (44/364 patients) and 0.6% (2/360 patients), respectively. Adverse drug reactions which led to study discontinuation in three patients or more included ejaculation disorder in 15 patients, diarrhea in four patients, and light-headed feeling in three patients, etc. The percent of patients whose dose was reduced to $4\,mg\,day^{-1}$ because of adverse drug reactions was 11.8% (43/364 patients), and dose reduction due to abnormal clinical laboratory test values occurred in 0.3% of patients (1/360 patients). Of these adverse drug reactions, ejaculation disorder disappeared in 3 of 17 patients, dizziness on standing up in 8 of 10 patients, thirst in four of six patients, light-headed feeling in four of six patients, and nasal congestion in two of five patients during the administration period. Of 91 patients who had ejaculation disorder, five could not be evaluated for resolution of the symptom due to lack of sexual activity and in two patients who underwent transurethral prostatectomy (TURP) after completion of the administration, but was confirmed in 73 patients after completion of administration and in 11 patients during administration.

Cardiovascular vital signs were recorded for any evidence of a CV effect. The systolic blood pressure (SBP) was 137.5 ± 18.1 mmHg at baseline, 134.7 ± 17.9 mmHg at week 28, and 134.6 ± 18.8 mmHg at week 52, and the diastolic blood pressure (DBP) was 80.1 ± 11.8 mmHg at baseline, 78.4 ± 12.0 mmHg at week 28, and 78.9 ± 12.1 mmHg at week 52; the pulse rate was 72.3 ± 11.4 beats/min at baseline, 72.8 ± 11.8 beats/min at week 28, and $74.3 \pm 12.3\,beats\,min^{-1}$ at week 52, showing only a little change in measurement, and not posing clinical concerns.

These study results demonstrated that silodosin improved urinary function and symptoms in the LUT associated with BPH starting soon after the first administration, without developing delayed adverse drug reactions or loss of efficacy, and confirmed that the efficacy is sustained over the course of the study.

14.8 SUMMARY: KEY LESSONS LEARNED

Pharmacologic therapy is the first-line therapy for BPH. α_1-AR antagonists are believed to improve the symptoms of BPH by relaxing the prostatic and bladder neck smooth muscle which reduces the degree of bladder outlet obstruction. There are currently three identified α_1-AR subtypes (α_{1A}, α_{1b}, and α_{1d}). All three subtypes exist in a wide range of human tissues, including the systemic vasculature, the prostatic smooth muscle and bladder neck. Primary subtype of prostate and urethra was α_{1A}-AR subtype. Thus, the α_{1A}-AR subtype is believed to play a primary role in mediating prostatic smooth muscle contraction. While, dominant subtype of blood vessels is α_{1B}-AR subtype.

The most significant safety concern with the selective α_1-AR antagonists is the occurrence of "vasodilatory" symptoms, such as dizziness, orthostatic hypotension, and syncope that result from nonselective alpha1 antagonists' activity on α_1-AR in the systemic vasculature. Theoretically, drugs that are pharmacologically "uroselective"—binding α_{1A}-AR subtype preferentially over α_{1B} or α_{1D}-ARs will have fewer vasodilatory effects.

Under these backgrounds, development of a α_{1A}-AR selective antagonist was started. Focusing on α_1-AR antagonists with the conventional quinazoline and phenylpiperazine motifs with low selectivity to α_{1A}-AR, amide group and trifluroethoxy group were introduced into their indoline structure to optimize the structure to increase the α_{1A}-AR blocking action and organ selectivity. Compounds were then assessed for their pharmacokinetics, to develop a drug product characterized by high intestinal absorption, long-lasting action, and less CNS penetration after oral administration. The eventual product was silodosin.

Nonclinical studies using silodosin included *in vitro* receptor binding studies, pharmacology and safety pharmacology studies, acute, subacute and chronic toxicology studies in rats and dogs, *in vitro* and *in vivo* genotoxicity assays, carcinogenicity bioassays in rodents, and reproductive and developmental toxicity in rats and rabbits. These studies showed that silodosin has higher affinity and superior selectivity for the α_{1A}-AR, higher selectivity of prostate and urethral smooth muscles, and demonstrated the safety profiles. Additionally, nonclinical pharmacokinetic studies of silodosin predicted the appropriation for its clinical use.

As a result, clinical studies showed that silodosin has useful for improving symptoms of BPH patients, and has good safety profiles. The importance and usefullness of α_{1A}-AR selectivity has been demonstrated.

After these developmental processes, silodosin is now using worldwide.

REFERENCES

1. AUA Practice Guidelines Committee. AUA guideline on management of benign prostatic hyperplasia (2003). Diagnosis and treatment recommendations. *J. Urol.* **2003**, *170*, 530–547.
2. Wasserman, N. F. Benign prostatic hyperplasia: a review and ultrasound classification. *Radiol. Clin. North Am.* **2006**, *44*, 689–710.
3. Thorpe, A. and Neal, D. Benign prostatic hyperplasia [published correction appears in Lancet. 2003;362: 496]. *Lancet* **2003**, *361*, 1359–1367.
4. Roehrborn, C. G. and McConnell, J. D. Benign prostatic hyperplasia: etiology, pathophysiology, epidemiology, and natural history. in *Campbell-Walsh Urology* (Wein, A. J., Kavoussi, L. R., Novick, A. C., Partin, A. W., Petes, C. A.), 9th ed. WB Saunders, Philadelphia, PA, **2007**, p 2727–2765.
5. Emberton, M., Cornel, E. B., Bassi, P. F., Fourcade R. O., Gomez, J. M. F., Castro, R. Benign prostatic hyperplasia as a progressive disease: a guide to the risk factors and options for medical management. *Int. J. Clin. Pract.* **2008**, *62*, 1076–1086.
6. Fine, S. R. and Ginsberg, P. Alpha-adrenergic receptor antagonists in older patients with benign prostatic hyperplasia: issues and potential complications. *J. Am. Osteopath. Assoc.* **2008**, *108*, 333–337.
7. Beduschi, M. C., Beduschi, R., and Oesterling, J. E. Alpha-blockade therapy for benign prostatic hyperplasia: from a nonselective to a more selective alpha1A-adrenergic antagonist. *Urology* **1998**, *51*, 861–872.
8. O'Leary, M. P. Lower urinary tract symptoms/benign prostatic hyperplasia: maintaining symptom control and reducing complications. *Urology*, **2003**, *62*(Suppl 1), 15–23.
9. Edwards, J. L. Diagnosis and management of benign prostatic hyperplasia. *Am. Fam. Physician* **2008**, *77*, 1403–1410.

10. Schwinn, D. A. and Roehrborn, C. G. Alpha1-adrenoceptor subtypes and lower urinary tract symptoms. *Int. J. Urol.* **2008**, *15*, 193–199.
11. Hieble, J. P., Bylund, D. B., Clarke, D. E., Eikenburg, D. C., Langer, S. Z., Lefkowitz, R. J., Minneman, K. P., and Ruffolo, Jr. R. R. International union of pharmacology. X. recommendation for nomenclature of alpha 1-adrenoceptors: consensus update. *Pharmacol. Rev.* **1995**, *47*, 267–270.
12. Hawrylyshyn, K. A., Michelotti, G. A., Coge, F., Guéninb, S-P., and Schwinn, D. A. Update on human alpha1-adrenoceptor subtype signaling and genomic organization. *Trends Pharmacol. Sci.* **2004**, *25*, 449–455.
13. Richardson, C. D., Donatucci, C. F., Page, S. O., Wilson, K. H., and Schwinn, D. A. Pharmacology of tamsulosin: saturation-binding isotherms and competition analysis using cloned alpha 1-adrenergic receptor subtypes. *Prostate.* **1997**, *33*, 55–59.
14. Schwinn, D. A., Johnston, G. I., Page, S. O. Mosley, M. J. , Wilson, K. H., Worman, N. P., Campbell, S., Fidock, M. D., Furness, L. M., and Parry-Smith, D. J. Cloning and pharmacological characterization of human alpha-1 adrenergic receptors: sequence corrections and direct comparison with other species homologues. *J. Pharmacol. Exp. Ther.* **1995**, *272*, 134–142.
15. Price, D. T., Lefkowitz, R. J., Caron, M. G., Berkowitz, D., and Schwinn, D. A. Localization of mRNA for three distinct alpha 1-adrenergic receptor subtypes in human tissues: implications for human alpha-adrenergic physiology. *Mol. Pharmacol.* **1994**, *45*, 171–175.
16. Price, D. T., Schwinn, D. A., Lomasney, J. W., Allen, L. F., Caron, M. G., and Lefkowitz, R. J. Identification, quantification, and localization of mRNAfor three distinct alpha 1 adrenergic receptor subtypes in human prostate. *J. Urol.* **1993**, *150*, 546–551.
17. Andersson, K. E., Lepor, H., and Wyllie, M. G. Prostatic alpha 1-adrenoceptors and uroselectivity. *Prostate.* **1997**, *30*, 202–215.
18. Smith, M. S., Schambra, U. B., Wilson, K. H., Page, S. O., and Schwinn, D. A. Alpha1-adrenergic receptors in human spinal cord: specific localized expression of mRNA encoding alpha1-adrenergic receptor subtypes at four distinct levels. *Brain Res. Mol. Brain Res.* **1999**, *63*, 254–261.
19. Malloy, B. J., Price, D. T., Price, R. R. Bienstock, A. M., Dole, M. K., Funk, B. L., Rudner, X. L., Richardson, C. D., Donatucci, C. F., and Schwinn, D. A. Alpha1-adrenergic receptor subtypes in human detrusor. *J. Urol.* **1998**, *160*, 937–943.
20. Ishizuka, O., Persson, K., Mattiasson, A., Naylor, A., Wyllie, M., and Andersson, K. Micturition in conscious rats with and without bladder outlet obstruction: role of spinal alpha 1-adrenoceptors. *Br. J. Pharmacol.* **1996**, *117*, 962–966.
21. Bouchelouche, K., Andersen, L., Alvarez, S., Nordling, J., and Bouchelouche, P. Increased contractile response to phenylephrine in detrusor of patients with bladder outlet obstruction: effect of the alpha1A and alpha1D adrenergic receptor antagonist tamsulosin. *J. Urol.* **2005**, *173*, 657–661.
22. Rudner, X. L., Berkowitz, D. E., Booth, J. V., Funk, B. L., Cozart, K. L., D'Amico, E. B., El-Moalem, H., Page, S. O., Richardson, C. D., Winters, B., Marucci, L., and Schwinn, D. A. Subtype specific regulation of human vascular α_1-adrenergic receptors by vessel bed and age. *Circulation.* **1999**, *100*, 2336–2343.
23. Souverein, P. C., Van Staa, T. P., Egberts, A. C. G., De la Rosette, J. J. M. H., Cooper, C., and Leufkens, H. G. M. C. Use of α-blockers and the risk of hip/femur fractures. *J. Int. Med.* **2003**, *254*, 548–554.
24. Shibata, K., Foglar, R., Horie, K., Obika, K., Sakamoto, A., Ogawa, S., and Tsujimoto, G. KMD-3213, a novel, potent, α_{1A}-adrenoceptor-selective antagonist: characterization using recombinant human α_1-adrenoceptors and native tissues. *Mol. Pharmacol.* **1955**, *48*, 250–258.
25. Yamazaki, Y. Development of silodosin. *Yakugaku Zasshi.* **2006**, *126*, 207–208.
26. Kitazawa, M., Ban, M., Okazaki, K., Ozawa, M., Yazaki, T., and Yamagishi, R. 1,5,7-Trisubstituted indoline compounds and salts thereof. U. S. Patent 5387603, **1995**.
27. Sorbera, L. A., Silvestre, J., and Castaner, J. GR-205171. *Drugs Future* **1999**, *24*, 254–260.
28. Zhu, J., Taniguchi, T., Takauji, R., Suzuki, F., Tanaka, T., and Muramatsu, I. Inverse agonism and neutral antagonism at a constitutively active alpha-1a adrenoceptor. *Br. J. Pharmacol.* **2000**, *131*, 546–552.
29. Muramatsu, I., Suzuki, F., Tanaka, T., Yamamoto, H., and Morishima, S. Alpha1-adrenoceptor subtypes and alpha1-adrenoceptor antagonists, *Yakugaku Zasshi* **2006**, *126*, 187–198.
30. Zhang, L., Taniguchi, T., Tanaka, T., Shinozuka, K., Kunitomo, M., Nishiyama, M., Kamata, K., and Muramatsu, I. Alpha-1 adrenoceptor up-regulation induced by prazosin but not KMD-3213 or reserpine in rats. *Br. J. Pharmacol.* **2002**, *135*, 1757–1764.
31. Tatemichi, S., Kobayashi, K., Maezawa, M., Kobayashi, M., Yamazaki, Y., and Shibata, N. α_1-Adrenoceptor subtype selectivity and organ specificity of Silodosin (KMD-3213). *Yakugaku Zasshi* **2006**, *126*, 209–216.
32. Ishiguro, M., Futabayashi, Y., Ohnuki, T., Ahmed, M., Muramatsu, I., and Nagatomo, T. Identification of binding site of prazosin, tamsulosin, and KMD-3213 with α_1-adreneergic receptor subtypes by molecular modeling. *Life Sci.* **2002**, *71*, 2531–2541.
33. Muramatsu, I., Ohmura, T., Kigoshi, S., Hashimoto, S., and Oshita, M. Pharmacological subclassification of alpha 1-adrenoceptors in vascular smooth muscle. *Br. J. Pharmacol.* **1990**, *99*, 197–201.
34. Murata, S., Taniguchi, T., Takahashi, M., Okada, K., Akiyama, K., and Muramatsu, I. Tissue selectivity of KMD-3213, an α_1-adrenoceptor antagonist, in human prostate and vasculature. *J. Urol.* **2000**, *164*, 578–583.
35. Morishima, S., Tanaka, T., Yamamoto, H., Suzuki, F., Akino, H., Yokoyama, O., and Muramatsu, I.

Identification of alpha-1L and alpha-1A adreno-ceptors in human prostate by tissue segment binding. *J. Urol.* **2007**, *177*, 377–381.

36. PRICE, D. T., SCHWINN, D. A., LOMASNEY, J. W., ALLEN, L. F., CARON, M. G., and LEFKOWITZ, R. J. Identification, quantification, and localization of mRNA for three distinct alpha 1 adrenergic receptor subtypes in human prostate. *J. Urol.* **1993**, *150*, 546–551.
37. NASU, K., MORIYAMA, N., FUKASAWA, R., TSUJIMOTO, G., TANAKA, T., YANO, J., and KAWABE, K. Quantification and distribution of α_1-adrenoceptor subtype mRNAs in human proximal urethra. *Br. J. Pharmacol.* **1998**, *123*, 1289–1293.
38. WALDEN, P. D., DURKIN, M. M., LEPOR, H., WETZEL, J. M., GLUCHOWSKI, C., and GUSTAFSON, E. L. Localization of mRNA and receptor binding sites for the α_{1a}-adrenoceptor subtype in the rat, monkey and human urinary bladder and prostate. *J. Urol.* **1997**, *157*, 1032–1038.
39. YAMAGISHI, R., AKIYAMA, K., NAKAMURA, S., HORA, M., MASUDA, N., MATSUZAWA, A., MURATA, S., UJIIE, A., KURASHINA, Y., IIZUKA, K., and KITAZAWA, M. Effect of KMD-3213, an α_{1a}-adrenoceptor-selective antagonist, on the contractions of rabbit prostate and rabbit and rat aorta. *Eur. J. Pharmacol.* **1996**, *315*, 73–79.
40. TATEMICHI, S., KOBAYASHI, K., MARUYAMA, I., KOBAYASHI, M., YAMAZAKI, Y., and SHIBATA, N. Effects of silodosin (KMD-3213) on phenylephrine-induced increase in intraurethral pressure and blood pressure in rats—study of the selectivity for lower urinary tract. *Yakugaku Zasshi* **2006**, *126*, 217–223.
41. AKIYAMA, K., HORA, M., TATEMICHI, S., MASUDA, N., NAKAMURA, S., YAMAGISHI, R., and KITAZAWA, M. KMD-3213, a uroselective and long-acting α_{1a}-adrenoceptor antagonist, tested in a novel rat model. *J. Pharmacol. Exp. Ther.* **1999**, *291*, 81–91.
42. TOMIYAMA, Y., TATEMICHI, S., TADACHI, M., KOBAYASHI, S., HAYASHI, M., KOBAYASHI, M., YAMAZAKI, Y., and SHIBATA, N. Effect of silodosin on intraurethral pressure increase induced by hypogastric nerve stimulation in dogs with benign prostatic hyperplasia. *Yakugaku Zasshi* **2006**, *126*, 225–230.
43. United State Food and Drug Administration (FDA)/ Center for Drug Evaluation and Research, Drug Approval Package, RAPAFLO (Silodosin) Capsules, Application No. 022206, *Pharmacology Review(s), U.S. FDA Website.* Available at: http://www.accessdata.fda.gov/drugsatfda_docs/nda/2008/022206s000TOC.cfm Accessed November 1, 2010.
44. SHIMIZU, T., MIYASHITAL, I., MATSUBARA, Y., IKEDA, M., and YAMAGUCHI, M. Pharmacokinetic profile of silodosin in clinical practice. *Yakugaku Zasshi* **2006**, *126*, 257–263.
45. KAWABE, K., YOSHIDA, M., and HOMMA, Y. Silodosin, a new α_{1A}-adrenoceptorselective antagonist for treating benign prostatic hyperplasia: results of a phase III randomized, placebo-controlled, double-blind study in Japanese men. *B. J. U Int.* **2006**, *98*, 1019–1024.
46. KAWABE, K., YOSHIDA, M., ARAKAWA, S., and TAKEUCHI, H. For silodosin clinical study group: long-term evaluation of silodosin, a new α_{1A}-adrenoceptor selective antagonist for the treatment of benign prostatic hyperplasia: phase III long-term study. *Jpn. Urol. Surg.* **2006**, *19*, 153–164.

CHAPTER 15

RALOXIFENE: A SELECTIVE ESTROGEN RECEPTOR MODULATOR (SERM)

Jeffrey A. Dodge and Henry U. Bryant

15.1 INTRODUCTION: SERMs

Research in the estrogen receptor (ER) field has attracted considerable attention over the last 15 years with significant events ranging from very basic discoveries such as resolution of the liganded ER crystal structure and identification of a second ER form (ER-β), to important clinical observations regarding estrogen use in postmenopausal women from studies such as the Women's Health Initiative or WHI trial. Estrogen exhibits a true "Jekyl and Hyde" therapeutic profile, as hormone replacement (estrogen + progestin) is associated with distinct benefits on the menopausal syndrome, including reductions in vasomotor symptoms and fracture incidence, as well as other benefits such as a reduction in colon cancer. However, these benefits are offset by significant increases in risk for coronary events (myocardial infarction and stroke) and breast and uterine cancer. In the early 1990s, research around the concept of selective estrogen receptor modulators, or SERMs—molecules that simultaneously agonized and antagonized estrogen action in different tissue types, offered a new way of looking at ER pharmacology and triggered renewed interest in estrogen research in the mid-1990s. While today there are several molecules with a SERM profile widely available for clinical use (Table 15.1), only one—raloxifene—has been globally approved and attained widespread use for prevention and treatment of postmenopausal osteoporosis, despite the fact that a number of pharmaceutical companies have invested heavily in the development of SERMs for use in various postmenopausal disorders. A listing of those SERMs which at least entered clinical evaluation for use in postmenopausal women and their outcome is shown in Table 15.2. While raloxifene was the first SERM specifically targeted for postmenopausal women and has been a highly successful molecule, one is struck by the high failure rate of other attempts at development of SERMs for postmenopausal-associated pathology. This chapter will focus on the unique properties of raloxifene that allowed the molecule to succeed where so many others have failed.

Prior to the development of the "SERM-concept," ER ligands were generally thought of as falling into either the category of full agonists, partial agonists or full antagonists across all tissue types (i.e., uterus, mammary, and bone). For example, steroidal hormones such as 17-β-estradiol were known to behave as full agonists both *in vitro* and *in vivo* across multiple tissue types while compounds such as fulvestrant (ICI-182,780) were known to be complete ER antagonists that bound tightly to the ER, but lacked intrinsic activity and therefore, completely blocked the action of full ER agonists like 17-β-estradiol. These "pharmacotypes" are depicted in Figure 15.1A and B, respectively. Conversely, compounds

Case Studies in Modern Drug Discovery and Development, Edited by Xianhai Huang and Robert G. Aslanian.

TABLE 15.1 SERMs (Scheme 15.1) Currently Approved for Human Use

SERM	Trade name	Approved indications	Daily dose
Clomiphene	Clomid®	• Induction of ovulation	50–100 mg
Raloxifene	Evista®	• Treatment and prevention of osteoporosis in postmenopausal women with osteoporosis. • Reduction in risk of invasive breast cancer in postmenopausal women with osteoporosis. • Reduction of invasive breast cancer in postmenopausal women at high risk for invasive breast cancer.	60 mg
Tamoxifen	Nolvadex®	• Metastatic breast cancer treatment • Adjuvant breast cancer treatment • Ductal carcinoma *in situ* • Breast cancer risk reduction in high risk women	20–40 mg
Toremifene[a]	Fareston®	• Metastatic breast cancer treatment	60 mg

[a]Toremifene (Fareston®) is currently not approved in the United States, but is approved for metastatic breast cancer treatment in Europe.

such as tamoxifen were known to, in the presence of estrogen, block estrogen action in estrogen-responsive tissues (i.e., breast cancer cells) but, in the absence of estrogen, mimic estrogen in bone and uterus in estrogen deficient animals and women, thus exhibiting a classical partial agonist profile (Figure 15.1C). While this profile held some attractive features for use in ER-dependent breast cancer, the profile was prohibitive for chronic use in postmenopausal women for noncancer indications (like osteoporosis) where even the potentially less robust uterine stimulation induced by tamoxifen's partial agonist action produced untenable side effects that created a risk/benefit ratio that was unfavorable for use in diseases like osteoporosis [1]. As a result, prior to the initial reports of the raloxifene SERM profile in animals [2] and humans [3], virtually no work was being done in the

TABLE 15.2 SERMs Entering Clinical Development for Postmenopausal Indications (Scheme 15.1)

SERM	Scaffold	Indication(s)	Outcome/Status
Raloxifene	Benzothiophene	Osteoporosis, breast cancer risk reduction	Approved globally for both indications
Droloxifene	Triphenylethylene	Osteoporosis	Terminated phase 3 (uterine stimulation)
Idoxifene	Triphenylethylene	Osteoporosis	Terminated phase 3 (uterine stimulation)
Levormeloxifene	Benzopyran	Osteoporosis	Terminated phase 3 (uterine stimulation)
Lasofoxifene	Triphenylmethane	Osteoporosis	Approved for osteoporosis in EU, under regulatory review in other geographies
Basedoxifene $(+/-E_2)$	Indole	Osteoporosis vasomotor symptoms	Under regulatory review
Arzoxifene	Benzothiophene	Osteoporosis breast cancer risk reduction	Terminated phase 3 (lack of nonvertebral fracture efficacy)
RAD1901	Triphenylethylene	Vasomotor symptoms	Currently in phase 2 development

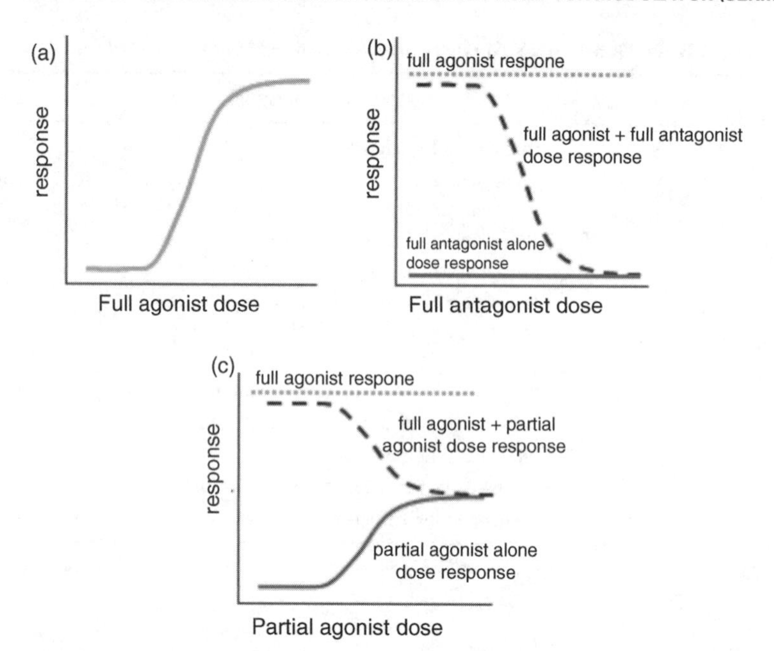

Figure 15.1 Potential pharmacotypes resulting from various ER-ligand interactions in the form of hypothetical dose response curves for a full agonist (panel A), a full antagonist (panel B) and a partial agonist (panel C).

pharmaceutical industry developing novel ER-ligands for osteoporosis, as the prevailing medical opinion at the time was that any molecule with sufficient estrogen agonism capable of producing a benefit in bone would also generate sufficient agonism (even if a partial agonist) in uterine tissue to create a risk that would unfavorably offset the bone benefit [4].

15.2 THE BENZOTHIOPHENE SCAFFOLD: A NEW CLASS OF SERMs

Many of the well-documented issues that are associated with the undesirable agonist properties of tamoxifen and analogs were addressed with a discovery of a new structural class of SERMs known as benzothiophenes (Scheme 15.2). This scaffold provided an improved side-effect profile in terms of estrogen antagonism on uterine tissue in rodents [5] and demonstrated differential interactions with the estrogen receptors [6]. Structure activity studies led to the landmark SERM raloxifene which showed antagonism of estrogen with minimal estrogen agonism in rodent uterine tissue [7]. Studies with raloxifene in ovariectomized rats showed a unique pharmacological profile in which protection against bone loss is observed without causing uterine hypertrophy, a significant differentiation from the pharmacology seen with tamoxifen [8].

15.3 ASSAYS FOR BIOLOGICAL EVALUATION OF TISSUE SELECTIVITY

Tissue selectivity for SERMs was assessed using a series of *in vitro* and *in vivo* assays. The *in vitro* assays included binding to ERalpha and ERbeta as a biochemical means of

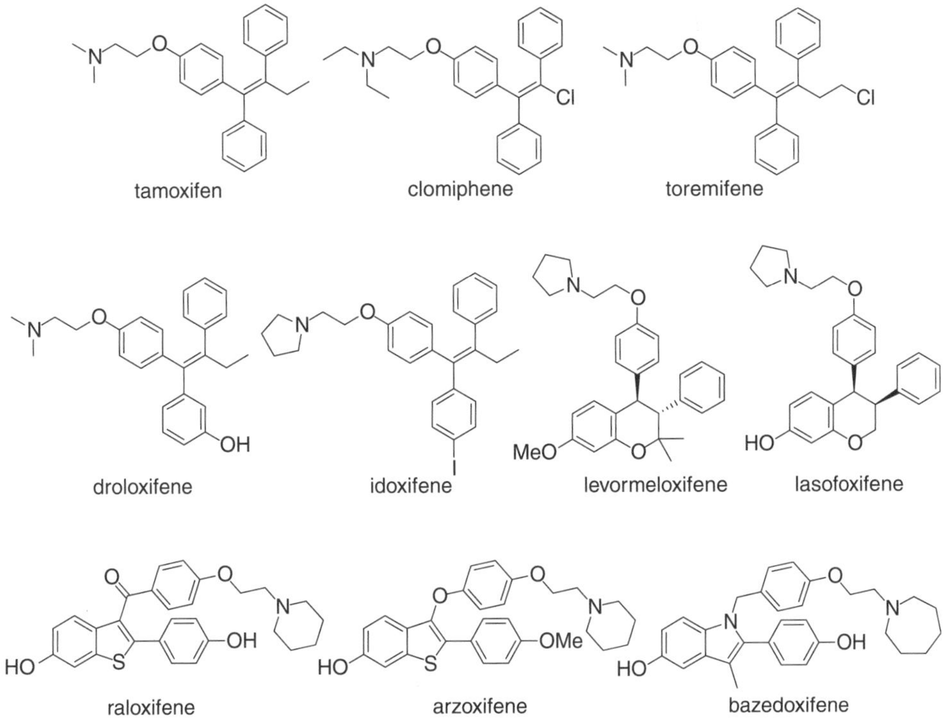

tamoxifen clomiphene toremifene

droloxifene idoxifene levormeloxifene lasofoxifene

raloxifene arzoxifene bazedoxifene

Scheme 15.1 Chemical structures for SERMS in Tables 15.1 and 15.3.

determining receptor affinity. Cellular activity in breast (MCF-7) and uterine cancer cells (Ishikawa) was determined in the presence and absence of 17beta-estradiol to assess agonist and antagonist effects in these tissue types. Uterine and bone parameters were assessed in the ovariectomized rat, a traditionally predictive model for postmenopausal osteoporosis.

15.4 BENZOTHIOPHENE STRUCTURE ACTIVITY

Crystal structures of various ligands bound to the ER indicate that small molecules can induce a spectrum of receptor conformations. As described below, the specific SERM-ER conformation has tremendous impact on cofactor recruitment and ultimate genomic activation or inhibition by the SERM. Key structural features of these molecules, which are indicated in Figure 15.2 for raloxifene versus 17-β-estradiol, are typical for the entire class with the most important features being: (1) the hydroxyl moieties and (2) the basic side chain.

The hydroxyl moieties on the "A" and "D" rings are required for the high affinity interaction with the ER [9] and align in the binding pocket of the ER in a manner that

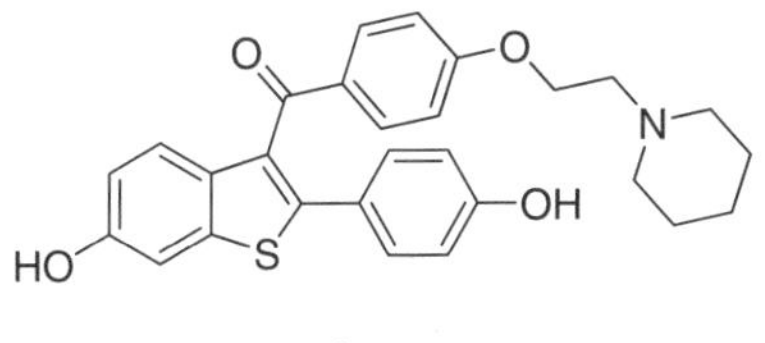

raloxifene

Scheme 15.2 Benzothiophene core represented by raloxifene.

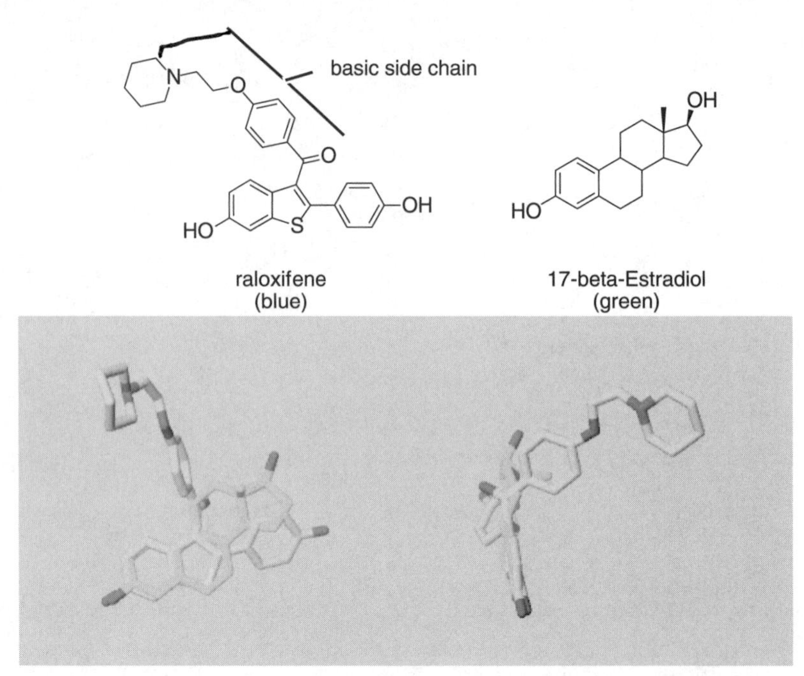

Figure 15.2 Key structural features and three-dimensional overlay of 17-beta-estradiol and raloxifene. (See color version of the figure in Color Plate section)

parallels the binding of the hydroxyl groups of 17β-estradiol, with the 3-hydroxyl on the "A" ring of 17β-estradiol being the most important [10]. As shown in Figure 15.2, the location of the hydroxyl groups for 17-β-estradiol and an energy-optimized orientation of raloxifene align very closely, allowing raloxifene to interact with the same peptide residues in the ER-binding pocket as those which bind estradiol. Note that those molecules lacking hydroxyl groups are likely hydroxylated *in vivo* as a result of cytochrome P-450 metabolism, such as tamoxifen to 4-hydroxytamoxifen, which is the likely active metabolite of this SERM.

The basic side is critical for determining the SERM-ER conformation that ultimately determines the tissue selective pharmacology of the various SERMs. Specifically, the basic side chain of raloxifene protrudes from the ER-binding pocket physically occupying the space helix 12 occupies when 17β-estradiol is bound to ER, thus forcing ER helix 12 to assume an orientation perpendicular to that which occurs with 17β-estradiol bound to the receptor [10,11]. Thus, not only is the chemical constituency of the basic side chain an important feature, but also the orientation of the basic side chain in space. For example, analogs of raloxifene with an orthogonally constrained basic side chain (fixed in the energy-optimized orientation as shown for raloxifene in Figure 15.2) show normal binding to the ER, the expected bone protective activity and lack of significant uterine stimulation, much as is observed with raloxifene in ovariectomized (OVX) rats [11]. This is in direct contrast to the orientation of the basic side chain in SERMs like tamoxifen in which the oxygen that provides the alkyl tether to the basic amine necessarily lies in the same plane as the stilbene core (Scheme 15.3).

Although the uterine pharmacology is strikingly different for raloxifene and tamoxifen, examination of the protein crystal structures of ER-α with raloxifene and 4-hydroxytamoxifen [10,12] reveal that these pharmacogical differences result from subtle differences in the spatial orientation of their respective basic side chains. Figure 15.3A shows a superimposition of the protein–ligand complexes for raloxifene and 4-hydroxytamoxifen,

raloxifene

4-hydroxytamoxifen

Scheme 15.3 Comparison of chemical constituency and orientation of the basic side chain in raloxifene and tamoxifen analog.

respectively, cocrystalized with the ligand binding domain (LBD) of ER-α. The tertiary structure of the protein is well-conserved between the two complexes. Figure 15.3B shows an overlay of the two ligands from these cocrystals. In their bound state, raloxifene (in green) and 4-hydroxytamoxifen (in teal), the two basic nitrogens (in blue) are separated in space by less than 1 Å distance.

The significance of the spatial orientation of the basic side chain is demonstrated by compound D in Figure 15.3. This analog is a single point mutation of raloxifene in which the carbonyl hinge has been removed, a structural modification that forces a more planar orientation of the basic side chain such that it directly overlaps with tamoxifen's basic side chain. This compound produced a profile in cells and rodents (OVX rats) that is very similar to that of tamoxifen: bone sparing, but uterine stimulatory [11]. Thus, very subtle differences in the structure of the ligand, such as the removal of one or two atoms, that is, compare compound 3D with 3C (raloxifene), can result in dramatic differences in tissue

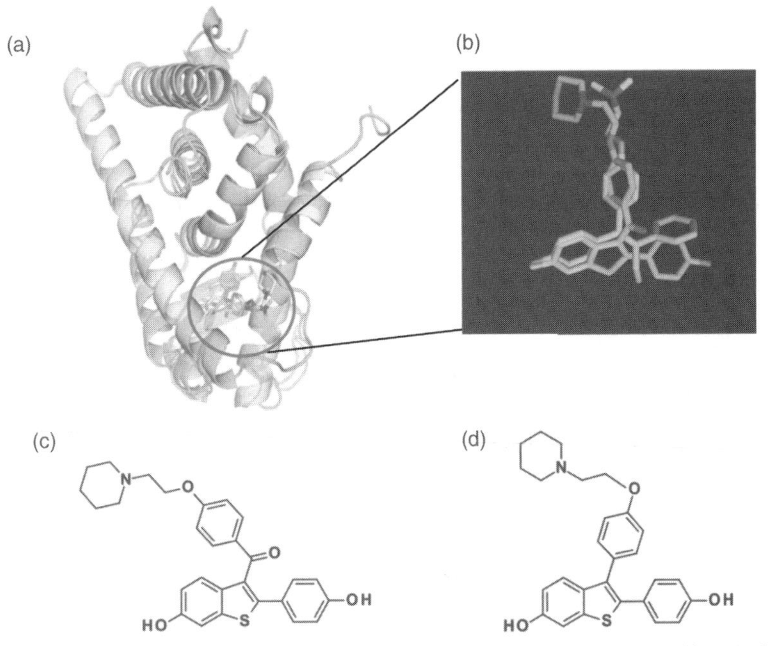

Figure 15.3 (A) Superimposed protein-ligand crystal structures of raloxifene (yellow) and 4-hydroxytamoxifen (teal) in the LBD of ERalpha. (B) Overlay of raloxifene (green) and 4-hydroxytamoxifen (teal) in their protein bound state. (C) Structure of raloxifene. (D) Structure of raloxifene analog with the hinge region removed. (See color version of the figure in Color Plate section)

selectivity. This data is consistent with broader SAR findings within the benzothiophene nucleus and highlights the empirical nature of determining a given SERM's overall tissue specificity.

Since protein crystallography provides only a static snapshot of protein–ligand interactions and does not interrogate the dynamic nature of this critical phenomenon, raloxifene and 4-hydroxytamoxifen have been studied using hydrogen–deuterium exchange, or HDX, a method more suited to quantifying the dynamics of protein–ligand interactions. Specifically, this mass spectrometry-based technology shows how a given ligand impacts the amide backbone of a protein by measuring the rate of exchange of hydrogen for deuterium in backbone amide NHs over time. For raloxifene and 4-OH-tamoxifen, HDX reveals significantly different stabilization profiles between the two SERMs [13]. The beta-sheet 1/beta-sheet 2 peptides experienced the largest change on binding with two-fold more stabilization observed in the 4-hydroxytamoxifen-bound complex than that in the raloxifene-bound complex. Other regions experience various degrees of stabilization and can be used in combination with the beta-sheet region to discriminate 4-hydroxytamoxifen and raloxifene. Comparison of these regions to the protein crystal structures, shown in Figure 15.4A and B, highlights the peptide region of the beta-sheet1/beta-sheet 2 region that experiences the most significant stabilization on binding with these two ligands. These differences result in unique molecular fingerprints that correlated well with the tissue specificity observed for these compounds [13]. Moreover, these fingerprints are distinct for ERalpha relative to ERbeta as the same HDX analysis with ERbeta LBD shows little correlation with tissue specific behavior [14].

In order to further investigate the role of the basic side chain of raloxifene, conformational restricted analogs were prepared. SERMs in which this side chain is held in an orientation which is orthogonal to the benzothiophene plane, illustrated by compound **1** in Figure 15.5, were shown to (1) bind the estrogen receptor, (2) antagonize estrogen-stimulated proliferation of MCF-7 cells *in vitro*, (3) stimulate TGF-β3 gene expression in cell culture, (4) inhibit the uterine effects of ethynyl estradiol in immature rats, and (5) potently reduce serum cholesterol and protect against osteopenia in ovariectomized (OVX) rats without estrogen-like stimulation of uterine tissue [11,15]. The impact of the orthogonal orientation of the basic side chain relative to planar core was confirmed by Wallace and coworkers [16]. For example, while compounds **2** and **3** (Figure 15.5) bind with similar affinity to the ERs, the analog with the basic side-chain coplanar to the benzothiophene, that is, **2**, is significantly less potent than **3** in its ability to inhibit uterine cell proliferation in Ishikawa cells. Likewise, naphthalene SERM **4** is less potent than **5** in functional assays.

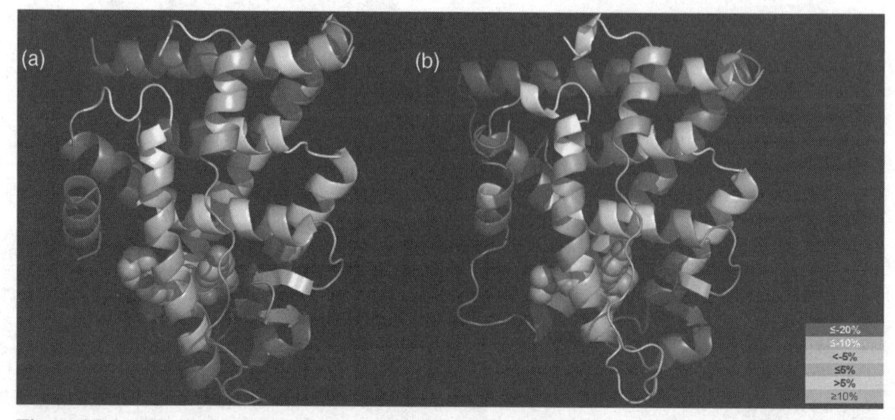

Figure 15.4 ER-ligand HDX profiles for raloxifene (A) and 4-hydoxytamoxifen (B) [13]. (See color version of the figure in Color Plate section)

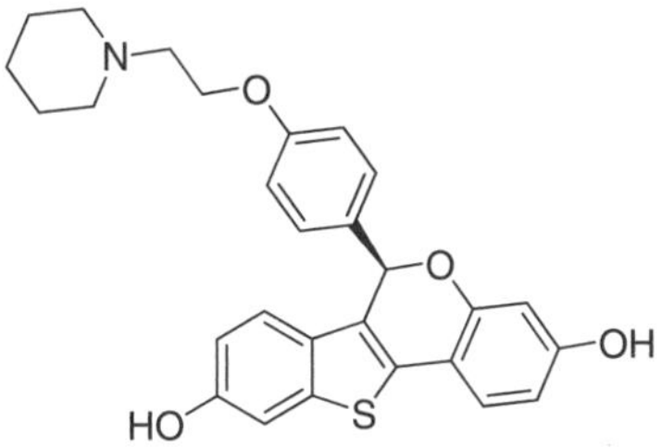

Figure 15.5 Conformationally restricted SERMs.

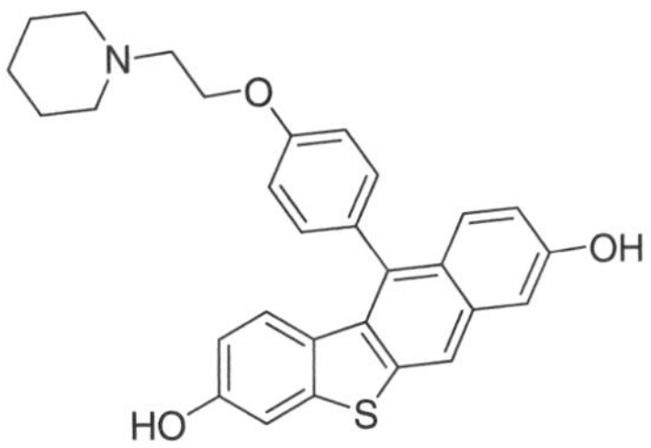

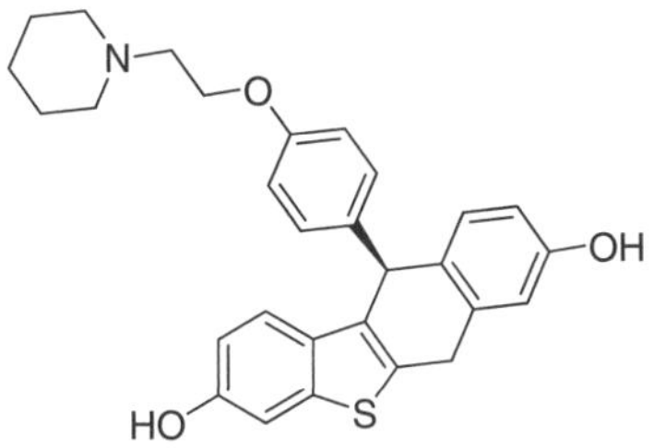

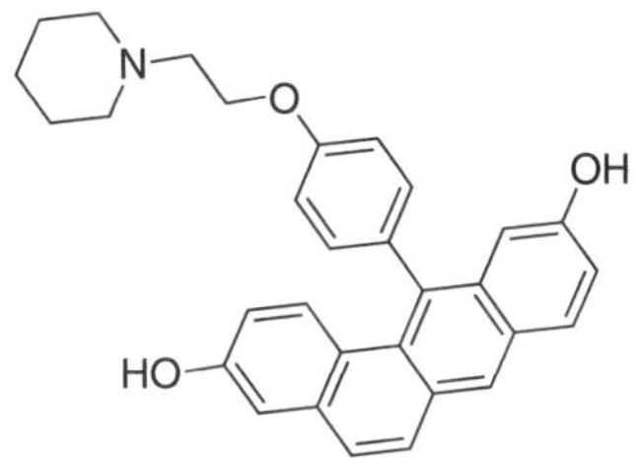

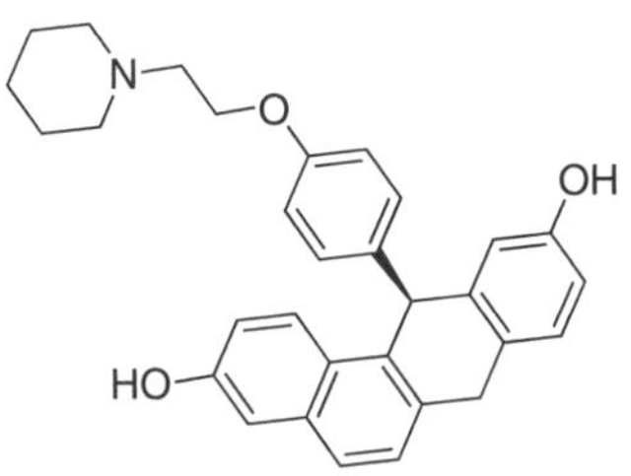

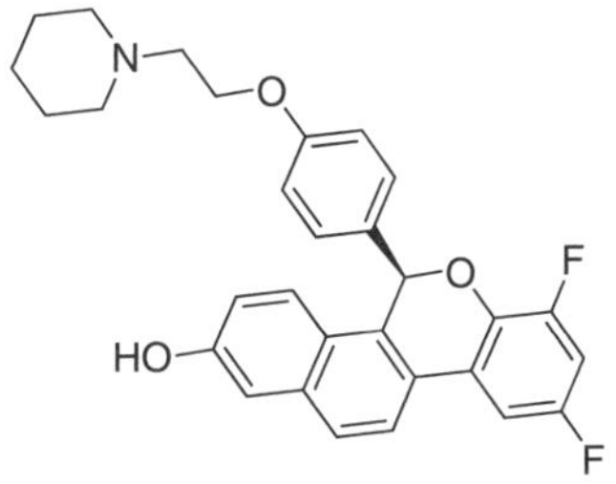

Other conformationally restricted analogs include replacement of the benzothiophene nucleus. For example, the benzopyran SERM **6** (Figure 15.5) displays dose-dependent activity in the morphine-withdrawal rat model of hot flush efficacy. This compound increases bone mineral density, lowers serum cholesterol, and exhibits minimal uterine agonist activity in OVX rats. SERM **6** binds with high affinity to both estrogen receptors and is an antagonist in breast and uterine cancer cell lines, MCF-7, and Ishikawa, respectively [17].

Structure-activity relationships of the 2-arylbenzothiophene core of raloxifene demonstrated that (1) the 6-hydroxy and, to a lesser extent, the 4′-hydroxy substituents of raloxifene are important for receptor binding and *in vitro* activity, (2) small, highly electronegative 4′-substituents such as hydroxy, fluoro, and chloro are preferred both *in vitro* and *in vivo*, (3) increased steric bulk at the 4′-position leads to increased uterine stimulation *in vivo*, and (4) additional substitution of the 2-aryl moiety is tolerated while additional substitution at the 4-, 5-, or 7-position of the benzothiophene results in reduced biological activity [11]. In addition, compounds in which the 2-aryl group is replaced by alkyl, cycloalkyl, and naphthyl substituents maintain a profile of *in vitro* and *in vivo* biological activity qualitatively similar to that of raloxifene. Several novel structural variants, including 2-methyl (**7**), 2-cyclohexyl (**8**), and 2-naphthyl (**9**) (shown in Figure 15.6),

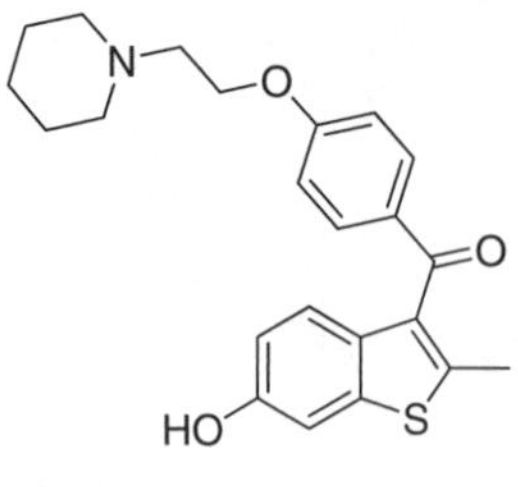

7

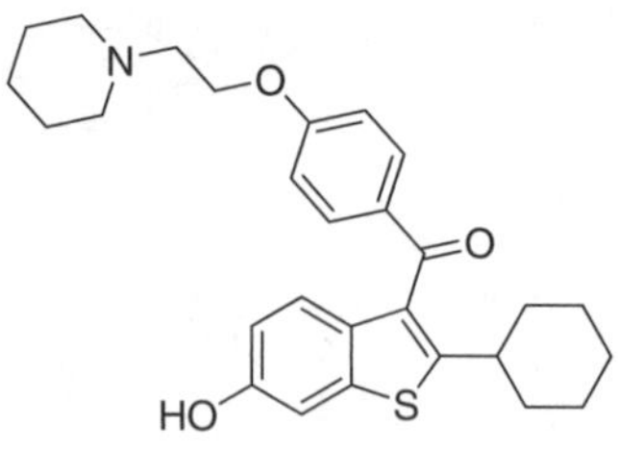

8

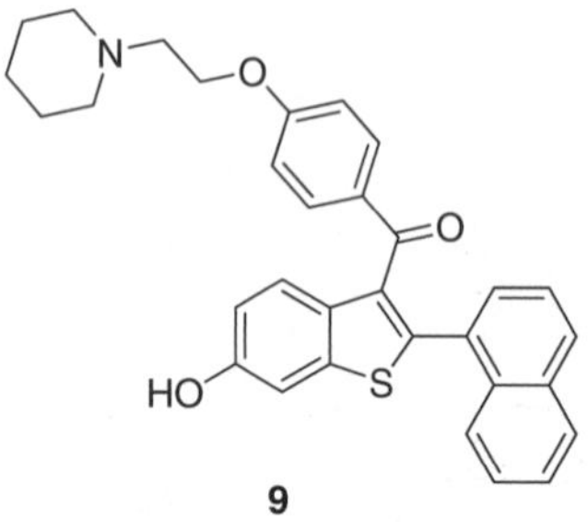

9

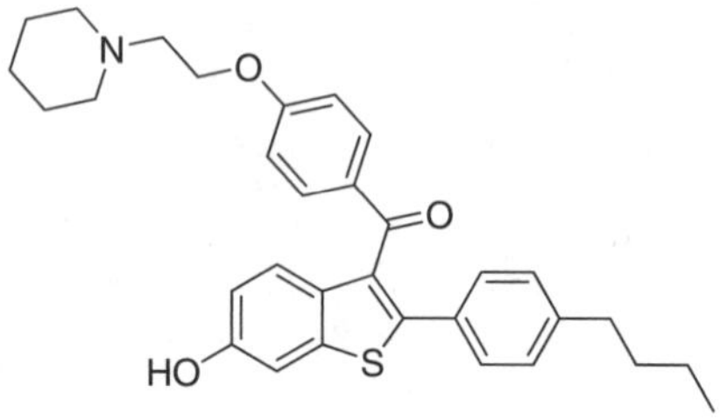

10

Figure 15.6 Representative 2-substituted benzothiophenes.

demonstrated efficacy in preventing bone loss in a chronic OVX rat model of postmenopausal osteopenia, at doses of 0.1–10 mg kg^{-1}. Improved selectivity for ERalpha is observed when *n*-alkyl substituents are added to the 4′-position. For example, the 4′-*n*-butyl SERM **10** is a high affinity ligand that is 140-fold selective for ERalpha relative to ERbeta. [18].

Substitution of the carbonyl hinge in raloxifene with an oxygen resulted in compound **11** (Figure 15.7) which had a substantial (10-fold) increase in estrogen antagonist potency relative to raloxifene in an *in vitro* estrogen-dependent cell proliferation assay ($IC_{50} = 0.05$ nM) in which human breast cancer cells (MCF-7) were utilized [19]. In addition, **11** potently inhibited the uterine proliferative response to exogenous estrogen in immature rats following both sc and oral dosing (ED_{50} of 0.006 and 0.25 mg kg^{-1}, respectively). In ovariectomized aged rats, compound **10** produced a significant maximal decrease (45%) in total cholesterol at 1.0 mg kg^{-1} (po) and showed a protective effect on bone relative to controls with maximal efficacy at 1.0 mg kg^{-1} (po). Other substitution at this position including nitrogen (**12**), sulfur (**13**), and methylene (**14**), (see Figure 15.7) was tolerated as well.

Recently, a SERM with improved selectivity for uterus and ovaries in rats was identified [20]. Naphthalene sulfone **15**, shown in Figure 15.8, bound with high affinity to both estrogen receptors and inhibited breast cancer cell proliferation. The effects on uterine tissue were assessed at the *in vitro* level in Ishikawa cells in the presence (antagonism) and absence (agonism) of the natural ligand 17beta-estradiol E2. In the antagonist mode, this

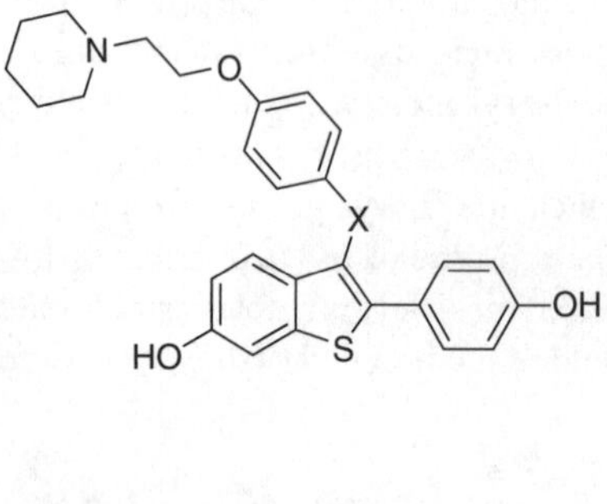

11, X =O

12, X = NH

13, X = S

14, X =CH_2

Figure 15.7 Oxy-hinge analogs.

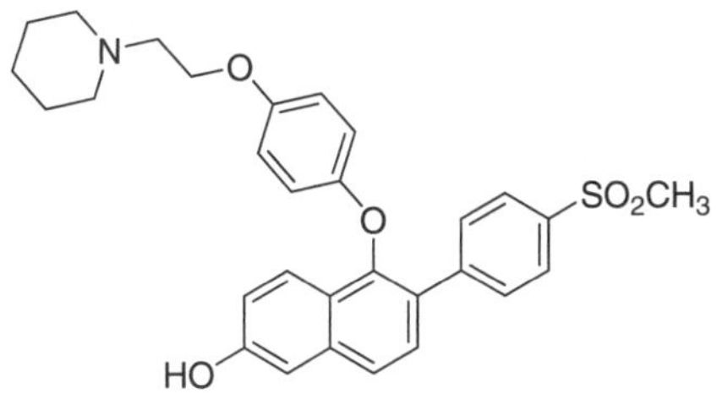

15

Figure 15.8 Ovarian selective SERM.

SERM blocked the effects of 1 nM E2 by >90% with an IC_{50} of 10.7 nM. When tested in rodents, this compound proved to be a highly potent, orally active uterine antagonist at blocking estrogen-induced uterine hypertrophy in immature, ovary-intact rats. In addition, it did not have agonist properties in the uterus when administered to OVX rats. The effects on the uterus and ovaries were studied in 6-month old ovary-intact female rats. Oral administration of **15** for 35 days resulted in a dose-dependent decrease in uterine weight. The effects on the ovaries were determined by measuring serum E2 levels and histologic evaluation of ovarian cross-sections. Treatment with **15** resulted in serum E2 levels that are similar to vehicle-treated animals while histological evaluation of the ovaries indicates minimal ovarian stimulation relative to untreated controls. This data collectively indicated that compound **15** is a potent uterine antagonist with minimal ovarian stimulation in rats [21].

Overall, traditional structure-activity studies coupled with biophysical analysis of benzothiophene SERMs using protein crystallography and HDX have led to a pharmacophore model illustrated in Figure 15.9. The two phenols in raloxifene-like SERMs provide an anchor to the receptor with the 6-OH phenol being the primary affinity determinant. The basic side chain provides the functional capacity for classical antagonist activity. Most significantly, however, the hinge region is the primary determinant of tissue selectivity, imparting the unique profile observed with raloxifene.

15.5 THE SYNTHESIS OF RALOXIFENE

The synthesis of raloxifene has recently been reviewed [22] in detail. As such, this review will not discuss the chemical synthesis but directs the readers to the referenced literature.

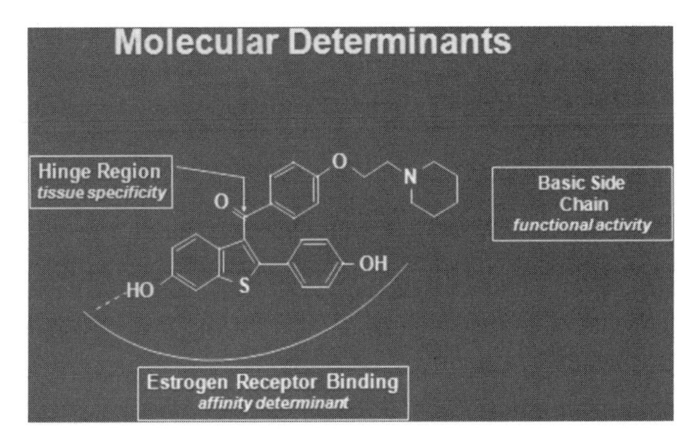

Figure 15.9 Molecular determinants of tissue specificity for benzothiophene SERMs.

15.6 SERM MECHANISM

The effects of SERMs on biologic systems are predominately mediated by specific, high-affinity, interactions with ERs that are primarily located in target cell nuclei [23]. Certainly non-ER-mediated effects (i.e., antioxidant properties) and nonnuclear ER-mediated effects (i.e., nitrous oxide production by cardiovascular endothelial cells [24]) have been described and may be important contributory factors to the overall pharmacology of SERMs. However, most attention has focused on the "nuclear hormone receptor" aspects of SERM mechanism. This nuclear hormonal action involves the complex interplay of a number of protein and genomic elements that allow SERMs to regulate gene transcription and subsequent protein production by the cell. Recent advances in understanding of the molecular biology of SERM action illuminate three key elements that distinguish estrogen and SERM effects. As depicted in Figure 15.10, these three elements include: (1) high-affinity interaction with the ER, (2) ER-ligand dimerization and the association with a tissue-specific set of coregulatory proteins, and (3) binding of the ER/adaptor protein complex to specific DNA response elements located in the promoter regions of nuclear target genes and ensuing regulation of gene transcription. Depending upon the cellular and promoter context, the DNA-bound receptor can induce or inhibit the transcription of specific genes within the tissue.

The ability to specifically bind to the ER is perhaps the single most important feature of all molecules with a SERM profile. The affinities of several of the more extensively studied SERMs are provided in Table 15.3. In the absence of ligand, the ER exists in a large protein complex, comprising the receptor bound to heat shock proteins [23]. Binding of a ligand to the ER induces a conformational change that results in dissociation of the heat shock chaperone proteins from the ER. One of the most important determinants of the ultimate pharmacological response is the shape of this ligand–ER complex, which is unique with each individual ligand [10,25]. The ligand-binding domain (LBD) of the ER consists of a hydrophobic core made up of parts of five distinct helices (helix-3, -6, -8, -11, and -12). When the LBD of ER-α is bound to estrogen, helix 12 adopts an orientation that lies over the

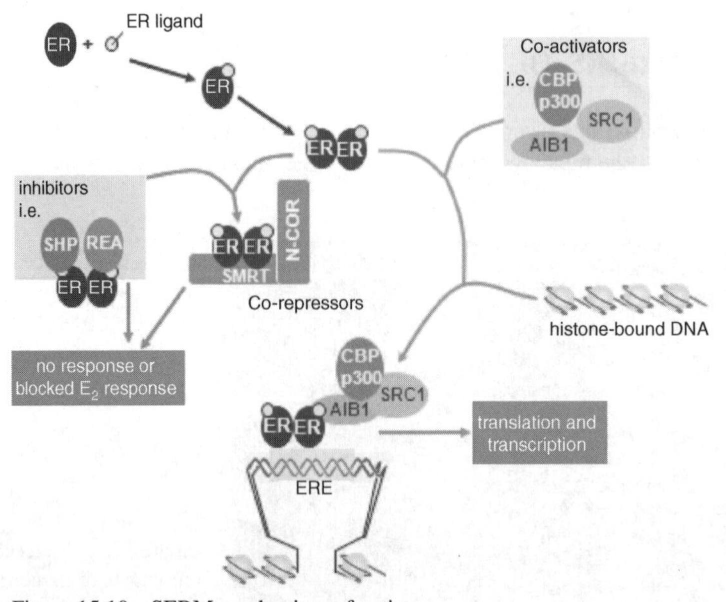

Figure 15.10 SERM mechanism of action.

TABLE 15.3 Affinities of Various SERMs for Human Estrogen Receptor (ER)-α and ER-β

ER Ligand	ER-α (IC_{50})[a]	ER-β (IC_{50})[a]
17-β-estradiol	0.3–0.8	0.9–2.5
Tamoxifen	72–138	173–1204
4-Hydroxy-tamoxifen	0.22–0.98	1.5–2.46
Raloxifene	0.4–1.31	5.6–13.0
Fulvestrant (ICI-182,780)	0.8–1.0	1.12–3.6

[a]All values are in nM.

binding pocket of the receptor and allows for interaction of cellular proteins with the coactivator recognition groove. In contrast, when the 4-hydroxy metabolite of tamoxifen (likely the active metabolite of tamoxifen at ER-α [26]) is bound to the ER-α, helix 12 adopts a distinct alignment from that of the estrogen bound receptor that occludes interactions with the coactivator recognition groove [12]. Raloxifene, when bound to the LBD of ER-α protrudes from the ligand-binding cavity and physically prevents the alignment of helix-12 over the binding cavity, thus shifting helix-12 away from the pocket it normally occupies when 17β-estradiol is bound [10]. Thus, the conformation or shape of the ligand–ER complex provides an important structural basis of SERM activity via determination of which particular subsequent protein–protein interactions are permitted. This is also a primary basis for the wide array of different pharmacological profiles produced by different SERMs, as the conformation of the ER–SERM complex is distinct for each molecule [25]. It is important to recognize that a second form of the ER is known to exist, ER-β [27], which may also form heterodimers with ER-α. ER-α and ER-β display unique patterns of tissue distribution typically with expression levels of one subtype dominating [28], although it should be noted that most tissues contain at least small amounts of both subtypes, and with the role of putative α:β heterodimers unknown, it is possible that low expression subtype, may be a key rate-limiting step in ultimate nuclear activity. ER-α and ER-β are also each known to have multiple isoforms that are splice variants [29], with the potential of further differences in ligand bound three-dimensional structures adding an additional layer of complexity to ER-mediated activation or inhibition of estrogen response genes. However, to date, all of the SERMs that have reached advanced clinical evaluation show high affinity for both ER-α and ER-β, with sufficient circulating and tissue exposure to insure binding of both subtypes indicating that, for these molecules at least, differential ER-α or ER-β activation does not explain the tissue selective pharmacological effects.

In addition to the ERs themselves, a number of other coregulatory proteins, such as coactivators (which enhance transcription) and corepressors (which reduce transcription) play an essential role in determining the ultimate response of an individual cell to liganded ER. The C-termini of both ER-α and ER-β harbor the ligand-dependent AF-2 domain. Specific interactions between amino acid residues within the ER and a distinct ER recognition groove of coactivator proteins [identified by a signature Leu-Xaa-Xaa-Leu-Leu (LxxLL) coactivator motif] are necessary for maximal ligand-dependent activation of estrogen target gene promoters [30]. Specific ER-associated coactivator proteins include various 160-kDa proteins, such as: SRC-1, TIF-2, AIB1, and ACTR [31–33], a 300-kDa protein (CBP) and an RNA coactivator (SRA-1 [34]).

Corepressors are the counterpart of coactivators, and possess a trans-repressor function. Corepressors also contain a signature motif related to the LxxLL sequence found in coactivators. This motif, known as the corner box (L/IxxI/V-I), mediates the interaction between the ER and specific corepressor proteins such as N-CoR, SMRT, REA, and SHP [35,36].

The relative expression of the different cofactors and the ability of the ER–ligand complex to interact with those cofactors play a major role in the tissue selective agonist/antagonist profile of the various SERM molecules, as despite the presence of numerous cellular proteins with transcriptional coregulatory activities, there are numerous examples of tissue selective activities [37,38]. An additional point of significance is that coactivators such as ACTR and AIB1 are amplified in various breast and uterine tumors [32,39]. The important nature of the tissue-relevant cofactor context was best demonstrated by Shang and Brown [40], who compared the effects of two SERMs, tamoxifen and raloxifene, to estrogen in two tissue contexts: a breast cancer cell line and a uterine endometrial carcinoma cell line. In the mammary cells, which are induced to proliferate in the presence of estrogen, 17β-estradiol recruited coactivators leading to increased gene expression. In these same cells, where tamoxifen and raloxifene both display estrogen antagonist pharmacology, the ligand–SERM complex with both molecules recruited corepressors and not the coactivators observed with 17β-estradiol on ER-mediated transcription. However, in a uterine cell line where tamoxifen exhibits estrogen agonist pharmacology and raloxifene behaves as a complete antagonist, tamoxifen was associated with the recruitment of a coactivator protein complex that included SRC-1, AIB1, and CBP that resulted in histone acetylation. SRC-1 in particular may be an important coactivator in the uterine cell stimulatory response to tamoxifen, as this coactivator is expressed at higher levels in uterine cells. Of note, the coactivator requirements for estrogen-stimulated gene expression in uterine cells were distinct from those for tamoxifen, indicating multiple signaling mechanisms even for the agonist response. Conversely, raloxifene failed to recruit a coactivator construct, rather inducing a corepressor construct associated with histone deacetylase activity in the uterine cell line [40]. Thus, the relative abundance of ER-associated coactivators and corepressors are an important factor in the tissue-specific pharmacology of SERMs.

The ligand bound ER-coactivator/repressor complex present in the transcriptionally active compartment of the nucleus faces its last hurdle in targeting cognate response elements on the promoter of the target gene. In addition to the layers of complexity provided by multiple ER–SERM conformations and tissue selective cofactor recruitment, the mechanism of tissue-selectivity of SERMs is further complicated by the existence of multiple DNA response elements. Many estrogen-responsive genes contain the classical estrogen response element (ERE), first observed in the chicken vitellogenin gene [41] and now including a number of DNA response elements, such as activator protein-1 and steroidogenic factor-1 response element [42]. The mechanism for SERM activation (or inactivation) of ER-mediated function is further complicated by the presence of novel DNA response elements that are more apparent following formation of the ER–SERM–cofactor complex. For example, the presence of unique response elements for SERM bound ER, which do not share sequence similarity to known EREs, was first demonstrated with studies employing raloxifene and activation of transforming growth-factor β3 gene promoter activity associated with raloxifene treatment [43].

While there has been considerable strides in understanding the molecular biology of SERM action in a general sense, with the critical role of the ER, specific cofactors that are recruited to the transcriptional complex and the specific DNA response elements activated, it is important to recognize that it is not clear at this point what distinguishes individual SERM molecules in the mechanism by which they arrive at their tissue selective pharmacology. It is clear that each SERM (even within a chemical class) produces a unique pharmacological fingerprint when all tissue types are considered. That is, varying degrees of agonism to antagonism are possible in each target tissue with different SERMs, creating the need to specifically characterize the precise mechanism of each SERM in each target tissue. Obviously, the important role of other factors, such as absorption, distribution, excretion, and metabolism of the SERM add another layer of complexity for the ultimate pharmacological response, creating the need to fully characterize the tissue-specific effects of each individual SERM in an *in vivo* paradigm.

15.7 RALOXIFENE PHARMACOLOGY

Given the wide distribution of ER and the pleiotropic nature of estrogen and its multiple metabolites, SERMs should be expected to likewise affect multiple organ systems, and this is indeed the case with raloxifene.

15.7.1 Skeletal System

15.7.1.1 Preclinical Studies Bone is a living, dynamic tissue that is continuously remodeled during the adult life of an individual. The remodeling process occurs in quantum units called bone-remodeling units through the action of osteoclasts and osteoblasts. Osteoclasts are the bone-resorbing cells which tightly adhere to the bone surface and then secrete acid which dissolves the hydroxyapatite mineral and proteolytic enzymes that degrade the organic matrix of bone. Osteoblasts are the bone-forming cells that synthesize a highly cross-linked, lamellar organic matrix (osteoid) which becomes mineralized by extracellular processes. Osteoblasts usually replenish the bone excavated by osteoclasts. Osteoporosis is a disease of the bone that leads to increased risk of fracture as a consequence of an imbalance between osteoclastic and osteoblastic activity, coupled with an increased rate of bone turnover observed. That is, a net loss of bone mass or inadequate architecture results due to either the excessive bone-resorbing activity of osteoclasts or the impaired bone-forming activity of osteoblasts, such that osteoblasts do not optimally replenish the lost bone. For women, this phenomenon is related to the decline of endogenous levels of the steroid hormone estrogen after menopause. Because the rate of remodeling is about 10 times higher in cancellous than cortical bone, bone loss following menopause is observed primarily in regions enriched for trabecular bone such as the vertebra and proximal femur. Gradually, perforations in or thinning of the trabecular bone spicules develop with the result that a weakened and inadequate architecture ensues.

Much as in postmenopausal women, estrogen deficiency in OVX animals leads to a rapid increase in bone turnover, where excessive osteoclast resorptive activity results in a marked decline in trabecular bone mass and strength, with concomitant increase in fractures. In rats, ovariectomy produces a rapid osteopenic response, which can be discerned within 5 weeks. In the OVX rat model, raloxifene [8] prevented the loss of bone in vertebrae, distal femur, and proximal tibia, all trabecular-rich bone sites. In addition to maintaining bone mass, raloxifene [44] also preserved bone strength through improvements in bone microarchitecture. For example, in OVX mice, administration of raloxifene not only improved vertebral bone mineral density (BMD), but increased trabecular thickness and maintained plate-like trabecular structures (versus rod-like), both of which correlate with improved biomechanical strength of bone [45]. As with estrogen, the primary activity of SERMs responsible for the beneficial effect on bone is antiresorptive. Mechanistic studies *in vitro* have demonstrated that raloxifene and estrogen exert their antiresorptive effects primarily as inhibitors of osteoclast differentiation, rather than as direct inhibitors of activated osteoclasts. Raloxifene suppressed mediators of osteoclast differentiation, such as the receptor activator of nuclear factor-κB (RANK), RANK-ligand, interleukin-6 and interleukin-7 [46–48] and increased endogenous antiresorptive factors such as TGFβ3 and osteoprotogerin [43,47]. *In vivo* studies demonstrated that biochemical markers of bone turnover (i.e., serum osteocalcin, urinary collagen crosslinks) were suppressed in a manner similar to that observed with estrogen [49]. Histomorphometric analysis of bone from raloxifene-treated OVX rats confirmed the antiresorptive mechanism of action for raloxifene [50]. Similar studies with the other SERMs discussed here indicate the same antiresorptive mechanism for bone protection. Of likely importance with respect to long-term safety in the skeleton is the finding that SERMs, like raloxifene, produce their inhibitory action on bone resorption with minimal suppressive effects on bone formation leaving bone formation rates at levels comparable to sham-operated control animals [50]. The molecular fingerprint of SERMs in estrogen-deficient rat trabecular bone, as assessed by DNA microarray, is unique for each SERM, although it is clear that some SERMs are less suppressive of bone formation. For example, in OVX rats raloxifene returned a cluster of genes associated with bone formation to ovary-intact control levels, as opposed to a bis-phosphonate (alendronate), estrogen or even another SERM (acolbifene), which exhibited a greater suppressive effect on bone formation-associated genes [51]. The overall SERM profile on bone then represents a sharp distinction from the marked suppression of bone formation that occurs with other bone antiresorptives, such as the bis-phosphonates [52]. The end result likely is greater opportunity for skeletal repair and remodeling with chronic SERM use, which permits the skeleton to retain its critical self-healing properties.

15.7.1.2 Clinical Studies The abundance of preclinical information on the effects of SERMs on bone has been matched by a plethora of long-term clinical trials that have been conducted on a number of different SERM molecules, either as the primary element of registration trials for postmenopausal osteoporosis or as part of the safety assessment for use in breast cancer. Certainly, the most extensively studied SERM on the human skeleton has been raloxifene, which has been investigated in nearly 40,000 clinical trial subjects enrolled in prospective, randomized trials (placebo or active comparator) that have ranged in duration from 1 to 8 years. As in the OVX rat studies, in postmenopausal women raloxifene (60 mg d^{-1}) exhibits an antiresorptive action as evidenced by reductions in the accelerated bone turnover as measured by biochemical markers of bone resorption [53], while only modestly suppressing bone formation. In calcium tracer kinetic studies in postmenopausal women, Heany and Draper [54] provided evidence for suppression of bone resorption with raloxifene, while bone formation was not affected in studies of up to 31 weeks duration. The observation of resorption inhibition with minimal formation suppression by raloxifene was confirmed by histomorphometric analysis of iliac crest bone biopsies [55,56]. This antiresorptive activity is associated with approximately a 2.5% increased vertebral BMD, relative to placebo-treated controls. This increase in spine BMD that occurs following raloxifene treatment in postmenopausal women is less marked than observed with a bis-phosphonate [57]. However, this magnitude of BMD improvement in the spine underestimates the mechanical improvement produced by raloxifene, as evidenced by the 30% reduction in new vertebral fractures (vs. placebo) in postmenopausal women without prevalent fractures and 55% reduction in new vertebral fractures in women with prevalent fractures [53], a rate comparable to that produced by other currently available antiresorptive agents for osteoporosis. This particular observation has led to an increased attentiveness to potential effects of raloxifene (and putatively other SERMs as well in the future) on bone quality and may be related to microarchitecural improvements as were observed in OVX mice [45]. The eventual resistance of bone to fracture is the result both of the content, or mass of the material (i.e., BMD), and the quality of that material. However, while BMD is a noninvasive, easily quantifiable, parameter in clinical trials, bone quality remains a more qualitative feature to date—only revealed by the eventual incidence of fracture. To that regard, a number of efforts have targeted better understanding, and quantifying, bone quality where raloxifene has shown some benefits over other antiresorptive therapies such as histomorphometric analyses of trabecular bone architecture and microcrack frequency in bone [58,59]. One area where some aspect of bone quality is beginning to be elucidated is the proximal femur, where imaging technologies have been applied to postmenopausal clinical trial subjects to show an increase in resistance to axial and bending stresses in raloxifene-treated women [60], indicating improved structural components of bone strength and stability with the SERM. Raloxifene does produce positive effects on hip BMD, which increased 2.1% versus placebo after 3 years in postmenopausal women [53], although without a significant effect on nonvertebral fracture rates [53]. Finally, in addition to reduction of vertebral fracture in osteoporotic women, raloxifene also provides fracture risk protection to osteopenic women [61]. Raloxifene did not lead to a significant overall reduction in nonvertebral fractures in the large, randomized, placebo-controlled registration studies that demonstrated the benefit on vertebral fractures. However, an interesting trend was noted in a subset of women who entered the trials with severe vertebral fractures. In this subset of more severely osteoporotic women, raloxifene produced a 50% reduction in nonvertebral fractures [62].

15.7.2 Reproductive System—Uterus

Atrophy of the uterus typically accompanies estrogen deficiency in both humans and most animal species, and cessation of menses is a hallmark feature of the menopause in women. A major side effect of most current estrogen receptor-based therapies is a stimulatory effect on the uterus. This uterine stimulating action of estrogen causes proliferation of uterine endometrial tissue. The cancer concern associated with this proliferative effect and the resumption of menses (when combined with progestin regimens as hormonal replacement therapy) are a major limitations to estrogen replacement therapeutic approaches The uterotrophic effects of estrogen historically have been an important detriment to the risk/benefit assessment of the decision for postmenopausal women to utilize, and remain compliant with, hormonal estrogen therapies for chronic use with diseases such as osteoporosis. A major and significant advantage of SERMs like raloxifene, for postmenopausal women, over hormonal estrogen therapies, is the lack of estrogen-like stimulation of the uterus with the SERM. However, not all SERMs share the same degree of uterine safety that is observed with raloxifene and thus, effects at the uterus also serve as an important distinguishing feature amongst various SERMs as well. To this regard, many of the SERMs that have failed to date in phase 3 clinical trials were associated with an untenable degree of uterine stimulation-related adverse events.

15.7.2.1 Estrogen Agonism in the Uterus Initial indication of the uterine estrogenic potential of SERMs can be demonstrated using Ishikawa cells, a human endometrial cancer cell line. Ishikawa cell proliferation is stimulated by 17β-estradiol, tamoxifen, or 4-hydroxy-tamoxifen (active metabolite of tamoxifen) but not by uterine sparing SERMs such as raloxifene [63,64]. More subtle changes amongst the various SERMs can be detected by evaluating ER-mediated alkaline phosphatase production, creatine kinase production, or expression of progesterone receptor following exposure to various compounds in cell culture [65]. Those SERMs known to possess greater uterine stimulatory potential typically produce greater induction of alkaline phosphatase and progesterone receptor expression, and are less effective antagonists of 17β-estradiol stimulated responses in Ishikawa cells [65]. Furthermore, while agents like raloxifene fail to stimulate activities like creatine kinase production by Ishikawa cells, raloxifene retains this activity in cell lines with an osteoblast background: consistent with the "SERM" activity profile [64].

Lack of biologically meaningful stimulation of the uterus in the estrogen-depleted state (e.g., postmenopausal women or OVX animals) is the crux of SERM uterine safety evaluation. The uterine effects of tamoxifen and raloxifene have been thoroughly evaluated in numerous clinical settings, as well as in a variety of preclinical models. Raloxifene does not produce estrogen-like stimulatory effects in the uterus of OVX rats [8] or monkeys [66]. In the OVX rat model, a slight, nondose-related elevation of uterine weight is frequently observed, however this phenomenon contrasts markedly from the robust, dose-related elevation of uterine weight produced by estrogen in these animals [8]. Raloxifene failed to stimulate other estrogen sensitive markers in the uterus of OVX rats, such as uterine eosinophilia, or uterine epithelial cell height [8]. In large-scale clinical trials after 8 years of chronic use in postmenopausal women, extensive uterine safety evaluation has revealed no significant uterine stimulatory effects of raloxifene in humans either [62]. Indeed, a significant reduction in endometrial cancer of the uterus has been noted in postmenopausal women using raloxifene [62].

15.7.2.2 Estrogen Antagonism in the Uterus The final component of importance in assessment of the uterine safety profile of SERMS relies primarily on preclinical data: the ability of SERMs to antagonize the uterine stimulatory effects of estrogen. Further insight into the uterine activity profile of SERMs can be gleaned from effects on the uterus in the presence of estrogen, as this allows assessment of the uterine estrogen antagonist potential for these compounds. As was the case in the estrogen deficient state, the various SERMs also produce one of two activity profiles in estrogen-replete animals: that of either complete estrogen antagonists or that of partial agonists at the ER. In the uterus of either estrogen-treated immature or adult-OVX rats, SERMs like raloxifene, arzoxifene, and bazedoxifene produce a complete estrogen antagonistic effect [52,67]. This effect is most clearly demonstrated in the estrogen-treated immature rat, a model classically used to determine uterine liability of ligands for the estrogen receptor. In this model, raloxifene blocks the uterotrophic effects of estrogen with an ED_{50} of 0.3 mg kg^{-1} [68]. A key feature of this antagonistic effect with SERMs like raloxifene in the immature rat uterus is the complete antagonism of the uterotrophic effect of estrogen. That is, uteri from estrogen-treated immature rats given doses of raloxifene exceeding 3 mg kg^{-1} are indistinguishable from those of nonestrogen-treated immature rats [67]. This is in dramatic contrast to other SERMs, best exemplified by tamoxifen, which behaves a classical partial agonist in the uterus. That is, tamoxifen does significantly antagonize the effects of estrogen in the immature rat uterus. However, in the case of tamoxifen, the maximal degree of this antagonism is only approximately 50% [67]. The primary reason for this incomplete antagonistic effect of tamoxifen is that at higher doses the inherent uterine stimulatory capacity of tamoxifen limits further suppression of the estrogen-induced uterotrophic response. Of note, in OVX rats the uterine stimulatory effects of tamoxifen can also be completely antagonized by raloxifene [69].

15.7.3 Reproductive System—Mammary

The effects of estrogens on mammary tissue in normal adult animals or women are not typically as clear and robust as those effects observed in the uterus. However, clearly a majority of mammary tumors are estrogen receptor positive, and respond favorably to estrogen antagonism [70]. The role of estrogen replacement in risk of breast cancer has been a topic of some controversy and clearly the concomitant use of progestins in most hormonal replacement therapy paradigms is confounding. In the Women's Health Initiative Trial, a significant increase in risk of breast cancer in postmenopausal women was a key finding [71], leading to dramatic reductions in the use of estrogen replacement strategies for various postmenopausal indications. The role of the progestin in this observation (either as a the direct contributor or through potential a combined effect with the estrogen) was suggested by a follow-up study in hysterectomized women using unopposed conjugated equine estrogens for over 7 years, where no increase in breast cancer risk was observed [72]. Thus, while there remains some controversy over the exact potential for increased risk of breast cancer with estrogen therapies, it is clear that concern over this risk has limited patient compliance with steroidal estrogen therapies. A major advantage of the SERM class of molecules is the lack of this cancer concern with respect to mammary tissue and the lack of a need for concomitant use of a progestin. Indeed, SERMs as a class have demonstrated a benefit in either treating or preventing breast cancer in animal models and women. To this regard, raloxifene has recently received approval for reducing the risk of invasive breast cancer in postmenopausal women with osteoporosis and in postmenopausal women at high risk for invasive breast cancer. After 8 years of following 4011 postmenopausal women with osteoporosis, a 66% reduction in the incidence of invasive breast cancer was observed with raloxifene use [73]. In the Study of Tamoxifen and Raloxifene (STAR) Trial, a head to head comparison of the two SERMs was conducted in 19,000 postmenopausal women at high risk of breast cancer, where tamoxifen and raloxifene were found to produce similar reductions in the incidence of invasive breast cancer [74], with the primary benefit being due to a reduced risk of ER-positive invasive breast cancers [75]. The most significant differences between raloxifene and tamoxifen in the STAR trial were significantly fewer uterine-associated adverse events with raloxifene (most notably the lack of endometrial cancer) while tamoxifen appeared to have a greater effect on noninvasive breast cancer incidence than raloxifene [74]. These differences between tamoxifen and raloxifene, although subtle indicate a difference from preclinical and even early clinical indicators, and as such, demonstrate the need for thorough clinical evaluation before accurate therapeutic risk/benefit assessment and approval of indications can be made for human use.

The mechanism by which SERMs such as tamoxifen and raloxifene inhibit breast cancer development or progression is likely the result of multiple beneficial effects of the pharmacological agents. Direct antagonism of estrogen action at estrogen target cells in breast tissue, as previously described, is a key component of the action of the SERMs, given the strong positive linkage of estrogen exposure to relative risk for developing breast cancer and the fact that SERMs are much more effective versus ER-positive breast cancers. However, it is also likely that antitumor effects to reduce estrogen bioavailability as well as effects independent of estrogen contribute to the ultimate antibreast cancer effect. Raloxifene is known to elevate levels of sex hormone binding globulin [76], which would be expected to reduce bioavailable estrogen levels and thereby further reduce the risk of estrogen-associated breast cancer. Other beneficial SERM effects that might be independent of estrogen include: (1) modification of signaling proteins with a role in tumor cell biology (i.e., as observed with tamoxifen on protein kinase C, TGFβ, calmodulin, ceramide, MAP-kinases [77]), (2) induction of apoptosis in mammary tumor cell lines, as with tamoxifen, raloxifene and toremifene [77–79] and/or (3) dampening of growth factor systems known to play a role in tumor progression. The latter of these indirect mechanisms may be the most important, as the contribution of growth factors in the pathogenesis of breast cancer is attracting considerable attention.

15.7.4 General Safety Profile and Other Pharmacological Considerations

15.7.4.1 Other Safety In addition to the adverse events of venous thrombolic events observed with all SERMs and uterine stimulation observed with some SERMs, this class of molecules is associated with other untoward effects that should be considered in the risk/benefit decision for each patient. Of these other adverse events observed in clinical trials, leg cramps and the induction of hot flushes are observed in women with all of the SERM molecules depicted in Table 15.1. Hot flushes, or vasomotor symptoms, are a hallmark indicator of the menopausal transition, occurring in up to 70% of US women [80]. The incidence of hot flushes is likely reflective of declining, or changing, estrogen status and typically abate when circulating estrogen levels reach their postmenopausal, steady-state, concentration. However, in a small percentage of women, vasomotor symptoms can be severe and extend well into the menopause. Estrogen replacement clearly is effective in relieving postmenopausal hot flushes [81]. With SERM use, however, it is likely that an estrogen withdrawal-like response is initiated producing a state similar to that experienced by women who are estrogen depleted with subsequent hot flushes, although it is unclear as to whether this phenomenon is due to estrogen antagonist or agonist properties of the SERM at ER in hypothalamic thermoregulatory centers. SERM-induced hot flushes are transient in nature, as with continued use in most cases this side effect subsides, typically within 6 months, likely as the thermoregulatory set-point re-establishes. Consistent with this proposed mechanism, proximity to the climacteric state may influence the incident rate, and severity, of SERM-induced hot flushes. In postmenopausal women over the age of 55, significantly fewer hot flushes are observed in response to raloxifene as compared to younger postmenopausal women and tamoxifen-induced hot flushes tend to be more severe in premenopausal breast cancer patients than in postmenopausal patients.

One problem in the assessment of the incident rate of hot flush induction following SERM administration is the relatively high placebo response rate in the postmenopausal population. In observational studies performed on randomized, placebo-controlled trials, the rate of reported hot flushes in postmenopausal women receiving placebo was 21% over a 30-month trial period [82]. In this study, the incidence of hot flushes in postmenopausal women using raloxifene was 28%. Others have confirmed an approximate 7% increase in hot flush incidence as a side effect of raloxifene use [83]. Of note, the hot flushes induced by raloxifene are in the mild to moderate category in terms of severity, as severe hot flushes in postmenopausal women using raloxifene occur at a rate indistinguishable from that of placebo controls. Finally, the increase in hot flush incidence with raloxifene is transient, as no differences relative to placebo controls are observed after 6 months [83].

15.7.4.2 Pharmacokinetic Pharmacokinetic properties of the SERMs are an important consideration in the overall effects of these molecules and have served as a focal point for development of novel, improved, agents. For example, the third generation SERMs arzoxifene, bazedoxifene, and lasofoxifene all have pharmacokinetic properties that represent improvements over raloxifene and tamoxifen. The ultimate advantage of these improvements to patients remains to be seen, as these molecules have yet to achieve registration approval. More information as to this impact will certainly be revealed in the upcoming years.

The pharmacokinetics of raloxifene presents some features similar to the triphenylethylenes but also some considerable differences. Like tamoxifen and its relatives, raloxifene is rapidly absorbed from the gastrointestinal tract following oral administration, with peak blood levels attained in approximately 6 h, and 60% of the oral dose absorbed [84].

Raloxifene is also highly bound to plasma proteins (approximately 95% [84]). However, in contrast to the triphenylethylenes, the elimination half-life of raloxifene is considerably shorter at 28 h and there are no known active metabolites of raloxifene in humans or rodents. While there is virtually no P450 metabolism of raloxifene in the liver, it is extensively metabolized by first pass hepatic glucuronidation, yielding an absolute oral bioavailability of only approximately 2% in humans [85]. Raloxifene is widely distributed, and as with the triphenylethylenes, very little is excreted in the urine with the bulk of clearance through biliary excretion and loss in the feces [86].

15.8 SUMMARY

SERMs are a diverse class of molecules that affect a broad spectrum of biological systems with potential therapeutic benefit for a variety of diseases. Concern over long-term use of estrogen-containing regimens created an opportunity for application of SERMs to chronic indications such as osteoporosis treatment or prevention. The profile of the SERM raloxifene allows for use in chronic indications of interest to postmenopausal women, most notably, osteoporosis treatment or prevention and breast cancer risk reduction. However, safety considerations are a very important consideration for SERM use in these chronic indications. The pleiotropic nature the ER and its role in numerous physiologic systems raise the importance of considering potential SERM benefits and/or adverse events in the cardiovascular system and other tissues.

REFERENCES

1. Kalu, D., Salerno, E., Liu, C. C., Echon, R., Ray, M., Gaza-Zepata, M., and Hollis, B.W. A comparative study of the actions of tamoxifen, estrogen and progesterone in the ovariectomized rat. *Bone Miner*. **1991**, *15*, 109–124.
2. Bryant, H. U., Black, L. J., Rowley, E. R., Magee, D. M., Williams, D. C., Cullinan, G. J., Kauffman, R. F., and Sato, M. Raloxifene (LY139481 HCl): bone, lipid and uterine effects in the ovariectomized rat model. *J. Bone Mineral Res*. **1993**, *8* (suppl 1), S123.
3. Draper, M. W., Flowers, D. E., Huster, W. J., and Neild, J. A. Effects of raloxifene (LY139481 HCl) on biochemical markers of bone and lipid metabolism in healthy postmenopausal women. *Proc. Fourth Int. Symp. Osteopor*. **1993**, 119–121.
4. Feldman, S., Minne, H. W., Parvizi, S., Pfeifer, M., Lempert, U. G., Bauss, F., and Ziegler, R. Antiestrogen and antiandrogen administration reduce bone mass in the rat. *Bone Miner* **1989**, *7*, 245–254.
5. Black, L. J. and Goode, R. L., Uterine bioassay of trioxifene, tamoxifen, and a new estrogen antagonist (LY117018) in rats and mice. *Life Sci*. **1980**, *26*, 1453.
6. Black, L. J., Jones, C. D., and Goode, R. L. Differential actions of antiestrogens with cytosol estrogen receptors. *Mol. Cell. Endo*. **1981**, *22*, 95.
7. Jones, C. D., Jevnikar, M. G., Pike, J., Peters, M. K., Black, L. J., Thompson, A. R., Falcone, J. F., and Clemens, J. A. Antiestrogens. 2. Structure-activity studies in a series of 3-aroyl-2-arylbenzo[b]thiophene derivatives leading to [6-hydroxy-2-(4-hydroxyphenyl) benzo[b]thien-3-yl]-[4-[2-(1-piperidinyl)ethoxy]phenyl] methanone hydrochloride (LY 156758), a remarkably effective estrogen antagonist with only minimal intrinsic estrogenicity. *J. Med Chem*, **1984**, *27*, 1057.
8. Black, L. J., Rowley, E., Bekele, A., Sato, M., Magee, D. E., Williams, D. C., Cullinan, G. J., Bendele, R., Kauffman, R. F., Bensch, W., Frolik, C. A., Termine, J. D., and Bryant, H. U. Raloxifene (LY139482 HCl) prevents bone loss and reduces serum cholesterol without causing uterine hypertrophy in ovariectomized rats. *J. Clin. Invest*. **1994**, *93*, 63–69.
9. Grese, T. A., Sluka, J. P., Bryant, H. U., Cullinan, G. C., Glasebrook, A. L., Jones, C. D., Matsumoto, K., Palkowitz, A. D., Sato, M., Termine, J. D., Winter, M. A., Yang, N. N., and Dodge, J. A. Molecular determinants of tissue selectivity in estrogen receptor modulators. *Proc. Natl. Acad. Sci*. **1997**, *94*, 14105–14110.
10. Brzozowski, A. M., Pike, A. C., Dauter, Z., Hubbard, R. E., Bonn, T., Engstrom, O., Ohman, L., Green, G. L., and Gustafsson, J. A. Molecular basis of agonism and antagonism in the estrogen receptor. *Nature* **1997**, *389*, 753–768.
11. (a) Grese, T. A., Cho, S., Finley, D. R., Godfrey, A. G., Jones, C. D., Lugar, C. W., Martin, M. J., Matsumoto, K., Pennington, L. D., Winter, M. A., Adrian, M. D., Cole, H. W., Magee D. E., Phillips, D. L., Rowley, E. R., Short, L. L., Glasebrook, A. L., and Bryant, H. U. Structure-

activity relationships of selective-estrogen receptor modulators: modifications to the 2-arylbenzothiophene core of raloxifene. *J. Med. Chem.* **1997**, *40*, 146–167; (b) Obata, T., and Kubota, S. Protective effect of tamoxifen on 1-methyl-4-phenylpyridine-induced hydroxyl radical generation in the rat striatum. *Neurosci. Lett.* **2001**, *308*, 87–90.

12. (a) Shiau, K., Barstad, D., Loria, P. M., Cheng, L., Kushner, P. J., Agard, A., and Greene, G. L. The structural basis of estrogen receptor/coactivator recognition and the antagonism of this interaction by tamoxifen. *Cell* **1998**, *95*, 927–937;(b) Sun, J., Meyers, M. J., Fink, B., Rajendran, R., Katzenellenbogen, J. A., and Katzenellenbogen, B. S. Novel ligands that function as selective estrogens or antiestrogens for estrogen receptor-α or estrogen receptor-β. *Endocrinology* **1999**, *140*, 800–804.
13. Dai, S. Y., Chalmers, M. J., Bruning, J., Bramlett, K. S., Osborne, H. E., Montrose-Rafizadeh, C., Barr, R. J., Wang, Y., Wang, M., Burris, T. P., Dodge, J. A., and Griffin, P. R. Prediction of tissue-specificity of selective estrogen receptor modulators by using a single biochemical method. *Proc. Natl. Acad. Sci. U.S.A.* **2008**, *105*, 7171.
14. (a) Dai, S. Y., Burris, T. P., Dodge, J. A., Montrose-Rafizadeh, C., Wang, Y., Chalmers, M. J., and Griffin, P. R. Unique ligand binding patterns between estrogen receptor alpha and beta revealed by hydrogen-deuterium exchange. *Biochemistry*, **2009**, *48*, 9668; (b) He, L., Xiang, H., Lu-Yong, Z., Wei-Sheng, T., and Hong, H. H. Novel estrogen receptor ligands and their structure activity relationship evaluated by scintillation proximity assay for high throughput screening. *Drug Discov. Res.* **2005**, *64*, 203–212.
15. Grese, T. A., Pennington, L. D., Sluka, J. P., Adrian, M. D., Cole, H. W., Fuson, T. R., Magee, D. E., Phillips, D. L., Rowley, E. R., Shetler, P. K., Short, L. L., Venugopalan, M., Yang, N. N., Sato, M., Glasebrook, A. L., and Bryant, H. U. Synthesis and pharmacology of Conformationally Restricted Raloxifene Analogues: Highly Potent Selective Estrogen Receptor Modulators. *J. Med. Chem.* **1998**, *41*, 1272–1283.
16. Wallace, O. B., Bryant, H. U., Shetler, P. K., Adrian, M. D., and Geiser, A. G. Benzothiophene and naphthalene derived constrained SERMs. *Bioorg. Med. Chem. Lett.* **2004**, *14*, 5103.
17. Wallace, O. B., Lauwers, K. S., Dodge, J. A., May, S. A., Calvin, J. R., Hinklin, R., Bryant, H. U., Shetler, P. K., Adrian, M. D., Geiser, A. G., Sato, M., and Burris, T. P. A selective estrogen receptor modulator for the treatment of hot flushes. *J. Med. Chem.* **2006**, *49*, 843–846.
18. Dodge, J. A., Bryant, H. U., Grese, T. A., Wang, Y., Sato, M., and Burris, T. B. Pharmacological characterization, SAR, and X-ray crystal structure of an estrogen receptor alpha selective SERM. *227th ACS National Meeting*, **2004**, abstract MEDI-219.
19. Palkowitz, A. L., Glasebrook, A. L., Thrasher, K. J., Hauser, K. L., Short, L. L., Phillips, D. L., Muehl, B. S., Sato, M., Shetler, P. K., Cullinan, G. J., Zeng, G. Q., Pell, T. R., and Bryant, H. U. Discovery and synthesis of 6-hydroxy-3-[4-(1-piperidinyl)-ethoxy-phenoxy]-2-(4-hydroxyphenyl)benzo[*b*]-thiophene: A novel, highly potent selective estrogen receptor modulator (SERM). *J. Med. Chem.* **1997**, *40*, 1407–1416.
20. Hummel, C. W., Geiser, A. G., Bryant, H. U., Cohen, I. R., Dally, R. D., Fong, K. C., Frank, S. A., Hinklin, R., Jones, S. A., Lewis, G., McCann, D. J., Rudmann, D. G., Shepherd, T. A. Tian, H., Wallace, O. B., Wang, M., Wang, Y., and Dodge, J. A. A selective estrogen receptor modulator designed for the treatment of uterine leiomyoma with unique tissue specificity for uterus and ovaries in rats. *J. Med. Chem.* **2005**, *48*, 6772–6775.
21. Geiser, A. G., Hummel, C. W., Draper, M. D., Henck, J. W., Cohen, I. R., Rudmann, D. G., Donnelly, K. B., Adrian, M. D., Shepherd, T. A., Wallace, O. B., McCann, D. J., Oldham, S. W., Bryant, H. U., Sato, M., and Dodge, J. A. A new selective estrogen receptor modulator (SERM) with potent uterine antagonist activity, agonist activity in bone, and minimal ovarian stimulation. *Endocrinology* **2005**, *146:* 4524–4535.
22. Piñeiro-Núñez, M. *Raloxifene, Evista: A Selective Estrogen Receptor Modulator (SERM), in Modern Drug Synthesis* (eds J. J. Li and D. S. Johnson), John Wiley & Sons, Inc., Hoboken, NJ. **2010**, doi: Slc.
23. Nilsson, S., Makela, S., Treuter, E., Tujague, M., Thomsen, J., Andersson, G., Enmark, E., Pettersson, K., Warner, M., and Gustafsson, J. A. Mechanisms of estrogen action. *Physiol. Rev.* **2001**, *81*, 1535–1565.
24. Simoncini, T., and Genazzani, A. R. Raloxifene acutely stimulates nitric oxide release from human endothelial cells via an activation of endothelial nitric oxide synthase. *J. Clin. Endocrinol. Metab.* **2000**, *85*, 2966–2969.
25. McDonnel, D. P., Clemm, D. L., Hermann, T., Goldman, M. E., and Pike, J. W. Analysis of estrogen receptor function *in vitro* reveals three distinct classes of anti-estrogens. *Mol. Endocrinol.* **1995**, *9*, 659–669.
26. (a) Jordan, V., Collins, M. M., Rowsby, L., and Prestwich, G. A monohydroxylated metabolite of tamoxifen with potent antioestrogenic activity. *J. Endocrinol.* **1977**, *75*, 305–316; (b) Furr, B. J. and Jordan, V. C. The pharmacology and clinical uses of tamoxifen. *Pharmacol. Ther.* **1984**, *25*, 127–205.
27. Kuiper, G. J. M., Enmark, E., Pelto-Huikko, M., Nilsson, S., and Gustafsson, J. A. Cloning of a novel receptor expressed in rat prostate and ovary. *Proc. Natl. Acad. Sci.* **1996**, *93*, 5925–5930.
28. (a) Saunders, P. T., Maguire, S. M., Gaughan, J., and Millar, M. R. Expression of oestrogen receptor beta (ER beta) in multiple rat tissues visualised by immunohistochemistry. *J. Endocrinol.* **1997**, *154*, R13–R16; (b) de Boer, T., Otjens, D., Muntendam, A., Meulman, E., van Oostijen, M., and Ensing, K. Development and validation of fluorescent receptor assays based on the human recombinant estrogen receptor subtypes alpha and beta. *J. Pharmaceutic. Biomed. Anal.* **2004**, *34*, 671–679.

29. Rey, J. M., Pujol, P., Dechaud, H., Edouard, E., Hedon, B., and Maudelonde T. Expression of oestrogen receptor-alpha splicing variants and oestrogen receptor-beta in endometrium of intertile patients. *Mol. Human Repro.* **2002**, *4*, 641–647.
30. McInerney, E. M., Rose, D. W., Flynn, S. E., Westin, S. E., Mullen, T. M., Krones, A., Inostroza, J., Torchia, J., Nolte, R. T., Assa-Munt, N., Milburn, M. V., Glass, C. K., and Rosenfeld, M. G. Determinants of coactivator LXXLL motif specificity in nuclear receptor transcriptional activation. *Genes Dev.* **1998**, *12*, 3357–68.
31. Onate, S. A., Tsai, S. Y., Tsai, M.-J., and O'Malley, B. W. Sequence and characterization of a coactivator for the steroid hormone receptor superfamily. *Science* **1995**, *270*, 1354–1357.
32. Chen, H., Lin, R. J., Schiltz, R. L., Chankravarti, D., Nash, A., Privalsky, M. L., Nakatani, Y., and Evans, R. M. Nuclear receptor coactivator ACTR is a novel histone acetyltransferase and forms a multimeric activation complex with P/CAF and CBP/p300. *Cell* **1997**, *90*, 569–80.
33. Voegel, J. J., Heine, M. J., Zechel, C., Chambon, P., and Gronemeyer, H. TIF2, a 160 kDa transcriptional mediator for the ligand-dependent activation function AF-2 of nuclear receptors. *EMBO J.* **1996**, *15*, 3667–75.
34. Lanz, R. B., McKenna, N. J., Onate, S. A., Albrecht, U., Wong, J., Tsai, S. Y., Tsai, M.-J., and O'Malley, B. W. A steroid receptor coactivator, SRA, functions as an RNA and is present in an SRC-1 complex. *Cell* **1999**, *97*, 17–27.
35. Smith, C. L., Nawaz, Z., and O'Malley, B. W. Coactivator and corepressor regulation of the agonist/antagonist activity of the mixed antiestrogen, 4-hydroxytamoxifen. *Mol. Endocrinol.* **1997**, *11*, 657–66.
36. Montano, M. M., Ekena, K., Delage-Mourroux, R., Chang, W., Martini, P., and Katzenellenbogen, B. S. An estrogen receptor-selective coregulator that potentiates the effectiveness of antiestrogens and represses the activity of estrogens. *Proc. Natl. Acad. Sci.* **1999**, *96*, 6947–52.
37. Xu, J., Liao, L., Ning, G., Yoshida-Komiya, H., Deng, C., and O'Malley, B. W. The steroid receptor coactivator SRC-3 (p/CIP/RAC3/AIB1/ACTR/TRAM-1) is required for normal growth, puberty, female reproductive function, and mammary gland development. *Proc. Natl. Acad. Sci.* **2000**, *97*, 6379–6384.
38. Smith, C. L., DeVera, D. G., Lamb, D. J., Zafar, N., Yong-Hiu, J., Beaudet, A. L., and O'Malley, B. W. Genetic ablation of the steroid receptor co-activator ubiquitin ligase, E6-AP, results in tissue selective steroid hormone resistance and defects in reproduction. *Mol. Cell. Biol.* **2002**, *22*, 525–535.
39. Bautista, S., Valles, H., Walker, R. L., Anzick, S., Zellinger, R., Meltzer, P., and Theillet, C. In breast cancer, amplification of the steroid receptor coactivator gene AIB1 is correlated with estrogen and progesterone receptor positivity. *Clin. Cancer Res.* **1998**, *4*, 2925–9.
40. Shang, Y. and Brown, M. Molecular determinants for the tissue specificity of SERMs. *Science* **2002**, *295*, 2465–2468.
41. Klein-Hitpass, L., Schorpp, M., Wagner, U., and Ryffel, G. U. An estrogen-responsive element derived from the 5′ flanking region of the Xenopus vitellogenin A2 gene functions in transfected human cells. *Cell* **1986**, *46*, 1053–61.
42. Vanacker, J., Pettersson, K., Gustafsson, J. A., and Ladet, V. Transcriptional targets shared by ERRs and ER alpha but not ER beta. *EMBO J* **1999**, *18*, 4270–4279.
43. (a) Yang, N. N., Hardikar, S., Sato, M., Galvin, R. J. S., Glasebrook, A. L., Bryant, H. U., and Termine, J. D. Estrogen and raloxifene stimulate transforming growth Factor-β3 expression in rat bone: a potential mechanism for estrogen or raloxifene-mediated bone maintenance. *Endocrinology* **1996**, *137*, 2075–2084; (b) Yang, N. N., Venugopalan, M., Hardikar, S., and Glasebrook, A. L. Identification of an estrogen response element activated by a metabolite of 17β-estradiol and raloxifene. *Science* **1996**, *273*, 1222–1225.
44. Turner, C. H., Sato, M., and Bryant, H. U. Raloxifene preserves bone strength and bone mass in ovariectomized rats. *Endocrinology* **1994**, *135*, 2001–2005.
45. Cano, A., Dapia, S., Noguera, I., Pineda, B., Hermenegildo, C., del Val, R., Caeiro, J. R., and Garcia-Perez, M. A. Comparative effects of 17β-estradiol, raloxifene and genistein on bone 3D microarchitecture and volumetric bone mineral density in the ovariectomized mice. *Osteoporos. Int.* **2008**, *19*, 793–800.
46. Bashir, A., Mak, Y. T., Sankaralingam, S., Cheung, J., McGowan, N. W. A., Grigoriadis, A. E., Fogelman, I., and Hampson, G. Changes in RANKL/OPG/RANK gene expression in peripheral mononuclear cells following treatment with estrogen or raloxifene. *Steroids* **2005**, *70*, 847–855.
47. Viereck, V., Grundker, C., Blaschke, S., Niederkleine, B., Siggelkow, H., Frosck, K.-H., Raddatz, D., Emons, G., and Hofbauer, L. C. Raloxifene concurrently stimulates osteoprotogerin and inhibits interleukin-6 production by human trabecular osteoblasts. *J. Clin. Endocrinol. Metab.* **2003**, *88*, 4206–4213.
48. Miyaura, C., Onoe, Y., Inada, M., Maki, K., Ikuta, K., Ito, M., and Suda, T. Increased B-lymphopoeisis by interleukin-7 induces bone loss in mice with intact ovarian function: similarity to estrogen deficiency. *Proc. Natl. Acad. Sci.* **1997**, *94*, 9360–9365.
49. Frolik, C. A., Bryant, H. U., Black, E. C., Magee, D. E., and Chandrasekhar, S. Time dependent changes in biochemical bone markers and serum cholesterol in ovariectomized rats: Effects of raloxifene HCI, tamoxifen, estrogen and alendronate. *Bone* **1996**, *18*, 621–627.
50. Evans, G., Bryant, H., Magee, D., Sato, M., and Turner, R. T. The effects of raloxifene on tibia histomorphometry in ovariectomized rats. *Endocrinology* **1994**, *134*, 2283–2288.

51. (a) HELVERING, L. M., ADRIAN, M. D., GEISER, A. G., ESTREM, S. T., WEI, T., HUANG, S., CHEN, P., DOW, E. R., CALLEY, J. N., DODGE, J. A., GRESE, T. A., JONES, S. A., HALLADAY, D. L., MILES, R. R., ONYIA, J. E., MA, Y. L., SATO, M., and BRYANT, H. U. Differential effects of estrogen and raloxifene on messenger RNA and matrix metalloproteinase 2 activity in the rat uterus. *Biol. Reproduct.* **2005**, *72*, 830–841; (b) HELVERING, L. M., LIU, R., KULKARNI, N. H., WEI, T., CHEN, P., HUANG, S., LAWRENCE, F., HALLADAY, D. L., MILES, R. R., AMBROSE, E. M., SATO, M., MA, Y. L., FROLIK, C. A., DOW, E. R., BRYANT, H. U., and ONYIA, J. E. Expression profiling of rat femur revealed suppression of bone formation genes by treatment with alendronate and estrogen but not raloxifene. *Mol. Pharmacol.* **2005**, *68*, 1225–1238.
52. SATO, M., BRYANT, H. U., IVERSEN, P., HELTERBRAND, J., SMIETANA, F., BEMIS, K., HIGGS, R., TURNER, C., OWAN, I., TAKANO, Y., and BURR D. B. Advantages of raloxifene over alendronate or estrogen on non-reproductive and reproductive tissues in the long-term dosing of ovariectomized rats. *J. Pharmacol. Exp. Ther.* **1996**, *279*, 298–305.
53. ETTINGER, B., BLACK, D. M., MITLAK, B. M., KNICKERBOCKER, R. K., NICKELSEN, T., GENANT, H. K., CHRISTIANSEN, C., DELMAS, P. D., ZANCHETTA, J. R., STAKKESTAD, J., GLUER, C. C., KRUEGER, K., COHEN, F. J., ECKERT, S., ENSRUD, K. E., AVIOLI, L. V., LIPS, P., and CUMMINGS, S. R. Reduction of vertebral fracture risk in postmenopausal women with osteoporosis treated with raloxifene. *J. Am. Med. Assoc.* **1999**, *282*, 637–645.
54. HEANY, R. P. and DRAPER, M. W. Raloxifene and estrogen: Comparative bone-remodelling kinetics. *J. Clin. Endocrinol. Metab.* **1997**, *8*, 3425–3429.
55. OTT, S. M., OLEKSIK, A., LU, Y., HARPER, K. D., and LIPS, P. Bone histomorphometric and biochemical marker results of a two year placebo controlled trial of raloxifene in postmenopausal women. *J. Bone Miner. Res.* **2002**, *17*, 341–348.
56. WEINSTEIN, R. S., PARFITT, A. M., MARCUS, R., GREENWALD, M., CRANS, G., and MUCHMORE, D. B. Effects of raloxifene, hormone replacement therapy, and placebo on bone turnover in postmenopausal women. *Osteoporos Intl.* **2003**, *14*, 814–822.
57. JOHNELL, O., SCHEELE, W. M., LU, Y., REGINSTER, J.-Y., NEED, A. G., and SEEMAN, E. Additive effects of raloxifene and alendronate on bone density and biochemical markers of bone remodeling in postmenopausal women with osteoporosis. *J. Clin. Endocrinol. Metab.* **2002**, *87*, 985–002.
58. ALLEN, M. R., IWATA, K., SATO, M., and BURR, D. B. Raloxifene enhances vertebral mechanical properties independent of bone density. *Bone* **2006**, *39*, 1130–1135.
59. LI, J., SATO, M., JEROME, C., TURNER, C. H., FAN, Z., and BURR, D. B. Microdamage accumulation in the monkey vertebrae does not occur when bone turnover is suppressed by 50% or less with estrogen or raloxifene. *J. Bone Miner. Res.* **2005**, *23*, 48–54.
60. UUSI-RASI, K., BECK, T. J., SEMANICK, L. M., DAPHTARY, M. M., CRANS, G. G., DESAIAH, D., and HARPER, K. D. Structural effects of raloxifene on the proximal femur: results from the multiple outcomes of raloxifene evaluation trial. *Osteoporosis Intl.* **2006**, *17*, 575–586.
61. KANIS, J. A., JOHNELL, O., BLACK, D. M., DOWNS, R. W. JR., SARKAR, S., FUERST, T., SECREST, R. J., and PAVO, I. Effect of raloxifene on the risk of new vertebral fracture in postmenopausal women with osteopenia or osteoporosis: a reanalysis of the Multiple Outcomes of Raloxifene Evaluation trial. *Bone* **2003**, *33*, 293–300.
62. DELMAS, P. D., GENANT, H. K., CRANS, G. G., STOCK, J. L., WONG, M., SIRIS, E., and ADACHI, J. C. Severity of prevalent vertebral fractures and the risk of subsequent vertebral and nonvertebral fractures: results from the MORE trial. *Bone* **2003**, *33*, 522–532.
63. SAKAMOTO, T., EGUCHI, H., OMOTO, Y., AYABE, T., MORI, H., and HAYASHI, S. Estrogen receptor-mediated effects of tamoxifen on human endometrial cancer cells. *Mol. Cell Endocrinol.* **2002**, *192*, 93–104.
64. KODA, M., JARZABEK, K., HACZYNSKI, J., KNAPP, P., SULKOWSKI, S., and WOCZYNSKI, S. Differential effects of raloxifene and tamoxifen on the expression of estrogen receptors and antigen Ki-67 in human endometrial adenocarcinoma cell line. *Oncology Rep.* **2004**, *12*, 517–521.
65. BRAMLETT, K. S. and BURRIS. T. P. Target specificity of selective estrogen receptor modulators within human endometrial cancer cells. *Steroid Biochem. Mol. Biol.* **2003**, *86*, 27–34.
66. LEES, C. J., REGISTER, T. C., TURNER, C., H. WANG, T., STANCILL, M., and JEROME, C. P. Effects of raloxifene on bone density, biomarkers, and histomorphometric and biomechanical measures in ovariectomized cynomolgus monkeys. *Menopause*. **2002**, *9*, 320–328.
67. ADRIAN, M. D., COLE, H. W., SHETLER, P. K., ROWLEY, E. R., MAGEE, D. E., PELL, T., ZENG, G., SATO, M., and BRYANT, H. U. Comparative pharmacology of a series of selective estrogen receptor modulators. *J. Bone Mineral Res.* **1996**, *11* (Suppl. 1), S447.
68. SILFEN, S. L., CIACCIA, A. V., and BRYANT, H. U. Selective estrogen receptor modulators: tissue specificity and differential uterine effects. *Climacteric* **1999**, *2*, 268–283.
69. FUCHS-YOUNG, R., MAGEE, D., COLE, H. W., SHORT, L., GLASEBROOK, A. L., RIPPY, M. K., TERMINE, J. D., and BRYANT, H. U. Raloxifene is a tissues specific anti-estrogen that blocks tamoxifen or estrogen stimulated uterotropic effects. *Endocrinology* **1995**, *136* (Suppl), 57.
70. WAKELING, A. E. and VALCACCIA, B. Antiestrogenic and antitumor activities of a series of non-steroidal antiestrogens. *J. Endocrinol.* **1987**, *99*, 455–464.
71. Writing Group for Women's Health Initiative Investigators. Risks and benefits of estrogen plus progestin in healthy postmenopausal women. *J. Am. Med. Assoc.* **2002**, *288*, 321–333.
72. (a) STEFANICK, M. L., ANDERSON, G. L., MARGOLIS, K. L., HENDRIZ, S. L., RODABOUGH, R. J., PASKETT, E. D., LANE, D.

S., Hubbell, F. A., Assaf, A. R., Sarto, G. E., Schenken, R. S., Yasmeen, S., Lessin, L., and Shlebowski, R. T. Effects of conjugated equine estrogens on breast cancer and mammography screening in postmenopausal women with hysterectomy. *J. Am. Med. Assoc.* **2006**, *295*, 1647–1657;(b) Leblanc, K., Sexton, E., Parent, S., Belanger, G., Dery, M.-C., Boucehr, V., and Asselin, E. Effects of 4-hydroxytamoxifen, raloxifene and ICI-182,780 on survival of uterine cancer cell lines in the presence and absence of exogenous estrogens. *Intl. J. Oncol.* **2007**, *30*, 477–487; (c) Boyd, N. F., Byng, J. W., Jong, R. A., Fishell, E. K., Little, L. E., Miller, A. B., Lockwood, G. A., Tritchler, D. L., and Yaffe, M. J. Quantitative classification of mammographic densities and breast cancer risk: results from the Canadian National Breast Screening Study. *J. Natl. Cancer Inst.* **1995**, *87*, 670–675.

73. Martino, S., Cauley, J. A., Barrett-Connor, E., Powles, T. J., Mershon, J., Disch, D., Secrest, R. J., and Cummings, S. R. Continuing outcomes relevant to Evista: Breast cancer incidence in postmenopausal osteoporotic women in a randomized trial of raloxifene. *J. Natl. Cancer Inst.* **2004**, *96*, 1751–1761.
74. Vogel, V. G., Costantino, J. P., Wickerham, D. L., Cronin, W. M., Cecchini, R. S., Atkins, J. N., Bevers, T. B., Fehrenbacher, L., Pajon, E. R., Wade, J. L., Robidoux, A., Margolese, R. G., James, J., Lippman, S. M., Runowicz, C. D., Ganz, P. A., Reis, S. E., McCaskill-Stevens, W., Ford, L. G., Jordan, V. C., and Wolmark, N. Effects of tamoxifen vs raloxifene on the risk of developing invasive breast cancer and other disease outcomes: The NSABP study of tamoxifen and raloxifene (STAR) P-2 trial. *J. Am. Med. Assoc.* **2006**, *295*, 2727–2741.
75. Barrett-Connor, E., Mosca, L., Collins, P., Geiger, M. J., Grady, D., Kornitzer, M., McNabb, M., and Wenger, N. Effects of raloxifene on cardiovascular events and breast cancer in postmenopausal women. *N. Engl. J. Med.* **2006**, *335*, 125–137.
76. Reindollar, R., Koltun, W., Parsons, A., Rosen, A., Siddhanti, S., and Plouffe, L. Effects of oral raloxifene on serum estradiol levels and other markers of estrogenicity. *Fertil. Steril.* **2002**, *78*, 469–472.
77. Mandlekar, S. and Kong, A. N. Mechanisms of tamoxifen-induced apoptosis. *Apoptosis* **2001**, *6*, 469–477.
78. Diel, P., Olff, S., Schmidt, S., and Michna, H. Effects of the environmental estrogens bisphenol A, o,p′-DDT, *p-tert*-octylphenol and coumestrol on apoptosis induction, cell proliferation and the expression of estrogen sensitive molecular parameters in the human breast cancer cell line MCF-7. *J. Steroid Biochem. Mol. Biol.* **2002**, *80*, 61–70.
79. Houvinen, R., Warri, A., and Collan, Y. Mitotic activity, apoptosis and TRPM-2 mRNA expression in DMBA-induced rat mammary carcinoma treated with anit-estrogen toremifene. *Intl. J. Cancer* **1993**, *55*, 685–691.
80. Fitzpatrick, L. A. and Santen, R. J. Hot flashes: the old and the new, what is really true? *Mayo. Clin. Proc.* **2002**, *77*, 1155–1158.
81. Barnabei, V. M., Cochrane, B. B., Aragaki, A. K., Nygaard, I. Williams, R. S., McGovern, P. G., Young, R. L., Wells, E. C., O'Sullivan, M. J., Chen, B., Schenken, R., and Johnson, S. R. Menopausal symptoms and treatment-related effects of estrogen and progestin in the Women's Health Initiative. *Obstet. Gynecol.* **2005**, *105*, 1063–1073.
82. Cohen, F. J. and Lu, Y. M. Characterization of hot flashes reported by healthy postmenopausal women receiving raloxifene or placebo during osteoporosis prevention trials. *Maturitas* **2000**, *34*, 65–73.
83. Davies, G. C., Huster, W. J., Lu, Y., Plouffe, L., and Lakshmanan, M. Adverse events reported by postmenopausal women in controlled trials with raloxifene. *Obstet. Gynecol.* **1999**, *93*, 558–565.
84. Heringa, M. Review on raloxifene: profile of a selective estrogen receptor modulator. *Int. J. Clin. Pharmacol. Ther.* **2003**, *41*, 331–345.
85. Snyder, K. R., Sparano, N., Malinowksi, and J. M. Raloxifene hydrochloride. *Am. J. Health Sys. Pharmacy.* **2000**, *57*, 1669–1678.
86. Knadler, M. P., Lantz, R. J., and Gillespie, T. A. The disposition and metabolism of 14C-labelled raloxifene in humans. *Pharm. Res.* **1995**, *12* (suppl), 372.

APPENDIX I

SMALL MOLECULE DRUG DISCOVERY AND DEVELOPMENT PARADIGM

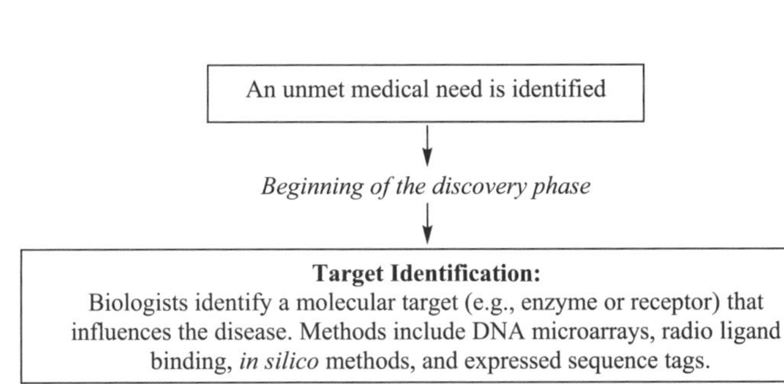

An unmet medical need is identified
Beginning of the discovery phase
Target Identification:
Biologists identify a molecular target (e.g., enzyme or receptor) that influences the disease. Methods include DNA microarrays, radio ligand binding, in silico methods, and expressed sequence tags.

Target Validation:
Confirm function and effects, and develop biological (*in vitro*/*in vivo*) assays

↓

Lead Identification:
A collection of molecules is screened for activity against the target. Methods include high-throughput screening, literature-based drug design, natural products and derivatives, structure-based drug design (X-ray crystallography, NMR studies, computer modeling), RNA interference (RNAi), genomics, and proteomics.

↓

Lead Optimization:
Medicinal chemists modify the structure of the lead to optimize the biological and pharmacokinetic properties with ADMET considerations. **Patent filing**

↓

Development Candidate Preclinical Studies:
Select development candidate, carry out nonclinical safety assessment, PK/PD studies in animals, and formulation and delivery system studies of the lead. Initial scale-up strategies investigated for delivery of tox/clinical supplies.

↓

Lead candidate compound recommended for development:
This concludes the discovery phase and initiates the development phase

↓

Beginning of the development phase

↓

Case Studies in Modern Drug Discovery and Development, Edited by Xianhai Huang and Robert G. Aslanian.

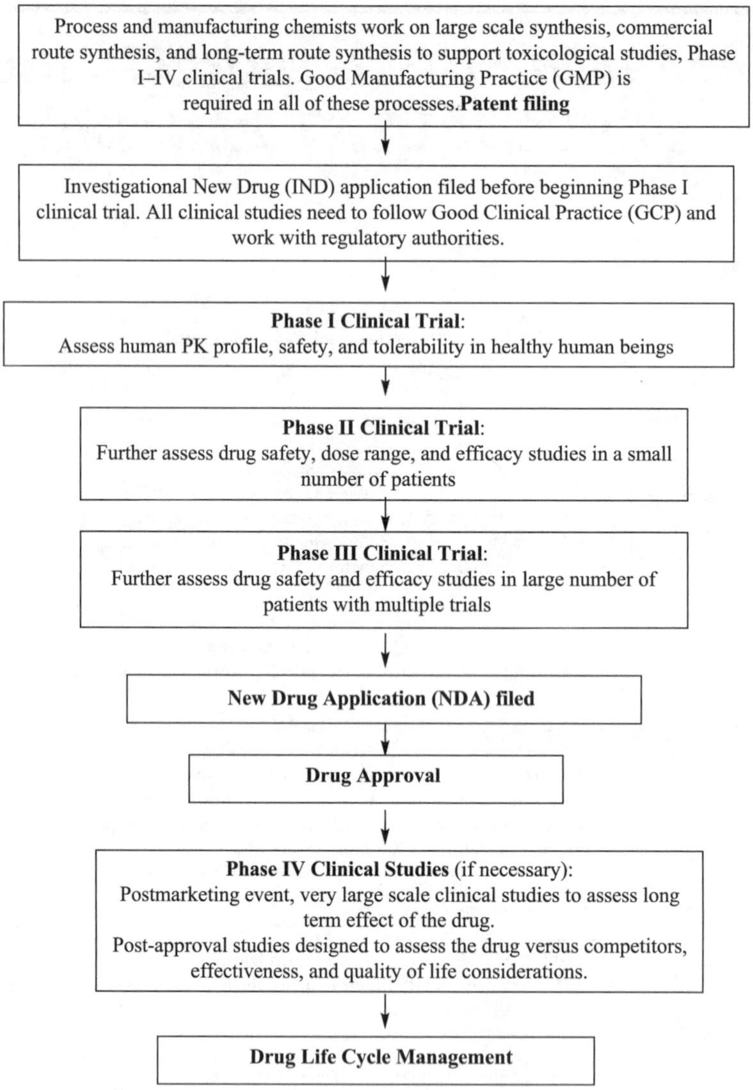

Process and manufacturing chemists work on large scale synthesis, commercial route synthesis, and long-term route synthesis to support toxicological studies, Phase I–IV clinical trials. Good Manufacturing Practice (GMP) is required in all of these processes. **Patent filing**

↓

Investigational New Drug (IND) application filed before beginning Phase I clinical trial. All clinical studies need to follow Good Clinical Practice (GCP) and work with regulatory authorities.

↓

Phase I Clinical Trial:
Assess human PK profile, safety, and tolerability in healthy human beings

↓

Phase II Clinical Trial:
Further assess drug safety, dose range, and efficacy studies in a small number of patients

↓

Phase III Clinical Trial:
Further assess drug safety and efficacy studies in large number of patients with multiple trials

↓

New Drug Application (NDA) filed

↓

Drug Approval

↓

Phase IV Clinical Studies (if necessary):
Postmarketing event, very large scale clinical studies to assess long term effect of the drug.
Post-approval studies designed to assess the drug versus competitors, effectiveness, and quality of life considerations.

↓

Drug Life Cycle Management

APPENDIX II

GLOSSARY

Accumulation factor: 1/fraction lost in one dosing interval = 1/(1 − fraction remaining).

Affinity: the ability of a drug to bind to a receptor.

Aglycone: the nonsugar component of a compound, for example anthracycline.

Agonist: a drug that produces a pharmacological response through binding to and then activating a receptor.

Allosteric antagonist: a molecule that does not compete with an agonists for the same binding site on the receptor, but instead binds to a distinctly separate binding site from the agonist to exert its action on the receptor. These antagonists can be noncompetitive antagonists or nonsurmountable antagonists.

Allosteric binding: a molecule that binds at an interface that is not within the active site of the protein. The binding is cooperative when the affinity for the native ligand rises as ligand concentrations increase and is noncooperative if the concentration of ligand has no effect on binding.

Allosteric effect: a change in the behavior of one part of a molecule caused by a change in another part of the molecule.

Alopecia: the lack or loss of hair from areas of the body where hair is usually found.

Ames test: the bacteria reversed mutation assay that is used to evaluate the mutagenic properties of test articles.

Antagonist: a molecule that attenuates the effect (blocks the action) of an agonist, but does not provoke a biological response itself upon binding to a receptor.

Antiapoptotic: acting to prevent apoptosis. Apoptosis is the process of programmed cell death that occurs in multicellular organisms.

Antiproliferative effect: inhibiting cell growth.

Area under the curve (AUC): as used in pharmacokinetics, the area under the plot of the plasma concentration of a drug against time after drug administration. It is used to measure drug exposure in humans or animals and is useful in estimating bioavailability and other parameters of a drug.

Asthenia: a condition in which the body lacks or has lost strength either as a whole or in any of its parts.

Ataxia: loss of muscle coordination.

Case Studies in Modern Drug Discovery and Development, Edited by Xianhai Huang and Robert G. Aslanian.

Bespoke screening cascade: a custom-made screening cascade to fit project needs.

Blind study: a study in which the experimenter is unaware of which test article the subject has received.

Blood–brain barrier: tight junctions that link the endothelial cells of the capillaries of the brain and spinal cord, which prevent direct contact between plasma and cells of the central nervous system.

Caco-2 cell line: a continuous line of heterogeneous human epithelial colorectal adenocarcinoma cells which can be used as a model system for intestinal epithelial permeability.

CACO2 permeability test: an assay used to estimate human intestinal permeability of a drug using Caco-2 cells for evaluating the potential for oral dosing of drug candidates.

CDC category C events: an event that causes illness or death in people by reagents characterized by the Centers for Disease Control and Prevention (CDC) as Category C agents such as emerging pathogens that might be engineered for mass dissemination because of their availability, ease of production and dissemination, high mortality rate, or ability to cause a major health impact.

Chemokines: a family of small cytokines, or proteins secreted by cells. The major role of chemokines is to act as chemoattractants to guide the migration of cells.

Chugg–Strauss Syndrome: this is a rare autoimmune-driven inflammation of small- and medium-blood vessels, mainly in the lung (but also involving other tissues including the heart), which may lead to necrosis.

CIC95: the values of CIC95 are defined as those which inhibited by 95% the spread of HIV infection in susceptible cell cultures in the presence of 10% FBS (fetal bovine serum).

cLogP: calculated Log P. a theoretical value (calculated) of Log P.

Cluster of differentiation 4: abbreviated CD4. This is a glycoprotein expressed on the surface of T helper cells, regulatory T cells, monocytes, macrophages, and dendritic cells.

Cmax: a pharmacokinetics term. The maximum (or peak) plasma concentration that a drug achieves after the drug has been administrated. It can be used to show bioequivalence between a generic and innovator drug products.

Cognate agonist: a drug (an agonist) that binds to different receptors.

Competitive antagonist: a molecule that binds reversibly to a region of the receptor in common with an agonist without activating the effector mechanism while occupying the site.

Complete response (CR): the disappearance of all signs of cancer in response to treatment.

Confidence limits: a statistical measure of the reliability of biological data. The higher the confidence limit, the closer the experimental data is to the true value.

Congestive heart failure: the physiological state in which cardiac output is insufficient in meeting the needs (supply sufficient blood flow) of the body and lungs, especially when the body becomes congested with fluid.

Coreceptor switch: over the course of HIV infection, the coreceptor usage of HIV changes from a preference for CCR5 to a preference for CXCR4 in ~50% of infected individuals. The switch is associated with accelerated CD4C T-cell decline and progression to AIDS.

Crossover design: a test in which two drugs (or a drug and placebo) are compared. The patient or animal is started on one treatment, and then changed to the other treatment after a specified time.

Cytochrome P450s (CYPs): a super family of heme-thiolate proteins widely distributed in living organisms. CYPs are involved in the metabolism of drugs and endogenous compounds. They function as a monooxygenase which introduce one oxygen atom into a substrate compound. Approximately 1000 CYPs are known, of which about 50 are known to function in humans.

Cytogenetic response: a response to treatment of CML that occurs in the marrow, rather than just in the blood.

Decatenation: the unlinking of a disk-shaped mass of circular DNA into free minicircles.

Design of experiments (DOE): experiments designed to gather information where variation is present, whether under the full control of the experimenter or not.

DFG-in conformation: a functional state of the kinases characterized by the conformation assumed by the DFG (asp-phe-gly) motif, conserved among most of proteins belonging to the kinase protein family and located in the activation loop (the DFG-loop). When the conformation adopts the buried location of the DFG-loop, it is called DFG-in conformation which can be ascribed both to an activated and to a nonactivated kinase.

DFG-out conformation: a functional state of the kinases characterized by the conformation assumed by the DFG (asp-phe-gly) motif, conserved among most of proteins belonging to the kinase protein family and located in the activation loop (the DFG-loop). When the conformation adopts a location that sterically interferes with ATP binding, it is the DFG-out conformation which is found as a nonactive form.

DNA topoisomerase II: a nuclear enzyme regulating DNA topology through strand breakage, strand passage, and ligation. Thus, it is extensively involved in DNA metabolism, including replication, transcription, recombination, and sister chromatid segregation.

Dose regimes: the amount of drug taken, expressed in terms of the quantity of a drug and the frequency at which it is taken. These include acute dosing (single dose), chronic dosing (repeated dosing), od dosing (once daily dosing), bds dosing (or bd, or bid, twice daily dosing), tds dosing (or td, or tid, thrice daily dosing), qds dosing (or qid, four-times daily dosing), nocte dosing (dosing at night).

Double-blind study: a clinical trial or experiment in which neither the investigators nor the patients know which treatment has been administered.

Double-dummy design: a form of double-blind study in which all patients are given both placebo and active doses in alternating periods of time during the study. When there is an active comparator in a drug evaluation trial, blinding can be ensured by the use of a so-called double-dummy design.

Drug–drug interactions: when an individual is prescribed more than two medications at the same time, the presence of one drug may alter the effect of another drug which may result in serious adverse events, reduced efficacy and side effects.

Dysuria: a voiding condition with lower urinary tract symptoms, especially voiding difficulties and painful voiding.

Eastern Cooperative Oncology Group (ECOG) Performance Status: A score system being used in publications by the WHO to quantify cancer patients' general well-being. The ECOG score runs from 0 to 5, with 0 denoting perfect health and 5 death. This measurement is used to determine treatment regiments (chemotherapy, dose adjustment, and intensity of palliative care).

EC_{50}: The molar concentration of a drug that produces 50% of the maximum possible response for that agonist. EC_{90} will be the concentration producing 90% of the maximum response.

ED_{50}: effective dose of a drug that produces 50% of its maximum response or effect.

Efficacy: the relationship between receptor occupancy and the ability to initiate a response.

Epidemiologic studies: studies of health-event patterns in a society for public health research. The results help to identify risk factors for preventive medicines and diseases, and to determine optimal treatment approaches and clinical practice.

Epigenetic changes: heritable changes in gene function that occur without a change in the sequence of the DNA.

Erythrocytic cycle: the life cycle of malarial organisms that takes place in the red blood cells at the pathogenic portion of the vertebrate phase.

Event-driven: a clinical trial in which the entry of patients is terminated when the occurrence of predefined events reaches a prespecified number. Increasing number of long-term, randomized, double blind clinical trials are event-driven in recent years for economical and other reasons.

Ex vivo test: experimentation or measurements carried out in or on tissues (such as from animal and human organs) outside the organism with the minimum alteration of natural conditions. These tests allow experimentation under more controlled conditions than possible in *in vivo* experiments.

Extensive disease: at the time of diagnosis, approximately 70% of patients with small-cell lung cancer will have tumors spread beyond the lung and regional lymphnodes. These patients are designated as having extensive-stage disease (ED).

Extracellular signal-regulated kinase (ERK): a protein kinase that is involved in the control of growth and division of cells. The cascade that consists of ERK and other kinases plays a central role in transmitting extracellular signals to the nucleus.

First-line therapy: initial treatment used to reduce a disease such as cancer.

First-pass metabolism: metabolism that occurs immediately after a drug is absorbed by the digestive system, enters the hepatic portal system and then the liver and before it reaches the systemic circulation. The major enzymes that affect first pass metabolism are from the gastrointestinal lumen, gut wall, bacterial, and liver.

Flaviviruses: a genus of the family Flaviviridae including the West Nile virus, dengue virus, Tick-borne Encephalitis Virus, Yellow Fever Virus, and several other viruses which may cause encephalitis.

Full agonist: agonists displaying full efficacy (full response) at a receptor.

Full antagonist: a drug that attenuates the full effect of an agonist.

Functional antagonism: reversal of the effects of a drug by an agent which, rather than acting at the same receptor, causes a response in the tissue or animal which opposes that induced by the drug.

Genetic polymorphisms: the simultaneous occurrence of two or more discontinuous forms (clearly different phenotypes) in the same population of a species in such proportions that the rarest of them cannot be maintained just by recurrent mutation. It is maintained in populations by natural selection

Geometric mean least square: the mean value for geometric random variables. The geometric distribution allocates only the nonnegative values. The mean value determines the mean for the geometric distribution in the probability distribution. The mean value is calculated by the probability of the success and the probability of the failures. The mean value is the ratio to the probability of failure to the probability of success.

Glucuronidation: the conversion of a drug to a glucuronide by linking glucuronic acid via a glycosidic bond, resulting in a metabolite which has much higher water solubility than the original substance and is eventually excreted.

G-protein coupled receptor (GPCR): membrane-bound proteins that possess seven transmenbrane helical domains. They are a large family of proteins consisting of approximately 800 different receptors. All receptors in the GPCR family share a common three-dimensional structure and mechanism of signal transduction, but the sequence homology of amino acids between different receptors is low. GPCRs are targets of about one-third of all marketed drugs. (GPCR X-ray structures background information: the crystal structure of bovine rhodopsin was determined first in 2000. Since then, almost all the homology models of GPCR were constructed using the bovine rhodopsin structure. Recently, that is, after 2008, structures for three different GPCRs were reported, in which transmembrane region were very similar to that of bovine GPCR. These studies have warranted the use of rhodopsin structure as a template for constructing structures of other GPCRs.)

Hematological response: increased hematocrit and decreased mean cellular hemoglobin content (blood counts go back to more normal levels following treatment). This is a way of describing how well a treatment has worked for some types of blood cancer.

HeLa cells: an immortal cell line used in research named after patient Henrietta Lacks. The cell line is very durable and prolific.

Hematemesis: the vomiting of blood.

hERG: the human Ether-à-go-go Related Gene, a protein known as Kv11.1 potassium ion channel. The hERG channel mediates the repolarizing IKr current in the cardiac action potential (the electrical activity of the heart that coordinates the heart's beating). If a drug inhibits hERG, it can result in a potentially fatal disorder (QT elongation) and create a concomitant risk of sudden death. Due to this potential undesirable side effect, hERG inhibition by a drug candidate must be avoided during drug development.

HGS004: an experimental anti-CCR5 monoclonal antibody for the treatment of HIV infection.

High-throughput experiments (HTE): also referred to as combinatorial chemistry. Several reactions are run simultaneously (in parallel) under different reaction conditions rather than carrying out single experiments one after another.

HIV-1 BaL: a prototype R5-using virus.

Homozygosity: the condition of having identical genes at one or more loci (genotype consisting of two identical alleles at a given locus) in homologous chromosome segments.

Human liver microsomal assay: an assay used to determine the clearance of a compound due to Phase I (including cytochrome P450) metabolism which are performed using pooled microsomes. In humans, variability in P450 expression is a significant factor, so a large number of liver microsome preparations are pooled to represent an average array of P450s.

Human liver microsomes: microsomes prepared from donor human livers using conventional homogenization and centrifugation techniques. Human liver microsomes (HLM2) are used widely to characterize the role of cytochrome P450s (P450) and other enzymes in drug metabolism.

Hyperglycemia: high blood sugar.

Hyponatremia: a common type of electrolyte disorder in which the sodium concentration in the serum is lower than normal. The common cause is excess body water diluting the serum sodium instead of sodium deficiency.

IC_{50}: the molar concentration at which a drug produces 50% of its maximum possible inhibition when the drug causes an inhibitory response. It can be measured by the displacement of 50% of the specific binding of the radioligand.

IK_r current: the cardiac "rapid" delayed rectifier current, a term related to hERG channels which mediates the repolarizing IK_r current in the cardiac action potential.

In vitro test: studies using cells and tissues outside the body in an artificial environment in order to permit a more detailed or more convenient analysis than can be done with whole organisms.

In vivo test: studies that are conducted with living organisms in their normal, intact state such as animal tests and human clinical trials to analyze the overall effects of an experiment.

Incretin effect: incretins are a group of gastrointestinal hormones that cause an increase in the amount of insulin released from the beta cells of the islets of Langerhans after eating, and inhibit glucagon release from the alpha cells of the islets of Langerhans. Incretins include two main peptide hormones, glucagon-like peptide 1 (GLP-1) and glucose-dependent insulinotropic polypeptide (GIP), which are secreted upon the ingestion of food from specialized enteroendocrine cells lining the GI tract. These "incretin" hormones are so-named because they powerfully stimulate insulin secretion and biosynthesis in the islets in response to the delivery of enteric rather than parenteral glucose—the so-called incretin effect. The stimulation of insulin secretion occurs in a glucose-dependent manner, which reduces the risk of hypoglycemia. In addition, both incretin hormones exhibit pleiotropic effects that modulate energy homeostasis. GLP-1 in particular decreases circulating levels of glucagon, a hormone that counters the glucose-lowering actions of insulin, and the pharmacology of GLP-1 includes delayed gastric emptying, increased satiety, and reduced food intake. Thus pharmacological activation of the GLP-1 receptor produces modest weight loss, which is of special benefit in treating T2DM patients, many of whom are obese.

Insurmoutable antagonist: in the presence of a surmountable antagonist, the dose–response curve for a ligand shifts to the right in a parallel fashion, where the degree of the shift depends on the concentration of the antagonist and the maximal response to the receptor is suppressed. On the other hand, in the presence of an insurmountable antagonist, the dose response curve for a ligand does not shift to the right and the maximal response to the ligand is suppressed. This does not necessarily mean that the insurmountable antagonist is bound to the receptor in an irreversible manner. (In the case of olmesartan, it has been proven by binding studies that the mode of binding to the AT1 receptor is reversible. Insurmountable feature of olmesartan's antagonism is accounted for by slow dissociation of the drug from the receptor.)

Inverse agonist: a drug acts at the same receptor as an agonist, but produces an opposite effect.

IRIS biomarker: a biomarker of immune reconstitution inflammatory syndrome. IRIS kills up to one-third of affected people. AIDS patients with cryptococcal meningitis who start HIV therapy are predisposed to IRIS. A panel of blood biomarkers can be used to stratify AIDS patients by risk for IRIS.

Irreversible antagonist: a drug that binds permanently to a receptor, either by forming a covalent bond to the active site, or by binding so tightly that the rate of dissociation is effectively zero at relevant time scales.

Isosteres: in medicinal chemistry, functional groups or moieties that have similar biological properties, also called bioisosteres.

Kaplan–Meier method: the method that tracks the survival of patients in the trial of an experimental drug.

K_i: the inhibition constant for a drug. The concentration of competing ligand in a competition assay which would occupy 50% of the receptors if no radioligand were present. It is a calculated value derived from IC_{50} using Cheng–Prusoff equation: IC50/(1 + ([L]/KD)).

Lacrimation: the production and secretion of tears.

Lipinsky guidelines: also named as Lipinski's Rule of Five. This is a rule formulated by Christopher A. Lipinski in 1997 to predict if a chemical compound has physical properties that would likely make it orally bioavailable in humans. According to this guideline, an orally active drug should have no more than one violation of the following criteria: (1) no more than five hydrogen bond donors (nitrogen or oxygen atoms with one or more hydrogen atoms); (2) no more than 10 hydrogen bond acceptors (nitrogen or oxygen atoms); (3) a molecular mass no greater than 500 Da; (4) $\log P$ no greater than 5.

Liver cirrhosis: a liver condition leading to loss of liver function caused by chronic liver disease characterized by replacement of liver tissue by fibrosis, scar tissue, and regenerative nodules.

Log P: a measure of lipophilicity of an organic compound. It is usually calculated through experiment by a formula: Log(concentration of nonionized compound in octanol/concentration of nonionized compound in buffer) at a pH at which the compound is nonionized. Higher value indicates higher lipophilicity of the compound. When the measurement is carried out at pH 7.4, the value is called Log D.

Lysine-aspirin: a soluble lysine salt of aspirin used for inhalation as a nebulized solution which is safer than oral aspirin for initiating bronchoconstriction.

MDS-Pharma PanLabs Screen: MDS Pharma Services (Panlabs)- a screen performed to assess potential off-target activities of a biologically active compound.

Melaena: abnormally dark tarry feces containing blood.

Michaelis constant (K_M): a constant representing the substrate concentration at which the velocity of an enzyme-catalyzed reaction is half maximal (1/2 the maximum velocity). A higher K_M number suggests the need for greater substrate concentrations to achieve maximum reaction velocity.

Microalbuminuria: this term does not relate to the molecular size of albumin but indicates a situation where a minute amount of albumin is detected in the urine (30–300 mg day^{-1}). Microalbuminuria serves as an early marker of glomerular disease which predicts glomerular injury in early diabetic nephropathy.

Micturition: urination, voiding.

Minimum efficacious dose: the minimum dose of a drug or other substance necessary to achieve sufficient efficacy (produce a desired or specified effect) against a target across the broad range of situations in which the product will be applied.

Mobility shift assay: a gel assay that is employed to analyze protein–DNA interactions, including the measurement of binding rates, affinity, and specificity based on the fact that protein bound to a small piece of DNA will alter the electrophoretic mobility of that DNA fragment. Bound and unbound DNA may be isolated from the gel and used for further types of analysis.

Molecular fingerprint: all cell types, depending on their functions, have unique, identifiable "signatures" with special characteristics such as which genes are active and what proteins or other cellular products are manufactured by the cell. For example, the signature changes during transformation of a normal cell to a cancer cell which can be a signal of the presence of cancer.

Molecular response: when a patient is diagnosed with CML or starting a new CML treatment, molecular tests (also called quantitative polymerase chain reaction or QPCR) will be carried out every 3 to 6 months to monitor how the treatment is working and how the patient is responding (molecular response) to the treatment.

Mucositis: a complication of some cancer therapies in which the lining of the digestive system becomes inflamed.

Mutagenesis: the induction of genetic change in a cell by the alterations (mutation) in the cell's DNA. This mutation can be inherited from one cell to the next.

Nephrotic syndrome: a condition in which a patient has very high levels of protein in the urine (proteinuria) and low levels of protein in the blood which results in swelling, especially around the eyes, feet, and hands.

Neutral antagonist: see inverse agonist section.

Neutral red assay: an assay using the pigment, neutral red, as a marker of cell injury.

Neutropenia: a condition in which there is a lower-than-normal number of neutrophils.

Nocturia: excessive night time voiding.

Occupancy: The proportion of receptors to which a drug is bound.

Open-label cross-over method: A crossover study (also referred to as a crossover trial) is a longitudinal study in which subjects receive a sequence of different treatments (or exposures). Open-label means that the administrated drug is not blinded to the patients and doctors.

Open-label extension of pivotal phase III study: open-label extension (OLE) studies are common, but they do not receive as much attention as traditional Phase I through Phase IV studies. Enrollment into an OLE study typically follows enrollment into a randomized, blinded, well-controlled main study. Participants are usually informed at the time they are recruited into the main study that they may elect to enroll in an OLE study after completing the main trial. The stated objective of most OLE studies is to obtain long-term safety and tolerability data.

Optimized background therapy (OBT): the therapy recommended for treatment experienced patients using a combination of antiretroviral (ARV) drugs which are most likely to increase CD4 count and decrease viral load based on patient retroviral (RV) history and resistance testing. Adding a new agent with a novel resistance profile or a new mechanism of action in the context of OBT can provide significant ARV activity.

Oral absorption: the gastrointestinal absorption of an orally administered drug.

Oral bioavailability: the ratio of the AUC after oral administration of a drug formulation to that after the intravenous injection of the same dose to the same subject and is used during drug development to assess a drug's pharmacokinetics.

p.o.: per os, latin for by mouth, meaning a drug that is taken orally.

Parandial: with food (meal)

Partial agonist: a compound (an agonist) that is unable to produce the maximal activation of the receptor no matter how high the concentration is.

Partial response (PR): a partial decrease in the size of a tumor, or in the extent of cancer in the body, in response to treatment.

Performance status: a measure of how well a patient is able to perform ordinary tasks and carry out daily activities.

Grade	Scales and criteria
0	Fully active, able to carry on all predisease performance without restriction.
1	Restricted in physically strenuous activity but ambulatory and able to carry out work of a light or sedentary nature, e.g., light house work, office work.
2	Ambulatory and capable of all self care but unable to carry out any work activities. Up and about more than 50% of waking hours.
3	Capable of only limited self care, confined to bed or chair more than 50% of waking hours.
4	Completely disabled. Cannot carry on any self care. Totally confined to bed or chair.

Pgp: refers to permeability glycoprotein (Pgp, ABCB1). It is part of a larger superfamily of efflux transporters (ABC-transporter of the MDR/TAP subfamily) which transports various molecules across extra- and intracellular membranes. It is extensively distributed and expressed in the intestinal epithelium, hepatocytes, renal proximal tubular cells, adrenal gland and capillary endothelial cells comprising the blood–brain and blood–testis barrier in organs such as the gut, gonads, kidneys, biliary system, and brain. It transports certain hydrophobic substances into the gut, urine, and bile and out of the brain. With a pgp substrate (inducer), the P-glycoprotein can reduce the absorption and bioavailability of a drug and its ability to cross the blood-brain barrier. A Pgp inhibitor may result in supratherapeutic plasma concentrations and drug toxicity.

Pharmacodynamic (PD) studies: the study of the biochemical and physiological effects of a drug, the mechanisms of drug action, and the efficacy studies of the drug under different dosages. Simply put, it is the study of what a drug does to the body.

Pharmacokinetic (PK) studies: the study of what happens to a drug after it is administered to an animal or human. These include the study of how the drug is absorbed and distributed within the body, the rate at which a drug action begins and the duration of the effect, the metabolism of the drug, and the effects and routes of excretion of metabolites of the drug.

Phenotypic tropism assay: an assay used to identify whether an HIV virus sample contains R5-only, X4-only, or dual/mixed virus.

pK_a: $-\log[K_a]$, the pH at which 50% of an acid dissociates into H^+ and base. A higher value indicates a weaker acid.

Placebo: a dummy treatment in a clinical trial, designed to assess the extent to which factors other than the drug under test affect the outcome of the disease.

Placebo-controlled trial: the use of a placebo (dummy treatment) in clinical trials to allow the researchers to isolate the effect of the study treatment.

Plasma protein bound: also called plasma protein binding (PPB) is that portion of a drug in blood that is bound to plasma protein. It is a measurement of a drug's affinity for plasma protein. Highly plasma protein bound drugs will have less free drug (unbound) in the blood. The unbound portion of the drug will exhibit pharmacologic effects and may be metabolized and excreted.

Pleiotropic effects: other effects of a drug which are not specifically intended for the drug. These effects (undesirable, neutral, or beneficial) are usually unanticipated and may be related or unrelated to the primary mechanism of action of the drug.

Polar surface area (PSA): the total surface area of all polar atoms including attached hydrogens of a biologically active compound. It is related to a drug's ability to permeate cells. Molecules with a PSA of >140 $Å^2$ tend to be poor at permeating cell membranes. Typically used to predict a compound's ability to cross the blood-brain barrier.

Pollakisuria: frequent daytime urination, see also nocturia.

Potency: the concentration of a drug at which it is effective (produce an effect of given intensity). A more potent drug evokes a larger response at low concentrations. EC_{50}, IC_{50}, K_A, or pD_2 are usually used for agonists, and pA_2, K_B, or pK_B for antagonist.

Pressor response: a rise in blood pressure; e.g. Ang II causes a pressor response when injected intravenously.

PRO-140: a humanized monoclonal antibody targeted against the CCR5 receptor found on T lymphocytes which is a potential therapy in the treatment of HIV infection.

Pro-apoptotic: leading to apoptosis

Prodrug: also called a probiodrug. A derivative of an active drug, which is inactive (or significantly less active), than the parent molecule. Once administered, the substance is metabolized *in vivo* into the active parent drug. A prodrug is usually designed to improve oral bioavailability (ADME profile).

Protein–protein interaction inhibitors: inhibitors that disrupt protein–protein interactions which play crucial roles in some biological processes such as the signal transduction pathways that regulate cellular function.

Ptosis: a condition that occurs when the muscles that raise the eyelid (levator and Müller's muscles) are not strong enough to do so properly.

QT study: a study to assess the effect of a compound on the QT interval.

Randomized study (or randomized trial): a study design in which each study subject is randomly assigned to receive either the study treatment or a placebo. The study result can provide the most compelling evidence that the study treatment causes the expected effect on human health.

RANTES: Regulated upon Activation, Normal T-cell Expressed, and Secreted, a cytokine (a protein) that is a member of the interleukin-8 superfamily of cytokines. It is also known as CCL5 which binds to CCR5 receptor.

Rapporteur state: an EU member state which is appointed by the EMEA to carry out the initial assessment of a new drug application for Marketing Authorisation. A second agency is appointed co-rapporteur. These countries remain responsible for taking the lead in the monitoring and assessment of safety of the product when it is subsequently marketed.

Routes of Administration: the route or course that a drug (an active substance) is applied to achieve its target effect. These are usually classified by application location which include intracerebroventricular (or icv, administered into the ventricles of the brain), intra-arterial (ia, administered into the lumen of an artery), intracerebral (or ic, administered into the brain), intradermal (or id, administered into the dermal layer of the skin), intramuscular (or im, administered into a skeletal muscle), intraperitoneal (or ip, administered into the peritoneal cavity), intrathecal (or it, administered into the spinal canal), intravenous (or iv, administered into a vein), oral (or po, administered by mouth), parenteral (any route other than by the alimentary canal), subcutaneous (or sc, administered under the skin), topical (administered on a surface such as skin).

S9 fraction: supernatant of liver homogenate centrifuged at 9000*g*, that contains many kinds of liver metabolic enzymes.

Salivation: the act or process of secreting saliva.

Second-line therapy: treatment that is given when first-line therapy does not work, or stops working.

Selectivity: relative potency of a drug between two receptors or receptor subtypes.

sGAW: specific airway conductance. It is reported as the reciprocal of resistance (conductance or 1/Raw) at the lung volume during measurements. In healthy adults sGaw ranges from about 0.125 to 0.33 $cmH_2O\,L^{-1}\,s^{-1}\,L^{-1}$.

Six Sigma: a business management strategy using a set of quality management methods such as statistical methods to improve the quality of process outputs (reducing defects and minimizing variability). 99.99966% of the products manufactured by a six sigma process should be statistically expected to be free of defects. This strategy was originally developed by Motorola in 1986.

Species homolog: also named as species variant. A receptor in similar tissue locations of different species that mediates the same physiological function. These receptors have small differences in their amino-acid sequences which result in differences in the affinity of some antagonist or the relative potency of agonists.

Specificity: relative potency of a drug between the receptors for two different endogenous ligands.

Sphyngomanometric method: the standard method for measuring systolic and diastolic blood pressure in clinical settings. In this method a cuff is placed around the forearm which is connected to a mercury manometer. The cuff is rapidly inflated near to 200 mmHg and slowly deflated while the sound of brachial artery (Korotkow sound) is monitored with a stethoscope. The sound first appears when the cuff pressure reaches the systolic blood pressure and disappears at the diastolic pressure.

Splenomegaly: an enlargement of the spleen.

Stand-alone open label study: a type of clinical trial in which both the researchers and participants know which treatment is being administered. This contrasts with single blind and double blind experimental designs, where participants are not aware of what treatment they are receiving (researchers are also unaware in a double blind trial).

Stevens–Johnson Syndrome: a serious and potentially life-threatening skin condition in which cell death causes the separation of the epidermis from the dermis. It is a hypersensitivity condition that affects the skin and mucous membranes, and can be idiopathic or may be caused by medications.

Structure-based drug design (SBDD): using X-ray crystallography and computation to design biologically active compounds.

Sub-G_1cell: cells undergoing apoptosis detected as a sub-G1 population. Using propidium iodide, the number of hypodiploid cells undergoing late apoptosis can be counted in the sub-G_1 region of DNA histogram.

Substrate walking approach: a fit-for-purpose approach to optimize the reactivity of a biocatalysts in chemical reactions. In this process, standard techniques such as direct evolution are used to gradually open up the binding site of the enzyme. Instead of using the target substrate from the outset, a series of proxy substrates which are catalyzed much more readily are used during the enzyme evolution process. Each substrate is more like the target substrate than the last so that the enzyme was gradually 'walked' towards the desired activity.

Subtype: receptors in a single species that are activated by the same family of endogenous ligands but exhibit sufficient differences in their pharmacological properties or molecular structure to justify being classified separately.

Sumoylation: the process in which a SUMO protein (small ubiquitin-related modifier) is conjugated to a target protein via an isopeptide bond between the carboxyl terminus of SUMO with an epsilon-amino group of a lysine residue of the target protein.

Surmountable antagonist: see competitive antagonist.

Tachyphylaxis: a reduction in the response to an agonist while it is continuously present at the receptor, or a progressive reduction in the response upon repeated presentation of the agonist.

The SF-12 quality of life measure: a short form health survey that is useful in monitoring outcomes of a drug in general and specific populations.

Therapeutic index: the ratio of the toxic dose of the drug to the dose which causes the desired therapeutic effect.

T_{max}: the time required for a drug to reach maximum concentration after its administration.

Transcriptionally active: being able to synthesize messenger RNA (mRNA).

Trigone: a smooth triangular region of the internal urinary bladder formed by the two ureteral orifices and the internal urethral orifice.

Tropism of the virus: viral tropism, a phenomenon in which different viruses/pathogens can evolve to preferentially target specific host species, or specific cell types within those species.

Vehicle: the medium used to dissolve drugs.

Viraemic: a medical condition where viruses enter the bloodstream and have access to the rest of the body.

Virologic escape: a phenomena in which a virus survives an antiviral treatment through mutants, thus resulting in treatment failure.

Volume of distribution: the distribution of a drug between plasma and the rest of the body after oral dosing. It is calculated by dividing the total amount of drug in the body by the amount of drug in the blood plasma.

Volume productivity: a measurement of the efficiency of production. It is calculated by the amount of product produced from the total volume of the reaction mixture, which includes starting materials and solvents.

Xenograft model: a cancer model in which human tumor tissue or cells are transplanted into animals typically mice followed by tumor treatment regimens.

β-agonist: a compound which binds to β-receptors on cardiac and smooth muscle tissues. These agonists (drugs) mainly affect the muscles around the airways (bronchi and bronchioles) and work by relaxing the muscles of the airways resulting in a widening the airways and easier breathing. These drugs can be short-acting or long-acting.

β-cells: a major cell type located in the islets of Langerhans in the pancreas. These cells make and release insulin to control the level of glucose in the blood. β cells can respond quickly to spikes in blood glucose by releasing stored insulin while simultaneously producing more.

APPENDIX **III**

ABBREVIATIONS

* numbers in parentheses are the chapter numbers.

ABL1	abelson 1 (5)
ACC	adrenocortical carcinoma (7)
AcCl	acetyl chloride (11)
ACE inhibitors	angiotensin-converting enzyme inhibitors (13)
ACE	angiotensin converting enzyme (3)
ACTG 5211	AIDS Clinical Trials Group 5211 (9)
ACTR	activin receptor (15)
AD	Anno Domini (10)
ADH	alcohol dehydrogenase (14)
ADME	absorption, distribution, metabolism, and excretion (1, 4)
ADPKD	autosomal dominant polycystic kidney disease (13)
AIB1	amplified in breast cancer 1 (15)
AIDS	acquired immunodeficiency syndrome (9)
AKR	aldo-keto reductase (6)
ALDH	aldehyde dehydrogenase (14)
AMC	aminomethylcoumarin (2)
AMP	adenosine-5′-monophosphate (4)
AMPDA	AMP deaminase (4)
Ang I	angiotensin I (3)
Ang II	angiotensin II (3)
ANOVA	analysis of variance (4)
AP	accelerated phase (5)
APD90	action potential duration at 90% repolarization (14)
API	active pharmaceutical ingredient (1, 11)
APL	acute promyelocytic leukemia (5)
APP	aminopeptidase P (2)
AQIP	*cis*-3-(3-azetidin-1-ylmethylcyclobutyl)-1-(2-phenylquinolin-7-yl) imidazo[1,5-a]pyrazin-8-ylamine (7)
AR	allergic rhinitis (8)
ARB	angiotensin receptor blocker (3)

Case Studies in Modern Drug Discovery and Development, Edited by Xianhai Huang and Robert G. Aslanian.

ARs	adrenergic receptors (14)
ARVs	antiretroviral drugs (9)
AT1	angiotensin I (3)
AT2	angiotensin II (3)
ATP	adenosine triphopshate (5)
AUA	American Urological Association (14)
AUC	area-under-curve (6, 12)
AVP	arginine vasopressin (13)
AZT	azidothymidine (9)
BA	bioavailability (14)
BC	Before Christ (10)
BCE	Before Common Era (10)
BCR	breakpoint cluster region (5)
BID	twice a day (4, 9)
BMD	bone mineral density (15)
BOO	bladder outlet obstruction (14)
BOP	benzotriazole-1-yl-oxy-tris(dimethylamino)phosphonium hexafluorophosphate (12)
BP	blast phase (5)
BPE	benign prostatic enlargement (14)
BPH	benign prostatic hyperplasia (14)
BUN	blood urea nitrogen (13)
CACO-2	colon carcinoma cell line (9)
CART	cocaine-and amphetamine-regulated transcript (2)
CAV	combination of cyclophosphamide, doxorubicin (adriamycin), and vincristine (6)
CBP	cyclic AMP response element-binding protein (15)
CBR1	carbonyl reductase 1 (6)
CCr	creatinine clearance (14)
CCR5	C-C chemokine receptor 5 (9)
CCyR	complete cytogenetic response (5)
CD4	cluster of differentiation 4 (9)
CDDP	combination chemotherapy including cisplatin (6)
CDK1	cyclin-dependent kinase 1 (5)
CHF	congestive heart failure (6, 13)
CHO	Chinese hamster ovary (3)
CHOP	cyclophosphamide, DXR (hydroxydaunorubicin), vincristine (Oncovin ®), and prednisone (6)
CHR	complete haematological response (5)
CI	confidence interval (10, 14)
CIs	combination indexes (6)
Cl_h	hepatic clearance (7)

Cl_{int}	intrinsic clearance (7)
CML	chronic myelogenous leukaemia (5)
COS	an acronym derived from the cells being **C**V-1 (simian) in origin, and carrying the SV40 genetic material (3)
CP	chronic phase (5)
CRC	colorectal carcinoma (7)
CROs	contract research organizations (1)
CRs	complete responses (6)
CSF	cerebro-spinal fluid (9)
CSF1R	colony stimulating factor 1 receptor (5)
CXCR4	CX chemokine receptor 4 (9)
CYP	cytochrome P450 (3, 7)
DAG	diacylglycerol (13)
DASH	DPP-4 activity- and/or structure-homologs (2)
DBP	diastolic blood pressure (14)
DBU	1,8-diazabicyclo[5.4.0]undec-7-ene (11)
DC	direct complementation (7)
DC	direct compression (2)
DCA	the dicyclohexylamine (8)
DDR1	discoidin domain receptor 1 (5)
DFG	asp-phe-gly (5)
DHA	dihydroartemisinin (10)
DHP	3,4-dihydro-2*H*-pyran (11)
DLT	dose-limiting toxicity (6)
DMA	*N*,*N*-dimethylacetamide (11)
DMAP	4-dimethylaminopyridine (2)
DMDO	(5-methyl-2-oxo-1,3-dioxol-4-yl)methyl (3)
DMF	dimethylformamide (11)
DMPK	drug metabolism and pharmacokinetic (7)
DMSO	dimethyl sulfoxide (2, 11)
DNA	deoxyribonucleic acid (6)
DNR	daunorubicin (6)
dNTPs	deoxyribonucleotide triphosphates; a generic term that refers to the four deoxyribonucleotides: dATP, dCTP, dGTP, dTTp (11)
DOCA	deoxycorticosterone acetate (3)
DOE	design of experiments (the technology for screening experiments.) (11)
DPP	dipeptidyl peptidase (2)
DRE	digital rectal exam (14)
DXR	doxorubicin (6)
E2	17 beta-estradiol (15)
ECF-A	eosinophil chemotactic factor of anaphylaxis (8)

ECG	electrocardiogram (6, 14)
ECL	extracellular loops (9)
ED	effective dose (10)
EDC	1-ethyl-3-(3-dimethylaminopropyl) carbodiimide (12)
ED-SCLC	extensive disease-SCLC (6)
EGFR	epidermal growth factor receptor (5, 7)
EIA	exercise-induced asthma (8)
EL	extracelluar loops (14)
ELISA	enzyme linked immunosorbant assays (5, 7)
EMA	European Medicines Agency (12)
EMCV	encephalomyocarditis virus (12)
EPHB4	ephrin type-B receptor 4 (5)
ER	estrogen receptor (15)
ER	extraction ratio (7)
ERBB2	the estrogen receptor kinase (v-erb-b2 erythroblastic leukemia viral oncogene homolog 2; also known as HER2/neu (Human Epidermal growth factor Receptor 2)) (5)
ERE	estrogen response element (15)
ERK	extracellular signal-regulated kinase (3)
EVR	early virological response (12)
EwS	Ewing's sarcoma (7)
FACO	fatty acyl Co-A oxidase (8)
FAP	fibroblast activation protein (2)
FBPase	fructose 1,6-bisphosphatase (4)
FBS	fetal bovine serum (11)
FDA	Food and Drug Administration (1, 5, 12)
FEV1	forced expiratory volume in the first second (8)
FLAP	5-lipoxygenase-activating protein (8)
FLIPR	fluorescent imaging plate reader (9)
FPG	fasting plasma glucose (4)
FQIT	*cis*-3-[4-amino-5-(8-fluoro-2-phenyl-quinolin-7-yl)-imidazo[5,1-*f*][1,2,4]triazin-7-yl]-1-methyl-cyclobutanol (7)
FTE	full time employee (1)
FVO	plasmodium falciparum, Vietnam Oak Knoll (10)
GAPDH	glyceraldehyde-3-phosphate dehydrogenase (12)
GEO	colorectal cells (7)
GH	growth hormone (2)
GHRH	growth hormone releasing hormone (2)
GI	gastrointestinal (2)
GIP	glucose-dependent insulinotropic polypeptide (2)
GK	Goto-Kakisaki (4)
GLP-1	glucagon-like peptide 1 (2)

GNG	gluconeogenesis (4)
GPCR	G-protein-coupled receptors (1, 3)
GRP	gastrin-releasing-peptide (2)
GSH	hydroxy-glutathione (12)
GSK	GlaxoSmithKline (11)
HAART	highly active antiretroviral therapy (9, 11)
HCC	hepatocellular carcinoma (7)
HCV	hepatitis C virus (12)
HDP	heme detoxification protein (10)
HDX	hydrogen-deuterium exchange (15)
HEK-293	human embryonic kidney 293 (9)
HeLa cells	Henrietta Lacks cells (13)
HER2	human epidermal growth factor receptor 2 (7)
hERG	human ether-a-go-go related gene (14)
HIV-1	human immunodeficiency virus 1 (9)
HLM	human liver microsomes (9)
HNE	human neutrophil elastase (12)
HOBt	1-hydroxybenzotriazole (12)
5-HPETE	5-hydroperoxyeicosatetraenoic acid (8)
HPLC	high performance liquid chromatography (8, 14)
HR	heart rate (14)
HRP	histidine-rich protein (10)
hsCRP	highly sensitive C-reactive protein (3)
5-HT	5-hydroxtryptamine (14)
HTE	high throughput experiments (the technology for screening experiments.) (11)
HTS	high throughput screen (1, 2, 13)
Huh7	human hepatoma cell line (12)
i.d.	intraduodonally (8)
i.v.	intravenously (8)
IFN	alpha-interferon (5)
IgE	immunoglobulin E (8)
IGF-1R	type I insulin-like growth factor receptor (7)
IGFBP3	insulin-like growth factor binding protein 3 (7)
IP	inositol phosphate (3)
IP3	inositol(1,4,5)-triphospate (13)
IPAc	isopropyl acetate (11)
IPM	[(isopropoxycarbonyl)oxy]methyl (3)
IPM	The International Partnership for Microbicides (9)
IPSS	international prostate symptom score (14)
IR	insulin receptor (7)
IRES	internal ribosomal entry site (12)

IRIS	immune reconstitution inflammatory syndrome (9)
IRIS	International Randomised Study of Interferon (5)
IRS-1/2	insulin receptor substrates 1/2 (7)
IUP	intraurethral pressure (14)
IV/PO	intravenous/oral (11)
JCOG	Japan Clinical Oncology Group (6)
JFH1	replicates (12)
KIT	stem cell factor receptor kinase (5)
K_M	Michaelis constant (2)
LAH	lithium aluminum hydride (12)
LBD	ligand binding domain (15)
LC/MS	liquid chromatography/mass spectrometry (2, 14)
LDA	lithium diisopropylamide (11)
LEVF	left ventricular ejection fraction (6)
LISN	NIH-3T3 cells over-expressing human IGF-1R (7)
5-LO inhibitors	5-lipoxygenase inhibitor (8)
LO	lead optimization (4)
LT	leukotriene (8)
LUTS	lower urinary tract symptoms (14)
LxxLL	Leu-Xaa-Xaa-Leu-Leu (15)
MAP	mitogen activated protein (15)
MBP	mean blood pressure (14)
MCC	microcrystalline cellulose (2)
MCF-7	Michigan Cancer Foundation—7 (a breast cancer cell line) (15)
MCP-1	monocyte chymoattractant protein 1 (3)
MCPBA	meta-Chloroperoxybenzoic acid (11)
MCyR	major cytogenetic response (5)
MED	minimum efficacious dose (2)
MEDEC	Medical Devices Association Canada (8)
2-MeTHF	2-methyltetrahydrofuran (a green solvent, which is produced from the fermentation of corn.) (11)
MHRE	maximum recommended human dose (14)
MinED	minimum efficacious dose (2)
MIP-1α	macrophage inflammatory protein-1 alpha (9)
MK	Merck (11)
MM	multiple myeloma (7)
MMR	major molecular response (5)
MOI	multiples of infection (11)
MPI	maximum percentage inhibition (9)
Ms_2O	methanesulfonyl anhydride (11)
MsCl	methanesulfonyl chloride (11)
MST	median survival time (6)

MTBE	methyl *t*-butyl ether (11)
MTD	maximum tolerated doses (6, 7)
mTOR	mammalian target of rapamycin (7)
MVC	maraviroc (9)
MW	molecular weight (4, 12)
NA	noradrenalin (14)
NADPH	nicotinamide adenine dinucleotide phosphate reduced form (3)
NBS	*N*-bromosuccinimide (7)
N-CoR	nuclear receptor corepressor (15)
ND	not determined (4)
NDA	new drug application (8, 12)
NeoR	neomycin resistance gene (12)
NHL	non-Hodgkin's lymphoma (6)
NHS	normal human serum (11)
NIR	near infrared (2)
NME	new molecular entities (1)
NMP	*N*-methyl-2-pyrrolidone (11)
NNRTIs	nonnucleoside reverse transcriptase inhibitors (9, 11)
NOAEL	no observable adverse effect level (8, 14)
NRTIs	nucleoside/nucleotide reverse transcriptase inhibitors (9)
NSCLC	nonsmall cell lung carcinoma (6, 7)
NTR	normotensive rats (3)
NVP	Novartis (2)
OATPs	organic anion transporters (4)
OBAV	oral bioavailability (4)
OBT	optimized background therapy (9)
OGTT	oral glucose tolerance test (2, 7)
OR	odds ratio (10)
ORIENT	olmesartan reducing incidence of endstage renal disease in diabetic nephropathy trial (3)
ORR	overall response rate (6)
OS	overall survival (6)
OvCa	ovarian carcinoma (7)
OVX	ovariectomized (15)
OXM	oxyntomodulin (2)
PACAP38	pituitary adenylate cyclase activating polypeptide 38 (2)
PAF	platelet activating factor (8)
PAMPA	parallel artificial membrane permeation assay (7)
PAP	4-phenylazophenyl (12)
PAT	process analytical technology (2)
PBMCs	peripheral blood mononuclear cells (7)
PCC	pyridinium chlorochromate (10)

PCR	polymerase chain reaction (5, 12)
PD	pharmacodynamic (2)
PDB ID	protein data bank ID (7)
PDGFR	platelet derived growth factor receptor (5)
PE	phenylephrine (14)
PEFR	peak expiratory flow rates (8)
pegIFN	pegylated α-interferon (12)
PEG-Intron	peginterferon alfa-2b (12)
PEP	prolyl endopeptidase (2)
PFS	progression-free survival (6)
PG biosynthesis	prostaglandins biosynthesis (8)
PHR	partial haematological response (5)
PHT	phthalidyl (3)
PI3	phosphoinositide 3 (5)
PI3K	phosphatidylinositol 3-kinase (7)
PIs	protease inhibitors (9)
PK	pharmacokinetic (2)
PKC	protein kinase C (5)
PKDs	polycystic kidney diseases (13)
PMB	*p*-methoxybenzyl (11)
PMBA	*p*-methoxybenzylamine (11)
POC	proof-of-concept (4)
PoC	proof-of-concept (7)
POM	pivaloyloxymethyl (3)
PPAR	peroxisome proliferator-activated receptor (2, 8)
PPB	plasma protein binding (8)
PPIs	protein–protein interaction inhibitors (1)
PPTS	pyridine *p*-toluenesulfonate (11)
PQIP	*cis*-3-[3-(4-methyl-piperazin-l-yl)-cyclobutyl]-1-(2-phenyl-quinolin-7-yl)-imidazo[1,5-a]pyrazin-8-ylamine (7)
PTBr	pyrrolidone hydrotribromide (14)
PTSA	*p*-toluenesulfonic acid (7)
QD	once a day (9)
QOL	quality of life (14)
QPP	quiescent cell proline dipeptidase (2)
QRS	Q wave R wave and S wave (6)
QTc	corrected Q wave and T wave (6)
QTcF	the QT interval corrected (for heart rate using) Fridericia's formulas (9)
R&D	research and development (1)
RANK	receptor activator of nuclear factor-κB (15)
RANTES	regulated upon activation, normal T cell expressed and secreted (9)

RAS GTPase	RAS guanosine triphosphate phosphohydrolase (5)
RAS	renin angiotensin system (3)
RBV	ribavirin (12)
RCTs	randomized controlled trials (10)
RdRp	RNA-dependent RNA polymerase (12)
REA	repressor of estrogen receptor activity (15)
Rh(COD)	rhodium(1,5-cyclooctadiene) (2)
RHR	renal hypertensive rats (3)
RIA	radio-immunoassays (8)
RI-HPLC	refractive index-HPLC detector (14)
RNA	ribonucleic acid (5)
ROADMAP	randomized olmesartan and diabetes microalbuminuria prevention (3)
RR	response rate (6)
RT	reverse transcriptase (11)
SAEs	serious adverse events (9)
SAR	structure–activity relationship (1, 2, 5)
SBDD	structure-based drug design (7, 12)
SBP	systolic blood pressure (14)
SCID	severe combined immunodeficiency disease (12)
SCLC	small-cell lung cancer (6)
SD rats	Sprague–Dawley rats (14)
SD	Sprague–Dawley (4)
SDF-1α	stromal cell-derived factor-1 alpha (9)
SERMs	selective estrogen receptor modulators (15)
SFC	supercritical fluid chromatography (1)
SH1	Src homology 1 domain (5)
SHP	small heterodimer partner (15)
SHR	spontaneously hypertensive rats (3)
SIADH	syndrome of inappropriate antidiuretic hormone (13)
SIOC	Shanghai Institute of Organic Chemistry (10)
Slc:ICR	secondary lymphoid tissue chemokine: imprinting control region (14)
SMRT	silencing mediator for retinoid or thyroid-hormone receptors (15)
SOC	standard of care (12)
SRA-1	specifically Rac1-associated protein-1 (15)
SRC	sarcoma (a proto-oncogenic tyrosine kinase) (5)
SRC-1	steroid receptor coactivator 1 (15)
SRS-A	slow reacting substance of anaphylaxis (8)
ssRNA	single-stranded RNA (12)
S-T	S wave and T wave (6)
STAR	study of tamoxifen and raloxifene (15)
STAT5	a signal transducer and activator of transcription 5 (5)

ST-T	ST segment and T wave (6)
STZ	streptozotocin (4)
SUMO	small ubiquitin-related modifier (5)
SVR	sustained viralogical response (12)
$T_{1/2}$	half-life (7)
T2DM	type 2 diabetes mellitus (2, 4)
3TC	2′,3′-dideoxy-3′-thiacytidine (also named epivir, lamivudine) (9)
TCM	traditional Chinese medicines (10)
TEMPO	2,2,6,6-Tetramethylpiperidine-1-oxyl (12)
TFA	trifluoroacetic acid (11)
TGFβ	transforming growth factor β (15)
TGI	tumor growth inhibition (7)
THF	tetrahydrofuran (8)
THP	tetrahydropyranyl (11)
TID	three times daily (2, 12)
TIF-2	transcriptional intermediary factor 2 (15)
TM	transmembrane (domains) (3, 14)
TMS	trimethylsilyl (12)
TRUS	transabdominal ultrasonography (14)
Ts_2O	*p*-toluenesulfonic anhydride (11)
TsCl	tosyl chloride or *p*-toluenesulfonyl chloride (11)
TT	genotype (12)
TURP	transurethral prostatectomy (14)
UDPG transferase	uridine diphosphate glucuronyl transferase (14)
UDP-GT	uridine diphosphate glucuronyl transferase (14)
UDS test	unscheduled DNA synthesis test (14)
UGT	UDP-glucuronosyltransferase (14)
UN	United Nations (10)
VEGF	vascular endothelial growth factor (3)
VEGFR	vascular endothelial growth factor receptor (7)
WHI	women's health initiative (15)
WHO	World Health Organization (10)
WRAIR	Walter Reed Army Institute of Research (10)
WT	wild type (3, 11)
ZDF	Zucker diabetic fatty rat (4)

INDEX

4-hydroxytamoxifen
  hydrogen–deuterium exchange studies 398
5-lipoxygenase activating protein 158
5-LO inhibitor 158
5α-reductase inhibitors 361
α1-adrenergic receptors 361
  description 361
  distribution 361
  subtypes 361
α1-AR antagonists 362
  in vitro functional activity 370
  in vivo activity
    dog 373 Table 14.5
    rat 371 Table 14.3, 372 Table 14.4
  structures 365 Figure 14.6
β-agonist 182
β-amino acid proline amide 22
β-barrel serine protease 299
β-cells 10

A
Abelson retrovirus 91
ABL kinase
  ATP bound structure 97 Figure 5.4
  imatinid bound structure 97 Figure 5.4
accelerated phase 89
ACE inhibitor 45
  temocapril 48
acid bioisosteres 22
acolbifene 406
acquired immunodeficiency syndrome 196
acute urinary retention 360
add-on therapy 38
adriamycin 103
aerosolized corticosteroids 183
age-specific prostatic hyperplasia 372
alendronate 406
Alfred Donné 89
alfuzosin 362
allergic rhinitis 185
allosteric antagonists 204
Alloxan-induced diabetes model 127
alpha-interferon 89
AMD070 198
AMD3100 198
amlodipine 62
AMN107 97 see nilotinib
amrubicin 106
  apoptosis 112
  cardiotoxicity 107
  combination studies 117
  dosing schedule 116
  dosing-limiting toxicity 118
  in vitro metabolism 116
  mechanism 111
  metabolic reduction 109
  metabolites 114
    in vitro activity 114
  MTD 109
    human 118
  myelosuppression 109
  pegylation 110
  pharmacokinetic parameters 122
  pharmacokinetic parameters, mice 109
  phase II
    combination studies 120
    survival rate 120
  second-line therapy 121
  summary of clinical studies 119 Table 6.3
  synergism with CDDP 117
  synthesis 108 Figure 6.2
  toxicity, human 118
amrubicin hydrochloride 106 see Calsed
amrubicinol 111, 113
  cell accumulation 114
  tissue distribution 115
Amylin 12
anesthetized guinea pigs 159
angiotensin
  converting enzyme 45
    inhibitors 336
  I 45
  II 45
anthracycline 104
  cardiotoxicity 107
  clinically approved compounds 106
  derivatives 104
  structures 104 Figure 6.1, 105 Figure 6.1
  toxicity 106
antihistamines 185
antioxidant properties 402
antitumor agents 112
aplaviroc 204
apoptosis 112
  induction mechanism 114
AQIP 129
aquaretics 336
AR subtypes 361
ARBs 46
  DuP 753 46
  insurmountable antagonism 60
  losartan 46
  marketed drugs 54 Figure 3.8
  PD-123177 46
  Saralasin 46
areas under curves 109
arginine vasopressin 336
  structure 337 Figure 13.1
arsenic trioxide 89
arteannuic acid 234
artemether
  auto-induction 249
  CYP profile 249
  meta-analysis 250

artemether (*Continued*)
 metabolism 249
 pharmacokinetics 249
 profile 248
artemisia annua 230
artimisinin
 alkyl and aryl derivatives 243 Figure 10.6
 analogs, antimalarial activity 239 Table 10.1
 cure rate 232
 dosing 232
 isolation 230
 structure 231
  assignment 230
  determination 231
 synthesis
  from arteannuic acid 234
  from arteannuin B 235
  from isopulegol 233
arzoxifene 393, 410
aspirin 170, 227
 intolerant asthmatics 170
AstraZeneca 99
asymmetric hydrogenation 29
ATA-117 31
atom-economy 28
AVP receptor
 cloned human, characteristics 351 Table 13.12
 V2 receptor antagonists 336
azidothymidine 196

B
Basedoxifene 393
basophils 185
bazedoxifene 410
BCR-ABL1 fusion gene 91
Ben Cao 228
 Gang Mu 228
Bengt Samuelsson 155
Benicar 63
 see olmesartan
benign prostatic
 enlargement 360
 hyperplasia 360
benzothiophenes 394
best-in-class 2
BI-201335 300
biguanides 67
BILN-2061 300
BILR-355 BS 262
biocatalysis processes 31
bioisostere 47, 52
bis(methanesulfonoxy)butane 89
bladder
 outlet obstruction 360
 stones 360
 trigone 369
blast phase 89
blend uniformity 34
blockbuster 1, 2
 drugs 1
BMS-378806 198
boceprevir 300
 in vitro profile 317
 isomerization of α-center 319
 pharmacokinetics 318
 RESPOND-2 319
 SPRINT-2 319
 synthesis 321 Scheme 12.5
 X-ray crystal structure with N3 protease 318 Figure 12.5
Boehringer Ingelheim 300
bone mineral density 405
BPH 360
 5α-reductase inhibitors 361
 description 360
 surgical intervention 361
 watchful waiting 361
 α1-adrenergic blocker 361
breast cancer 409
bronchodilators 187
busulphan 89
Byetta 12

C
Calsed 106
Capravirine 260
CAPRISA 0004 trial 215
captopril 45
cardiac glycosides 336
cardiovascular vital signs 388
caspase 112
cause of resistance 95
CCR5
 and flaviviruses 207
 and malignancies 207
 antagonist, additional indications 217
 bespoke screening cascades 200
 cognate agonists 198
 computer docking model 205
 HTS 199
 MIP-1α 198
 RANTES 198
 Δ32 deletion 198
CCR5 gene 197
CD4 197
CDDP 103
Celsentri 205
chemokine receptor 197, 198
 4 197
 5 197
chemotaxis 198
chiral molecules 7
chronic asthma 182
chronic myelogenous leukemia 89
chronic phase 89
Chugg-Strauss Syndrome 184
CIC95 266
cisplatin 103
clinical development 37
Clomid 393
Clomiphene 393
CML 89
 arsenic trioxide, treatment of 89
 complete hematological response 89
 evolution of treament 90 Table 5.1
 major cytogenetic response 89
 partial hematological response 89
 phases
  chronic 89
  accelerated 89
  blast 89
 treatment of 89
coactivators 403
Codexis Inc. 31
combination indexes 117
combinatorial chemistry 6
complete hematological response 89
complete responses 103
computational chemistry 7
congestive heart failure 336
contract research organizations 3
coreceptor "switch" 203
corepressors 403
covalent trap 300
croscarmellose sodium 33
CV-2198 47
CV-2961 47
CX chemokine receptor 4 197
CXCR4 197

CXCR4-using viruses 213
cyclophosphamide 103
cyst fluid accumulation 356
cystgenesis 356

D
danoprevir 300
Delavirdine 257
delayed adverse drug reactions 388
dexamethasone 157
DFG-in conformation 96
DFG-out conformation 96
diabetes 67
  complications 67
dibasic calcium phosphate 33
digitoxin 227
dihydroxy-leukotriene 156
direct compression 33
diuretics 336
DNA topoisomerase 110
  mechanism 110 Figure 6.3
docetaxel 103
dopamine receptors 369
doxazosin 362
doxorubicin 103, 104
DPP-4 11
  acid bioisosteres 22
  activity and/or structure homologue 16
  crystal structure 20
  deficient mice 12
  high-throughput screening 22
  inhibitor 16, 67
    pre-clinical tox 16 Table 2.2
  medicinal chemistry synthesis 27
  piperazine 24
  process synthesis 27
  β-amino acid proline amide 22
DPP
  8 17
  9 18
Droloxifene 393
DuP 753 46 see losartan
DXR
  metabolic reduction 109

E
Efavirenz 257
Eli Lilly 186
emerging nations 4
enamine amide 29
Encyclopedia of Chinese Materia Medica 228
endometrial cancer 408
enfuvirtide 197
enteroendocrine cells 11
eosinophil 156, 185
  chemotactic factor of anaphylaxis 156
equipment design 34
ER
  coactivator 403
    recognition groove 403
  corepressors 403
  ligand binding domain 402
erlotinib 99
ER-α 397
  ER-β heterodimers 403
  ligand binding domain 397
essential hypertension 45
estrogen 99, 392, 408
  depleted state 408
  induced uterotrophic response 408
  receptor 392
    kinase 99
Etoposide 103
Etravirine 258
European Caucasians 198
Evista 393
Ewing's sarcoma 127
Exenatide 12
exercise-induced
  asthma 182
  bronchoconstriction 181
EXP3174 60
extensive disease –SCLC 103

F
Fareston 393
fast followers 2
fatty acyl Co-A oxidase 173
FBPase 68
  crystal structure, inhibitor bound 72 Figure 4.4, 73 Figure 4.5, 79 Figure 4.7
  glucose lowering in ZDF rats 76 Figure 4.6
  inhibitor 68
  interactions with critical amino acids 70 Scheme 4.2
  phosphate surrogate 70
  phosphonic acids analogs 71
  prodrug approaches 80
    phosphonic diamides 81
    phosphoramidate 81
  regulation 68
  SAR
    of C8 analogs 71 Table 4.1
    of phosphonic acid analogs 72 Table 4.2
    of prodrugs 81 Table 4.6
    benzimidazole analogs 75 Table 4.4
    thiazole analogs 75 Table 4.5
  selectivity 74 Table 4.3
  structure-aided drug design 71, 73
  X-ray crystallographic studies 69
formulation attributes 34
FPL-55712 159
FQIT 132
  AMES 149
  blood glucose 148
  CYP450 inhibition data 144 Table 7.8
  drug-drug interactions 144
  effect of plasma protein on IC50 142 Table 7.5
  formulation 144
  GEO mouse xenograft model 146
  in vitro profile 140 Table 7.3
  inhibition of cellular signaling pathways 141 Figure 7.8
  kinase selectivity 149
  microsomal stability 143
  model with IGF-IR 150 Figure 7.15
  mouse biomarker study 147 Figure 7.13
  OGTT 148
  permeability 140 Table 7.4
  pharmacokinetics
    rat 145
    mouse 145
    rhesus monkey 145
    tissue distribution 146
  PK/PD
  plasma protein binding 143 Table 7.6
fragment-based hit identification 6

Friedrich SertÜmer 227
full time equivalent 4
fulvestrant 392
Fuzeon 197

G
gastrin-releasing peptide 14
gefitinib 99
gemcitabine 103
genomic positive-strand RNA 297
GEO mouse xenograft model 146
GeorgeW.Merck 2
GIP 11
GlaxoSmithKline 1
Gleevec 94
glipizide 38
Glivec 88
GLP-1 11
glucagon-like peptide 10, 11, 15
  1 10
  2 15
gluconeogenesis pathway 68
glucose-dependent insulinotropic polypeptide 11
glutathione S-transferase activity 374
glycemic control 38
glyceraldehyde-3-phosphate dehydrogenase 303
gp120 197, 198
  CD4 198
green chemistry 28
GW-695634 261

H
Halofantrine 229
HbA1c 38
HCV
  chimpanzee model 298
  genome 297
  replication 297
  replicon assay 298
  SCID mouse model 298
  virus life cycle 297
heart rate 371
heat shock proteins 402
hematuria 360
heme detoxification protein 229
hemozoin 229
hepatic gluconeogenesis 67
hepatitis C virus 296
hepatocellular carcinoma 127
highly active antiretroviral therapy 196, 257
high-throughput 6, 22
  screening 6, 22
  synthesis 6
histidine-rich protein 229
HIV Protease inhibitor 261
HIV-1 196
  age-related problems 216
  antiviral targets 197 Figure 9.1
  cell entry process 197 Figure 9.1
  host cell infection 197
  resistance 203
Hoffmann-La Roche 233
hormone releasing hormone 15
Huang hua hao 230
Human
  Genome Project 1, 6
  immunodeficiency virus 196
  neutrophil elastase 302
  tumor xenograft models 107
    effect of amrubicin and doxorubicin 107 Table 6.1
Huperzine A 228
Hydrea 89
hydroxydaunorubicin 106
hydroxypropyl-b-cyclodextrin 144
hyperglycemia 10
hypogastric nerve 372
hypoglycemia 11
hypoglycemic agents 67
  biguanides 67
  DPP4 inhibitor 67
  PPAR-γ agonists 67
  structures 68 Figure 4.2
  sulfonylureas 67
hyponatremia 336
hypotension 385

I
ICI-182,780 392
Idoxifene 393
IGF-IR & IR
  co-crystal structure 135 Figure 7.6
  compensatory signaling 128 Figure 7.1
  research operation plan 133
  signaling cascade 128 Figure 7.1
  structure-based drug design 129
imatinib 88, 94
  binding mode 96
  crystal structure with ABL kinase 95 Figure 5.3, 98 Figure 5.5
  DFG conformation 96
  human PK 94
  resistance 95, 96
    rates 95
    causes 95
  salt form 94
immune reconstitution inflammatory syndrome 216
incretin
  effect 11
  hormones 11
inhibitors of virus entry 196
inmitochondrialmembrane potential 112
insulin receptor 127
integrase inhibitors 196
Intelence 258
Interleukin
  6 405
  7 405
InterMune 300
International Partnership for Microbicides 215
intraurethral pressure 371
IRES 298
Iressa 99
irinotecan 103
Ishikawa cells 399, 400
isopulegol 233

J
Janus kinase 91

K
K103N mutation 257
Karolinska Institute in Stockholm 155
kidney
  accumulation 377
  diseases 356
kinins 46
KMD
  3213 363
  3241 377
  3250 375
  3289 377

3293 374
3310 375
KwaZulu-Natal 215

L
L-648,051 163
L-649,923 162
L-660,711 166
Labelle 186
LAF237 17
lasofoxifene 393, 410
left ventricular ejection fraction 109
leukotrienes 154
biological effects 157
biosynthesis 156 Figure 8.2
history 154
in vivo models
anesthetized guinea pigs 159
squirrel monkeys 159
allergic sheep 160
Levormeloxifene 393
ligand-binding domain 402
Lilly 12
lipoxygenases 154
Liraglutide 12
losartan 46, 47
metabolite 60
lower urinary tract symptoms 360
LTB4 156
LTC4 156
LTD4 156
binding mode 161
first generation antagonists structures 160 Figure 8.3
initial screening 163
plasma-protein binding 166
PPAR activity 173
protein shift 174
LTE4 156
LTs 157
LY-171,883 163

M
magnesium stearate 33
major cytogenetic response 89
malaria
morbidity and mortality 228
occurance 229
pathology 229
mammary tumors 408
maraviroc 198
allosteric antagonists 204
and dapivirine combinations 215
bioavailability 208
clearance profile, animals 201
CNS penetration 201
counter-screening 206
CYP profile 201
dissociation from CCR5 202
drug-drug interaction studies 208
hERG data 206
histology 207
human
ex vivo studies 208
PK profile 202 Table 9.1
QT study 208
immune selectivity profile 203 Table 9.2
immunotoxicology 207
MERIT study 212
MOTIVATE study 210
Phase 2a viral load reduction 209 Figure 9.7
process synthesis 206 Figure 9.5
QT prolongation 202
receptor modeling using rhodopsin 204
T1/2 207
Tmax 207
treatment failure 213
UK-427857 201
Marketing Authorization Application 356
mast cells 185
materia medica 228
maximum tolerated doses 109
MB06322 68
clinical studies 84
in vivo studies 83
pharmacokinetics 82 Table 4.7
toxicology profile 83
MCF-7 399
MD127 375
mean blood pressure 371
medicinal chemistry synthesis 27
Medivir 300
Mefloquine 229
menopausal transition 410
Merck 1, 156
Frosst 156
methanesulphonate salt 94
microcrystalline cellulose 33
MinED 37
minimum efficacious dose 37
mixed tropism 197
MK-0476 174 see montelukast
MK-0591 158
MK-0697
aspirin-intolerant asthmatics 170
enzymetic hydrolysis 169
process synthesis 169 Scheme 8.3
serum transaminase elevation 170
MK-1107 265
MK-571 166
enantiomers 168
and liver toxicity 169
human
doses 168
plasma concentrations 168
liver effects 168
process synthesis 167 Scheme 8.2
profile 166
MK-7009 300
MK-866 158
montelukast 158
bioavailability 179
chronic asthma 182
Chugg-Strauss Syndrome 184
combination with β-agonist 182
comparison to corticosteroids 183
effect
on eosinophils 185
on nitric oxide 185
exercise-induced
asthma 182
bronchoconstriction 181
first launch 183
human
pharmacokinetics 181
Tmax 181
LD_{50}
mouse 180
rat 180
LTD4 challenge in humans 181
metabolites 179

MK-866 (*Continued*)
  mouse MTD 180
  NOAEL 180
  P450 isozymes 180
  pharmacokinetics 179
  phototoxicity 180
  rat MTD 180
  teratogenicity studies 180
  tumorigenic activity 180
morphine 227
mozavaptan 347
  biological data 347
  Ki, human and rat AVP receptor 352 Table 13.13
multiple myeloma 127
multiples of infection 266
muscarinic receptor 369
mutant viruses 262
myelosuppression 109
Myleran 89

N
naftopidil 370
  in vitro functional activity 370
  in vivo activity, rat 371 Table 14.3, 372 Table 14.4
NA-induced contraction 369
narlaprevir 300, 326
  co-crystal structure with NS3 protease 327
  co-dosing with ritonavir
  improved synthesis 329 Scheme 12.9
  in vitro profile 326
  pharmacokinetics 326
  synthesis 328 Scheme 12.8
Nelfinavir 261
neutral antagonist 362
neutral lipids 379
neutrophils 185
Nevirapine 257
N-hydroxyurea 89
nilotinib 97
  comparison with imatinib 98 Table 5.3, 99
  crystal structure with ABL kinase 98 Figure 5.5
  kinase selectivity 97
  plasma concentrations 99
nocturia 360
Nolvadex 393
noncovalent inhibitors 300
non-Hodgkin's lymphoma 106
  standard of care
nonnucleoside reverse transcriptase inhibitors 196
nonnucleoside reverse transcriptase inhibitors 257
Non-small-cell lung cancer 103
  occurance 103
Novo 12
NS2 297
NS3 297
  depeptization structures 306
  macrocycle strategy 306
  P1 side chain SAR 312 Table 12.3
  P2 residue modifications 308 Table 12.1
  P3
    capping SAR 315 Table 12.5
    residue optimization 313 Table 12.4
  protease 298
    covalent trap 300
    crystal structure 299 Figure 12.3
    HTS 303
    inhibitor
      structures 301 Scheme 12.1
      noncovalent 300
  Sch-6 crystal structure 309 Figure 12.4
NS4A 297
NS4B 297
NS5A 297
NS5B 297, 298
  polymerase 298
nuclear hormone receptor 402
nucleoside/nucleotide reverse transcriptase inhibitors 196
NVP-728 13
NVP-LAF237 13

O
Office 523 231
oligomycin 112
Olmetec 63
  see olmesartan
olmesartan 45
  antagonist activity 54
  binding interactions 56, 57
  bioavailable rat 48
  characteristics 54
  computer modeling 57
  drug-drug interaction 62
  elimination 62
  esterase cleavage 58
  insurmountable antagonist activity 54
  inverse agonist activity 55, 56
  medoxomil 58
  metabolic stability 55
  mutant receptors 56
  prodrug
    mechanism 58
    of 48
  renal protection in humans 63
  vascular contraction assay 59
  vascular inflammation in humans 63
  vs. amlodipine 62
  vs. other ARBs 62
Oncovin 106
OPC
  21268 342
    in vivo antagonism of pressor response 342 Figure 13.5
    structure 342 Figure 13.5
  31260 347
  41061 350
operating parameters 34
oral glucose tolerance test 37, 148
OSI-906 129
  back-up criteria 131
  binding interactions 130 Figure 7.2
  biomarkers 129
  clinical studies 130
  molecular modeling 130 Figure 7.2
osteoblasts 405
osteopenic women 407
osteoporosis 411
osteoprotogerin 406
Otsuka 336
overall response rate 103, 120
overall survival 103
OVX
  mice 406
  rats 397
Oxyntomodulin 14

P
P. falciparum 244
P. vivax 250
P236L 266
P32/98 15
paclitaxel 103
parallel and high-throughput synthesis 6
parent transamination enzyme 31
partial hematological response 89
particle size 35
patent expirations 1
peak expiratory flow rates 182
pegylated α-interferon 296
peroxysome proliferator-activated receptor 173
PF-232798 204
Pfizer 1
pharmacological modulation 109
phenylephrine 371
Philadelphia 90
phosphate surrogate 70
Physuline 347
PI3 kinase 91
pilocarpine 227
piperazine 24
pituitary adenylate cyclase activating polypeptide 38 14
placebo response rate 410
plasmodium 229
platinum-based combination chemotherapy 117
plerixafor 198
pobilukast 161
polymerase chain reaction 303
postmenopausal osteoporosis 392
postmenopausal women 406
postural hypotension 362
PPAR-γ agonists 11, 67
PQIP 129
pranlukast 162
prazosin 362
  in vitro functional activity 370
  in vivo activity, rat 371 Table 14.3
Prednisone 106
Prescriptions and formulations for fifty-two diseases 228
pressor responses 342
Prix Galien
  Canada 185
  MEDEC 185
  Portugal 185
Probiodrug GmbH 15
Process Analytical Technology 34
prodrug 52, 80
Project 523 229
prostatic hyperplasia 372
protease inhibitors 196
protein
  kinase 91, 92
  shift 174
  protein interaction inhibitors 6
pyridine N-oxides 271

Q
Qin hao 230
Qin Hao Su 231
QTcF interval 208
quality of life 5
quinine 227, 229

R
R5
  CCR5-tropic 197
R5/X4
  dual-tropic 197
RAD1901 393
radioligand-binding assays 199
raloxifene 392
  basic side chain orientation and selectivity 396
  cofactor recruitment 404
    uterine cells 404
    breast cancer cell line 404
  conformationally restricted analogs 398
  crystal structure with ERalpha and 4-hydroxytamoxifen 397 Figure 15.3
  effects 405
    on bone 405, 406
    on osteoblasts differentiation 405
    on uterus 407
  hydrogen–deuterium exchange studies 398
  metabolism 411
  overlay with 17β-estradiol 396 Figure 15.2
  pharmacokinetics, human 410
  plasma protein binding 411
  reduction in endometrial cancer 408
  use in breast cancer 409
RANK-ligand 405
RAS GTPase 91
rates of resistance 95
receptor activator of nuclear factor-κB 405
renal failure 360
renal insufficiency 360
renal protection 63
renin angiotensin system 45, 46 Figure 3.1
replicase 298
replicon assay 302
reverse transcriptase 197
rhodopsin 204
ribavirin 296
rilpivirine 259
rituximab 106
RNA-dependent RNA polymerase 298
Roche 197

S
S-1153 260
S-8308 47
salbutamol 157
Samsca 356
saralasin 46
SCH
  503034 317
  900518 300
Schiperine 228
S-cysteine 156
S-cysteinyl-glycine 156
selective estrogen receptor modulators 392
Selzentry 205
serine ectopeptidase dipeptidyl peptidase IV 11
SERM-ER conformation 396
SERMs 392
  approved for human use 393 Table 15.1
  chemical structures 395 Scheme 15.1
  clinical developments, postmenopausal indications 393
  comparison with antiresorptive agents 406

SERMs (*Continued*)
conformationally restricted, structures 399
DNA response elements 404
hot flushes 410
hypothetical dose-response curves 394 Figure 15.1
inhibition of breast cancer, mechanism 409
mechanism of action 402 Figure 15.10
side effect profile 410
tissue selectivity assay 394
serotonin (5-HT1) receptor 369
serum sodium concentrations 355
S-glutathione 156
Shanghai Institute of Organic Chemistry 231
Shen Nong Ben Cao Jing 228
Shennong Herbal 228
Shi-Zhen Li 228
Signal Transducer and Activator of Transcription 91
silodosin 362
^{14}C labeled 374
accumulation 378
adverse events, Phase III 385, 387, 388
AMES study 380
bioavailability, rat, dog 376
carcinogenicity studies 380, 381
distribution 377
drug-drug interaction 376
enzyme induction 374
excretion 378
fertility study 381
food effect 382
glucuronide metabolite, toxicology 380
in vitro functional activity 370
in vivo activity, rat 371 Table 14.3
long term study results 387
metabolism
enzymes responsible 375
mouse 376
metabolites 369, 374
human 383
molecular modeling studies 367
NoAEL 380
pharmacokinetics, human 382
phototoxicity 381
primary outcome measures 385
QoL scores 384
receptor binding
profile 369
studies 365
reprotox study 381
secondary outcome measures 384, 386
site of absorption 376
subtype selectivity 366
synthesis 364
toxicology, rat, dog 379
whole blood autoradiography 378
single-stranded RNA 297
Singulair 185
sitagliptin 10, 29
add-on therapy 38
asymmetric hydrogenation 29
biocatalysis processes 31
blend uniformity 34
clinical development 37
Codexis Inc. 31
comparison with glipizide 38
enamine amide 29
equipment design 34
formulation attributes 34
minimum efficacious dose 37
OGTT in healthy human subjects 38
operating parameters 34
oral glucose tolerance test 37
particle size 35
substrate walking 31
weight reduction with 38
Six Sigma 3
SKF
101926 337
105494 337
slow reacting substance of anaphylaxis 154
SM-5887 106
small-cell lung cancer 103
occurance 103
standard of treatment
cisplatin 103
etoposide 103
irinotecan 103
sodium
cromoglycate 157
stearyl fumarate 33
sphygmomanometric method 45
Sprague–Dawley (SD) rats 371
squirrel monkeys 159
SRS-A
biosynthesis 155
structure 155
Stevens–Johnson syndrome 259
structural
biology 7
guided drug discovery 71
Study of Tamoxifen and Raloxifene 409
sub-G1 112
substance P 15, 46
substrate walking 31
sulfonylureas 11, 67
syndrome of inappropriate antidiuretic hormone 347
secretion 356

T
T-20 197
Tamoxifen 393
tamsulosin 362
in vitro functional activity 370
in vivo activity, rat 371 Table 14.3, 372 Table 14.4
molecular modeling studies 368
Taqman 303
Tarceva 99
Tasigna 97 see nilotinib
telaprevir 300
temocapril 48
tenofovir 215
teratogenicity studies 180
terazosin 362
theophylline 157
therapeutic plateau 120
therapeutic ratio 5
three-dimensional space 7
thyroid follicular cell hypertrophy 381
Tibotec 300
TMC-125 258
TMC-278 259
TMC435 300
tolvaptan 350
autosomal dominant polycystic kidney disease 356
binding affinity for V1a and V2 350
cAMP assay 352

carcinogenicity 354
CYP inhibition 355
genotoxicity 354
in vivo activity 350
rat 352
Ki, human and rat AVP receptor 352
Table 13.13
metabolism 355
pharmacokinetics, human 355
phototoxicity 354
reproductive and development tox 354
serum parameters, rat 353
Table 13.14
toxicology 353
topo 109
topotecan 103
Toremifenea 393
Traditional Chinese Medicines 228
Trappsol 144
Trimeris 197
tumorigenic activity 180
type 2 diabetes 67
mellitus 10
type I insulin-like growth factor receptor 127
cancer types involved with 127
mechanism of action 127

U
UGT isoforms 375
UGT2B7 microsomes 375
UK-372673
CYP activity 200
profile 200
UK
408026 205
408027-15 205
427857 201 see maraviroc
453453 205
453464 205
453465 205
urethra 369
urgency 360
uridine diphosphate glucuronyl transferase 374
urinary frequency 360
urinary tract infection 360
uroflowmetry 384
uroselectivity 371

V
V106A 266
V1a receptors 336
V2 receptors 336
Vaniprevir 300
vascular contraction 59
vascular inflammation 63
vasomotor symptoms 410
vasopressin receptors
antagonists
screening 338
mechanism 338 figure 13.3
Ventolin 187
verlukast 170
Vertex 300
vicriviroc 204
Victoza 12
vildagliptin 13, 17, 18
vincristine 103
vinorelbine 103
Vioxx 4
viral breakthrough 257
viral resistance
of HAART 196
voiding symptoms 384
VX-950 300

W
W229 259
WalterReedArmyInstitute of Research 229
water diuretics 336
Women's Health Initiative 392
Wu Shi Er Bing Fang Lun 228

X
X4
CXCR4-tropic 197

Y
Y181C 259, 264
Y188L 265
Yinzhaosu 231
Young 186

Z
Zamboni 186
ZDF rats 75
Zhong Yao Da Ci Dian 228
zidovudine 196
zileuton 158
Zyflo 158

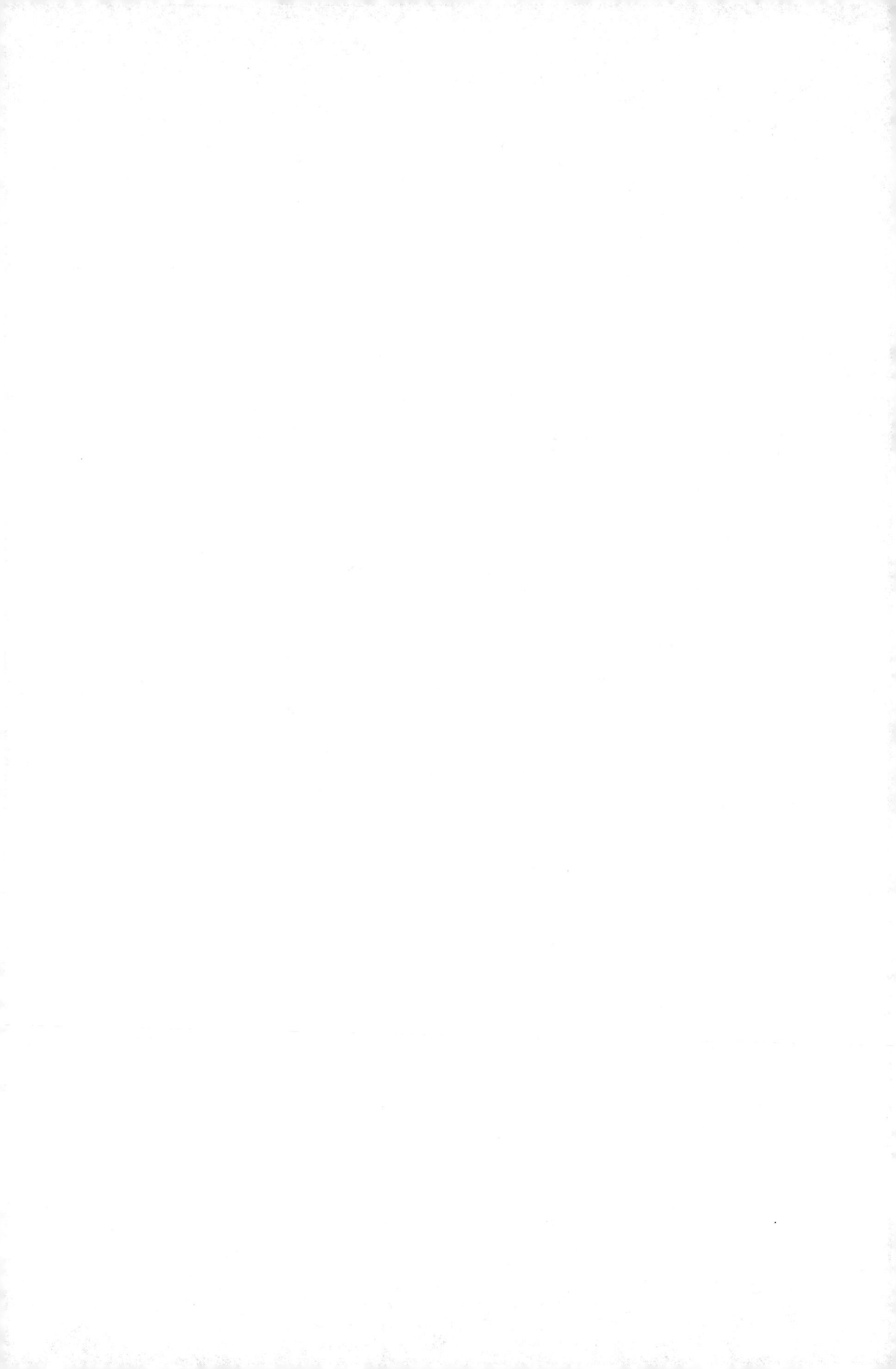